Third Edition

Clinical Textbook for VETERINARY TECHNICIANS

DENNIS M. McCURNIN, DVM, MS

Diplomate, American College of Veterinary Surgeons
Professor, Department of Veterinary Clinical Sciences
Associate Dean for Clinical and Public Services
Hospital Director, Veterinary Teaching Hospital and Clinics
School of Veterinary Medicine
Louisiana State University
Baton Rouge, Louisiana

W.B. SAUNDERS COMPANY

A Division of Harcourt Brace & Company

PHILADELPHIA LONDON TORONTO MONTREAL SYDNEY TOKYO

W.B. SAUNDERS COMPANY
A Division of
Harcourt Brace & Company

The Curtis Center
Independence Square West
Philadelphia, Pennsylvania 19106

Library of Congress Cataloging-in-Publication Data

Clinical textbook for veterinary technicians / [edited by] Dennis McCurnin. — 3rd ed.

    p.   cm.

Includes bibliographical references.

ISBN 0–7216–3792–2

1. Veterinary medicine.   I. McCurnin, Dennis M.

SF745.C625 1994

636.089—dc20   93–10417

Clinical Textbook for Veterinary Technicians, 3rd edition   ISBN 0–7216–3792–2

Printed in the United States of America.

Last digit is the print number: 9   8   7   6   5   4   3

This textbook is dedicated to the people most responsible for my professional success. **Dr. Don E. Sceli**, my role model, who first introduced me to veterinary medicine and was my practice partner; **Dr. Philip T. Pearson**, who trained me in surgery and was my major professor in graduate school; **Dr. John L. Mara** who opened the door to the world of consulting, lecturing, and travel; to all the **Veterinary Technicians** who have taught me so much about our clients, profession, and the true meaning of dedication; and to my wife, **Jeri,** and my son, **Brad,** who have allowed me to take the time needed to complete my work.

Dennis M. McCurnin, DVM

CONTRIBUTORS

R. JOHN BERG, D.V.M., M.S., Diplomate, American College of Veterinary Surgeons

Associate Professor, Tufts University School of Veterinary Medicine, North Grafton, Massachusetts

Wound Management and Bandaging

CHARLES BLASS,* D.V.M., Diplomate, American College of Veterinary Surgeons

Instrumentation and Principles of Aseptic Technique

SANDRA S. BRACKENRIDGE, M.S.W.

Coordinator of Counseling Services, School of Veterinary Medicine, Louisiana State University, Baton Rouge, Louisiana

Client Bereavement and the Grief Process; Stress and Its Management

DANIEL J. BURBA, D.V.M.

Assistant Professor of Equine Surgery, Department of Veterinary Clinical Sciences; Equine Clinician, Veterinary Teaching Hospital and Clinics, School of Veterinary Medicine, Louisiana State University, Baton Rouge, Louisiana

Wound Management and Bandaging

SHAREE A. CHAVIS, R.R.A.

Director of Medical Records, Veterinary Teaching Hospital and Clinics, School of Veterinary Medicine, Louisiana State University, Baton Rouge, Louisiana

The Medical Record

JOHN M. CHENEY, D.V.M., M.S.

Associate Professor, Diagnostic Laboratory; Clinical Parasitologist, Veterinary Teaching Hospital, College of Veterinary Medicine and Biomedical Sciences, Colorado State University, Fort Collins, Colorado

Parasitology and Public Health

M. S. CLAXTON-GILL, D.V.M., M.S., Diplomate, American Board of Veterinary Practitioners

Associate Professor of Food Animal Medicine and Surgery, Department of Veterinary Clinical Sciences; Food Animal Clinician, Veterinary Teaching Hospital and Clinics, School of Veterinary Medicine, Louisiana State University, Baton Rouge, Louisiana

Food Animal Medicine and Surgery; Preventive Health Program

JANYCE L. CORNICK, D.V.M., M.S., Diplomate, American College of Veterinary Anesthesiology and American College of Veterinary Internal Medicine

Assistant Professor, Anesthesiology, Department of Veterinary Clinical Sciences; Anesthesiologist, Veterinary Teaching Hospital and Clinics, School of Veterinary Medicine, Louisiana State University, Baton Rouge, Louisiana

Veterinary Anesthesia

---

*Deceased

STEPHEN W. CRANE, D.V.M., Diplomate, American College of Veterinary Surgeons

Adjunct Professor of Surgery, North Carolina State University, Raleigh, North Carolina; Director of Veterinary Science Group, Mark Morris Associates, Topeka, Kansas

Clinical Nutrition

SHARON M. DIAL, D.V.M., Ph.D., Diplomate, American College of Veterinary Pathologists

Assistant Professor of Pathology, Department of Veterinary Pathology; Clinical Pathologist, Veterinary Teaching Hospital and Clinics, School of Veterinary Medicine, Louisiana State University, Baton Rouge, Louisiana

Clinical Pathology

KRISTA DICKINSON, C.V.T.

Head Oncology Nurse, Veterinary Teaching Hospital, College of Veterinary Medicine and Biomedical Sciences, Colorado State University, Fort Collins, Colorado

Veterinary Oncology

DOO-YOUN CHO, D.V.M., Ph.D.

Professor of Veterinary Pathology, Department of Veterinary Pathology; Chief, Surgical Pathology and Necropsy Service, Veterinary Teaching Hospital and Clinics, School of Veterinary Medicine, Louisiana State University, Baton Rouge, Louisiana

Basic Necropsy Procedures

ERICK L. EGGER, D.V.M., Diplomate, American College of Veterinary Surgeons

Associate Professor of Surgery, Department of Clinical Sciences; Orthopedic Surgeon, Veterinary Teaching Hospital, College of Veterinary Medicine and Biomedical Sciences, Colorado State University, Fort Collins, Colorado

Surgical Assistance and Suture Material

STUART D. FORNEY, R.Ph., M.S.

Director of Pharmacy, Veterinary Teaching Hospital, College of Veterinary Medicine and Biomedical Sciences, Colorado State University, Fort Collins, Colorado

Pharmacology and Pharmacy

SHEILA R. GROSDIDIER, B.S., R.V.T.

Senior Paraveterinary Educator, Hill's Pet Nutrition, Inc., Topeka, Kansas

Clinical Nutrition

SUZANNE HETTS, B.S., M.S., Ph.D.

President, Animal Behavior Associates, Inc; Certified Applied Animal Behaviorist, Littleton, Colorado

Animal Behavior

RICHARD J. HIDALGO, D.V.M., M.S., Ph.D., Diplomate, American College of Veterinary Microbiology

Professor of Veterinary Microbiology, Department of Veterinary Microbiology and Parasitology; Director of Veterinary Computer Resources, School of Veterinary Medicine, Louisiana State University, Baton Rouge, Louisiana

Computer Applications in Veterinary Medicine

ROBERT A. HOLMES, D.V.M., M.S., Ph.D.

Associate Professor of Veterinary Radiology, Department of Veterinary Clinical Sciences; Adjunct Associate Professor of Veterinary Microbiology and Parasitology, Department of Veterinary Microbiology and Parasitology; Chief, Veterinary Medical Information System, Veterinary Teaching Hospital and Clinics, School of Veterinary Medicine, Louisiana State University, Baton Rouge, Louisiana

Computer Applications in Veterinary Medicine

GISELLE HOSGOOD, B.V.Sc., M.S., F.A.C.V.Sc, Diplomate, American College of Veterinary Surgeons

Assistant Professor of Surgery, Department of Veterinary Clinical Sciences; Surgeon, Veterinary Teaching Hospital and Clinics, School of Veterinary Medicine, Louisiana State University, Baton Rouge, Louisiana

Wound Management and Bandaging

JOHNNY D. HOSKINS, D.V.M., Ph.D., Diplomate, American College of Veterinary Internal Medicine

Professor, Internal Medicine, Department of Veterinary Clinical Sciences; Internist, Veterinary Teaching Hospital and Clinics, School of Veterinary Medicine, Louisiana State University, Baton Rouge, Louisiana

Parasitology and Public Health; Neonatal Care of Puppy, Kitten and Foal; Preventive Health Programs

JUDY L. HUTTON, M.R.T.

Medical Records Technician, Veterinary Teaching Hospital and Clinics, School of Veterinary Medicine, Louisiana State University, Baton Rouge, Louisiana

The Medical Record

ROBERT L. JONES, D.V.M., Ph.D., Diplomate, American College of Veterinary Microbiology

Professor of Microbiology, Department of Microbiology; Assistant Dean, College of Veterinary Medicine and Biomedical Sciences, Colorado State University, Fort Collins, Colorado

Clinical Microbiology

M. LYNNE KESEL, M.A., D.V.M.

Assistant Professor of Clinical Sciences, Department of Clinical Sciences, College of Veterinary Medicine and Biomedical Sciences, Colorado State University, Fort Collins, Colorado

Restraint and Handling of Animals

ANTHONY P. KNIGHT, B.V.Sc., M.S., M.R.C.V.S., Diplomate, American College of Veterinary Internal Medicine

Professor and Head, Department of Clinical Sciences, College of Veterinary Medicine and Biomedical Sciences, Colorado State University, Fort Collins, Colorado

Food Animal Medicine and Surgery

JACK L. LEBEL, D.V.M., M.S., Ph.D., Diplomate, American College of Veterinary Radiology

Professor, Department of Radiology and Radiation Biology; Clinical Radiologist, Veterinary Teaching Hospital, College of Veterinary Medicine and Biomedical Sciences, Colorado State University, Fort Collins, Colorado

Diagnostic Imaging

MERLYN J. LUCAS, D.V.M., M.S., Diplomate, American College of Theriogenology

Clinical Research Scientist, Worldwide Animal Health Clinical Research and Product Development, The Upjohn Company, Kalamazoo, Michigan

Diagnostic Sampling and Treatment Techniques

SUSAN E. LUCAS, A.H.T.

Private Practice Consultant, Kalamazoo, Michigan

Diagnostic Sampling and Treatment Techniques

MICHAEL L. MAGNE, D.V.M., M.S., Diplomate, American College of Veterinary Internal Medicine

Assistant Clinical Professor of Oncology, Veterinary Medical Teaching Hospital, School of Veterinary Medicine, University of California–Davis, Davis; Staff Internist, Animal Care Center, Rohnert, California

History and Physical Examination

GEORGE S. MARTIN, D.V.M., M.S., M.B.A., Diplomate, American College of Veterinary Surgeons

Associate Professor, Department of Veterinary Clinical Sciences; Ancillary Service Chief, Equine Surgeon, Veterinary Teaching Hospital and Clinics, School of Veterinary Medicine, Louisiana State University, Baton Rouge, Louisiana

Equine Medical and Surgical Nursing

HOWARD D. MARTIN, D.V.M.

Exotic Animal Practitioner, Agoura, California

Birds, Reptiles, Ferrets, Rabbits and Rodents

DENNIS M. McCURNIN, D.V.M., M.S., Diplomate, American College of Veterinary Surgeons

Professor, Department of Veterinary Clinical Sciences; Associate Dean for Clinical and Public Services; Hospital Director, Veterinary Teaching Hospital and Clinics, School of Veterinary Medicine, Louisiana State University, Baton Rouge, Louisiana

Hospital Practice Management

C. WAYNE McILLWRAITH, B.V.Sc., Ph.D., Diplomate, American College of Veterinary Surgeons

Professor of Surgery, Veterinary Teaching Hospital, College of Veterinary Medicine and Biomedical Sciences, Fort Collins, Colorado

Wound Management and Bandaging

T. MARK NEER, D.V.M., Diplomate, American College of Veterinary Internal Medicine

Associate Professor of Medicine, Department of Veterinary Clinical Sciences; Chief and Internist, Small Animal Clinic, Veterinary Teaching Hospital and Clinics, School of Veterinary Medicine, Louisiana State University, Baton Rouge, Louisiana

Small Animal Medical Nursing

DAVID NEIL, B.V.Sc., M.R.C.V.S.

Director of Laboratory Animal Care, Heritage Medical Research Center, University of Edmonton, Edmonton, Alberta, Canada

Restraint and Handling of Animals

ASHLEY B. OAKES, D.V.M.

Veterinary Associate and Veterinary Dentist, All Pets Clinic, Boulder, Colorado

Small Animal Surgical Nursing and Dentistry

MATT G. OAKES, D.V.M.

Chief Resident, Companion Animal Surgery, School of Veterinary Medicine, Louisiana State University, Baton Rouge, Louisiana

Small Animal Surgical Nursing and Dentistry

MAURA G. O'BRIEN, D.V.M., Diplomate, American College of Veterinary Surgeons

Fellow, Surgical Oncology, Department of Clinical Sciences, College of Veterinary Medicine and Biomedical Sciences, Colorado State University, Fort Collins, Colorado

Veterinary Oncology

BETH PAUGH PARTINGTON, D.V.M., M.S., Diplomate, American College of Veterinary Radiology

Assistant Professor of Veterinary Radiology, Department of Veterinary Clinical Sciences; Clinical Radiologist, Veterinary Teaching Hospital and Clinics, School of Veterinary Medicine, Louisiana State University, Baton Rouge, Louisiana

Diagnostic Imaging

JILL E. SACKMAN, D.V.M., Ph.D., Diplomate, American College of Veterinary Surgeons

Assistant Professor, Division of Vascular and Transplant Surgery, Department of Surgery, University of Tennessee Medical Center–Knoxville; Assistant Professor, Department of Urban Practice, College of Veterinary Medicine, University of Tennessee, Knoxville, Tennessee

Pain Management

DON E. SCELI, D.V.M.

Private Practice Consultant, Phoenix, Arizona

Hospital Practice Management

PETER D. SCHWARZ, D.V.M., Diplomate, American College of Veterinary Surgeons

Associate Professor of Surgery, Department of Clinical Sciences; Surgeon, Veterinary Teaching Hospital, College of Veterinary Medicine and Biomedical Sciences, Colorado State University, Fort Collins, Colorado

Instrumentation and Principles of Aseptic Techniques

TOM L. SEAHORN, D.V.M., M.S., Diplomate, American Academy of Veterinary Internal Medicine

Assistant Professor of Equine Medicine, Department of Veterinary Clinical Sciences; Equine Internist, Veterinary Teaching Hospital and Clinics, School of Veterinary Medicine, Louisiana State University, Baton Rouge, Louisiana

Preventive Health Programs

HOWARD B. SEIM, III, D.V.M., Diplomate, American College of Veterinary Surgeons

Associate Professor of Surgery, Department of Clinical Sciences; Small Animal Surgeon, Veterinary Teaching Hospital, College of Veterinary Medicine and Biomedical Sciences, Colorado State University, Fort Collins, Colorado

Small Animal Surgical Nursing and Dentistry

TERRY R. SPRAKER, D.V.M., Ph.D., Diplomate, American College of Veterinary Pathology

Associate Professor, Diagnostic Laboratory, College of Veterinary Medicine and Biomedical Sciences, Colorado State University, Fort Collins, Colorado

Basic Necropsy Procedures

CYPRIANNA E. SWIDERSKI, D.V.M.

Graduate Assistant, Department of Veterinary Microbiology and Parasitology, School of Veterinary Medicine, Louisiana State University, Baton Rouge, Louisiana

Neonatal Care of the Puppy, Kitten and Foal

JOSEPH TABOADA, D.V.M., Diplomate, American College of Veterinary Internal Medicine

Associate Professor, Department of Veterinary Clinical Sciences; Internist, Veterinary Teaching Hospital and Clinics, School of Veterinary Medicine, Louisiana State University, Baton Rouge, Louisiana

Euthanasia; Client Bereavement and the Grief Process

THOMAS N. TULLY, D.V.M., M.S.

Assistant Professor, Department of Veterinary Clinical Sciences; Exotic Animal Clinician, Veterinary Teaching Hospital and Clinics, School of Veterinary Medicine, Louisiana State University, Baton Rouge, Louisiana

Birds, Reptiles, Ferrets, Rabbits and Rodents

A. SIMON TURNER, B.V.Sc., M.S., Diplomate, American College of Veterinary Surgeons

Professor, Department of Clinical Sciences, College of Veterinary Medicine and Biomedical Sciences, Colorado State University, Fort Collins, Colorado

Equine Medical and Surgical Nursing

STEVEN L. WHEELER, D.V.M., M.S., Diplomate, American College of Veterinary Internal Medicine

Staff Internist, Animal Medical Specialists, Veterinary Referral Center of Colorado, Denver, Colorado

Small Animal Emergency Care

STEPHEN J. WITHROW, D.V.M., Diplomate, American College of Veterinary Surgeons

Professor of Oncology, Department of Clinical Sciences; Chief, Clinical Oncology, Veterinary Teaching Hospital, College of Veterinary Medicine and Biomedical Sciences, Colorado State University, Fort Collins, Colorado

Veterinary Oncology

PREFACE

As we approach the 21st century, it is appropriate to look ahead and attempt to anticipate the needs of the professional veterinary technician. With this in mind, this third edition has again grown in subject areas. New chapters dealing with Pain Management, Stress Management, and Neonatal Care of the Puppy, Kitten, and Foal have been added. The majority of existing chapters, such as Diagnostic Imaging, Computer Applications, Clinical Nutrition, and Clinical Pathology, have been extensively revised and updated. Twenty-six new contributors have been used in this edition.

This textbook continues to attempt to meet the basic clinical needs of the technical student and practicing technician as their professional roles expand. A single book can not possibly provide all the needed information; however, this book has been translated into several languages and adopted by many training programs and practices worldwide.

The third edition continues to be dedicated to its many loyal users and each edition has been a labor of love for the technical and veterinary medical professionals. We all must continue to work together to achieve excellence in patient care and client satisfaction.

Dennis M. McCurnin, DVM

CONTENTS

1

Restraint and Handling of Animals

M. LYNNE KESEL and DAVID H. NEIL

INTRODUCTION

Most people who enter the field of veterinary medicine have had experience in handling animals, and some are even experts in handling and training certain species (e.g., dogs or horses). There is a tendency to think that if one has developed a good rapport with one species of animal the same knowledge can be transferred directly to other species. Unfortunately, handling techniques may have little transferability among different animals; sometimes the techniques are merely inefficient, and sometimes they are dangerous when applied to other animals. Few people would dream of trying to restrain a cow as they would a dog, but those unfamiliar with horses might assume that they can be handled with the same techniques used for cattle, which is not true because of their radically different personalities. Certain behavioral signs may have different meanings in different animals. For instance, a horse pawing the ground is displaying *ennui* or nervous energy, whereas a bull pawing the ground may be making an aggressive threat or may be merely flipping dirt onto his shoulders to discourage flies.

This chapter is intended to be a guide to the behavior, handling and restraint of animals commonly encountered in veterinary medical practice. It is not intended to be an exhaustive text but to provide a broad range of confidence and competence. A list of recommended readings follows the text for the individual with special interest in animal behavior or restraint of exotic animals. Restraint of exotic species has not been included. However, material on certain rodents, rabbits and birds, which are becoming increasingly prevalent as pets (especially for people living in multiple dwellings or places in which dogs and cats are not allowed), will be reviewed briefly. These small animals have their own special handling needs, which are often overlooked.

INDICATIONS FOR RESTRAINT

What are the reasons for restraining an animal? The most obvious is to control it for a procedure. Most diagnostic and therapeutic procedures performed on animals are unpleasant for them, and naturally they resist. The restraint itself often has aspects of unpleasantness for animals. In order to avoid excess discomfort for an animal, one should strive to apply the *minimum effective restraint*. It is not necessary, for instance, to "stretch" the average cat to examine its mouth; cats generally have a better attitude and cooperate more with minimal restraint. Conversely, it would be foolhardy to attempt a jugular venipuncture on anything but a moribund cat with someone loosely cradling it. It is obvious, then, that the procedure determines the degree of restraint, and good judgment is necessary for deciding exactly how much restraint is needed.

A second important reason for effective restraint is to prevent the animal from harming itself. This is immediately evident in the use of restraining devices (e.g., Elizabethan collars, neck cradles, and so forth) to prevent self-mutilation or tearing of bandages. However, there are other ways animals may harm themselves while reacting to an unpleasant procedure (or merely avoiding people) if they are not adequately restrained. There are environmental factors to be considered. Dogs and cats are generally examined atop tables, and scrambling off the table may result in a damaging fall. Large animals are often held in potentially hazardous environments. A barbed wire fence or protruding nails can cause cuts or punctures in a horse's skin. Horses often panic if their feet get tangled in wire and will severely cut their lower legs while thrashing around. Horses do occasionally rear, and rearing in a low barn or shed can result in severe damage to the head. Stocks and runways for cattle may have dangerously splintered boards sticking out. These are only examples—the point is that veterinary personnel must try to make the examination and treatment areas as safe as possible. The client will blame you if the animal is injured.

Animals must also be restrained so that they do not harm themselves because of the procedure itself. A simple venipuncture can result in torn vessels, hematomas, and free-flowing blood if the animal moves at the wrong time. A struggling animal might cause a rectal tear during palpation. Sutures are impossible to place correctly on a moving target.

One of the most important reasons for adequate restraint of animals is the protection of personnel. The veterinarian and the technician rely on their own functioning body parts to do their job and make their living. Relatively slight injuries may result in significant loss of income or efficiency. A badly bitten, swollen and bruised hand cannot assist in, or perform, surgery. The use of crutches severely retards one's effectiveness around hoofed stock—especially the effectiveness of the technician, who is expected to provide the restraint. More severe injuries are generally incurred while working with large animals, which may kick, bite or body-slam personnel. However, small animal bites may cause facial disfigurement requiring plastic surgery, or they may even cause septicemia. It should be noted that the veterinarian may be legally responsible if a client is hurt by his own animal during a veterinary procedure.

The bottom line is that effective restraint is essential for the success of the procedure and the health and safety of animals and people.

ANIMAL PERCEPTION AND BEHAVIOR

Human evolution is inextricably tied to our successful use of animals. Early humans learned enough of animal behavior and ability to prey successfully on small, then larger, animals. As time passed, certain groups of people adopted a nomadic existence depending on and following great herds of ungulates, as the Lapps follow the reindeer even today. Early partnership with the dog may have been inspired by the dog's ability to flush, chase or bring down game—useful activities for the partner hunter. True domestication of food and service animals—in which man controls all, or nearly all, aspects of the animals' existence (feed, range, reproduction)—gradually arose from early, tentative uses of animals.

Humans have always been avid students of animal behavior, with the sometimes unacknowledged intent of using the knowledge so acquired to better control and maneuver animals to their own advantage. This involves an interspecies communication system, which usually is silent or, at least, nonverbal.

Body language, "discovered" in humans a number of years ago, is in fact as old as humans and animals. The unspoken language of gesture and touch of human beings is in part the language of the silent hunter.

All of us possess an innate ability to control and manipulate animals, which can be consciously developed according to interest or occupation. It is indeed gratifying, but not surprising, to see how rapidly an adequate degree of competence in manipulating animals may be attained by the majority of us. However, before you rush out to wrestle your first bull, bursting with dangerous overconfidence, remember that most of the detailed knowledge required to prevent injury to the animal or yourself during restraint and handling must be acquired by study (observing animals and reading or listening to expert advice) and extensive practice. You must learn to analyze each handling and restraint situation carefully, being concerned with the environment in which an animal is to be brought under control and the typical behavior of that species within that environment. For example, what sex are the animals, or are both sexes present? Are they young and unaccustomed to being herded? Are there young, unweaned animals still with and under the obvious protection of their mothers? As you progress through this chapter, you will see the relevance of these and additional observations. Having carefully assessed the situation, you may then apply your knowledge of species behavior, along with the appropriate equipment, to bring the animal (or animals) under control.

Perception in Domestic Animals

All animals are aware of their environment and the changes occurring in it through their five senses, particularly those of smell, sight and hearing. One or more of the senses may be more developed in animals than in humans. Domestic and laboratory animals retain to a considerable degree the acute senses that are so important to their wild counterparts in social interaction, defense, reproduction and the detection and selection of food. The question of how the animal senses your encroachment on its environment must be a primary consideration in approaching the various species.

Smell or Olfaction

The sense of smell, or olfaction, consists of the detection of odor molecules by the olfactory epithelium on the surface of the nasal turbinate bones. The turbinates are scrolls of bone (like loosely rolled paper) situated in the nasal cavity and covered with a vascular epithelium that provides a large warming surface for incoming air. The system is well developed in all domestic mammals but is poorly developed in domestic fowl. In the rabbit and the cat, olfaction is improved by a larger area of olfactory epithelium, which covers an area 14 times greater than that found in humans.

Domestic mammals all demonstrate sniffing behavior. They initially identify their own young in herds and flocks by olfaction. When an attempt is made to foster an orphaned lamb onto another ewe, one may try to render the lamb acceptable by smearing it with secretions of the ewe or her dead lamb and by temporarily bottle feeding the fostered lamb with the ewe's milk. All these measures are attempts to render the fostered lamb acceptable as judged by the ewe's sense of smell.

Smell plays an important part in the identification of places and people. This is most highly developed in the dog, which marks its territory with urine, thus creating a personal odor boundary. Tracking dogs have an exquisite sense of smell; a few seconds of exposure to a personal object will establish a tracking scent of a human. The cat marks its territory and familiar objects by rubbing scent glands on the side of its face on outdoor marking posts and furniture in the house. Rabbits and rodents similarly mark territory by rubbing glandular skin on objects in their environment.

Pheromones are odors secreted by animals to convey messages to other animals via the sense of smell. They are unique from other odors, however, in that the response of the recipient animal is unconscious or automatic. Female mice, which become anestrous when deprived of the presence of males, return to estrus at almost exactly 72 hours after being reintroduced to males or their excreta. The male horse will curl up the upper lip after smelling mare urine (Flehman response); males and other horses will respond to other strong odors (e.g., garlic) with a similar automatic response. Pheromones seem to be primarily associated with reproductive behavior, but the full extent of pheromone communication is not yet understood.

It is sometimes said "animals can smell fear." Many behaviorists have pointed out that your "body language" is more likely to convey your lack of confidence and that this may be misconstrued as the "smell of fear." However, the "language" of smell clearly has a more extensive vocabulary in animals than in humans.

Hearing

Humans are deaf to the high-frequency sounds that are important in the awareness and communication of the domestic and laboratory animal. All domestic mammals have well-developed methods for collecting sound waves into the external ear. The skin-covered, cartilaginous sound collectors that most people call the ear or ear flaps are properly called *pinnae*. Domestic animals, including the rabbit, are able to move the pinnae with muscles, thus focusing on the source of the sound. The pinnae are also excellent behavioral indicators, apart from their sound-collecting function. A horse with the ears back is upset, even aggressive; a dog when dominant or actively aggressive pricks the ears forward, whereas a submissive dog wrinkles and flattens the ears.

Sounds are produced by vibration, and the greater number of vibrations or cycles per second (hz), the higher the sound or note becomes. Humans hear 20 hz at the lower end of the scale and up to 20,000 hz at the highest limit. The dog hears sounds at 40,000 hz and probably up to 60,000 hz. Incredibly, bats catch flying insects by echolocation of sounds they emit at up to 98,000 hz. The laboratory rat can hear sounds of 60,000 hz to 80,000 hz. It has been demonstrated that social communication between rats and their young is carried out in the ultrasonic range.

Since we are unaware of the communication of animals at frequencies above our hearing capabilities, its significance at this time is in emphasizing that the sensory world of animals must not be judged by our standards.

We have used our knowledge of the perception of ultrasound by the dog to good effect. The "silent" dog whistle in fact emits a mixture of ultrasonic frequencies, which commands the animal's attention. Ultrasonic devices consisting of flat metal shapes threaded on a metal chain are commercially available. When shaken or thrown, they emit an extremely brief sound at 34,200 hz, which will rivet the attention of a dog. It elicits such a strong orienting reaction that it is found to be extremely useful as a distractant when treating behavioral problems in dogs, especially dangerously aggressive ones.

Vision

Domestic animals (except the pig) have a reflective layer behind the sensory part of the eye (retina), which, by reflection, intensifies the perception of light entering the eye. This reflective layer, the tapetum, permits better vision at low light intensity, giving night vision that is superior to that of humans. Everyone is familiar with the way the eyes of animals reflect, in different colors depending on the animal's pigmentation, a car's headlights at night. What is visible is the tapetum, reflecting through fully dilated pupils.

Whether mammals perceive color has still not been determined. The nerve components of the retina that are responsible for color vision in humans are called cones, in comparison with the other components, which are called rods. All domestic mammals have some cones in the retina, so it is reasonable to believe that some color vision exists.

The field of vision in herbivorous domestic mammals tends to be wide, enabling them to more readily detect the encroachment of predators from various angles. This is particularly evident in the horse and rabbit, both of which enjoy almost complete all-round vision without having to move the head. The position of the eyes in the head of the rabbit is such that the only place not covered is the area immediately behind the head and a small area in front of the nose. It has a visual field of 215 degrees for each eye, overlapping in front with the blind area being immediately behind, resulting in an almost 360-degree visual field. When we describe how to approach a horse later in this chapter, we specifically warn against moving up immediately behind a horse in its blind area, and then suddenly appearing by moving out to the left or the right rear. This is a certain way to put the animal in a state of alarm, and a good occasion to cause flight, a kick or both.

The eyes of the domestic animal focus by means of muscles controlling the shape of the lens. Most animals accommodate, or focus, the eye on near objects, much less readily than humans. The horse has a particularly sluggish accommodation. What some handlers may take for fractious head raising may be nothing more than the horse attempting to visually accommodate, this particularly happens when a horse perceives a quick movement nearby.

Horses, apparently, have acute vision at middle and far distances, not surprising for a prey species. Many of the behavioral displays of horses are visual, and they can pick up subtle cues from human body language. Clever Hans, a 19th century equine prodigy, was thought to be able to do arithmetic problems by pawing. Instead, he was perceiving movements of his trainer, like depth of breathing, that were imperceptible to human observers. Some stories assert that Hans' trainer was unaware he was giving the cues.

The dog is thought to be poor in the discrimination of form and pattern compared with human ability. In spite of this, there are obvious breed differences. The sight hounds (greyhounds, borzois, salukis, afghans) were bred to hunt by vision rather than by scent and are highly perceptive of movement. Herding dogs can act on human hand signals from as far away as 1.5 km.

Cats have excellent night vision that is consonant with their nocturnal habits. They are acutely aware of the slightest movement, which facilitates the precision of their rush after stalking their prey. Regrettably, it also facilitates the "nailing" of those who move too suddenly or find themselves in close proximity to a fearful or vengeful feline patient!

Touch

Although we tend to discount the sense of touch in the behavior of animals, contact of different body parts may be very important in the communication between animals and among animals and humans. Huddling is common in herd animals as a response to perceived threat or cold. Dogs and other pack animals may pile upon each other to sleep. Mutual grooming may occur between friendly cats or between horses, which chew at each other's withers. All of these behaviors are socially solidifying in an altruistic mode.

There are also contact behaviors that appear to result from or to resolve conflict. Biting, scratching, kicking and striking may be used to resolve a hierarchy conflict. Other, dominant animals may also use these, or moderations of these, to teach youngsters proper behavior. Canids will bite or hold the scruff of puppies' necks, hold their muzzles, or force them prone by weight over the withers if their behavior is unacceptable. This is why hanging dogs or shaking them by the scruff or collar is often a potent punishment. Horses may slam a shoulder into another or kick or strike to make the point, "I'm the boss." Some people successfully use blows of the fist or knee to correct unacceptable equine behavior. However, one must carefully choose a target and possess a measure of physical strength to be effective.

A word about how people should touch animals should be inserted here. Tentative, light touching or patting makes many species nervous or apprehensive. A steady, firm stroke or hearty slap (after proper introduction, of course) are reassuring to most species. Scratching and stroking the hair and skin is also relaxing to most animals.

Agonistic Behaviors

Agonistic behaviors are those associated with conflict. Many animals have to be maneuvered into a position in which restraint is possible, or they must be restrained from the outset as a safety measure. Such maneuvering is perceived by the animal as conflict, and in order to understand the principles of maneuvering each species, it is wise to familiarize oneself with the predominant forms of agonistic behavior in the different species. Agonistic behaviors cover the range of response to conflict—from passive avoidance, through the assertion of dominance, to the extreme of aggression and fighting. In nature, overt aggressive attacks that lead to fights with other animals of the same or different species are not common outside sexual or predatory behavior. Dominance and submissive behavior is the more common method of resolving disagreement over things such as territory and favors.

Flight or Fight

When an animal is approached by a stranger, the same basic principles apply whether it is a domestic or a wild animal. Each species in a given environment has its own degree of response, but the factors or cues giving rise to the response are common to all animals in varying degrees. Each animal has a flight distance. If a person encroaches on that distance, which is measured visually, the animal goes into a state of alert. This has been referred to as being "adrenalinized," because the signals from the brain via the sympathetic nervous system cause the secretion of adrenaline from the adrenal gland. This is what causes the pounding of one's heart and the tingling, alert sensation one feels when scared or apprehensive before competition or before speaking to a large audience. In the flight mode, the animal's muscles prepare for movement, the heart rate increases and the available blood is routed to body parts that are essential for dealing with emergencies, namely, skeletal muscles, lungs, and brain.

Further movement toward the animal, particularly if it is unable to maintain a safe distance between itself and you, will lead to action that may take the form of avoidance or aggressive action referred to as "fight or flight."

Effects of Domestication

Domestic animals have been selected by humans for certain characteristics, such as the ability to be socialized and handled. It must have been obvious to our early ancestors that certain species of animals were more suitable for domestication than others.

The characteristics of wild species deemed suitable for domestication would be that (1) they herded or flocked easily, (2) males cohabited alongside females, (3) males would mate with any female in heat, (4) they bred and reared young easily, (5) they were easily approached within a relatively short flight distance and (6) they adapted well to containment and different feedstuffs. Animals unsuitable for domestication would be those that are strongly territorial, with the males and females living separately or pair bonding, thereby requiring one male for each female. Unsuitable species would also have a strict diet, not being adaptable to a new environment, and show fear of humans by having a large flight distance.

Aggressive Behavior

Aggressive behavior is the form of agonistic or conflict behavior that leads to and includes fighting. Aggression is not the result of a single cause. The different forms of aggression are classified according to the stimuli or circumstances giving rise to ferocity.

Irritable or Pain-Induced Aggression

Inevitably, irritable or pain-induced aggression is a common problem in the veterinary hospital. Injections and certain manipulations, such as treatment of minor wounds, cause a certain degree of pain and discomfort. Even the initial injection of a local anesthetic can be most uncomfortable, no matter how skillful the anesthetist. The state of mind of the patient may have a lot to do with an aggressive outcome. If the animal is apprehensive and nervous initially, the probability for aggression is higher. It is for this reason that calming and familiarization of the patient is practiced whenever possible.

Maternal Aggression

All female domestic animals suckling their young are sensitized to interference with their offspring by strangers. The calmest, gentlest old mare in the herd may be particularly protective of her foal. The bitch can be aggressive with strangers or even less familiar family members whom she perceives to be a threat to her pups. The sow remaining in earshot of her piglets during their restraint for castration can become one of the most dangerous animals encountered. In fact, the screaming of any young pig as it is manipulated can galvanize all the sows in the farrowing house.

Predatory Aggression

Aggressive activity displayed by chasing and killing prey, which is observed in the predatory domestic animals (i.e., dog and cat), is called predatory aggression. It does not usually pose a threat to the animal handler, though the sight hounds or large dogs of other breeds may pull you off your feet to chase a cat.

Territorial Aggression

All domestic mammals are territorial, in that they will protect the area over which they range from intruders, and they may exhibit territorial aggression. Separate groups of horses may share feeding sites and watering holes, but they remain apart from one another and retain control of their home range.

Dogs retain the innate characteristic of territoriality of their ancestor, the wolf. The domestic dog regards the yard as its territory, or at least the territory of its pack—its family. Thus, members of the family go about their business without hindrance, whereas strangers are treated with suspicion, which may lead to barking or even an attack. Dogs harassing mail carriers and meter readers are behaving within the norms of canine behavior. The fact that this is not socially acceptable to humans is a different matter.

The female rabbit is strongly territorial in the captive situation. If the buck rabbit is taken to her cage, she will attack him very aggressively, often causing serious injury. Thus, the doe is always taken to the buck's cage for mating. This strong female territoriality may be associated with a maternal aggression that continues even when the nesting box is empty and that can be directed at humans as well as other animals. The image of an "attack rabbit" is laughable until you must reach into the cage of an obstreperous female who thumps, growls, strikes or even bites in response.

Fear-Induced Aggression

When an animal is fearful of the environment and the people in it, and it feels that it cannot avoid the situation, it will resort to aggression. Fear is a common cause of aggression in dogs in such circumstances. Fear biting is the most commonly encountered type of attack in veterinary clinics. The attack is not overtly dominant. The dog is usually giving classic signs of intimidation, avoiding direct eye contact with head down, lips pulled back horizontally, ears flattened, tail between the legs and perhaps emitting a low growl. If you enter the personal space of such a dog in an attempt to placate it, a sudden attack may ensue. This is fear biting, and as might be expected, this attack is usually confined to the proffered hand or forearm.

Intermale Aggression

Aggression occurring between males, or intermale aggression, can be a problem, particularly when stud animals are being kept. Boars can be particularly vicious when confronting each other, and great care for one's own safety should be taken when dealing with them.

Sexually Induced Aggression

Sexual fighting in the presence of females in estrus is well recognized.

Dominance Aggression

The domestic dog, as we have said before, is descended from the wolf, and like the wolf it is a pack animal. The dog recognizes a hierarchy in the family and knows the pack leader. Pack leadership is established by the owner, as a result of providing food, shelter, play and companionship, exercise and authority. Certain dogs, however, establish their authority over the family, other animals and strangers, and do so quite aggressively. Alternatively, a dog may accede to dominance from one family member but attempt to assert itself aggressively with others. Such animals are a menace in the clinic, as they will not merely fear bite but will attack you. Persuasion will be of little value in handling these dogs. Forget your canine charisma and use reliable restraint from the start.

Other species housed in groups also develop hierarchies. Horse owners recognize the "pecking order" of their animals and learn to avoid being in the escape path of a submissive animal when it is challenged by an aggressively dominant one.

Typical Behavior of Domestic Animals in Aggression and Avoidance

Horses

Blatant aggressive behavior in the horse is not common. Certain horses, however, are known to be nasty, and, of course, mares with foal at foot and stallions with brood mares may be aggressive for the reasons we have just discussed. Aggression is characterized by lunging forward and biting, by kicking with the hind legs, or by striking with the forelegs. Striking is invariably accompanied by squealing. Although the field of vision for a horse is almost 360 degrees, the binocular field of vision is only 60 to 70 degrees in front. Binocular vision is essential for judging distance; therefore, vision outside the 60-degree to 70-degree binocular vision field will detect objects and movement and will result in a change of the head position, or sometimes the body position, for further investigation.

When approaching a horse, it is obvious that one does not creep up on its blind spot from immediately behind and suddenly appear from the left or right rear. When a horse detects a new object or person in its environment, it raises its head and observes. If it is satisfied that it is a nonthreatening person or object, it will resume its previous activity. If it is anxious, it will turn its head toward the object or person, raising the neck, focusing its ears and dilating its nostrils, thereby using its keen senses to analyze the situation. The tail is elevated, the legs are poised for flight and, occasionally, if startled, the horse will snort, rapidly exhaling through tensed nostrils. This alarm signal will alert other horses to your approach and signal them to get ready to run from danger. A mare with a foal will usually give a warning nicker, and the foal will move in close to her side in response. If one approaches further and the horse is alarmed, it will move rapidly away to avoid the object or person. If there is more than one horse, they will move together.

Cattle

The primary concern is with the bull, regardless of size. The smaller Channel Island dairy breed bulls are particularly unpredictable. Aggressive behavior is characterized by pawing the ground with the forefeet while holding the head with the frontal area almost vertical with the ground and snorting. A bull, after charging and knocking a person down, will then make continued attempts to toss the victim, which may lead to goring if the bull has horns. In addition, he may attempt to kneel on a victim. Since little can be done to thwart a determined bull, the gory details given are merely to emphasize that bulls should *always* be treated with the utmost respect and with the appropriate means of restraint and containment. There are special handling considerations for those who may work with semen donors at artificial insemination centers. Insensitive handling prior to and during coitus may give rise to reproductive behavior problems. Suffice to say that bad handling may lead to considerable economic loss.

Aggressiveness in the heifer and the cow seems to be directly related to breed and socialization. Dairy breed cows are generally very docile because they are handled a great deal. Beef breeds that are handled frequently are very manageable. However, the more cattle are left to themselves and the more frequently they are reared as calves with little human contact, the more aggression they will demonstrate in the situations described earlier.

The flight or fight distance for a herd of cattle will vary tremendously, depending upon the previous degree and type of contact with humans. There is a vast difference between handling a herd of dairy cows and herding range cattle. The flight distance for dairy cattle is very short, with the animals only veering away as their personal space is entered. The other extreme is cattle that attempt to maintain a long flight distance by gradually moving farther away. In situations in which this is no longer effective, the animals may break into a run. It is amazing how few people it can take, either on foot in a fenced situation or on horseback in a range situation, to maneuver cattle at the walk. If cattle break into a run, control is much more difficult, if not impossible. Part of the secret to maneuvering cattle is body extension. Using a staff or stock whip when on foot is perceived by the cattle as an extension of the body. If the cattle are kept calm, such body extension is a good visual barrier to them. A person on horseback has the substantial advantage of the body extension of the horse, in addition to increased mobility.

Calves

The calf is invariably inquisitive and will become very attentive to your presence with the head stretched toward you. If you *dart* forward, the calf may panic, veer and run away. Calves remember rough handling and, after such experiences, will be harder to approach in the future. If your approach is quiet, deliberate and unruffled, the calf will turn slowly to avoid you. You then move to one side or the other to cut off the escape. The calf should thus be negotiated into a corner and the lower face or jaw should be grasped, pulling the head over to one side against you.

Adult cattle may be held by the nose, but this is too severe and inhumane for calves and may lead to handling problems later in life.

Pigs

Aggressive behavior in the domestic pig may have serious economic and physical consequences. Two strange adult boars in one another's presence will circle each other, obviously using olfaction as a principal means of perception. Threats will be made by jaw snapping and barking grunts. Fighting commences in the side to side, head to head position, with sideways pushing and slashing at one another with tusks. Such fights may, if not stopped, result in significant wounding. Only foolhardy people would use their body parts to break up a boar fight. Solid or heavyweight wire panels or plywood may be inserted between the combatants.

Pigs are mostly reared in groups, which provides opportunity for fighting. Pigs more than 2 weeks of age will fight, and hierarchies or pecking orders are established on the basis of dominance and submission. When new pigs are introduced to the group, fighting may occur, particularly if living space and trough space are limited. A sow introduced into an established group may be attacked savagely and even killed. Aggression in pigs may be reduced by allowing more space and/or diversions (such as playthings). Chemical manipulation (tranquilizers) may reduce initial fighting when unfamiliar swine are put together.

The fully grown sow is capable of killing a human and is most dangerous when raising her litter. In our description of maternal aggression, we cited the sow as a prime example. We repeat, when handling unweaned pigs always remove the sow to a secure area, out of earshot, if possible.

Avoidance behavior in young pigs in confined spaces usually involves running into corners and huddling, shoving and even climbing over one another. When pigs are approached and some are caught, the rest may run again and huddle in another corner. This tendency continues as they get older. If kept calm, pigs in the open will move well as a herd.

Sheep

Intermale aggression in rams can lead to injury and fatal gangrenous lesions of the head from butting. An aggressive ram may be formidable to handle and, because of a willingness to challenge and butt people, should be treated with respect.

Avoidance behavior in sheep is the basis of maneuvering the flock. When sheep are approached, they will form a tight bunch and move together. This herding or flocking behavior is well understood by the sheep dog. Sheep dogs by breeding and training have had the canine predatory behavior modified to herding. By carefully controlling their posture, speed of movement, and distance from the flock, they can use ovine avoidance behavior precisely enough to maneuver the flock into an enclosure. The combined results of the observation and use of the behavior by shepherd dog and flock is undoubtedly one of the most fascinating, complex interspecies relationships in domestic animal management.

Dogs

Overt viciousness is not a common occurrence in the dog. Aggressive behavior, however, is a significant social problem. It has been estimated that there are more than 1 million dog bites in the United States annually and that close to 40 percent of the animals identified in biting incidents have not been vaccinated against rabies. The number of human deaths occurring as a result of dog attacks has not been accurately determined, but the number is considered to be significant, particularly among small children.

Dominance and submission are important in communication between two dogs in a conflict situation. *Dominance* is signaled by fixing the other animal in a direct stare; the ears are raised and angled forward. The front end of the body is held high, and the hackles raised. The head is held up and lips curl to reveal the incisor and canine teeth, and the tail is raised. A *submissive* role is shown by lowering the front end of the body and avoiding direct eye contact, with the tail held between the legs. The animal may squat and urinate or defecate. The backbone may adopt an S shape, and the animal may lie down on its side or on its back, raising the upper legs and exposing its undefended belly.

It should be noted that the "clinical stare" of veterinary personnel, as they examine a dog, can be taken as a dominance challenge by the dog.

When treated by a person, the dog may demonstrate potential aggression by adopting the dominantly aggressive posture already described or by adopting a submissive or intimidated stance. In this case, the dog lowers the front of the body and head. The ears are flattened back on the head, and the lips are pulled back at the corners in a "grin." The tail is held between the legs. A dog in the active or dominant aggressive posture may attack if the threat is not removed from its fight or flight distance. The dog in the intimidated posture will bite only if you attempt to encroach on its personal or intimate distance. This, of course, is the pattern of fear biting.

Certain dogs do not attempt to resolve potential conflict by dominance or aggression, preferring to avoid and circumvent it completely whenever possible. Dogs that tend to face conflict situations are said to have an active defense reflex (ADR), whereas those that skillfully avoid conflict are described as having a passive defense reflex (PDR). These two major categories of canine agonistic behavior were recognized as militarily important in selecting dogs. These dogs having highly developed ADRs were selected as guard dogs, and those with strong PDRs, which would carefully avoid being captured, were selected to be message-carrying dogs.

Cats

Aggressive behavior in the cat should never be underestimated. The use of the claws of all four feet and teeth makes the cat a formidable patient in a situation of conflict. Handling cats in all moods is discussed later in this chapter. Note that the cat stalks its prey and runs short distances to pounce. It is a stealthy aggressor. The cat's true speed never becomes apparent until it is actively avoiding conflict. In the clinic, to prevent its escape, all doors and windows must be closed before an attempt is made to handle a cat.

Management Ethology

Ethology is the study of animal behavior. What we are discussing in this chapter is sometimes called "management ethology," which is the study of animal behavior as a means of determining how best to maneuver and control animals. A complete discussion on animal behavior is found in Chapter 26.

What follows is a detailed description of standard methods of approaching and handling animals that have been developed over the years. You will see that the approach and handling techniques are essentially in harmony with the behavior of the various species, and the physical methods of restraint are compatible with their anatomy. The unique powers of humans to observe, and a great deal of trial and error, have brought us to the present state of the art. You must acquire that knowledge to attain competency, but nothing can substitute for keen perception, alertness and the ability to comprehensively observe and analyze each situation. The only way to learn the art is to prepare yourself mentally and then do it, with confidence and the knowledge that you have made a sound assessment of the particular situation.

Capture and Restraint of Horses

Horses may pose interesting problems in their capture. Most horses soon learn that capture leads to work or unpleasantness and therefore practice avoidance to a greater or lesser degree. Let us begin with the horse that does not readily avoid people.

One thing that must always be kept in mind when handling horses is their innate antipathy to close confinement. Horses do not do well in "squeeze"-type situations, although most can be trained to accept them. Whereas most cattle will accept tight quarters for capture, this situation is liable to make a horse nervous or anxious. Close quarters may well lead to an attempt at escape and may result in injuries to the horse, people or both.

A cardinal rule when approaching almost any animal, but *especially* a horse, is not to startle it. One should always make one's presence known by talking, calling, whistling, singing, thumping feed buckets and so forth before entering the flight distance of the horse. For the normal domesticated horse, the flight distance is probably between 6 meters (m) and 15 m. Things that occur outside this radius are usually of little concern to the horse as threats, but once within this area sudden movements or sharp noises may easily startle it. Always be sure that the horse is observing you as you approach. If it suddenly is aware of you already inside its danger zone, it will be startled, which usually results in its jumping away from you, but it may also result in your getting kicked as the intruder.

It should be obvious to anyone that approaching a horse from the rear should be avoided if at all possible. Given the horse's zone of vision and its blind spot behind, the horse is less likely to see the person and is therefore likely to "spook" when the person's presence is discovered; in addition, the person becomes dangerously vulnerable to a kick. Horses approached from the front or side may whirl and kick, but the extra 1.5 seconds that the horse takes to turn is well used to effect a rapid retreat.

A horse's kick zone extends 1.8 m to 2.5 m behind him. The furthest extension of his heels is the most dangerous and is the area of potentially fatal kicks to the head. Horses usually kick to the rear, rather than to the side as the cow kicks. Therefore, the prudent person will circle at least 3 m to 3.5 m behind a horse or else directly behind and in physical contact with him. Grasping the tail as one walks around the rear of the horse may discourage a kick. Staying close to the rear end of the horse will not allow the full force of a kick and will keep the blow low on the person's body. This is not to suggest that a short-range kick is not painful or dangerous—it very well may be—but a fractured tibia is of much less importance than a fractured skull.

It should also be noted than one should never stand directly in front of a horse whether the animal is loose or on a lead. The rare horse (often a stallion or gelding) may strike with a foreleg, which can be as damaging as a kick.

The best approach to a horse is from the front and slightly to the left side. The left side is, in horseman's terminology, the "near" side, the side from which the horse is usually handled because of convention and because most people lead horses with the right hand. The horse's right side is called the "off" side. The reason for approaching somewhat from the side is to give the horse the option of turning slightly away. At the first indication of the horse turning away (the head turning away from you), you should stop or even back off a step. The horse will usually stop turning away and your standing there talking to him will pique his curiosity. Many "shy" horses may be approached this way, in increments, with each pause assuring the horse that you do not intend to hurt him. The worst thing one can do when the horse starts to move away is to proceed toward him, because he will assume you are giving chase and will keep moving off. Once you are behind the horse and he cannot see you well, you become even more of a threat from which to flee.

The approach to a horse should be unhurried and without sudden movements. Horses may be wise to the purpose of halters or ropes, so it is often sensible to conceal these items under the clothing. One may also use a small-diameter catch rope or piece of baling twine hidden in the hand to loop around the neck before trying to halter the animal. Presenting the hands empty may help to gain the horse's confidence. Sometimes horses, especially foals, will walk right up to a person who squats on the heels. The shorter stature probably makes the figure less threatening, as well as an object of curiosity.

Once you have gotten up to a horse, it is worth a moment's attention to reward it for standing still. Most horses like to be scratched on the side of the face behind the lips. One may then work backward along the side of the jaw, to the base of the neck, which is a favorite scratching spot. Some horses are "head-shy" and should be scratched on the neck first. If the horse stands quietly for these operations, it will probably accept a rope around the neck. The rope is best applied by bringing the rope end in the left hand from under the neck

on the off side and grasping the end with the right hand, which has been slipped over the neck (Fig. 1–1). An alternate method on quiet horses is to have the right arm over the neck and to pass the crown strap of the halter to the right hand. While giving the horse the impression that it is restrained by the right arm, one manipulates the halter noseband over the nose, and the crown strap is then fastened (Fig. 1–2). The type of halter that does not unfasten to go behind the ears will require that the horse be restrained by a neck rope while being haltered. This is usually best accomplished by standing on the near side and holding the neck rope with the left hand while the right hand glides the halter over the face and ears. The horse is usually "caught" when the crown piece is behind the ears. Some horses are gentle and good-natured and may allow someone to walk up to them and throw a rope around their necks or halter them without ceremony, but after the veterinarian's truck pulls into the yard it is more often not the case. The veterinarian's truck usually signals (whether by acute vision, memory of previous contact, medicinal smells or a combination) the arrival of strangers who will draw blood, administer medication by stomach tube and/or injection and so forth.

What does one do with the horse that moves off as soon as he sees a person approach? The usual answer is bribery. A handful of grain, hay or grass, or a bucket of grain may entice the horse to approach or be approached. It is best to hold the bribe in the left hand and to turn at right angles to the horse so that the neck and shoulder are within easy reach of the right hand for scratching. When confidence has been established through scratching the neck, the right hand may be placed around the neck for restraint. Some horses are cagey and cooperate up to the point of restraint with the arm, whereupon they will whirl away. These horses may be candidates for roping or trapping.

Many horses that are impossible to catch in a large field "give up" in an enclosed space. Some animals, however, may become exceptionally nervous in a small area and may be prone to kick or to try to break out in panic when approached. A pole syringe or capture gun with tranquilizer is sometimes the only answer. Luring cagey but tame animals into a corral or stall with feed may work well. It may be necessary to leave

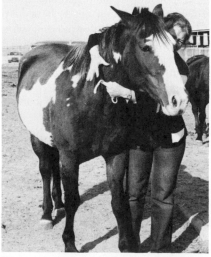

FIGURE 1–1. Placing the rope around the horse's neck.

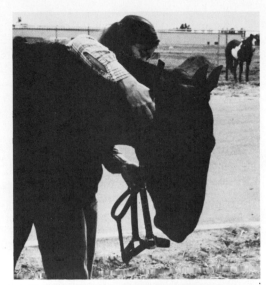

FIGURE 1–2. Putting the halter on the horse. Do not bump the horse's nose with the noseband.

the bait inside and then sneak up and close the gate after the horse has entered.

Exciting the horse at any point is a self-defeating act. An excited horse loses its common sense and in fear can try to go over, under, around or through whatever is containing it.

Roping the horse is impossible (except for an expert on a roping horse) unless the horse is in a reasonably small enclosure. Again, it is important to keep the horse as quiet as possible. Therefore, whirling the rope overhead is not desirable, as it will be frightening to the average horse that is unacquainted with such cowboy tactics. Instead, one needs to cultivate a low, backhand roping technique. A loop is made that just brushes the ground when the loop and rope are held at waist level (Fig. 1–3). A generous amount of excess rope (yet not enough to touch the ground) is played out from the coils, which are held loosely in the left hand so as to peel them off with a light pull. The right hand holds the loop on the left side of the body, palm facing the body, and the roper situates himself or herself 2.5 to 3 m from a fence on his or her right side. The horse (facing the roper) is then driven past, between the roper and the fence. The roper, anticipating when the horse will go past, flips the loop backhanded for the horse to run into. The fence keeps the horse from ducking away from the movement, and strong driving from behind will force it into the loop. This technique is surprisingly successful for amateurs.

It should be stressed that one should not attempt to rope a horse without wearing gloves, for the obvious reasons. The right hand initially will be holding the rope. The coils could tighten around the left hand if they are held fast. If the horse is charging through at such a rate that it cannot be held, one should release the rope before being jerked off balance and dragged. One may always pick up the loose end of the rope after the horse has stopped running.

Horses that show signs of dangerous vices or viciousness (such as charging or threatening to kick) should not be given the opportunity to harm you by physical proximity. There are means of tranquilization or anesthetization that do not require being close to the horse (i.e., pole syringe, capture gun). However, they are seldom used in veterinary practice.

Restraining and Catching Foals

Foals pose different problems of capture than do adult horses. Being without any previous knowledge of humans, newborn foals act from instinct in avoiding strange creatures and will hide behind the mother for safety.

Before approaching the foal, one must have the mare securely restrained. When her foal starts to struggle or vocalize in fear, or both, a mare may try to attack whatever threatens her baby. The most docile mare may be the most protective of her foal.

When capturing a foal, one must be careful not to let it harm itself in trying to escape. The ideal situation is to crowd the foal into a corner of a stout solid fence or solid wall. The barrier must not have holes that the youngster may try to climb through and possibly hurt itself. One should never crowd a foal into a barbed wire fence or other flimsy barrier. If that is all that is available, one should use enough people to surround and capture the foal. Obviously, catching a foal is at least a two-person job, except when the mare and foal are in a stall in which the mare is tied.

The easiest way to catch a foal is to back the mare snugly against the wall about the length of the foal from the corner, which will form a box in the corner of the barrier. The person who is to catch the foal then enters the box at its open end and slowly approaches the foal. Almost inevitably the foal will cower against the opposite wall with its head close to the mother's rump. The foal should be approached "amidship," with the knowledge that the nearness of hands or actually touching it will be a signal to bolt. A foal almost always bolts forward and toward its mother, and the person should be ready to catch it under the neck with one arm when this occurs, to be followed immediately by the other arm around the rump or the hand around the tail (the tail is grasped from underneath, with the palm facing the underside of the tail). Grasping the tail is the most secure way to hold the hindquarters but, bear in mind that it is more uncomfortable for the foal, so it may struggle longer. Also, some owners may object to their foals being han-

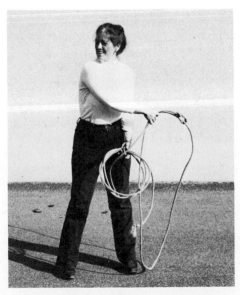

FIGURE 1–3. The method of holding the lariat for roping a horse.

dled this way because it is a more negative experience for the foal, with long-term effects on behavior. There is also a rare chance that the tail could be injured.

If one grabs only the foal's neck, its reaction will be a rapid reverse and the foal will escape, becoming harder to catch the next time. Veterinary personnel should not contribute unduly to the negative experiences of the foal. Extra attention to scratching and getting the foal to develop trust in people is appreciated by clients and will make the youngster easier to deal with the next time.

Having grabbed the foal fore and aft, the handler may have need to push it against the fence until it stops struggling. There is a tendency to lift a foal off its feet when doing this, which is poor technique. If the foal loses its footing, it may become more frightened and struggle more vigorously, and it may severely batter your shins with its hooves.

As soon as the foal is securely caught one should take pains to reassure it and its mother that no harm is meant. One way is to position the mare and foal so that they face each other. They should be as close as possible without the mare becoming a nuisance in whatever procedure is being carried out on the foal. It is generally a poor practice to separate mare and foal, as both will fret until they are close again.

Halter and Chain Lead

The halter is the basic restraint tool for horses, but it is inadequate for some tasks. Halters that have rings at the side of the nosepiece may be made more effective if a chain lead is passed from one side to the other. The lead is snapped on the side of the halter that is away from the handler after being passed through the loop near the handler, usually on the near side. This arrangement allows finer control of the direction of the horse's nose and, if squeezed when pulled, puts some authority into the restraint because of the discomfort it causes. If at all possible, the chain lead should come in contact with the horse very lightly, or not at all, unless the horse misbehaves. Constant pressure is worrisome to the animal and does not leave any reserve.

There are three possible positions for the chain lead on the halter. The least authoritative is under the jaw, at which point it mainly causes a squeeze around the nose. Horses with very tender chins or those who are not accustomed to a chain lead may throw their heads or lunge backward when the lead is pulled. Horses that sense a squeezing of the nose as a signal to back up must be carefully retrained to respond correctly. It is often necessary to *release* pressure to allow the horse to stop its reverse. The chain over the nose is very effective (Fig. 1–4). The top of the nose is sensitive, and a pull there will make the horse drop the nose and stop forward progress. Very few stallions should be led about by a plain halter; the chain over the nose is essential. Finally, a more severe treatment would be the chain passing through the mouth. However, many stallions are hand-bred with the chain lead through the mouth, so they might associate it with breeding and become sexually excited.

Tying the Horse

There are a few simple rules to follow when a horse must be tied. First, all equipment must be strong and sound. This includes the halter, the rope and whatever the rope will be tied to. If the halter is suspect, the rope may be passed through the

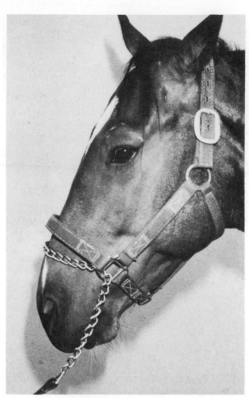

FIGURE 1–4. The chain lead used to increase control of the halter.

nose of the halter and tied around the horse's neck with a nonslip knot, preferably a bowline. Snaps on ropes are suspect, because all but the heaviest will break when a strong horse jerks back on them with all its weight. If something breaks, the horse will be free (and may learn to pull back as an escape whenever tied), but perhaps more importantly it may throw itself over backward and sustain serious harm. The second rule is that the horse be tied to something at its shoulder height or higher. There should be about only 60 centimeters (cm) of rope between the halter and the tie post (i.e., a little longer than the length of the horse's head) to prevent the horse from pawing over the rope, panicking and pulling back. Third, there should be no hazardous objects in the tie area (i.e., children, dogs) that might spook the horse. Finally, a horse should never be left unobserved.

In general, one should be holding rather than tying horses for veterinary procedures, since horses can get into trouble while tied. It is also a general rule that the holder should stand on the same side of the horse as the veterinarian, because the head, rather than the body or hindquarters, will therefore be directed toward the practitioner if the horse should move around.

The Twitch

The twitch is a nerve-stimulating device that can immobilize horses and is therefore helpful in veterinary restraint. Most twitches are applied to the upper lip of the horse. The most innocuous is the so-called humane twitch, which is a hinged pair of long handles that squeeze down over the sides of the lip and may then be secured at the bottom by a thong and snapped back to the halter. The advantage of this twitch is that once applied it need not be held in place (Fig. 1–5). The

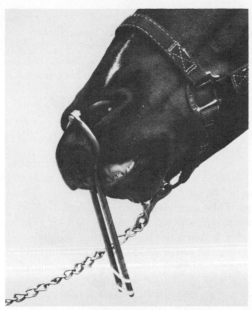

FIGURE 1–5. The humane twitch in place on the horse's lip.

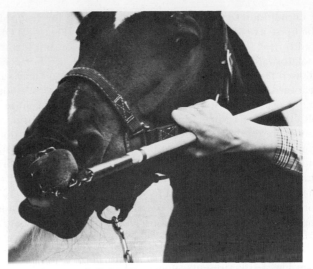

FIGURE 1–6. The correct way to hold the chain twitch.

disadvantage is that the pressure is fairly mild and some horses ignore it. More traditional twitches rely on a loop and a leverage device. The loop of chain or rope is placed on the lip and tightened by twisting the leverage device. The leverage may be from a piece of wood or pipe about 50 cm long. The loop needs to be seated on the lip behind the heavy gristle pad at its tip and ahead of the nostrils. On some thick-nosed horses this area may be hard to find. Horses that have been twitched are wise and will throw their heads and tighten the lip when one attempts to apply the twitch.

To apply the twitch, place the loop over the back of three fingers and the thumb (leaving one finger, the first or second, out of the loop to keep the twitch from sliding back on the hand or wrist). Grasp the end of the horse's lip, slide the loop off your fingers, and twist the handle until the twitch is snug and starts to elongate and distort the horse's lip. It is best to have someone hold the horse's halter as the twitch is applied. This will allow the second hand of the person applying the twitch to keep the handle from flinging around if the horse should throw its head. If the horse is to stand still, the twitch should be tightened until the horse responds. The average person probably cannot twist enough to damage the horse. Once the twitch has been applied, the person holding it should also be holding the halter (Fig. 1 6). To keep the long handle of the twitch from being in the way, it should be held with the cheekpiece of the halter alongside the horse's face. After removing the twitch, the horse's nose should be rubbed vigorously to counteract the discomfort and numbness present. This will feel good to the horse and may keep it from avoiding hands on the nose after the twitching experience. In the absence of a twitch, a person with a firm grip can hold the upper lip.

Whenever applying or holding a twitch of any kind do not stand directly in front of a horse. Sometimes twitches will encourage a horse to strike. There are people who twist horses' ears for restraint. Ear twisting is a poor practice because the supporting structures of the ear may be damaged, causing disfigurement.

Lifting the Foreleg

Some horses will stand still if a foreleg is picked up and held. When one foreleg is held up, the horse will usually leave the other three legs on the ground.

To lift up a horse's foreleg, one stands next to the horse slightly forward of the leg, facing toward the horse's rear (Fig. 1–7). It is easier to lift any leg if the horse's weight is first pushed off that leg. You may lean against the horse or push with the hand near it to effect the shifting of weight. The leg itself is grasped at the same time by running thumb and forefinger down on either side of the suspensory ligament, just behind the cannon bone. Squeezing the suspensory ligament between the cannon bone and the flexor tendons is uncomfortable to the horse if it has weight on its foot, and the horse will therefore cock its knee and fetlock joint. The foot may then be picked up by the fetlock hair or by cradling the anterior aspect of the fetlock. The forefoot may then be inserted between one's legs from behind to be held between the thighs just above the knees, which frees both hands.

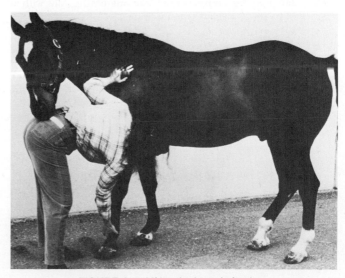

FIGURE 1–7. Lifting the horse's foreleg.

Lifting hind feet is almost the same as lifting forefeet; shift the horse's weight, then grasp the leg and foot (Fig. 1–8). One stands near the horse's stifle or further anterior and lifts the foot forward to get it off the ground. Once the horse has allowed the leg to be lifted and is holding it up, one may walk rearward with the leg, staying quite close to the horse's body and proceeding rearward until the lower leg nestles comfortably across one's upper thigh, with the hoof on the inside of the thigh, the horse's hock at about waist level and the tibial region of its leg snug against one's side. The leg should stay braced in this position without the use of hands. The horse that threatens to kick or refuses to let its hind leg be held up may have it dragged up and forward with a scotch hobble. A foreleg may be tied up by passing a strap or rope around forearm and lower leg in a loop and doubling up the leg. A horse could fall and seriously injure the knee with a foreleg tied up. Having the hind leg pulled up with a scotch hobble (see Fig. 1–10) presents similar concerns of instability, especially if the horse is struggling. Legs should never be pulled up like this if the horse is not on a "soft" surface.

Stocks

Horses have an innate fear of being enclosed. In some horses this fear is pathological, and they will kick their way out of close situations. Therefore, the use of stocks with horses should be approached with caution, and every effort should be made to calm the horse and accustom it to the situation. The best horse stocks are heavy pipes or poles in a single row that are the height of the point of the shoulder. It is best if they have some quick-release mechanism, particularly for the piece at the rear, in case the horse should throw a fit. Horses should not be left unsupervised in stocks. Stocks are often used for rectal palpations. If no stocks are available, one might wish to stand a horse next to a wall or stout pole fence and back it up to a couple of bales of hay or straw, which might deflect or discourage kicks. Some veterinarians prefer to palpate standing unprotected tight behind the horse (especially if the veterinarian has short arms).

Tail Tie

During rectal palpations and vaginal examinations, the horse's tail may be conveniently tied out of the way with a small cord tied to the hair. The end of the rope must *never* be tied to anything but the horse itself. Tying the free end around the neck is best. If the horse gets loose with the tail tied to a stationary object, serious injury could result. The tail tie is a simple quick-release knot using a small rope placed across the tail just below the fleshy portion (Fig. 1–9). The long end of the rope can be tied with a quick-release knot around the neck.

Hobbles

Horses are very seldom hobbled or cast (thrown to the ground) since the advent of chemical restraint. However, breeding hobbles are still used to prevent a horse from kicking effectively. These are hobbles fitted around the hocks with web or leather straps, which are tied to a neck strap or neck rope after passing between the forelegs. They should be adjusted to snugness with the horse standing in a normal position.

The scotch hobble is a means of drawing up the hind leg (Fig. 1–10). It is often used, with or without a figure-eight on the lower leg, for holding the "up" leg for a castration procedure. A heavy rope should be used to avoid rope burn. Before the animal is anesthetized, a loop is tied with a bowline (nonslip knot) around the base of the horse's neck. Once the horse is down, a loop to catch the hindleg is passed through the neck loop and is placed behind the pastern. The leg is drawn up and forward by pulling the end of the rope, using the neck loop as a pulley. To avoid rope burn of the pastern, the leg can be pulled up by hand at the same time the rope is tightening.

Restraint While Lying Down

There are times when a horse must be held lying down. Control of the head is the key, because in order to get up the horse must first lift its head. Therefore, sitting or kneeling on the neck near the head will keep it down. In addition, to keep the horse from waggling its head and possibly damaging the down eye, one should pull the horse's nose off the ground by the nosepiece of the halter. The head can be held at almost 45 degrees to the neck. One always climbs on the neck from the back of the horse. Any activities performed on a lying horse should be done from the back, not from the belly side, in which position a thrashing leg could strike you. A horse that is lying down should either have its head held up or have its lateral face and eye cushioned to prevent eye and facial nerve damage. A gunny sack or coat can be folded and tucked under the halter, or an inner tube can be pushed under the head.

Other Head and Mouth Restraints

Horses sometimes mutilate themselves or tear bandages. There are devices to restrict the movement of the head laterally. One is the cradle, a device of wooden slats that buckles over the horse's neck to brace it straight (Fig. 1–11). These devices restrict lateral movement but allow the horse to eat. A wire muzzle may be put on a horse that is to be held off feed to prevent it from eating bedding while giving it access to water.

There are at least two kinds of gags for horses' mouths. One is a simple wedge (Fig. 1–12), which is pushed up between the upper and lower cheek teeth with the handle hanging out of the side of the horse's mouth. The other, a large hinged spec-

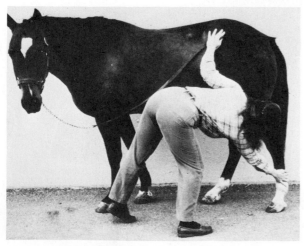

FIGURE 1–8. Lifting hind leg.

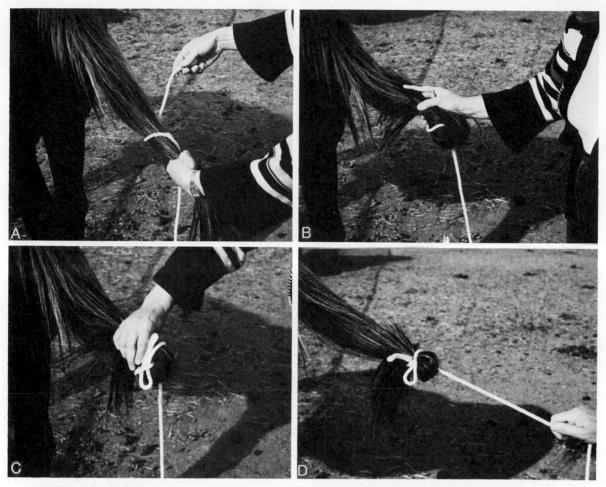

FIGURE 1–9. The steps in making a secure tail tie. A, The rope is placed around the tail. B, The tail is folded back on itself and on the rope. C, The short end of the rope passes over the folded tail, and a loop is pushed under the tail-encircling portion of the rope. D, Tension on the long end of the rope makes the knot snug. Pulling the short end of the rope will release the knot.

ulum, fits over upper and lower incisors and hangs from the halter. The mouth can be cranked open. Although this device is effective in getting the mouth open, it is, unfortunately, heavy and cumbersome. The horse's tongue may be pulled out of the side of the mouth in the interdental space and held, usually by the clinician. Some veterinarians prefer to hold the tongue to the opposite side when examining the mouth or floating the teeth, rather than using a gag.

Blindfolding a pushy horse that insists on charging around and walking all over its handler may make it reluctant or hesi-

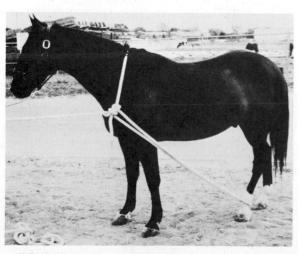

FIGURE 1–10. The scotch hobble on a standing horse.

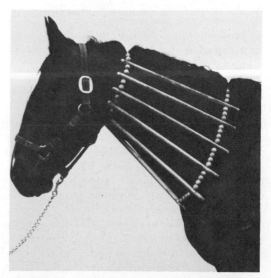

FIGURE 1–11. The horse wearing a neck cradle.

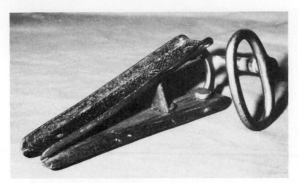

FIGURE 1–12. The wedge gag. The wedge is slid between upper and lower cheek teeth, and the handle comes out of the corner of the mouth.

tant to move. A blindfold may also make the horse kick at painful or unfamiliar sensations around the hindquarters.

Chemical Restraint

Manual casting of horses has been largely replaced by chemical restraint and anesthesia. Casting has always held inherent danger for both horse and handler. One of the common injuries for the horse is damage to the knees when the forefeet are pulled out from under it. The thrashing around that tends to accompany casting can cause a variety of injuries.

The most commonly used chemical restraint for horses is xylazine hydrochloride (Rompun) in tranquilizing dosages, but many people have been dismayed by some horses that can and will kick readily under the influence of xylazine. Some practitioners use morphine with xylazine, which generally leaves horses standing stolidly in a saw-horse stance, unwilling to move. Whenever a horse has been anesthetized or tranquilized, it should be observed until it is steady on its feet. It may be necessary for several people to steady a wobbly horse so that it does not fall and hurt itself. Anesthesiology and chemical restraint are discussed in Chapter 11.

Capture and Restraint of Cattle

Cattle are less difficult to capture than are horses. Generally, except for "pet" cattle and some dairy cattle, they are not directly approachable for haltering and leading. However, they are easier to drive into chutes and stocks.

Cattle are less discriminating than horses about what (or whom) they step on or bump into. Domestic cattle have much of the natural avoidance bred out of them and are very curious. They may stand still and ogle as a person approaches, especially if there is something odd about the person (e.g., a limp or strangely shaped clothing). They will then bolt when the person gets too close. Unfortunately, they may choose to bolt over the person if there are obstacles to other routes. If cattle do not move away as they are approached within 9 m to 12 m, drivers should attempt to agitate them into avoidance behavior, that is, wave arms, ropes or other objects, jump around and shout to make them start off. There is a difference between mobilizing a herd and stampeding it, however.

Cattle are tremendously herd-oriented, so they will crowd and bunch together as they are driven, even climbing onto others' backs if they are pushed too hard from behind. Herding cattle too fast (generally they should not be herded faster than a walk or a slow jog) should be avoided because of bruising or other injuries the cattle may incur.

It must be stressed that herding cattle into weak barriers must be avoided. Most beef cattle will walk through a loose barbed wire or smooth wire fence completely unconcerned and apparently unscathed, leaving the wire somewhat looser but often still in place. Calves become adept at slipping through the lower strands of the pasture fence. Horses, in contrast, tend to see fences as psychological barriers, and the more visible fences are, the more formidable they seem as barriers.

Cattle are usually less spooky than horses about strange surroundings, but they may balk and then bolt suddenly. Generally the balking occurs just as the cattle reach the open gate of a holding corral after being driven off an 80-acre pasture. Smart people avoid having strange things (e.g., stray dogs, raincoats flapping in the breeze) where they expect to drive the cattle.

A good cow dog is an invaluable asset in herding cattle. It is incredible how the calculated nipping at the heels and yapping of a small dog can whip a whole herd of cattle into line. It is also incredible how an undisciplined dog or two can stampede a quiet group of cattle.

Cattle, being herd animals, generally follow the leader, and so a tractable animal may be used to lead them places they might ordinarily find frightening. The leaders in a herd of cattle may prove the making or unmaking of one's attempt to drive the group. If they turn around, they may either turn the whole bunch in another direction or simply mill around in the security of the group, unconcerned at the efforts to drive them from the rear. Cattle chutes are built just wide enough for one animal, to prevent the animals from turning around. A person on foot may follow cattle in a chute to drive them through but should always be cautious and ready to climb out of the way. Never enter a chute that cannot be readily evacuated.

Chutes are funneled from larger areas. They are usually arranged so that posts or boards may be slipped behind animals to prevent their moving backward. *Tailing* may be used to push a cow ahead of you. Tailing is simply grasping the tail 7.0 cm to 15 cm from the base and pushing it up and forward over the back. This is uncomfortable and encourages the animal to move forward. A word of caution: When inside a chute, never underestimate the ability of a cow to get frightened and run backward, possibly causing serious crushing injuries. Cattle prods, sticks or electrical shock devices have the advantage of being used from outside a chute. If chutes are not available, cattle may also be roped if they are in a small area.

A single bovid in a small stall sometimes may be haltered without resorting to a head catch or stock. It becomes a matter of maneuvering the animal until the head is between you and a wall, with the hindquarters in a corner. After loosening the chin loop of a rope halter, the crown loop can be flipped over the back of the ears with the right hand (animal facing to one's left) while the left hand guides the nosepiece over the nose; then the right hand can quickly take up the slack in the chin rope once it is under the jaw. Cattle are less head-shy than horses, and this relatively rough means of haltering does not seem to bother them.

Calves are captured much the same as foals are. One should watch for the mother, though she will probably be too frightened to charge.

Bulls are quite another story; aggression is always there, even if hidden. They should *never* be trusted. One should avoid driving bulls while afoot. Some breeding bulls (i.e., dairy bulls) can be enticed by food to a "squeeze" area, where gates and stocks may be found. They can be caught with head catches or squeeze gates or by poles with hooks for the nose ring.

Head Catch

The head catch or stock is often the final capture and restraining device for cattle (Fig. 1–13). Cattle usually will not put their heads through willingly. Most have had negative experiences with stocks previously, and unless the opening is large enough to make them think they can escape through it, they will not enter. It takes precise timing to close the head catch after the head and before the shoulders. The spring-loaded head catches in commercial stocks make capture easier but may be dangerous to personnel. Many careless people have lost teeth or have been knocked down by rapidly swinging handles. One should be absolutely certain how to operate a stock or head catch before working near it or trying to operate it.

In a suitably small enclosure, the use of a tranquilizer in a pole syringe can be attempted with an animal that is vicious and cannot be caught with a stock. Pole syringes are available commercially or may be fabricated. They discharge their contents when pressed against the animal. Capture guns are also a possibility but are seldom used with cattle. They probably should not be used by anyone who is not expert in their use or without such a person's supervision.

Restraint of the Head

The halter may be used as an adjunct to a head catch to tie an animal's head up and to the side (e.g., to expose the jugular vein for venipuncture). A strong person can grasp over the

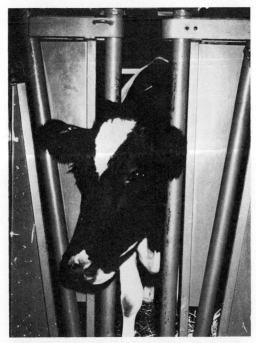

FIGURE 1–13. A cow in a head catch, or stock.

muzzle or around the lower jaw and into the mouth and effect the same restraint. The nasal septum may be pinched with thumb and forefinger in the nostrils, or nose tongs may be placed in the nose to stabilize the head. The horn or ear should be held in the other hand for leverage. The most common type of mouth gag for cattle is a block of wood about 15 cm long and 7.5 cm wide at the middle tapering toward the ends. There is a hole in the middle of the block to allow the passage of a tube. This gag is placed in the interdental space and is held in place by a strap behind the head. Large, metal hinged speculums may also be used for oral examinations. The tongue may be grasped and held as with the horse.

Tail

A cow's tail may be tied up just as a horse's can. Again, the tail should be tied only to the animal itself or held; it should not be attached to an inanimate object. The cow's tail may also be tied up slightly differently, with the tail on one side of the cow and the tail rope passing over the back to be secured around the foreleg near the elbow on the opposite side.

Kicking Restraints

Cattle usually kick to the side and forward with a hooking action rather than to the rear. There are several devices to prevent kicking and to restrain the hind legs. Milking hobbles, or hock hobbles, are flat metal hooks with a chain in between. The hooks are placed over the tendons of the hind leg just above the hock, with the open end of the hooks to the inside of the leg and the chain passing around the front of the limbs. Once the hooks are in place, the chain can be drawn up until the hocks are close together. If the brush of the tail is placed under one hook, the tail will also be restrained.

Pressure on the flank seems to discourage cows from kicking. A commercial metal device shaped like gigantic ice tongs may be squeezed over the flank, or a rope may be tied snugly around the abdomen just anterior to the udder. A hock twitch may be used to immobilize one hindleg. It is made out of heavy rope and is twist-tightened much like a tourniquet around the Achilles tendon just above the hock.

Lifting Feet

Cattle are very reluctant to lift up their feet, and to get their feet up requires an expenditure of energy. To raise a foreleg, a noose is tied around the pastern, and the end of the rope is passed over the cow's back as a pulley. The hind leg is more of a problem, as there is no portion of the cow's anatomy to use as a pulley. The limb may be tied using a beam overhead. Unfortunately, this treatment may result in injury to the cow. It is probably better if there is a strong enough person available to pick up and hold the hind leg much as with a horse, bearing in mind that it is simply a matter of forcing the leg up by brute force. To accomplish this feat it helps to have the cow's head turned away from the leg by means of nose tongs.

Casting

Casting a cow is usually simple. The first point is to always tie the haltered cow to a sturdy anchor. There are several variations of the rope "harness" fashioned on the cow. The simplest technique consists of a noose around the neck, a half-hitch around the girth and a half-hitch around the abdomen just anterior to the udder. The free end of the rope comes off the cow's back with all knots positioned dorsally. Once the rope harness is secure, a strong pull toward the rear of the cow will make her lie down. Two average-sized persons can usually cast a large cow easily.

If a cow is cast about 1.0 m or 1.5 m from a fence and parallel to it, she may be rolled onto her back up against the fence with a bale of hay wedged beside her to hold her up. Her legs should then be stretched to the front and rear with stout rope. To prevent bloating, cattle should be maintained on their backs or their bellies, in which positions they may continue to eructate (belch), rather than their sides. It is vital to remember that a standing cow, if in danger of going down (such as might be the case during calving), should always be tied by the halter and never by the neck. If she goes down with a rope or chain at the neck, she may well strangle and asphyxiate before she can be freed.

Small calves may be thrown by reaching over their backs to grab the forelegs and hind legs next to your body and lifting the legs up and away, letting the calves' bodies slide down your legs to the ground. Larger calves may be "flanked," which means to stand on one side and reach over the back to grab hair and skin in the lower flank and behind the elbow, then to lift and roll the calf up off its feet and drop it to the ground. A calf or cow can be restrained in lateral recumbency by weight on the neck.

Most bulls wear a nose ring, and not only may they be captured by it, but they may also be led by it. It is best not to depend upon the nose ring entirely for leading, as the ring can rip through the cartilage. A bull should not be tied fast with the nose ring. Leading a cantankerous bull is at least a two-person job, with the leaders ranging to the side well out of the bull's way, keeping the ropes taut to avoid his hurting the other person. Any combination of halter ropes, ropes to the nose ring, or nose ring pole with hooks may be used to effect the leading of the bull. Bulls may be hooded or blindfolded for easier leading into areas where they do not wish to go.

Xylazine is the standard chemical restraint for cattle. It should be remembered that cattle and other ruminants are sensitive to xylazine. The dose for cattle is one tenth of the equine dosage.

Driving Sheep and Goats

Sheep and goats are also herd-conscious animals and can be driven in bunches. Dogs are an excellent adjunct to working sheep, though some goats will challenge dogs. Goats are less timid and more adventurous than sheep. Sheep and goats commingle and herd together easily, and a goat trained to follow a person or to go to a certain place can be used to lead sheep into an enclosure (the "Judas" goat). Goats and sheep seldom stand staring and then bolt as cattle may when a person approaches.

Sheep can be worked in chutes, and though they will climb on each other like cattle, they do less damage to each other because of their smaller size. Interestingly, despite their greater agility, sheep do not seem to climb on chute walls when driven (unlike cattle). Although they may spring nearly straight up into the air twice their height and well above chute walls, they seldom jump out of the chute. Temporary fencing, like slatted snow fence, may serve as effective barriers for sheep.

Kids and lambs may be acrobatic and climb or jump on fences or other structures to avoid being caught. Jumping or falling from heights can cause injury, especially leg fractures, so handlers should be alert to avoid these situations.

Goats and sheep can be caught in small enclosures in the same way as foals or calves are caught, with a hand under the neck and one under the rump. In goats that are wearing collars, but that may not lead, it is probably preferable to catch the whole body rather than just the collar until they have stopped struggling.

One must never grab the wool to catch or restrain a sheep or mohair goat. The fleece itself may be damaged, or, in meat animals, a subcutaneous bruise may develop at the site.

Restraint

Sheep and goats resist being held by their horns and will only struggle if restrained this way. They can be held like foals or calves, set up on their rumps for hand restraint or held in miniature stocks. Goats may be trained to lead and tie.

Setting Up Sheep

Sheep are often set up on their rumps for several different procedures (i.e., shearing, vaccination, examinations, hoof trimming). There are several different ways to end up with the sheep on its rump with its back leaning against the holder, who is holding the forelegs (Fig. 1–14). The easiest method is for the person to begin on the sheep's left side. Reach under the base of the neck with the left hand and over the back to the right hind leg with the right hand. The sheep is gently lifted off the ground and upturned, after which the right hand

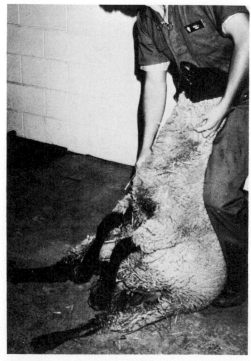

FIGURE 1–14. Holding the sheep set up on its rump.

moves to the right foreleg, the left hand moves to the left foreleg and the sheep is held on its rump facing away from you. One person can shear a sheep or perform several other procedures unassisted with the sheep on its rump by steadying its upper torso between the arms and the lower torso between the legs as one works.

Castration and Docking

Lambs are usually docked and castrated at the same time. The method of holding the legs is the same whether one rests the torso in one's lap, on a bench or fence or allows it to hang in front of one. The lamb is held head upright, facing away from the holder. The holder holds the two legs of each side together in each hand. The straightened hind legs are grasped between hock and fetlock, and the forelegs are held just below the elbows.

Drenching

Drenching, or oral administration of liquids, may be accomplished by one person. The sheep is backed into a corner and the person straddles the sheep above its shoulders, squeezing the forequarters with the knees. With one hand the handler lifts the head by the lower jaw, holding loosely around the muzzle, while inserting the dose syringe into the interdental space of the mouth on the opposite side with the other hand. One must be careful not to lift the jaw above a line parallel to the ground and to administer the substance slowly enough so that the sheep can swallow it. The nozzle of the syringe or gun should be inserted well back into the mouth between the cheek teeth, or the sheep will be liable to dribble the substance out of the mouth.

Goat Collars and Leading the Goat

Many of the sheep restraint techniques can be used on goats. Goats also often wear collars, which are usually leather straps with buckles. They probably should be laced closed rather than buckled to prevent the goat from rubbing the buckle loose. Goats that are trained may be led or tethered by their collars. A buck may be handled by leading him by the collar and beard, but if he does not like and respect his handler, he can be difficult.

Capture and Restraint of Swine

Catching Swine

Small piglets or pigs can be crowded into corners, and as they dart away, they can be grasped by a hind leg or two. The hind leg hold should be rapidly changed to holding in both hands around the torso for the comfort and reassurance of the pig. The technique is not applicable to full-grown swine.

Swine, especially boars and broody sows, can be very aggressive. One way to herd aggressive swine somewhere is to use a fence panel or large piece of plywood (at least a few inches taller and longer than a single animal) to "haze" them. Apparently, the larger barrier looks more formidable than a person and also provides some protection. When "planting" a panel to prevent animals from pushing through it, the foot should be used to steady the bottom corner, where swine will try to

"root" out. Always make sure you have an escape route when entering a pen with potentially aggressive swine. Most swine can be driven by people on foot, which is to say that they avoid people getting near them. Swine are also intelligent and individualistic and may be difficult to direct in a large area. Swine tend to dart through small openings for escape. A cane may be used to tap swine on the side of the face or neck to direct them while driving. Gentle swine may also be individually directed by pushing or slapping lightly on the rump or side of the neck or face.

Swine can sometimes be enticed into a small, secure enclosure by a food trail or food placed inside. Once inside a small enclosure that they cannot break out of, swine may be caught by a snubbing rope (a lariat, in essence) or by some variation of the hog snare, which is usually an adjustable metal cable loop at the end of a rigid handle (Fig 1–15). The loop is slipped over the upper jaw of the animal from behind (usually swine will hide their heads in a corner when they are trying to get away from you), and it is tightened after it is behind the incisors. The snare has the advantage of the rigid handle for directing the snout, whereas the snubbing rope is useful only for pulling. Generally, swine brace themselves by pulling backward when caught by the snout and are immobilized but are not stifled by it. The discomfort of a snare usually results in nonstop shrieking until it is removed. Swine can be tied by a snubbing rope, which may also be combined with hobbles or ropes on the hind legs to stretch them out and hold them in a lateral reclining position. These techniques are rough and should be avoided, if possible. Some procedures can be accomplished by squeezing the pig tightly with hog panels.

Body Restraints

Pigs can be restrained on their backs in a vee trough. The legs can be tied or held. A sling of canvas with holes for the legs has been used with great success in research laboratories and veterinary hospitals to cradle swine comfortably for certain procedures. The farrowing crate is essentially a restraint device for sows to keep them from lying on their pigs. The sow is restrained in a narrow corridor with areas on the sides for the young.

Pigs can be restrained for castration or vaccination by hold-

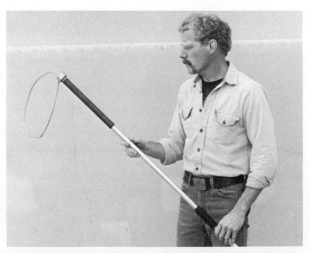

FIGURE 1–15. The swine snare or "rabies" pole for dogs.

ing them off the ground by the hind legs with their backs against one's legs. Large pigs will struggle less if their forefeet rest on the ground. Pigs can be held for oral administration by holding them up by the forelegs and leaning their backs against one's legs while they stand on their hindlegs. Giving a sweet feed to nibble before and after a capsule will encourage them not to spit it out.

Humane Restraint of Pet Swine

The reader is probably struck by the apparent (and real) brutality of some of the above-mentioned handling techniques with swine. The hog snare and the vee trough, for instance, are despised by swine. The pig is an intelligent animal that can be trained to tolerate minor discomforts and lie willingly in a sling, for instance. Unfortunately, the time involved to train swine is often "unprofitable" in agricultural animals, although it quickly pays for itself in the research or pet situation.

Miniature swine kept as individual pets are most often seen these days in small animal practices. Many of these pets are spoiled, willful creatures that run the household. Owners who allow pets to run their lives will not be impressed by rough handling, yet it is difficult to be firm and effective, but not abusive. The support sling is the best method for restraint, as it causes the animal no discomfort yet provides immobilization. In the absence of a sling, they may be held like a watermelon, with one forearm under the neck, but the holder will be gouged by the hind foot nearest his body when the pig struggles. Pigs have incredibly powerful jaws and some will bite readily, especially if in pain or uncomfortable. These can be muzzled with a small rope used like gauze in a dog, but pigs will fight them, and they may be more trouble than they are worth. Muzzling, or holding the jaws closed, may be used to cut down the noise of a vocalizing pig as well.

Once a pig is restrained, its mouth can be opened by means of a gag. The gag is a U-shaped device with a handle at the bottom of the U and two bars, separated by a space, near its top. The bars are inserted into the mouth behind the canines, and the gag then is rotated to spread the jaws. Many miniature swine readily allow stomach tubing and do not bite down on a hand inserted into the mouth over the incisors to place the tube; however, fingers straying between cheek teeth are in harm's way. Never put fingers into the side of a pig's mouth.

Many pet swine are inordinately fond of having people scratch their backs, and they may even stand or lie quietly for an examination if this is done for them. Scratching the belly, especially of a gilt or sow, will often induce her to flop down on her side to expose the belly. It is always worthwhile to ask an owner if his or her pig leads on a leash, or how he or she gets it to do things. Sometimes the owner has worked out ingenious ways to make the pig do things it would not normally do willingly.

Finally, it should be mentioned that even though a miniature pig may live in the house and be trained to lead and to void and defecate outdoors, it is in the end still a pig. And one of the things pigs do most readily is to vocalize when uncomfortable or painful or just dissatisfied with what is being done to them. Do not be surprised when that 15-kg porker emits an ear-piercing shriek as it is first picked up and continues unrelenting until it is set free. Swine can be tranquilized with acepromazine or azaparone, if necessary, but both have fairly long effects (24 to 36 hours).

Capture and Restraint of Dogs

Catching Dogs

Since most veterinarians do not make house calls for animals, the only time one usually needs to catch a dog that is not in a cage or run is if the animal has escaped. Dogs are often motivated by terror in the animal hospital, so personnel should learn to deal with fear in dogs, which results in two types of behavior. One is avoidance (running away) with abject submissiveness when cornered, and the other is avoidance until cornered, then aggression (fear biting). Unfortunately, the two types of dogs are often discriminated between only at the last moment, as one's hands approach. Almost any dog will turn around and snap if it is grabbed as it runs past, though it is difficult, if not impossible, to avoid the temptation to grab at the dog on his way to freedom.

How does one catch an elusive dog in the great outdoors? Animal control officers deal with this problem daily. Obviously, a person is not going to outrun any but the smallest and most debilitated dogs. Like horses, dogs that feel they are being chased will run. It is best to try to keep a dog in sight at a less threatening distance until there is an opportunity to corner it or until the dog decides the pursuer is not that much of a threat. Sometimes, especially if the fugitive is male, it may help to have a canine companion to entice the dog to approach you. It never hurts to have a pocketful of bait of some sort to gain the dog's favor.

An apprehensive dog, whether it is in the examination room or in a backyard, needs reassurance that no one will harm it. Do not grab the dog's collar or try to pick it up before some reassurance is given. Most dogs respond favorably to being talked to. The higher voice usually gets better results, which may be because of the higher range of hearing and vocalization in dogs. With many dogs it helps to "hunker down"—squat—in front of them to appear less large and overbearing. Without moving quickly or awkwardly, offer your hand for the dog to sniff at or below the level of its nose. Sometimes the point at which the hand is proffered is the first indication that the dog will bite.

Some people say that one should offer the back of the hand to a strange dog, rather than the palm, because the palm may appear to be threatening a slap. Whether the slap notion is true or not, the fingers are a little more out of the way with a loosely cupped hand held with the palm down, and the dog will be forced to make more of an effort to bite the whole hand, possibly giving you more time to withdraw. However, a dog's bite is lightning-fast, even in the large ponderous breeds, and, unless warned, you will not be able to move your hand in time.

A dog tells by body language whether it has accepted your introduction. If it is prone to think you are all right, the body will relax and the dog will actively sniff your hand. This may be followed by wagging the tail, losing interest in the hand, and approaching. If these things occur, one may begin to make friends by reaching below the ear for a scratch, starting gently and then scratching more vigorously. The next best scratching place is on the chest. Once a dog has accepted your scratching its ears or chest it may indicate that it would just as soon have you finish the job, scratching neck, shoulders, top of hips. It is a good idea to run the hands all over the dog in a friendly fashion before taking liberties with its body, like trying to lift it. Some dogs are naturally gregarious and trusting and require little in the way of preliminaries. There are a few dogs whose natural temperament is not so positive but that are well enough trained that they may be handled less carefully than their personalities warrant. Evaluating dogs may require evaluation of the client. Some clients have obviously been trained by their dogs rather than the reverse, and you are on your own to make your peace with the pooch. (Clients may help or hinder your efforts with dogs. Those that have no control over their animals may undermine any authority you might have with the dog by virtue of your being a stranger, so these people are best sent politely to the waiting room, if possible.)

Many times dogs may act reasonably in an initial examination with the owner present, and then, after being held in a cage or run, threaten to bite when approached. Whenever faced with a dog that will obviously bite if given the chance, the only sensible thing to do is to keep your hands out of the way. For small dogs, the answer may be heavy leather gauntlets. Sometimes these dogs will work out their aggression snapping at the gloved fingers of one hand (flesh fingers carefully withdrawn) while the other hand approaches and grabs them at the neck. Most dogs will give up as soon as they feel restrained, but some will not.

For larger dogs that want to bite, the first step is to catch them by the neck. Always remember to keep cage doors closed as far as possible when trying to catch biters (or any other dog, for that matter), as they will be more trouble if they escape. Sometimes a lead rope with a slip knot can be tossed over a dog's head, but sometimes a rope snare similar to a hog catcher is required. Most dogs will give up when caught by the neck. A few, the truly vicious or confirmed fear biters, will continue to try to bite, and even attack. In these cases, you may apply a muzzle (described later), keep the teeth a safe distance by keeping a tight grip behind the head, or use both of these methods. Sometimes vicious little dogs may be dragged out of cages snarling and snapping and can be held off the ground by the choke rope for a few moments to subdue them. There is a slight chance of permanent tracheal damage with this technique, and it is not the way to win friends. Some of these dogs are incorrigible and will hate you regardless, so there is sometimes justification in forcing them to respect you.

A truly vicious large dog is a real challenge. It should never be approached except by a snare, and even then, if it is very strong, two leads may be required (two snares or a snare and a rope) to stretch the dog between two people for leading.

A dog at large that will not allow approach may require the use of a capture gun or even a pole syringe. Animal control officers may be experienced with the capture gun and may be able to provide assistance. Inexperienced persons should not try to use capture guns. Occasionally, the darts malfunction or strike some poorly absorbing portion of the body, and the animal will not succumb in the time expected. Note that it is dangerous to repeat the dose in such an animal without knowing how much of the drug it has received. Drugs often used with capture guns include ketamine, xylazine and nicotine.

Lifting Dogs

Dogs are generally examined on a table, and lifting them onto that table is usually the first order of business. Small dogs may be lifted by grasping on either side of the thorax behind the elbows. Medium-sized dogs are lifted by putting the arms around them, in front of the chest and behind the rump and

pulling them to your chest. Unfortunately, that position places your face uncomfortably close to their teeth, but there really is no other way, except for lifting tables or prior muzzling.

Large dogs are harder to lift for at least three reasons. First, of course, is their weight, which may be prohibitive. Second, their large size makes them more awkward to lift. The third reason is that large dogs are not accustomed to being lifted, which makes them uneasy, if not downright panicky. One person may be able to lift a large dog by forklifting him, with the arms behind the forelimbs and in front of the hind legs. However, if the animal struggles it can fall forward or backward easily. Two people can lift a dog together by one person's placing the arms around the forequarters and the other person placing the arms around the hindquarters. They should both be on the same side of the dog, away from the table, of course. Some dogs, especially males, object to being lifted from under the flank area, where the male genitalia terminate. If this is the case, they will definitely need two people to lift the dog, with the person at the rear placing the arm or hand well forward of the prepuce. If a large dog is unduly nervous about being lifted or being on top of the table, it should be dealt with on the floor.

Never let a dog jump down from a table. Most tables and floors have slick surfaces that invite slips and fractures. Lift the dog off the table in the same manner as it was placed there.

Injured or sick animals may pose different problems in lifting. Usually, it means providing more hands for more even support. A limb with a fracture, for example, requires separate support to prevent additional soft tissue damage and pain to the animal. An animal with a painful abdomen should not be lifted under the posterior abdomen. There are times when a stretcher may be required for lifting a badly injured dog. Lifting injured animals calls for judgment in the particular situation.

Table Restraint

The degree of restraint required for a dog on the table depends on what is being done. Regardless, however, the forequarters and hindquarters must be controlled at all times to prevent the dog from jumping or falling off the table.

The form of restraint most often used is to have the arms behind the rump and in front of the chest, pulling the dog inward, much as in lifting. In addition, one may wish to pull the head against the chest with the hand on the neck, which is adequate restraint for most dogs for examination and subcutaneous or intramuscular (thigh or forequarters) vaccinations or injections.

A rectal examination is common in male dogs, and only a slight adjustment need be made from the position just described. The holder's arm or hand should not be behind the hindquarters, as it will interfere with the examination. The arm used to restrain the hindquarters can be placed over the dog's back to stabilize lateral movement by drawing the dog's body toward the handler. A hand supporting the ventral abdomen may be required to prevent the dog from sitting down.

Whenever puppies are examined, vaccinated, have dewclaws removed and so forth, the bitch should be out of the room. When her puppies cry, she may be inclined to attack; this is especially true when the pups are newborn. If the bitch must be in the same room, it might be worthwhile to slip her into a crate while the procedures are carried out. The pups could then be taken away from her one at a time. Dogs cannot count, and unless attention is paid when the pup is removed or the pup makes noise, she will not notice when one puppy out of several is gone.

Restraint for Venipuncture

Venipuncture, for drawing blood or administering substances, requires most exacting restraint. The animal must not be allowed to move, because movement is the most common cause of "blowing" a vessel. The resultant hematomas are painful and unsightly and obscure the vessel for future use. It should be noted that the primary reason that an animal struggles during venipuncture is anxiety. Calm, affectionate handling with lots of petting and soothing words will go far to relieve anxiety. The most painful portion of the venipuncture is usually when the vessel is pierced, although puncturing the skin and administering certain substances may also be unpleasant. At these times restraint should be the most secure. Positioning, apart from preventing movement, is the most critical part of venipuncture because without good positioning the vessel cannot even be located.

For cephalic venipuncture, the holder must restrain the dog's body, present the forelimb, and occlude the vessel to make it fill and stand up under the skin. The animal is placed on the table near one end, facing the edge. The holder stands beside the table, facing the same direction as the dog, and nestles the animal on the table under the arm; the handler's forearm, upper arm and elbow will exert pressure to bring the animal snugly to the person's side and down to a sternal reclining position on the table. The hand of the same arm cradles the animal's elbow with the palm and fingers while the thumb clamps down on the cephalic vein. In order to be sure that the vein is under the thumb and on the top (front) of the forearm,

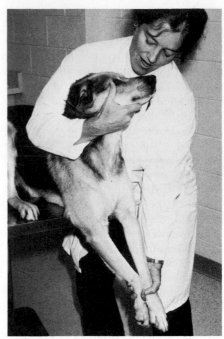

FIGURE 1–17. Method of holding the dog for jugular venipuncture. Note the straight line from the ramus of the mandible to the feet.

the holder grasps the limb just below the elbow with the thumb as far inside the limb as possible, then, with pressure applied, rotates the skin outward (Fig. 1–16). The fingers should rest on the table, and the dog's elbow be pushed slightly forward to stabilize the leg. The elbow should be at or near the edge of the table to allow good access to the vein.

The free hand is used to restrain the animal's head, and for most dogs this is best accomplished by pressing the head to your chest by reaching under the neck and placing the hand behind the jaw. The hand may also go around the dog's muzzle to prevent biting, when necessary. The holder must remember to release the thumb when the other person is ready to perform the injection. Failure to release the vessel will not allow a substance to be injected into the general circulation; it may also result in the rupture of the vessel.

A large dog can be restrained on the floor for cephalic venipuncture with the handler kneeling or squatting behind the sitting dog to prevent its backward movement. Most dogs submit well to cephalic venipuncture, and their cephalic veins are large and straight enough to hit easily. However, in chondrodystrophic short-legged dogs and in certain other circumstances, the preferred site may be the jugular vein. Dogs that are gentle and phlegmatic may submit well to cephalic venipuncture while sitting up (Fig. 1–16).

For jugular venipuncture (Fig. 1–17), the dog is placed further forward on the table, the edge of which should be just behind the forelegs. The holder stands alongside and puts the arm over the animal as in the cephalic technique, pressing the animal to the table. However, the hand of the arm over the animal is the one that restrains the head; the hand away from the table restrains the forefeet, with a finger between the feet for a secure grip. For the head restraint, the hand grasps the muzzle with the fingers under the jaw (one or two fingers may fit between the mandibles of the jaw for a more secure grip) and the thumb is over the nose. Care is taken to avoid cutting off the animal's breathing by holding the muzzle too near the

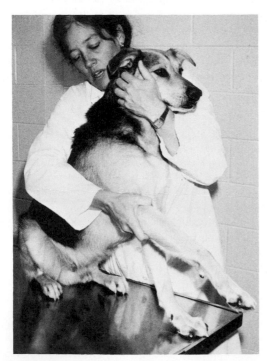

FIGURE 1–16. Method of holding the dog for cephalic venipuncture. This dog is being held in a sitting position rather than in a position of sternal recumbency.

nose. Also, if the fingers are too far back under the jaw, they may occlude the jugular vein so that it will not fill and therefore will not be located.

The main advantage of this position is to provide a nearly straight plane from the angle of the dog's jaw to the forefeet for easy access to the jugular vein. The dog is somewhat "stretched" to achieve this effect. Common errors in this position are to have the dog's forelegs or shoulders too far forward, interfering with the angle of entry for the syringe, or to pull the head too far backward, stretching the skin and vessel and collapsing the vein. The dog's head should be lifted no more than slightly above 90 degrees from the neck. The head may be directed toward the handler to rest on the chest, but in this position only the vessel away from the handler is available for venipuncture. A large dog can be restrained on the floor for jugular venipuncture with the handler kneeling or squatting behind the sitting dog while steadying the chest with one hand and the muzzle with the other.

The saphenous vein, on the lateral aspect of the hind leg, is an alternate venipuncture site, for which the dog must be held in lateral recumbency. To hold a dog on its side, the handler stands behind the dog, with one forearm pressed across the animal's neck and the hand holding the forelegs (with a finger between the legs). The other forearm presses across the dog's flank, with the hind legs held in a similar manner, except that when venipuncture is being attempted, only the down leg is held; the other is stabilized by the person making the puncture.

Muzzles and Mouth Gags

There are commercial muzzles available that are made of a variety of materials. The problem with most commercial muzzles is that they are not very adjustable, and several sizes need to be kept on hand. Therefore, one usually resorts to the gauze or rope muzzle.

Nylon rope (6.35 mm) choke leads are sometimes very handy as muzzling devices for snapping dogs. The dog must first be caught by the neck, possibly with a snare. A loop of rope, made with a single overhand knot, is positioned from above the dog's nose until it is in place over the muzzle. Once the rope is in place, it is rapidly tightened. A smart dog will try to push the rope loop off its nose with its forepaw. The first knot must be held snugly while a second knot is made with the ends under the nose. The second knot may be a single overhand knot or a double knot (preferably a square knot). The two free ends are then passed behind the dog's head and tied again; this knot will hold the muzzle on the dog and must be secure. It may be tied for fast release by using a bow knot in case the dog cannot breathe.

Gauze roll bandage (7.5 cm to 15 cm) may be used as a muzzle in the same fashion as the rope (Fig. 1–18). Gauze is used more often and has an advantage over rope in that it is less slick. Gauze, however, makes a less rigid loop to apply to a recalcitrant dog. For most dogs, the piece of gauze needs to be about 90 cm long.

Pug-nosed dogs are difficult to muzzle, and they can be determined biters. For them, the gauze bandage is tied first around the nose with the first knot tied underneath the jaw. The ends are then passed behind the head and tied with a square knot. Finally, one of the free ends of the gauze is passed over the forehead and under the loop on top of the nose and

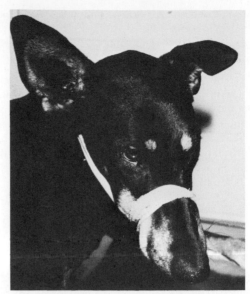

FIGURE 1–18. The gauze muzzle.

is then tied back to the other side. This keeps the loop from slipping off the top of the short nose (see Fig. 1–20).

Sometimes a dog's mouth can be restrained manually, by bringing the hands from the rear on both sides of the face; thumbs are placed on the forehead, and fingers are looped under the mandibles. The palms should be below the ears.

A variety of mouth gags can be used in dogs. A simple dowel may be pressed to the back of the mouth, to rest on the carnassial teeth. The dowel can be tied in place behind the ears or can be handheld by the assistant. Dogs can undergo insertion of a stomach tube with the dowel in place. The commercial spring type of mouth gag has a hole on either end for the canine teeth, and it is inserted on one side of the mouth for a variety of procedures. However, this gag hangs outside the mouth, is heavy, and can fracture teeth to which it is attached. It is much better to cut off the end of an appropriately sized plastic syringe cover to place over opposing canine teeth. This is especially useful when a mouth gag is needed for dentistry.

Mobility-Limiting Devices

Self-mutilation and tearing of bandages can be prevented by means of several devices. The most common mobility-limiting devices are variations of the Elizabethan collar, which is so named because of its resemblance to the wide, stiffly starched collars popular in 17th century England. The idea is to place a stiff material to the tip of the dog's nose so that it cannot chew on or lick its body. There are commercial plastic cone-shaped collars, or similar appliances can be fashioned from buckets, large bottles or sheets of heavy plastic. It is most important with these collars to ensure that no sharp edges are present and to secure the Elizabethan collar to the neck by gauze or fasten it to the dog's neck collar. Make sure the dog knows how to eat and drink with the collar on. Commercial collars can be worn with the wide part of the cone over the body rather than over the head if the affected area is on the forequarters.

Another type of device that limits the movement of the head is made by fastening a pole along the body to a snug collar high on the neck. Usually, tape is used to keep the device from shifting.

Chemical Restraint

There are drugs that can be used for chemical restraint in dogs. The most common are acepromazine and xylazine. Both have tranquilizing effects that may vary from dog to dog. Dogs may still be capable of biting when tranquilized. The main reason for tranquilization is to remove anxiety, which is one of the main reasons dogs bite. More information on chemical restraint is found in Chapter 11.

Catching Cats

Cats are often more apprehensive than dogs with strange people and surroundings. An escaped cat will often search out a hiding place, whereas a dog that escapes will look for a route to run. This is probably because of the lower endurance that cats have for running when compared with dogs and the security that cats feel in enclosed spaces. A cat that is "treed" or trapped (as in a cage) may well respond with flattened ears, hissing and scratching and biting at an extended hand. Heavy leather gauntlet gloves may be used to subdue them as with small dogs. Grasp the scruff of the neck to lift the cat. This may be followed by a rapid "stretch" restraint by also grasping the hind legs. Certain cats are too fast and smart to succumb to the glove technique. These cats may sometimes be caught by neck rope or snare, but they react poorly to a choke as compared with the scruff of the neck. Another technique worth trying may be ketamine oral spray. Although injectable ketamine can be irritating to muscle tissues, it does not seem to cause trauma to the eyes (in case some is accidentally sprayed into the eyes). The plan is to spray a syringe containing ketamine or ketamine and acepromazine into the mouth of a hissing cat, using the intramuscular tranquilizing dose. The drugs are effective orally, but of course they take longer to take effect than if injected intramuscularly or subcutaneously.

A cat may also be "lassoed" with the end of the rope passed between the cage bars, the cage rapidly closed and the cat brought to the front of the cage with the noose. Ketamine may then be injected intramuscularly or subcutaneously into whatever body part is closest.

Restraint for Examination

Much of the table restraint of cats is similar to that of dogs, except that cats tend to use their claws (unless declawed) as the first line of defense rather than their teeth. When there is no reason for holding them still, cats should be allowed supervised movement. Some cats are so terrified that they are best held or cuddled with the head buried under one's arm. Cats are not necessarily malicious when they climb onto a person's chest or clamp nails into a forearm. It is a good idea to wear protective gowns or laboratory coats with long sleeves when dealing with cats and not to wear knit clothing that will snag. A free nail clip at the beginning of an examination can be a practice-builder and save some scratching of personnel, especially if blood is to be drawn.

Restraint for Venipuncture

Cephalic and jugular venipuncture restraint can be applied to cats much as with dogs. Cats tend to engage their three relatively unfettered sets of claws and their teeth in an effort to get away from the hold. When they are thus inclined, they are impossible to hold like dogs, and one is forced to use other restraints. The positioning for jugular venipuncture is more appropriate for cats, as it restrains the head and forefeet more securely than in the cephalic technique. Also wrapping the hind feet with a towel disarms all but the most persistent cat. The cat's head is held with the hand over the top of the head, and the jaw or the zygomatic arch (the bony arch under the eyes) is grasped with the thumb on one side and two or three fingers on the other side. This leaves the index finger free for scratching, since many cats will be thoroughly distracted from the venipuncture if the handler strokes the bridge of the nose vigorously while talking to them. The other hand then restrains both forelimbs as in the dog.

Besides the technique described for holding dogs, there are other ways to hold cats for jugular venipuncture. They all involve the cat's being placed on its back with the holder occluding the jugular vein and the person using the syringe pushing the chin down toward the table to make the head move backward to get a straight shot at the jugular. The holder can hold all four legs (two in each hand, with a finger in between the legs), while pushing the cat down on the table and using the little finger to press on the thoracic inlet to occlude the jugular vein. A cat can also be rolled in a towel to engage its feet, or it can be placed in a cat bag for this type of jugular venipuncture. When a towel or cat bag is used, the handler need only steady the cat on its back and occlude the vessel or vessels. Some cat bags are made with zippers, so that a single limb can be withdrawn, and could thereby be used for cephalic venipuncture.

Carrying Cats

Cats feel more secure in close quarters, and seldom resist being put in a bag or rolled in a towel. They are best carried from place to place in a cat carrier or a small cardboard box with a lid. They can also be carried in one arm if they are not particularly nervous. To carry a cat, its hindquarters are placed under the elbow area and are pressed securely to the holder's body with the forearm. The cat lies in a sternal position along the forearm while the forelegs are pinioned by the hand—again, with one finger between the legs. The cat may still use his hind claws to gouge the abdomen of the holder, so you should be prepared to grab the scruff of the neck and hold the cat at arm's length if it becomes wild. Also, quickly grasping the hind legs and pulling away from the scruff of the neck will effectively immobilize almost any cat. Although this is not a comfortable position for the cat to be carried, it is safer for the handler.

Lateral Recumbency

Stretching the cat from the scruff of the neck and the hind feet is generally effective for immobilizing a cat on its side (Fig. 1–19). Most cats do not seem to realize that they can use their forefeet to scratch the hand on their neck. Some cats can be restrained on their sides as with dogs, but this is generally less effective than a stretch.

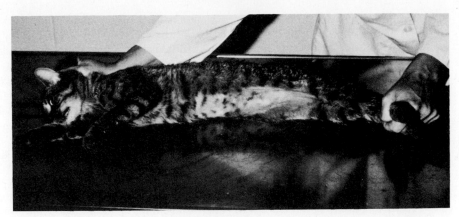

FIGURE 1–19. Stretching a cat on its side.

A modification of the stretch allows access to the medial saphenous vein of the thigh. The holder has the scruff of the neck securely in one hand while the other holds the "up" rear leg flexed. The little finger can be used to hold off the vein for the venipuncturist, who stretches the "down" leg with one hand while handling the syringe with the other.

Bathing

Cats' antipathy to water is a cliché, but true nonetheless. Bathing a cat may therefore be a trying experience for both the cat and the person. Most cats will try to climb up the person's arms to escape standing water or a spray. Cats should be bathed on top of a screen suspended over a tub (any metal window screen in a sturdy frame will do) and washed with a light spray of warm water. Almost always the cat will clamp all four sets of claws into the screen and stand like a statue for the entire bath.

The Muzzle

The cat may be muzzled with gauze in the same way as pug-nosed dogs (Fig. 1–20).

Chemical Restraint

The most common chemical restraint for cats is ketamine, which can be used at a tranquilizing or an anesthetic dose. The eyes of cats under the influence of ketamine should be treated with ophthalmic ointment to avoid corneal drying from the lack of blinking while the drug is being taken. Combining acepromazine with ketamine reduces the ketamine rigidity. Cats can also be given tranquilizing doses of acepromazine alone. Both drugs can be administered intramuscularly or subcutaneously.

Ferret Restraint

Noncooperative ferrets are a restraint challenge. Unless the ferret is exceptionally "mellow," you are probably well advised to wear heavy gloves, as almost all ferrets will bite when frightened or hurt. Ferrets may be "stretched," in a similar manner to cats, or they may be grasped with both hands around the forequarters, using one hand on the scruff of the neck and the other holding the forelegs down.

Ferrets are subject to "hypnosis," although it is less likely to be effective if the animal is apprehensive or in strange hands. The ferret is hung by the scruff with one hand and stroked around and the length of its torso with the other. After repeated stroking, the susceptible animal will begin to yawn and its eyelids will droop or close. The effect is not long-lasting, and animals are easily startled out of the trance.

Short periods (10 to 20 minutes) of chemical restraint in ferrets can be achieved by intramuscular injection of xylazine (1 mg to 4 mg per kg) and ketamine (20 mg to 30 mg per kg).

Rabbit Restraint

Rabbits have some peculiarities for restraint with which one should be familiar. First, rabbits have a very high muscle to skeleton ratio. Their bones are very small and light for animals of their size. In addition, they have tremendously powerful hind limbs. Uncontrolled kicking by a rabbit may result in too much torque in the lumbosacral area, resulting in "broken back," an imprecise lay term that means loss of neural function in the hindquarters resulting from spinal cord trauma. Not only are the rabbit's hind legs paralyzed, but bladder and anal function are also lost. The prognosis for recovery is grim in cases of total paralysis, and although anti-inflammatory treatment, as for dachshunds with disc disease, may be undertaken,

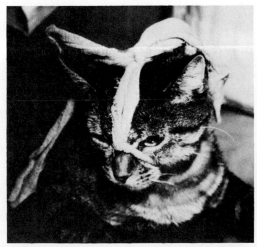

FIGURE 1–20. The gauze muzzle on a cat. It may also be used on a pug-nosed dog.

the most humane thing to do is to perform euthanasia if response is not seen within a week or two. Invariably, the rabbit traumatizes his spinal cord while being put back into his cage. He is familiar with the cage, and he will make a premature leap. Paralysis may be immediate or may be delayed until hemorrhage and edema compress the spinal cord.

How do you avoid this unhappy situation? There are essentially two ways to carry a mature rabbit, in a "hanging" carry or nestled in the arms. The nestled carry is esthetically more pleasing, and is probably more comfortable, but the hanging technique does not appear to be damaging or painful to even large rabbits, and *it suppresses the inclination to kick*. Although small bunnies may be safely lifted by the scruff of the neck, large, heavy rabbits are best lifted by two generous handfuls of skin over the neck and shoulders and the hindquarters (Fig. 1–21). Held this way they usually hang quite immobile. They can be carried short distances this way without undue discomfort. Lifting by the scruff of the neck, with the second hand cradling the rump (not grabbing the hind feet, which will cause resistance), is also very practical and probably more acceptable to clients. One may also grasp the rabbit about the middle to pick it up, but many rabbits readily struggle when lifted this way.

To carry rabbits longer distances, they may be set down on a table or other surface and then gathered to your body by the forearms. This snugly supports the hindquarters. Rabbits will often tuck their heads under your elbow when carried in this way. They seldom bite, and leaving the head free is therefore not a problem. The best way to replace a rabbit in a cage is by holding its skin fore and aft, placing it well inside the cage but facing outward (so that it must turn before leaping into the safety of the cage) and pressing its body down to the floor for a few moments before releasing it. One should never lift a rabbit, young or old, by its ears.

Rabbits have extremely formidable, sharp, straight nails on their rear feet, which can gouge severe scratches on your abdomen or arms if one struggles while being carried in your forearms. Although long-sleeved protective garments should always be worn, the best way to avoid being scratched is to avoid carrying rabbits for any distance in the forearms. Rabbits' nails may be trimmed easily by pressing the rabbit to the table with the forearm and chest. Hind feet are trimmed by pulling

them out to the rear, as with horses' feet. Forefeet are lifted up off the table.

Rabbits do not like slick surfaces, and losing their footing on them may encourage them to struggle and kick. It is best to set them down on something on which they will have good traction, like a rubber mat, during examination or treatment.

Rabbits have sensitive whiskers and will flinch whenever the sensitive hairs of the muzzle or eyelids are touched or the mouth is approached. Therefore, the head must be firmly held before attempting to examine the mouth or put something into it. To steady the head in order for someone to examine the mouth, the rabbit is placed facing away from the person holding it with the forearms pressing down on the length of the body, the thumbs behind the ears, and the fingers lifting the head from below the mandible. Incisor teeth may be trimmed with the rabbit in this position.

Rabbits may be chemically restrained by ketamine and acepromazine, and this combination may be used for induction for gas anesthesia.

Occasionally, rabbits, especially females, may be aggressive and may growl and try to scratch with the forelegs at your hand when you reach into the cage. As already mentioned, rabbits seldom bite, so medium-weight gloves to prevent scratches are all that is needed to subdue them. Normally, the fight goes out of these rabbits when their forequarters are pressed to the floor and their bodies are restrained from free movement.

Rabbits may be restrained in boxes with a head-catching device, parallel sides, and some sort of rump board. The rump board should be tight against the hindquarters to push the rabbit into the head restraint. Under no circumstances should the rabbit be left with only its head restrained, because it will try to back out of the box and may possibly injure itself struggling.

Rabbits can be held for ear venipuncture by use of the same technique as described above for the oral examination.

Restraint of Hamsters and Gerbils

Hamsters and gerbils may be handled with gloves if they are wild and want to bite. Gerbils have long tails (with hair on them), so they may be caught by the tail. The tail must be grasped at its base to pick up a gerbil, not near the tip, where the hair and skin may easily be pulled off, leaving the naked flesh. A scruff of the neck hold is moderately effective on gerbils and hamsters, though hamsters have a lot of redundant skin from cheek pouches, which must be gathered up in the hold. Hamsters have insignificant tails, so they must be caught in hands cupped over their bodies. This technique is also more comfortable for gerbils and should be used on them unless they are biters. These small rodents may be restricted from movement on a surface by placing the hand over them to form a cage, the head protruding between the first and second fingers. Hamsters may be caught and restrained by "hazing" them into a small can, as they readily enter holes. Rodent restraint tunnels in several sizes are available. They are usually made of Plexiglas and have several ports available for injection.

Ketamine may be used in any of the rodent species. Light gas anesthesia may also be used for restraint, but many gerbils seem to have adverse reactions to gas anesthesia, and once they have ceased breathing, they usually die despite attempts at resuscitation.

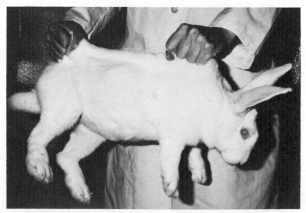

FIGURE 1–21. The hanging carry position for a rabbit. Even adults tend to "freeze" in this position much like neonates while carried in the mother's mouth.

Guinea Pig Restraint

The guinea pig is a docile creature that rarely bites, even when extremely fearful or when being hurt. They seldom jump, unlike most other rodents, but they scurry and dart around rapidly. They can be quite vocal during restraint. In a cage, they can be trapped in a corner or along the wall with hands, and they should be picked up by both hands encircling the body (fingers cradling underneath, thumbs on top), one hand partially behind the other to support the entire abdomen. Pregnant guinea pigs get enormously pendulous bellies, and they may be lifted by grasping around the thorax with one hand and placing the other hand behind and under the rump to hold them upright.

Guinea pigs can be easily held for restraint in the same fashion that they are picked up for most procedures, or the shoulder and pelvic girdles can be held in your two hands. Teeth can be clipped by holding the head with one or two hands, with the forefinger under the jaw and the thumb behind the head. The guinea pig tolerates being placed upside down in a vee trough with legs tied down much like swine.

Ketamine may be used on guinea pigs for restraint, though it is seldom necessary.

Bird Restraint

Caged birds are captured either by hand or with a net. When using a net one must take care not to strike the bird with the hoop or remove the bird roughly, as bones of the wings and legs are easily fractured. It is evident that the bird's wings must be restrained and that it must be prevented from biting. Small birds, like the budgerigar (parakeet), should be held with the hand cupped around the back to restrain the wings, and the thumb and forefinger should grasp the nape of the neck. The fingers should not completely encircle the body but should stay on the sides of the bird. Care should be taken to hold the head straight so that the thumb does not slip to the anterior part of the neck and occlude the trachea. A lot of the unexplained deaths of small birds while being held probably result from suffocation, since the sternum (or keel) must be able to move up and down for respiration to occur. Larger caged birds are held essentially in the same way as the smaller ones are, but heavy gloves may be required.

Predatory birds (raptors) may use their talons as defenses and must, therefore, be grasped first by the feet and then by the head. The movement and aggression of raptors may be curtailed by blindfolding or hooding. Wings may be wrapped.

Never release a bird in midair, as it might be disoriented, stiff or injured and, therefore, fall and hurt itself. Birds should be held squatting on the ground or the floor of the cage before the hands are removed to release it. Wild birds can be given a nudge to make them move off as their heads and feet are released. You must be cautious of the possibility of being raked by the talons of raptors upon their release. It may be necessary to restrain the wings of wild birds to keep them from damaging feathers in the cage. Wings and body can be encircled with adhesive tape to temporarily effect this purpose.

Ketamine is the standard for chemical restraint and anesthesia in birds and is usually administered intramuscularly in the breast. Xylazine has also been used successfully in parakeets but may cause prolonged sedation. Birds may be maintained on gas anesthesia. Methoxyflurane and halothane are widely used.

TRANSPORTATION AND SHIPPING

Traveling with or transporting animals presents some challenges in restraint and in paperwork.

Cats are often nervous when riding in cars and usually are best transported in carriers. If they are particularly nervous, they may be given one of the promazine tranquilizers, which also have an antiemetic effect. Excessive nervousness or nausea may also result in profuse salivation, which can be controlled with atropine or a similar drug. Dogs can be treated with the same drugs in appropriate doses.

Most dogs and cats do not need tranquilization when shipped on airlines, as they feel secure enough in their shipping containers if accustomed to them before the trip. Even if the animals tend to be nervous in their crates, they are probably better off untranquilized in this situation of minimal supervision. Airlines have strict codes regarding acceptable crates for animals. Commercial shipping crates of an acceptable size for the dog or cat are useful not only for shipping but also for containment at home if needed. All animals in air freight must be accompanied by a current health certificate. Different states have different requirements for vaccination, quarantine, and so forth, and these guidelines may be found in the United States Department of Agriculture (USDA) State-Federal Health Requirements and Regulations handbook or learned by calling state veterinarian's offices (state regulations may have changed since the USDA handbook was printed, so it is a good idea to call for confirmation of regulations).

Most states require health certificates for any animal entering or traveling within their boundaries, and many people who travel by car with their small pets are not aware that they are breaking the law by not having health certificates for their cats and dogs.

Some states require negative results from a current Coggins or brucellosis test for entering horses or cattle. In addition, whenever livestock are transported, they should be accompanied by brand inspections.

Recommended Reading

Clutton-Brock J: Domesticated Animals from Early Times. The British Museum (Natural History), 1981.

Craig JV: Domestic Animal Behavior. Englewood Cliffs, NJ, Prentice-Hall, Inc., 1981.

Dunbar I: Dog Behavior: Why Dogs Do What They Do. Neptune, NJ, T.F.H. Publications, 1979.

Fox MW: Understanding Your Cat. New York, Bantam Books, Inc., 1974.

Fox MW: Understanding Your Dog. New York, Coward, McCann and Geoghegan, 1972.

Fowler ME: Restraint and Handling of Wild and Domestic Animals. Ames, IA, Iowa State University Press, 1978.

Fraser AF: Farm Animal Behavior. London, Balliere Tindall, 1974.

Hafez ESE: The Behavior of Domestic Animals, 3rd ed. London, Balliere Tindall, 1975.

Hart BL: Canine Behavior. Santa Barbara, Veterinary Practice Publishing Company, 1980.

Hayes MH: Illustrated Horse Training. Reprinted from 1889 edition. Hollywood, CA, Wilshire Book Co., 1973.

Kiley-Worthington M: The Behaviour of Horses in Relation to Management and Training. London, JA Allen, 1987.

Leahy JR and Barrow P: Restraint of Animals. Ithaca, NY, Cornell Campus Store, Inc., 1953.

Ryland LM and Bernard MS: A Clinical Guide to the Pet Ferret. Compendium for Continuing Education 5(1): 1983.

2

History and Physical Examination

MICHAEL L. MAGNE

INTRODUCTION

Large animal and small animal practices both require personalized, detailed, thorough and accurately performed services. The veterinary technician can greatly enhance the overall quality of service through initial contact with the client (history taking) and gathering routine physiological parameters (physical examination). Many veterinarians in today's busy practices occasionally take shortcuts in the diagnostic approach. Experience allows for most shortcuts to slide by with little or no consequence. However, if enough routine procedures are overlooked on a consistent basis, costly mistakes will eventually be made.

Veterinary medicine has only begun to tap the resources of practice quality enhancement that can be provided by the veterinary technician. Increased utilization of the technician for preliminary patient-herd evaluation allows the practicing veterinarian to concentrate more energy on the problem or problems at hand and yet not overlook an important piece of information. Therefore, the technician must be meticulous about history taking and the general physical examination. All pertinent information must be recorded in the medical record for further evaluation by the veterinarian. Examples of a history form and physical examination form that can become part of the medical record are found in Figures 2–1 and 2–2.

HISTORY

History taking is the first, and often most important, step in the diagnosis of a specific ailment. On first encountering the client, it is important to introduce oneself and to verify the name of the owner as well as the name and gender of the animal. Use vocabulary that the client understands; fancy, scientific jargon is useless if it is beyond the client's comprehension. Neutral, nonleading questions should be used, for instance: "How much does Fifi drink daily?" rather than "Does Fifi drink more water now?" Used appropriately, the history can be a source of much useful information and often directs the course of further patient evaluation, including acquisition of laboratory data, specific clinical tests and even therapy.

The patient signalment (age, breed, sex, reproductive status), though technically not a part of the history, may be important in determining the course of questioning and physical examination. Young animals are often presented for gastrointestinal parasitism, foreign bodies, intussusceptions or communicable or congenital diseases. Older animals are more commonly seen with degenerative or neoplastic diseases. Breed predisposition should always be considered, e.g., patellar luxations in poodles, respiratory problems in brachycephalic breeds, neoplasia in boxers, cerebellar hypoplasia and congenital immunodeficiencies in Arabian foals. The patient's sex and reproductive status may be important, as certain conditions are sex-limited (pyometra in intact females, retained testicles in males).

Chief Complaint

The initial step in history taking is to identify the chief complaint—that is, what does the owner perceive the animal's problem to be? Specific signs exhibited by the patient should

HOSPITAL NAME

ADDRESS

OWNER INFORMATION

HISTORY

HOSPITAL REGULATION: ALL POSITIVE AS WELL AS NEGATIVE FINDINGS SHALL BE RECORDED

DATE _____ HOUR _____ [A.M.] [P.M.]

**ORDER
OF
RECORDING**

1. (CC) CHIEF
   COMPLAINT

2. (HPI) HISTORY
   OF PRESENT ILLNESS

3. (PH) PAST
   HISTORY
   A. MEDICAL
   B. SURGICAL
   C. TRAUMA
   D. VACCINATIONS
   E. Coggins

4. (EH) ENVIRONMENTAL
   HISTORY

5. (SR) SYSTEM
   REVIEW
   A. GENERAL
   B. SKIN
   C. HEAD/NECK
   D. (EENT) EYES-EARS-
      NOSE-THROAT
   E. RESPIRATORY
   F. CARDIOVASCULAR
   G. (GI) GASTRO-
      INTESTINAL
   H. URINARY
   I. REPRODUCTIVE
   J. MUSCULOSKELETAL
   K. NERVOUS

6. SIGNATURE

ATTENDING CLINICIAN

MR 125 Rev. 3/77

HISTORY

14786

FIGURE 2–1. History-taking form.

PHYSICAL EXAMINATION

(1) GENERAL APPEARANCE ☐ Normal ☐ Abnormal	(2) INTEGU-MENTARY ☐ Normal ☐ Abnormal ☐ Not examined	(3) MUSCULO-SKELETAL ☐ Normal ☐ Abnormal ☐ Not examined	(4) CIRCU-LATORY ☐ Normal ☐ Abnormal ☐ Not examined
(5) RESPIRA-TORY ☐ Normal ☐ Abnormal ☐ Not examined	(6) DIGESTIVE ☐ Normal ☐ Abnormal ☐ Not examined	(7) GENITO-URINARY ☐ Normal ☐ Abnormal ☐ Not examined	(8) EYES ☐ Normal ☐ Abnormal ☐ Not examined
(9) EARS ☐ Normal ☐ Abnormal ☐ Not examined	(10) NEURAL SYSTEM ☐ Normal ☐ Abnormal ☐ Not examined	(11) LYMPH NODES ☐ Normal ☐ Abnormal ☐ Not examined	(12) MUCOUS MEMBRANES ☐ Normal ☐ Abnormal ☐ Not examined

DESCRIBE ABNORMAL: (Use numbers above) T _____ P _____ R _____ Wt. _____

TEMPORARY PROBLEM LIST	Initial Plan	
(1)	Dx	Rx
(2)		
(3)		
(4)		

STUDENT SIGNATURE   CLINICIAN SIGNATURE

PHYSICAL EXAMINATION

FIGURE 2–2. Physical examination form.

be determined. It is important at this point that clinical signs, and not the owner's diagnosis, be recorded—that is, diarrhea rather than enteritis, vomiting rather than gastritis, and so forth. The onset and progression of signs should be noted: When did the problem first begin, and how has it progressed? Has there been a change (improvement or deterioration) in the signs seen? Any precipitating events (travel, change in environment, relationship to eating, exercise) should also be recorded. Previous therapy and response to that therapy should be noted, because this may alter further diagnosis and therapy.

Medical History

The patient's past history must be thoroughly reviewed. Have there been previous medical problems, surgeries or per-

haps trauma, and when did these occur? What is the animal's vaccination status? (Always inquire about specific dates of vaccination; do not merely ask whether the animal has had recent vaccinations.) Have specific diagnostic tests been performed on the animal in question: Coggin's test in horses, Knott's test for heartworm in dogs, *Brucella* testing, fecal examinations or feline leukemia in cats?

Environmental History

The environmental history may reveal valuable clues pertaining to the current illness. If the animal is large, has it been shipped recently (shipping fever)? Have the owners traveled with the animal through areas endemic for particular diseases, such as heartworm or systemic fungal diseases? Has there been a recent move to a new household or geographical area? What composes the patient's diet; how much and how often is it fed? Have there been recent dietary changes or is any supplementation (vitamins-minerals, table scraps) added? How is the animal used? (The problems of the working or racing animal are very different from those of a breeding animal.) Even among pets, different problems are seen in indoor and outdoor animals. If there are other animals in the same environment, determine whether any have exhibited similar clinical signs; this may suggest a communicable or perhaps environmental disease. Have there been similar problems with litter-mates or parents, suggesting a genetic or congenital problem? Where was the animal obtained—sale barn, pet shop, breeder, humane society?

Specific Systems History

The next step in the history-taking process is referred to as a specific systems history and is designed to provide in-depth information concerning current or previous problems with specific body systems. As with any portion of the history or physical examination, the order in which one proceeds is not critical; the important thing is that no system be overlooked.

Integumentary System

With problems of the integumentary system (skin), one of the most important questions is whether or not there has been pruritus, or itching. If so, where does the animal scratch? How frequently is scratching seen, and does it occur in a particular season? Has there been hair loss (alopecia)? If so, what is the pattern of alopecia, and is it associated with any particular activity or stressful event? Have there been previous ectoparasite problems such as fleas, mites or lice? Are there any skin lumps—when were they first noted and what is their location and growth rate? Have other skin lumps been removed in the past? Is the patient an indoor or outdoor pet, and where does the patient sleep? Have there been recent environmental changes, such as new carpeting or new bedding? Have skin problems been seen with other animals or family members, suggesting a communicable disease? When was the skin problem first noticed? At what location did it start on the animal? What did it first look like, and how has it progressed? Has there been any bathing or medication administered, and what was the clinical response?

Head and Neck

Have there been problems with the head and neck area, such as head tilt, head shaking, rashes or bald spots? Has there been excessive tearing or other discharges from the eyes? Has the animal been blinking, squinting or pawing at the eyes? Have visual deficits been noted? If so, are they more obvious at night or during the day? Has the animal suffered from cataracts or other eye diseases, such as recurrent uveitis in horses or conjunctivitis ("pink eye") in cattle? Has there ever been trauma to the eyes? Is there any discharge or unusual odor associated with the ears? Head shaking often indicates a problem with the ears. Has discharge or bleeding from the nose been noted, or are there any abnormal respiratory sounds? Gagging, retching or difficulty in swallowing may indicate problems in the throat or pharyngeal area.

Respiratory System

Coughing is a cardinal sign of respiratory system disease. It is important to determine whether the cough is productive or nonproductive, and when it occurs. A cough occurring at night or during sleep is suggestive of heart disease. Other signs of respiratory disease include sneezing, nasal discharge, exercise intolerance or cyanosis. Has the animal exhibited dyspnea (difficulty in respiration) or tachypnea (rapid respiration), and are they seen at rest or after exercise? Is there a history of exposure to other animals, which may indicate a contagious respiratory disease, such as kennel cough, in the dog? Has there been travel through or residence in areas endemic for lungworm, heartworm or systemic fungal disease?

Cardiovascular System

Coughing is also commonly seen with diseases of the cardiovascular system. Other signs that may be seen are fainting (syncope), dyspnea or ascites ("bloated" abdomen). Have murmurs been previously diagnosed in the patient, or has previous treatment been instituted for heart problems? Has the patient traveled or resided in heartworm endemic areas?

Gastrointestinal System

Problems of the gastrointestinal system often present with vomiting or diarrhea as the major clinical sign. How often is the patient vomiting, and is there any relationship to eating? What are the color and consistency of the vomitus; does it contain digested or undigested food? Similarly, with animals showing diarrhea, it is important to determine the number of stools passed daily, the volume of each stool and the color of the feces. The presence of blood or mucus is an important characteristic to note. The dietary history should not be overlooked. Is there a history of "garbage" eating? Has there been exposure to toxins (rat poison, ethylene glycol) or infectious agents (parvovirus) that might cause vomiting or diarrhea? Have there been recent changes in the animal's diet? With small animals, do the owners routinely feed table scraps? In large animals, have they overeaten on a specific feedstuff? Has the patient had previous parasite problems? When was the last fecal examination performed, and when was the last worming? What type of routine worming program does the owner utilize?

Urinary System

Problems of the urinary system can present with a wide variety of signs, and careful questioning is important to localize disease. What does the urine look like, and how does it smell? Has there been blood, pus or any discoloration in the urine? Has the animal been drinking excessively (polydipsia) or urinating excessively (polyuria)? Has there been pollakiuria (small amounts frequently), dysuria (difficulty), or stranguria (straining), or has the animal shown incontinence (dribbling, accidents)? Have there been previous urinary tract infections or urinary calculi? If so, what was the treatment, and how did the condition respond? If stones were involved, were they analyzed for mineral content? Is there any history of trauma (hit by car, gunshots, falls) that may have involved the urinary tract or perhaps the pelvis? With cats showing urinary tract problems, always determine whether the animal has had previous bouts of feline urological syndrome ("blocked" cat, bloody urine, and so forth).

Reproductive System

The reproductive history should be elicited. Have there been previous breedings, and, if so, what was the outcome? Did the animal have a normal gestation and parturition, or were there any problems such as dystocia (difficult birth), abortions or stillbirths? Has the patient been cycling normally, and when was the last heat cycle? Has there been any vaginal discharge? What were the color, consistency and odor? Have there been previous false pregnancies, hormone therapy or mammary gland problems? Has *Brucella* testing been performed, or have vaginal cultures been done? With males, determine whether there has been abnormal penile discharge or any trauma to the penis or scrotum. Also, has the animal had a complete semen evaluation?

Musculoskeletal System

Diseases of the musculoskeletal system are common in veterinary medicine, and many can be diagnosed accurately with a thorough history and physical examination. The use of the animal (working versus racing horse, racing hound versus house pet) is very important, for characteristic orthopedic problems occur in these groups. Breed predispositions must also be remembered, for example, hip dysplasia in German shepherd dogs or Old English sheepdogs, congenital orthopedic problems in giant breeds. Has there been previous lameness, and what were the diagnosis and treatment? Is there any history of trauma, with possible fractures or luxations? If lameness is present, when was it first noticed? Did the lameness show a sudden, acute or more gradual, insidious onset? Does it occur at a particular time or perhaps at rest or after exercise? Does the animal "warm out" of the lameness? Are single or multiple limbs affected? Does the lameness shift from one limb to another; is it continuous or intermittent?

Central Nervous System

A thorough history is of utmost importance in the diagnosis of neurological problems, for often physical examination yields nonspecific findings. If seizures are the presenting problem, determine the duration and character (localized or generalized, urination-defecation?). Is the animal normal between seizures? Are the seizures related to eating? Has the frequency increased or decreased? Has there been exposure to possible neurotoxins, such as strychnine (rodenticides), lead (paint), ethylene glycol (antifreeze), or infectious agents, such as rabies, canine distemper, toxoplasmosis, equine encephalomyelitis or listeriosis? Have there been changes in the animal's behavior, for example, aggressiveness, depression, lethargy or abnormal responses to stimuli? Does the animal still recognize family members? Does the animal have a history of disk disease or other neurological problems? With any neurological problem, it is important to determine when the abnormality was first noted and whether it has improved or deteriorated. Are there any changes in vision, hearing or smell, or any problems with eating or drinking? Does the animal show problems in walking, head tilt or arching of the back?

Systems Review

After the detailed history specific to the particular problem system has been elicited, it is helpful to briefly review all other body systems. This *systems review* can add useful information to the history, and it also avoids exclusion of significant problems. The first step is simply to inquire if the owner has noted any other problems with the animal. Has there been scratching, hair loss or any skin rashes? Have there been any problems seen around the head and neck, or has there been any nasal or ocular discharge? Has there been coughing, sneezing, shortness of breath, fainting or a decreased exercise ability? Has there been any vomiting or diarrhea? Is the animal's appetite normal? Is the animal urinating normally, and is water consumption normal? Have the owners noticed bloody urine, or have there been any "accidents" in the house? Has lameness been seen? Have there been seizures or any abnormal behavior?

PHYSICAL EXAMINATION

The physical examination is the single most cost-efficient diagnostic tool available, and many diagnoses can be established with a thorough history plus a complete physical examination. Findings of the physical examination also serve to guide the course of later diagnostic testing. Remember the three "Ps" of physical examination: patience, perseverance and practice.

Visual inspection and observation is the oldest approach to physical examination. Observe the animal at a distance first. Temperament can be evaluated by the animal's response to the immediate environment and by appropriate reactions to strangers. Apprehension, fear and excitement may be perfectly normal in an animal subjected to a strange setting. Dullness and lethargy are abnormal and may indicate underlying central nervous system or metabolic disease. The general condition can be assessed by noting the condition of the haircoat, any hair loss, or abnormal pigmentation. Is the animal emaciated (cachectic) or, conversely, obese? Observe the animal's gait for lameness, weakness or neurological deficits. Head tilts may also be observed from a distance. Visual function can be assessed by noting the ability to negotiate doorways and other obstacles. Hearing can be difficult to evaluate; observe the animal closely for responses to auditory stimuli outside the visual field.

To inspect the patient more closely, approach slowly in a friendly manner. Offer the back of your hand and allow the animal to smell it. This establishes contact with the animal in a nonthreatening fashion. Animals with aggressive tendencies require appropriate restraint; however, it is important to avoid over-restraint, as this may aggravate certain animals' fractious behavior (see Chapter 1). Simple methods of minimal restraint are the muzzle for dogs, a towel or bag for cats, twitching for horses, and the nose twitch for cattle (see Chapter 1). If these methods are unsuccessful, chemical restraint may be necessary.

Techniques in Physical Examination

Palpation

Palpation is the application of touch to determine the character of deeper, underlying body structures. It may be direct by using the fingers or indirect by using a probe. When palpating, *trace* structures with the fingertips, do not grab internal structures! Certain terms should be used when describing

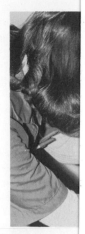

FIGURE 2–3. Exa
metry of nares, lips

ellipse in the cat
lens for opacitie!
ine the muzzle b
symmetrical and
slight serous disc
of the nares ca
nares or by noti
amination table.
visible swellings.

Examination
for inflammatio
or anatomical d
membranes for
cerations or tur
should be exam
and fractured, r
rior of the ora
technique for o|
Elevate the muz
one hand over
thumb into the
jaw (Fig. 2–6). /
upper finger an
with the other

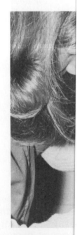

FIGURE 2–4. Ey
cornea, conjuncti

structures palpated. *Doughy* implies a soft feel, which can be impressed with the fingertips. *Firm* refers to normal organ consistency (e.g., liver), whereas *hard* refers to structures that are bone-like in consistency. *Fluctuant* structures are soft and elastic and undulate under pressure; cysts, abscesses and ascites are good examples. *Emphysema* refers to the presence of air or gas in tissues, which lends a characteristic crackling sound (like cellophane) to the tissues.

Superficial palpation is especially important in longhaired animals, as visual inspection may be limited. The skin, superficial muscles and skeletal structures should be thoroughly palpated for abnormalities. The throat area and thoracic inlet should be palpated for masses (thyroid tumor, thoracic tumors) and structural abnormalities, such as megaesophagus.

Abdominal palpation is a technique applicable only to small animals. In cats and small dogs, it may be performed with a single hand, whereas in large dogs two hands work best. Palpation can begin either caudally or cranially. Starting dorsally, allow the abdominal viscera to slip through the fingers as you move your hands ventrally. Repeat this procedure until the entire abdomen is palpated. The colon, uterus, bladder, prostate and small intestine are palpable in the caudal abdomen; the small intestine, kidneys and spleen are palpable in the midabdomen; and the liver, spleen and small intestine are palpable cranially. The left kidney is normally more easily palpated because it is located more caudally and is more freely movable. The stomach is not normally palpable unless it is distended with gas or food. The liver may also be unpalpable in normal animals. In the horse and cow, rectal palpation will be commonly done by the veterinarian. Because of the legal liability, the veterinary technician will be required to perform rectal examination under direct supervision only. Rectal tears and lacerations may occur even with experienced hands.

Auscultation

Auscultation is the art of listening with the stethoscope to sounds produced by the function of various body organs. It is most applicable in the evaluation of cardiovascular and respiratory systems, though in the equine and the bovine it is of considerable use in evaluating gastrointestinal sounds. Intestinal *hypermotility* results in increased intensity and frequency of intestinal sounds, whereas *hypomotility* (ileus) causes a decreased intensity or absence of normal intestinal sounds. Auscultation should be performed in a quiet environment. The bell portion of the stethoscope is used for low-pitched sounds, and the diaphragm is designed for high-pitched sounds. The earpieces should be directed anteriorly to align with the ear canals, and the stethoscope should be held firmly and flatly on the area to be auscultated. Auscultation requires frequent practice because cardiovascular, respiratory, gastrointestinal and extraneous environmental sounds may all impinge on your ears at one time.

Auscultation of the respiratory system should include sinuses, trachea and thorax. The sinuses and trachea are normally relatively silent, and abnormal sounds indicate the presence of fluid or obstruction. Fluid accumulation may result from sinusitis or may be secondary to pulmonary edema or pneumonia. Laryngeal obstruction (paralysis, tumor, foreign body) produces a characteristic wheezing sound on inspiration known as *stridor*. Normal lung sounds are categorized as either *vesicular* or *bronchial* sounds. Vesicular sounds are heard over

normal lung parenchyma and are caused by air movement through small bronchi, bronchioles and alveoli. Vesicular sounds occur during both inspiration and expiration, but they are usually louder during the inspiratory phase. They have been likened to the sound of "rustling leaves." Bronchial sounds are produced by air movement through the trachea and larger bronchi. They are louder on expiration and are usually heard over the trachea and carina.

Two general categories of abnormal lung sounds are recognized: crackles and wheezes. Crackles, or *rales,* have been compared to the crackling sound of cellophane. They occur as either coarse or fine crackles and are most commonly heard with fluid accumulation in alveoli or bronchioles, as occurs in pulmonary edema or bronchopneumonia. Crackles can also occur in certain "dry" lung diseases, such as pulmonary fibrosis. *Wheezes*, or *rhonchi*, are "musical" sounds produced by airway obstruction and result from air flow through a decreased airway lumen. Wheezes can be low pitched (*sonorous*) or high pitched (*sibilant*), and they occur in a variety of pathological states; for example, laryngeal obstruction, bronchospasm (feline asthma) or pneumonia, or in the presence of pulmonary masses, such as tumors, abscesses or granulomas. The absence of sounds in places they are normally heard is also abnormal and most commonly occurs with consolidation of lung tissue in pneumonia conditions. Pleural friction sounds are produced by movement of dry, roughened pleural surfaces over each other. Friction rubs have been compared to the sound of "creaking leather" and usually represent previous pleural effusion or pleuritis.

The goal of cardiac auscultation is to detect the presence of murmurs, abnormal heart sounds or arrhythmias. The areas of maximal intensity for the normal cardiac valvular sounds are as follows: The pulmonic valve is auscultated in the left second to fourth intercostal space just above the sternal border; the aortic valve area is auscultated in the left third to fifth intercostal space at the midthorax; the mitral valve is heard in the left fourth to sixth intercostal space just above the sternal border; and the tricuspid valve is auscultated in the right third to fifth intercostal space at the midthorax.

Sinus arrhythmia is a fluctuation in the heart rate concurrent with respiration; a decreasing heart rate is seen with expiration, and an increasing heart rate is seen with inspiration. Sinus arrhythmia is a normal finding in the dog but is rare in other species. The peripheral pulse should always be determined while auscultating the heart. A *pulse deficit* is said to occur when the pulse rate is less than the heart rate, and it implies a primary cardiac problem that warrants further investigation (an electrocardiogram [ECG] and so forth).

Several normal heart sounds are recognized in domestic animals. The first heart sound, or S1, represents closure of the atrioventricular (mitral, tricuspid) valves and is a loud, long, low-pitched sound. The second heart sound (S2) represents closure of the semilunar (aortic, pulmonic) valves. The interval between S1 and S2 represents *systole* or the period of active cardiac contraction. Conversely, the interval between S2 and S1 represents *diastole* or the resting phase of the cardiac cycle. Normally, systole is much shorter than diastole. The third heart sound (S3) is felt to represent ventricular filling. S3 is commonly heard in the horse and is felt to be of no clinical significance. However, in the dog, the presence of a third heart sound is thought to be pathological and reflects underlying cardiac disease. *Cardiac murmurs* are abnormal heart sounds

and repre
Murmurs
and point

A fixed
tion is of
all patien
specific te
and thorc

Immatu
tions or
closely fo
cleft pala
ture or ag
problem (
physical e
complaint
nonspecif
preclinica

Assessr
of every e
early indi

Evaluat
step in ph
to ''accor
permits t
response
with infec
mune) or
perature
common
The pulse
and with
mandible

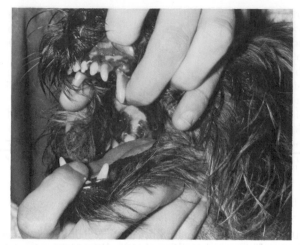

FIGURE 2–7. Mouth may be opened by slowly depressing the mandible.

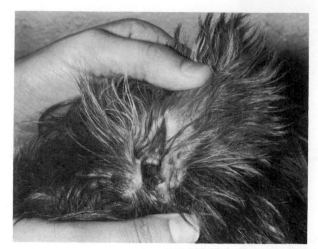

FIGURE 2–9. Examine the external ear canals for exudate, wax accumulation, inflammation or foreign bodies.

induce a cough. The thoracic inlet should also be palpated for abnormal masses.

At this time, the animal's haircoat and skin should be inspected for alopecia, ectoparasites, inflammation, crusts, scales or masses (mast cell tumors in dogs, sarcoid in horses, and so forth).

Proceed with the examination to the trunk and extremities. Palpate all lymph nodes, especially the prescapular, axillary and popliteal, for size and consistency. Muscles and bones of the rib cage, forelimbs and hind limbs should be palpated for swelling, atrophy, tumors or pain on palpation. Flex and extend all joints, noting any swelling, crepitus or pain. Lateral recumbency may facilitate orthopedic examination in smaller animals (Fig. 2–10). The condition of the feet should be evaluated. Check the interdigital spaces and the nails in dogs and cats (Fig. 2–11). Evaluate the hooves in horses and cows, checking for hoof cracks, bruised or abscessed soles or poor trimming or shoeing (Fig. 2–12).

Mammary glands should be evaluated individually, and any tumors, cysts or possible mastitis (swelling, heat, pain, abnormal-appearing milk) should be noted. Milk should be ex-

pressed from the mammary glands of lactating animals. Note the color, consistency and odor. The California Mastitis Test (CMT) should be performed on any cow suspected of having mastitis (see Chapter 8).

Evaluate the vulva for size, inflammation or discharges (Fig. 2–13). *Lochia,* a normal vaginal discharge, may be present for several weeks post partum and is usually a clear, odorless, serosanguineous fluid. The penis must be prolapsed to be examined (Fig. 2–14). A preputial exudate (*smegma*) may be normal in the dog and in the equine stud. Note any discharge, bleeding or masses. Palpate the scrotum, especially checking for testicles in intact males. Retained testicles are often palpated in the inguinal area. Note any swelling or pain of the scrotum, suggesting orchitis or epididymitis. The inguinal lymph nodes should be palpated for size and consistency.

Examine the perineal area for the presence of masses, perianal fistulas, perineal hernias or rectovaginal fistulas in mares. Rectal examination should be a normal part of the physical examination. Evaluate the rectum, bony pelvis, uterus, and vagina, urethra, prostate and anal sacs. Perineal hernias and

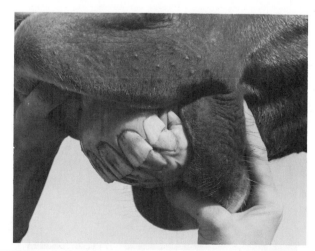

FIGURE 2–8. Dental examination in the horse enables one to determine the horse's age.

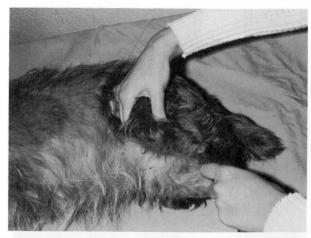

FIGURE 2–10. Lateral recumbency often facilitates examination of the limbs for musculoskeletal or neurological abnormalities. Palpate thoroughly, and put each joint through range of motion, noting pain, crepitus or resistance to manipulation.

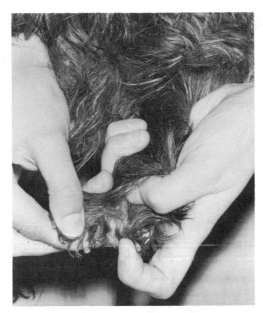

FIGURE 2–11. Always examine between the toes for foreign bodies, abscesses, and so forth. This is a favorite hiding place for grass awns.

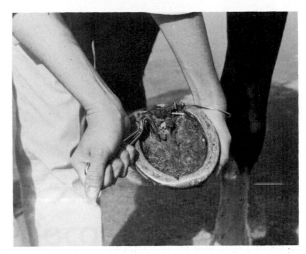

FIGURE 2–12. The feet, or hooves, should be examined for bruising, abscesses, and so forth. Picking may be necessary beforehand.

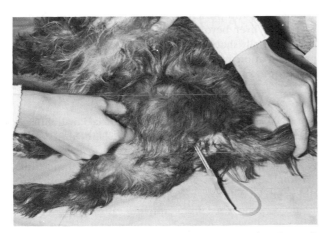

FIGURE 2–13. While taking the temperature, examine the perineal area, popliteal lymph nodes and vulvar area in females.

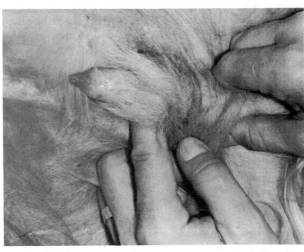

FIGURE 2–14. The prepuce must be pushed posteriorly for adequate visualization of the penis.

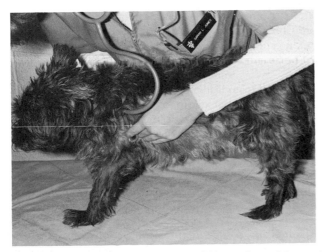

FIGURE 2–15. Thoracic auscultation should be performed thoroughly in a quiet environment.

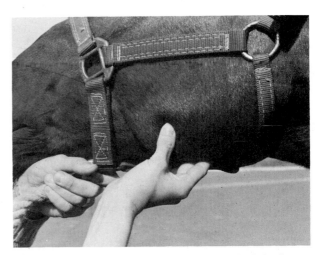

FIGURE 2–16. The facial artery pulse is palpated (with the fingers not the thumb) at the point at which it crosses the mandible. The facial artery is similarly located in both the horse and the cow.

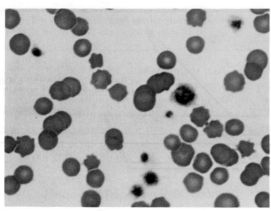

FIGURE 4–5. Feline erythrocytes and platelets. The platelets vary greatly in size.

increased numbers of large platelets may indicate an increased output from the bone marrow (Fig. 4–5). After the platelets have been evaluated, the erythrocytes should be studied. First of all, their size should be noted. The RBCs of different domestic species normally differ in size, with the dog having the largest diameter (7 μ), followed by the horse, cow and cat (5.8 μ), the sheep (4.5 μ) and the goat (3.2 μ). Some species have RBCs that vary in size more than others or show *anisocytosis*. Cows normally have more anisocytosis in the size of their RBCs than do other species. In other species, extreme anisocytosis implies either that many of the RBCs are smaller (microcytic), which may indicate iron deficiency, or that many are larger (macrocytic), which may indicate increased production by the bone marrow. Some poodles normally have larger RBCs than do other dogs. Some Japanese Akita dogs normally have smaller RBCs. These are genetic traits and do not indicate a change in RBC dynamics.

RBCs can vary in shape and appearance as well as in size. *Leptocytes* are RBCs with an increased surface area that makes them highly deformable. Target cells and cells with a transverse fold are two common forms of leptocytes. Since leptocytes can occur for many reasons, they are rarely diagnostic of any specific condition. The most common condition associated with leptocytes is polychromatophilia. Young polychromatophilic RBCs are often leptocytes.

Acanthocytes are RBCs with a membrane abnormality that causes them to develop multiple club-shaped projections from the cell surface. Acanthocytes are usually associated with disorders of lipid metabolism and some neoplasms (especially splenic hemangiosarcoma). *Schistocytes* are fragmented RBCs that are produced by the trauma of colliding with intravascular fibrin strands. Hence, schistocytes are associated with disseminated intravascular coagulopathy (DIC), heartworm disease and occasionally diseases of the spleen or liver that involve fibrin deposition within the vasculature of those organs. *Spherocytes* are small, dense RBCs that show no central pallor. They are spherical because they have a reduced amount of membrane but no loss of volume. Spherocytes are most commonly seen in immune hemolytic anemia. Spherocytes can also be seen following blood transfusions. They are most easily identified in canine blood, since normal canine RBCs have a distinct zone of central pallor. In other species that do not normally have RBCs with central pallor, spherocytes are difficult to confirm. Figure 4–6 illustrates normal dog RBCs and spherocytes.

Nucleated RBCs, or *metarubricytes,* may be seen in peripheral blood films. An occasional nucleated RBC may be found in a normal animal, but increased numbers are a significant finding and should be reported as the number of NRBCs per 100 WBCs. Remember to correct the WBC count if more than 10 NRBCs per 100 WBCs are found (see earlier discussion of Leukocyte Determination).

The color of erythrocytes should be noted during examination of the blood film. *Polychromatophilic* RBCs (Color Plate IA) are bluish, though this is not as consistently evident with Diff-Quick stain as it is with Wright's stain. The presence of polychromasia in anemias indicates that the anemia is regenerative; in other words, the bone marrow is responding to a need for RBCs. If no polychromasia is detected on a blood film from an anemic animal, the anemia is nonregenerative; the bone marrow is not responding and, hence, is primarily responsible for the anemia.

Polychromatophilic RBCs are the same cells that show up as *reticulocytes* when the blood is stained with new methylene blue. Two drops of blood and two drops of stain are mixed in a small tube and are left to stand for 5 to 10 minutes; a blood film is then made from the mixture. Stain kits (Retic-Set, Curtin Matheson Scientific, Inc., Houston, TX) are available for reticulocyte counts that eliminate the need to use liquid stain. Three to five drops of whole blood are added to a stain-coated plastic tube and agitated. The sample is then treated as explained above.

Normal RBCs appear yellowish, whereas reticulocytes contain bluish dots or strands. Cats have two types of reticulocytes. Only the reticulocytes that have prominent clumps of reticu-

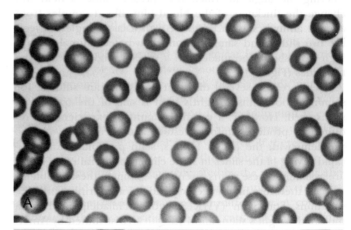

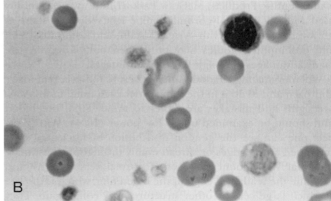

FIGURE 4–6. A, Normal canine RBCs. Note the distinct central pallor. B, Blood from a dog with immune-mediated hemolytic anemia. Note the lack of central pallor in several cells, the large polychromatophilic cell and a NRBC.

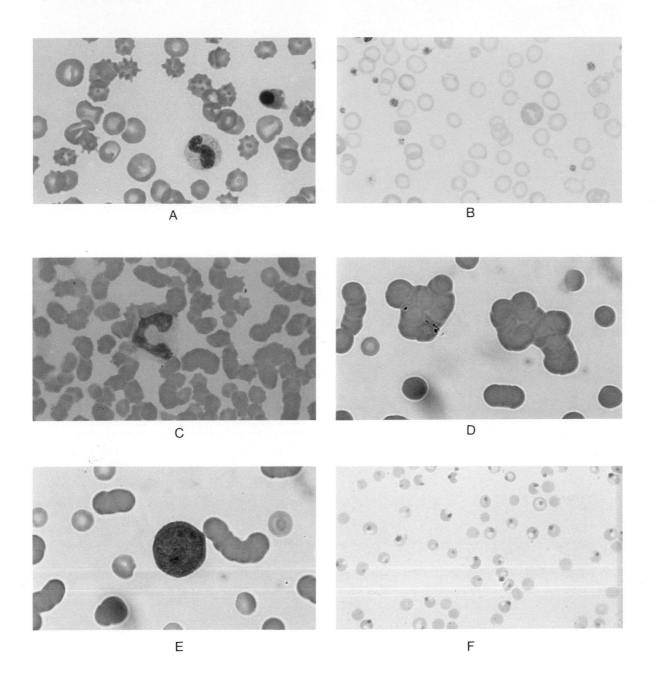

COLOR PLATE I. A, Canine blood film displaying several polychromatophilic erythrocytes and one nucleated erythrocyte. A segmented neutrophil is also present. B, Canine blood film showing hypochromic erythrocytes with increased central pallor. C, Equine blood film showing rouleau formation. D, Feline blood film showing agglutination. E, Feline blood film showing rouleau formation. F, Feline blood film, new methylene blue stain, showing dark-staining Heinz bodies on the periphery of the erythrocytes.

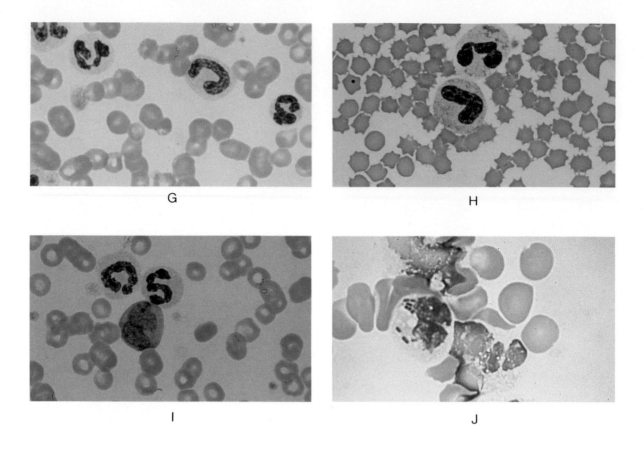

COLOR PLATE I *Continued.* G, Canine erythrocytes, segmented neutrophils, and one band neutrophil. Several platelets are also present. H, Feline blood film with two toxic neutrophils. The toxic changes evident are increased basophilia of the cytoplasm and Döhle bodies. I, Canine blood film showing two segmented neutrophils and one monocyte. J, Equine abdominal fluid showing a neutrophil with intracellular rod-shaped bacteria. Two smudged cells are also present.

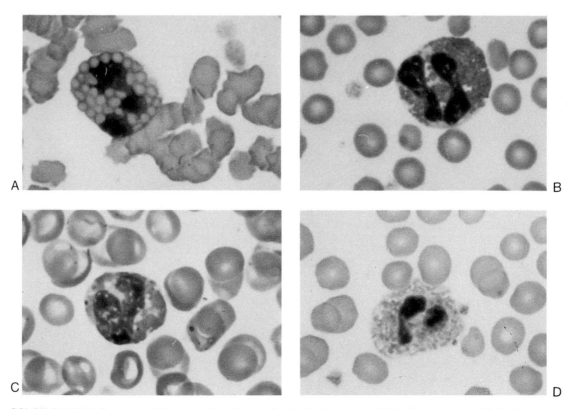

COLOR PLATE II. Species variation in eosinophil granules. A, Equine eosinophil. B, Bovine eosinophil. C, Canine eosinophil. D, Feline eosinophil.

lum (aggregate reticulocytes) are counted. The RBC with small single dots (punctate reticulocytes) are not included in the count, but their presence should be noted. A reticulocyte count is the number of reticulocytes noted in a count of 500 RBCs expressed as a percentage (20 reticulocytes out of 500 RBCs = 4 percent reticulocytes). Horses do not release immature RBCs from the bone marrow even when they are severely anemic; therefore, polychromasia or reticulocytosis is not seen in equine peripheral blood.

Hypochromic RBCs have an increased area of central pallor resulting from an abnormally low amount of hemoglobin within the cell. The most common cause of hypochromasia is iron deficiency. Hypochromasia can be confirmed by a low MCHC. True hypochromic RBCs (Color Plate IB) must be differentiated from "punched out" RBCs. Punched out cells are normochromic but have a distinct central pallor with a thick dense rim of hemoglobinized cytoplasm. These cells are an artifact of blood film preparation, not a significant pathological change. Hyperchromasia or increased hemoglobin content in RBCs does not occur.

Rouleaux are groupings of RBCs that resemble stacked coins. Marked rouleaux formation is normal in horses (Color Plate IC) and, to a lesser extent, in cats. In dogs, rouleaux formation may occur in inflammatory or neoplastic diseases. It is important to differentiate rouleaux from true *agglutination* (clumping) of RBCs. Agglutinated RBCs tend to appear as clumps rather than as stacked coins (Color Plate ID and E). Often, agglutination of RBCs can be noted on the side of the blood tube as well as on the blood film. If there is some question in determining whether a blood sample is exhibiting rouleaux or true agglutination, a saline test can be performed. The blood cells are washed, that is, one drop of blood is added to 5 ml of saline and this mixture is centrifuged for 3 minutes. The supernatant is poured off, the RBCs are resuspended in saline, and a wet mount preparation is made. Rouleaux will disperse, but agglutinated RBCs will remain clumped together.

The evaluation of erythrocytes under oil immersion should also include a search for RBC parasites, particularly in cases of anemia. *Haemobartonella felis*, the parasite responsible for feline infectious anemia, appears as small coccoid or rod-like structures on the surface of RBCs. A careful search for *H. felis* organisms should be performed on any anemic cat. *Eperythrozoon* spp., found in cattle, sheep and swine, may appear similar to *Haemobartonella* or may occur as ring forms on the RBCs. *Anaplasma marginale*, a parasite of bovine RBCs, appears as a small spherical body within the RBC, close to the cell margin. Another RBC parasite is *Babesia*, which has various species that can infect any domestic animal. *Babesia* spp. are larger and lighter-staining than the previously mentioned parasites, and they tend to occur as piriform structures (often paired) within the RBCs. *Babesia* can cause intravascular hemolysis of RBCs, whereas *Haemobartonella*, *Eperythrozoon* and *Anaplasma* cause anemia by extravascular phagocytosis of RBCs.

Other RBC morphological abnormalities associated with anemia include *Howell-Jolly bodies, basophilic stippling* and *Heinz bodies*. Howell-Jolly bodies are small, often singular, deeply basophilic nuclear remnants that are occasionally seen on normal blood films. Increased numbers of Howell-Jolly bodies can be seen with regenerative anemias. Basophilic stippling is due to staining of small amounts of cytoplasmic RNA in RBCs. These inclusions are multiple tiny, lightly basophilic dots in the RBC cytoplasm. They can be found in markedly regenerative anemia (especially in cows) and, occasionally, in lead poisoning.

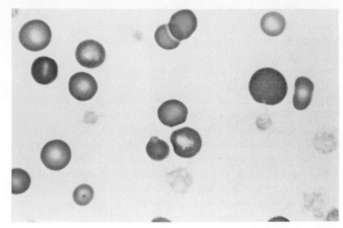

FIGURE 4–7. Feline blood film showing Heinz body formation. Note the small RBC with a distinct pale rounded projection from its surface (Wright's stain; see Color Plate).

The most consistent finding in lead poisoning is increased numbers of NRBCs with mild to no anemia. Heinz bodies are denatured hemoglobin that has fused to the RBC membrane and appear as refractile projections from the RBC cell membrane (Fig. 4–7). These inclusions are most readily seen on the reticulocyte stain, where they appear as distinct darkly staining inclusions (Color Plate IF).

Neutrophils

In most species, the predominant WBC is the neutrophil (Fig. 4–8). Neutrophils have phagocytic and bactericidal capabilities, which means they have an important role in inflammatory conditions. The average time spent by the neutrophil in the blood is only about 10 hours, so it is clear that the neutrophil can rise or fall in a matter of hours, depending on the stimuli present. Normal neutrophils have segmented nuclei. Horse neutrophils have more segmentation than dog neutrophils. The cytoplasm is usually clear but may show a faint granularity.

A morphological change in neutrophils that should be noted is band-shaped nuclei, which indicate release of imma-

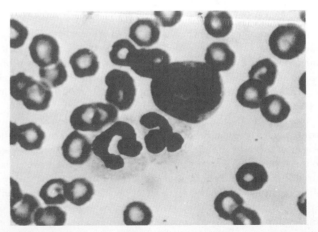

FIGURE 4–8. Canine blood film. Two segmented neutrophils and a monocyte are present.

ture neutrophils from the bone marrow. A band nucleus has no segmentation as seen in the mature segmented nucleus but instead has parallel borders (Color Plate IG). Even more immature cells, with oval or bean-shaped nuclei, may be seen in cases of extreme tissue demand for neutrophils. Neutrophils may show evidence of systemic toxemia by certain cytoplasmic characteristics. Cats seem to show toxic neutrophils during many kinds of illnesses (Color Plate IH), but in other species toxic changes usually imply severe bacterial infections. One cytoplasmic change includes *Döhle bodies,* which are small bluish-gray inclusions in the cytoplasm and usually indicate mild toxemia. Generalized *basophilia* of the cytoplasm, or *cytoplasmic vacuolation,* is a slightly more severe toxic change. In contrast to these cytoplasmic changes, *nuclear hypersegmentation* (nuclei with 5 or more lobes) is a feature that implies a prolonged life span of a neutrophil and is frequently seen in steroid or stress leukograms, in which neutrophils remain in circulation longer than is normal. Inflammatory leukograms are frequently accompanied by an increased number of band or other immature neutrophils, and the total number of neutrophils in the blood stream actually increases.

Neutropenia, a decrease in circulating neutrophils, may occur when tissue demand exceeds the bone marrow's ability to supply neutrophils. If this is the case, there will probably be an increased proportion of immature neutrophils along with the decreased number of neutrophils, indicating the bone marrow's vain attempt to meet tissue demands.

Monocytes

Monocytes (Fig. 4–8 and Color Plate II) are derived from the bone marrow and circulate in the blood briefly before entering the tissues in which they become *macrophages.* Macrophages phagocytize (ingest) large particles and cellular debris that neutrophils cannot handle. Monocytes have gray-blue cytoplasm and a variable-shaped nucleus. The nucleus can be round, oval or lobed. The monocyte is usually larger than the lymphocyte or neutrophil. The most common problem associated with the identification of monocytes is the tendency to confuse monocytes, which have a bean-shaped nucleus, with a band neutrophil. This is especially a problem when there is toxic change present in the neutrophils. The cytoplasm of the monocyte is usually a darker blue than the band neutrophil.

Eosinophils

Eosinophils help to control allergic or anaphylactic hypersensitivity reactions. They are attracted to the sites of these reactions by substances released from sensitized mast cells; therefore, eosinophils tend to occur at the same locations where mast cells congregate. The eosinophil is characterized by distinct red-staining granules in the cytoplasm. Their nuclei are segmented.

The morphological appearance of eosinophil granules varies from species to species, so that they can be used to identify the origin of a blood sample. The eosinophils of cats contain rod-shaped granules. The eosinophilic granules of dogs are more variable in size and shape and are less numerous. The eosinophilic granules of horses are extremely distinctive, being very large and round and a much brighter orange than those of small animals. Cattle eosinophilic granules are also bright orange but are much smaller and more numerous than the

horse's. Greyhounds often have eosinophils that have degranulated and appear vacuolated. Color Plate IIA to D illustrates the diversity of eosinophil granules found in various domestic species.

Basophils

Basophils are not the same as mast cells (morphologically the most distinct difference is the segmented basophil nucleus, compared with the mast cell's round or oval nucleus), but they are similarly involved in hypersensitivity reactions. Basophils are relatively rare in blood films. Cat basophils have light lavender granules rather than the dark purple granules seen in other species.

Lymphocytes

Lymphocytes are usually small to medium-sized mononuclear cells with a thin rim of cytoplasm that ranges from light blue to dark blue. Their cytoplasm may or may not contain azurophilic granules. Cattle are notorious for their often bizarre-looking lymphocytes. In normal cattle, lymphocytes outnumber neutrophils and may be quite large, with indented (rather than round) nuclei, increased cytoplasm and perhaps azurophilic cytoplasmic granules. During periods of antigenic stimulation in all species, some of the lymphocytes in the blood film may have extremely basophilic cytoplasm with a pale perinuclear zone (the site of the Golgi apparatus) and possibly azurophilic granules. These cells are referred to as reactive lymphocytes.

Occasionally, evaluation of the blood film reveals abnormal circulating cell types, such as mast cells, lymphoblasts, myeloblasts and erythroblasts. The number and type of abnormal cells should be noted, as they may indicate leukemia or systemic mastocytosis. Blood films with unusual or abnormal cells can be sent to a reference laboratory for evaluation.

Electronic Cell Counters

Currently several instruments are available for automated cell counting. These instruments range in price from $10,000 to more than $100,000. A veterinary practice must have a significant daily sample volume to justify their expense. The most widely recognized instruments are those made by Coulter Electronics, Inc. (Hialeah, FL) for use in human laboratories. These instruments must be specially calibrated for use with veterinary samples due to the wide variation in blood cell size among the different species. Recently, several instruments have been introduced specifically for veterinary medicine (Fig. 4–9). These instruments are computer-driven with species options, which automatically change the instrument settings for multiple species use. The major advantages of electronic cell counters is their speed, accuracy and reproducibility. In addition to providing red and white blood cell counts, some cell counters will measure hemoglobin and calculate the red blood cell indices (such as mean corpuscular hemoglobin concentration and mean corpuscular hemoglobin). Mean corpuscular volume is measured directly by these instruments.

The disadvantage of electronic cell counters is their quality control and maintenance requirements. The veterinary technician must be able to recognize when the instruments are not

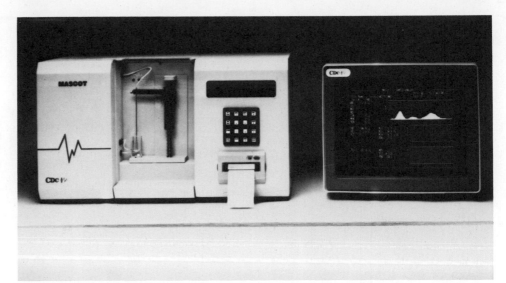

FIGURE 4–9. The CDC Mascot multispecies hematology unit with specific program settings for the common domestic species. (CDC Technologies, Inc., Oxford, CT.)

functioning properly and determine the problem. The manufacturer should be willing to train the technician to perform quality control and calibration procedures, keep adequate quality control records, and handle minor adjustments. In addition, the manufacturer should be available for service calls if needed. In some practices, consideration should be given to the purchase of a service contract. This should be discussed prior to investing in a major instrument. The operating principle involved in electronic cell counting is based on a type of flow cytometry (the counting of particles as they flow past a detection device). This technology allows the instrument to count blood cells and measure their size. Most instruments use a simple orifice through which an electrical current passes. As particles (such as blood cells) move through the orifice, they disrupt the current by increasing the resistance proportional to the size of the particle. The instrument is set to detect and count only those particles that produce a signal that exceeds a specific resistance or threshold. The threshold settings will determine what particles are counted, based on their size. This principle is important when an instrument is evaluated for use in veterinary medicine. Many instruments developed for human medicine do not accurately count red blood cells with a volume less than 55 femtoliters (fl). The cat, horse, cow, goat and pig red blood cells all have mean cell volumes below this value.

White blood cells from different species also have varying sizes after exposure to red cell lysing solutions. Total white cell counts on some instruments can be falsely decreased in the dog owing to the small size of their leukocytes. The reverse is true in the cat. The cat's platelets tend to form large clumps that are counted as leukocytes, thus falsely elevating the white blood cell count. Close inspection of the blood film will help the technician to identify this problem.

Whole blood can be diluted for counting either before introducing the sample into the machine (pre-dilution) or by the instrument as part of the sampling cycle. In the newer instruments, whole blood is aspirated and diluted for the red blood cell count, and a portion of the sample is lysed to remove the red blood cells and allow the white blood cells to be counted. The lysed sample is often used for hemoglobin determination. The counters that determine hemoglobin often will provide a calculated hematocrit and the RBC indices.

Occasionally there is a discrepancy between the spun PCV and the calculated hematocrit. This is most commonly seen in blood samples from collection tubes that have an inadequate volume of blood (less than 1 ml in a 5-ml tube or less than 0.5 ml in a 2-ml tube). The excess anticoagulant causes the RBCs to shrink, erroneously decreasing the PCV. When the blood is diluted by the electronic cell counter, the diluent re-expands the RBCs to their true size, providing the true value for the hematocrit. The MCH and MCHC calculated by an electronic cell counter will be artifactually affected by hemolysis and lipemia and therefore cannot be interpreted on such samples. The early Coulter instruments are simple particle counters, require pre-dilution of the sample and do not provide a hemoglobin determination.

A basic understanding of the principles of electronic cell counting is useful for the veterinary technician regardless of whether the practice has an in-clinic laboratory. Many practices find it convenient to use human reference or hospital laboratories. Because of the aforementioned differences in veterinary samples, the veterinary technician may be of assistance in helping these laboratories to provide accurate data.

Quantitative Buffy Coat Analysis

Quantitative buffy coat (QBC) analysis is currently used in many veterinary practices for measurements of PCV, total WBC count, platelet count, and a limited leukocyte differential. The QBC instrumentation consists of large-bore capillary tubes fitted with a free-floating plastic cylinder slightly smaller in diameter than the tube, a centrifuge and a reading instrument that converts buffy coat band lengths into numerical readings. The tubes are coated with acridine orange, a dye that allows the differentiation of the granulocytes, mononuclear cells (monocytes and lymphocytes) and platelets. Figure 4–10 illustrates the expansion of the buffy coat by the plastic float and where the specific cell layers are found. The QBC instrument is relatively inexpensive compared with the electronic cell counters and provides much the same information. It is important to remember, however, that the limited differential obtained should not replace the blood film examination. Blood cell morphology is important in evaluating the numbers ob-

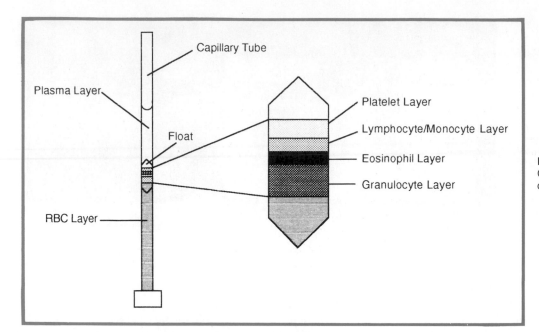

FIGURE 4–10. Illustration of the QBC buffy coat layers following centrifugation.

tained in the blood cell counts. The QBC instrument cannot tell the technician whether band neutrophils, polychromatophilic RBCs or NRBCs are present. One important advantage to using the QBC instrument is improved detection of circulating microfilaria.

Plasma Protein Determination

To complete the routine CBC, the plasma protein concentration should be measured. The simplest method is to take the capillary tube that was used for the PCV determination, break the tube at a point slightly above the *buffy coat* (layer of WBCs and platelets just above the RBCs) and allow the plasma to run through the unbroken end onto the prism of a refractometer by capillary action. It is best not to lift the cover and tap the hematocrit tube on the prism, as this may scratch the surface of the prism. Plasma protein values obtained on a refractometer are accurate as long as the plasma is clear; if the plasma is lipemic, hemolyzed or otherwise cloudy, the refractive index will be increased and provide an erroneously high protein measurement.

The plasma *fibrinogen* determination may be useful in the detection of inflammatory processes in cattle and horses. Two capillary tubes of blood are centrifuged; the first is used for the PCV and plasma protein determination, as already described. The second is placed in a 56° C to 58° C water bath for 3 minutes to cause the precipitation of the fibrinogen. The tube is then centrifuged again so that the fibrinogen settles just above the buffy coat. The tube is broken above the fibrinogen, and the remaining plasma is placed on the refractometer for the protein determination. The difference between the protein concentration of the first tube and the protein concentration of the second tube is the fibrinogen concentration.

Fibrinogen is usually expressed in milligrams per deciliter; therefore, if the first tube had a protein concentration of 7.3 g/dl and the second tube has a protein concentration of 6.9 g/dl, the plasma fibrinogen concentration is 0.4 g/dl or 400 mg per dl. Plasma from cattle with markedly increased fibrin-

ogen may completely coagulate during incubation. When the specimen is re-spun the fibrinogen does not settle out, and a fibrinogen value cannot be determined.

URINALYSIS

Urinalysis is the one clinical laboratory procedure that should be done in all veterinary practices. It is an important diagnostic test that should be done on fresh urine whenever possible. The techniques involved are simple and require no special instrumentation. Urine samples should be collected into clean glass or plastic containers. In general, no preservatives are used. The best time to collect urine for urinalysis is usually first thing in the morning; this is especially true of house-trained animals. Urine that accumulates during the relative inactivity of the night is less likely to be influenced by feeding or exercise. It is generally concentrated, and therefore abnormal constituents, if present, are more easily detected.

Urine Collection

Urine may be collected by several methods. The simplest (if the animal will cooperate) is to catch a free-flow sample as the animal voids. If this method is used, the initial stream of urine should not be caught, as the first portion may contain cells and debris from the urethra and lower genital tract, which may interfere with interpretation. It is better to collect a "midstream" sample; that is, try to avoid the very beginning or the very end of a voided urine sample.

A second method that may be used to collect urine is called *cystocentesis*. This procedure involves placing a needle (with a syringe attached) through the ventral abdominal wall into the lumen of the bladder and aspirating urine. Aseptic technique must be used. By performing cystocentesis, the secretions and debris of the lower urogenital tract are avoided and interpretation of urinalysis findings is simplified. Cystocentesis is routine in many animal hospitals. Iatrogenic hemorrhage can occur during cystocentesis; therefore, it is not unusual to have a widely variable number of RBCs in the sediment of samples obtained by this method.

Another method for collecting urine is by catheterization of the bladder. This procedure must be done as aseptically as possible to prevent introduction of bacteria into the urinary tract. Extreme care should be taken to avoid traumatizing the lining of the urethra with the catheter, or the sample may contain increased numbers of erythrocytes and epithelial cells. Additional information on cystocentesis and catheterization is found in Chapter 8.

No matter how the urine sample is collected, it should be analyzed as soon as possible. Many changes begin to occur immediately: Any bacteria present in the urine will multiply, cells will autolyze, casts may dissolve (especially if the urine is alkaline) and bacteria that produce urease will convert urea to ammonia, causing the pH to increase. If there is to be any delay at all in performing the urinalysis, the sample should be refrigerated to slow these processes. However, refrigeration may cause a change in urine specific gravity (SG) and interfere with some of the chemistry reactions on the chemistry reagent strip. Before a urinalysis is performed on refrigerated urine, the specimen should be allowed to come to room temperature.

Urine Evaluation Procedure

The parameters evaluated in most routine urinalyses include color, appearance, SG, pH, protein, glucose, ketones, blood, bilirubin and a microscopic examination of sediment. As with all laboratory procedures, it is wise to follow the same routine protocol with every urine sample analyzed. First, after making sure the sample is mixed well, assess its color and appearance. Next, reagent strip chemistries should be performed, unless the urine is very turbid (cloudy). If it is turbid, the chemistry tests may be done after the sample has been centrifuged. The SG can also be determined either before or after centrifugation, depending on the turbidity of the sample. The material that settles out during centrifugation has almost no effect on SG. Finally, the sediment should be prepared for microscopic examination. Pour 10 ml of urine into a conical tip centrifuge tube. If the sample available is smaller than 10 ml, use all that is left after the reagent strip chemistries and SG determinations have been completed. Centrifuge the urine at 1500 rpm for 5 minutes. Decant the supernatant, leaving the sediment in the bottom. Gently tap the tube to resuspend the sediment in the small amount of urine remaining in the bottom of the tube. With a small pipette, transfer a drop of suspended sediment to a glass slide and place a coverslip on it.

A phase-contrast microscope is ideal for examining unstained urine sediment. A more practical and highly satisfactory alternative is to lower the condenser of the light microscope and reduce the intensity of the light itself (as for the manual mammalian WBC count). The slide should first be examined at 10× magnification to get an overall impression of how much and what type of sediment is present. The 40× to 45× power ("high dry") is then used to make the final identification and count of various structures. At least 10 microscopic fields must be evaluated, and the average number of various cells and casts per high-power field is reported. The presence and relative amounts of other components are also noted.

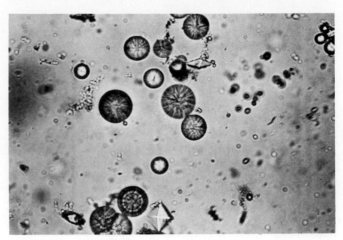

FIGURE 4–11. Equine urine sediment. Photomicrograph showing the round calcium carbonate crystals with distinct radiating striations.

Urine Color

Normal urine is yellow to amber, depending on its concentration and constituents. Bright red urine indicates *hematuria* (RBCs in the urine) or *hemoglobinuria* (hemoglobin in the urine). A reddish-brown color usually suggests hemoglobinuria or *myoglobinuria* (myoglobin in the urine); note that these two pigments cannot be distinguished from one another solely on the basis of color. High concentrations of bilirubin or urobilin cause yellowish-brown urine that, when shaken, produces yellowish foam. Whenever an unusual discoloration of the urine occurs, the history of any drug therapy should be evaluated, as there are many drugs that can produce oddly colored urine. For example, methylene blue causes greenish urine.

Fresh urine is normally transparent, but as it cools, some salts may precipitate, causing the urine to become cloudy. Except for horse urine, fresh urine that is cloudy is often pathological, and it must be examined microscopically to identify the cause: pus, blood, mucus, bacteria, casts or crystals. Fresh horse urine is normally cloudy because it contains mucus and calcium carbonate crystals (Fig. 4–11). Clear urine should also be examined microscopically because some abnormal constituents may be present in small amounts and may not cause the urine to be cloudy.

Specific Gravity

Specific gravity determination is one of the most important parts of a urinalysis. The SG value depends on the number and the size of particles in solution. The refractometer is the current method of choice for measuring SG, and it requires only a drop of urine. If the urine sample is turbid, the SG may be determined from the supernatant following centrifugation.

The normal range for SG is extremely wide: 1.001 to 1.060 in dogs and 1.001 to 1.080 in cats. The major determinant of urine SG is salt concentration, because of the large number of particles involved. Protein, in contrast, has little influence on SG, because although the particles are large, they are few in number. Glucose, likewise, has relatively little effect on SG. Both of these components, when found in large amounts in the urine, will increase the SG about 0.001 to 0.002 refractive index units. Specific gravity provides a very good indication of how well the kidneys are able to function in maintaining the body's water and osmotic balance. In addition, SG is important in interpreting other tests: for instance, because of the usual inverse relationship between SG and volume, a "2+" protein in dilute urine (SG <1.012) suggests a greater loss of protein than a "2+" protein in concentrated urine (SG >1.050).

Isosthenuria is the continued excretion of urine at the SG of glomerular filtrate (1.008 to 1.012). Isosthenuria indicates that the tubules have not attempted to concentrate urine. A single, routine urine sample with an isosthenuric SG is not necessarily abnormal, since this is within the normal range and could be a chance occurrence. However, if an animal is dehydrated, azotemic or uremic, the renal tubules are under pressure to concentrate urine, and under those circumstances, a SG lower than 1.035 in cats, 1.030 in dogs and 1.025 in large animals indicates that the kidneys are not functioning appropriately.

Urine Protein

Many commercial urine reagent strips include a test for protein. The strips rely on color changes in tetrabromophenolphthalein blue to detect protein levels that are above a very small amount (>10 mg/dl) present in normal urine. The test reaction is usually graded "trace" or "1+" through "4+," which supposedly corresponds to various protein concentrations; for instance, 1+ indicates 30 mg/dl and "4+" indicates 1000 mg/dl. However, as with most reagent strip chemistry tests, results are at best only semiquantitative and are subject to several types of error. First, false-positive trace values may occur when urine is very alkaline. Second, the strips are more sensitive to albumin than to globulins and therefore can give false-negative readings when proteinuria is caused by globulins. Finally, different technicians may make different readings on the same urine sample. As previously mentioned, a positive protein reaction in a dilute urine implies a greater protein loss than the same level of reaction in a concentrated sample.

Even though it is often stated that normal urine contains no protein, the truth is that almost all urine contains a small amount of protein, which is due to normal leakage and secretion from the urinary tract lining. However, this normal amount of protein is not detected by routine methods.

Protein loss into urine can be a significant drain on the body's protein stores. One can make subjective evaluation of the amount being lost by comparing the results to the SG, as previously mentioned; however, a more exact method is to collect all urine produced in a 24-hour period and calculate its total protein content. Collection of 24 hours' worth of urine generally requires a metabolism cage and is not very practical. The ratio of urine protein to urine creatinine (P/C ratio) in any single sample is a good index of protein loss in the urine. A urine P/C ratio of less than 1.0 is considered normal; greater than 2.0 indicates abnormal urinary protein loss; between 1.0 and 2.0 is suspicious. Urine samples with a sediment that indicates inflammation are not suitable for urine P/C ratios. The inflammation must first be successfully treated. If the patient still has proteinuria once all evidence of inflammation is gone, a urine P/C ratio can be requested. Urine P/C ratios are usually done at a reference laboratory because they require a sensitive protein determination.

In interpreting the cause for a positive urine protein test, one must also consider the results of the test for blood and the microscopic examination of sediment. These results may aid in identifying the source of proteinuria. Proteinuria without a positive blood reaction or significant cells accompanies glomerular disease, in which defective glomeruli allow the passage of albumin into the urine, often resulting in protein readings of 3+ or 4+. There are some extrarenal factors that may temporarily alter glomerular permeability to protein and result in proteinuria. They include fever, severe exercise, shock, cardiac or central nervous system disease and the postcolostral period in neonates.

When hemorrhage into the urinary tract occurs, tests for urine protein and blood will be positive. Erythrocytes will be seen in the sediment. Possible causes for urinary tract hemorrhage include trauma, neoplasia and inflammation. Hemoglobin or myoglobin in the urine will cause a positive protein test as well as a positive blood test. In either case, intact RBCs are not a significant part of the sediment. Hemoglobinuria and myoglobinuria will be discussed further under Urine Blood.

When proteinuria occurs in conjunction with increased leukocytes in the urine sediment, inflammation of the urinary tract should be suspected. Inflammation rarely causes a urine protein test greater than 2+, unless hemorrhage is associated with the inflammatory process. In some urinary tract infections, bacteria may be seen in the sediment. The location of the problem is difficult to determine from urinalysis alone.

Urine Glucose

In addition to urine protein, another common reagent strip test for urine is the test for glucose. The reagent strips generally utilize glucose oxidase to detect glucose, and for this reason they are quite specific for glucose. However, as with all reagent strip tests, they are not quantitative. Tablets that detect glucose are available; they are somewhat more quantitative, but they are not specific. The tablets utilize a copper reduction method that detects many sugars and reducing agents besides glucose. Normally, urine contains no detectable glucose. Glucose is filtered by the glomerulus, but the body preserves this energy source by reabsorbing it in the proximal renal tubules. This resorption ability is exceeded once the blood glucose level rises above 180 mg/dl in most species or above 100 mg/dl in the cow. This is the so-called "renal threshold" for glucose, above which it will "spill" into the urine. The primary cause for *glycosuria*, therefore, is *hyperglycemia*. To confirm this, the blood glucose level should be determined at the same time as the urine glucose. Diabetes mellitus is a common cause of hyperglycemia and glycosuria.

Urine Ketones

A test for urine *ketones* is included on many reagent strips. Tablets are also available. Both use a nitroprusside method that detects acetone and acetoacetic acid but does not detect beta-hydroxybutyric acid, so that false-negative results are possible. Ketones will appear in the urine before they build up to a detectable level in the blood stream; hence, *ketonuria* may occur before a detectable *ketonemia* occurs. Ketonuria indicates excessive fat metabolism, a deficiency in carbohydrate metabolism or both.

Urine Bilirubin

Bilirubin in urine can be crudely detected by the "foam test." Shake a sample of urine, and if the foam that forms is yellow, bilirubin is present. There are reagent strips and tablets for detecting *bilirubinuria*, both of which utilize a similar reaction (diazotization), but the tablets are less subject to interference by urine color. The tablets are also highly sensitive so that a 1+ reading, especially in concentrated urine, may not be significant. Both strips and tablets react mainly with conjugated bilirubin and less with unconjugated bilirubin. If there is much delay between obtaining the urine sample and performing the urinalysis, false-negative results may occur, as bilirubin may be oxidized on exposure to light. Many normal dogs and cattle have a certain degree of bilirubinuria because the kidneys, as well as the liver, have an enzyme that can conjugate bilirubin.

Urine Blood

The designation "blood" is somewhat misleading because this test actually detects intact RBCs, hemoglobin and myoglobin. Both reagent strips and tablets make use of the peroxidase property of free hemoglobin or myoglobin, which oxidizes orthotoluidine to a blue-colored derivative. If the urine is red and cloudy and shows erythrocytes in the sediment and there is not evidence of anemia or muscle disease, *hematuria* is the reason for the positive blood reaction.

Hemoglobinuria (hemoglobin pigment in the urine) results in red to brown urine with no erythrocytes in the sediment, a positive urine protein test and a positive urine blood reaction. Because of the high renal threshold for hemoglobin, *hemoglobinemia* will cause the blood serum or plasma to turn pink or red by the time hemoglobinuria is detectable.

Myoglobinuria (myoglobin pigment in the urine) results in red to brown urine with no erythrocytes in the sediment, a positive urine protein test and a positive urine blood reaction, which are all findings that are also typical of hemoglobinuria. However, during myoglobinuria, the blood serum or plasma generally remains clear. Myoglobin is a smaller molecule than hemoglobin and does not bind to serum proteins; thus it is rapidly excreted into the urine before reaching levels high enough to produce discoloration of the serum. Animals with myoglobinuria generally do not show evidence of anemia but have some type of muscle disease, such as exertional myopathy in horses ("tying up syndrome"), trauma, electrical shock or pressure necrosis from prolonged recumbency.

Urine pH

Urine pH is detected by reagent strips with chemical indicators. The symbol pH is used to express the hydrogen ion concentration (acidity) of a fluid. The pH of 7 is the neutral point; above 7, alkalinity increases, and below 7, acidity increases. It is imperative that a fresh sample be used, because as urine stands it loses carbon dioxide and bacteria present may produce ammonia, both of which result in increased alkalinity (raising the pH). The body's acid-base status may affect urine pH, but it is a mistake to use the urine pH to evaluate the systemic acid-base balance. Too many other factors influence urine pH, and in fact the urine pH may be completely contrary to the body's pH. For example, some cows with metabolic alkalosis have a paradoxical aciduria because the kidney attempts to maintain electrolyte balance at the expense of acid-base balance.

Urine Sediment

Urine sediment examination may reveal extremely useful diagnostic information. A few cells and a few casts may be found in normal urine, but increased numbers of certain elements indicate certain diseases. The *Handbook of Canine and Feline Urinalysis,* by Osborne and Stevens, has excellent illustrations of elements commonly found in the urine sediment examination (see Recommended Reading list).

Two main types of *epithelial cells* can be found in urine sediment: squamous and transitional. Squamous epithelial cells are very large, with angular borders and small nuclei. They come from the lining of the distal urethra and vagina or prepuce and are not generally indicative of disease. Transitional epithelial cells are medium-sized and oval, spindled or caudate in shape. They may occur in groups, especially if the urine was obtained by catheterization. Transitional cells line the proximal urethra, bladder, ureters and renal pelvis.

Other cells found in urine sediment are those derived from blood. Erythrocytes in unstained sediment appear round and slightly refractile, with no internal structure. They may be confused with fat droplets, but erythrocytes are fairly uniform in size and do not float in and out of planes of focus as fat droplets do. If there is doubt, a drop of dilute acetic acid will lyse erythrocytes, helping to differentiate them from fat droplets. In concentrated urine, erythrocytes may lose fluid and become *crenated* (shrunken and notched); in dilute urine, they may imbibe water and swell or even lyse, becoming so-called *ghost cells.* Leukocytes in urine sediment are round and granular and are larger than erythrocytes but smaller than epithelial cells. More than five to eight WBCs per high-power field indicates inflammation of the urogenital tract, and when this occurs, a careful check for bacteria should be made.

Casts are another prominent feature of urine sediment. Casts are elongated structures composed of protein from plasma and mucoprotein from the renal tubules. Generally they form in the distal tubules, in which the urine is more concentrated and acidic. Any structures that happen to be in the tubules at the time the casts form (erythrocytes, leukocytes or epithelial cells) become embedded in the casts. The presence of increased numbers of casts helps to localize the renal disease to the tubules, but the numbers do not necessarily correlate with the severity of disease. For instance, severe chronic nephritis may be accompanied by just a few casts. There are five main types of casts: (1) *Hyaline casts* are colorless, homogeneous and semi-transparent. They may be difficult to see unless the light is reduced. They indicate mild glomerular leakage. (2) *Cellular casts* may be epithelial cell casts that contain sloughed tubular epithelial cells, erythrocyte casts that indicate renal hemorrhage or leukocyte casts that indicate renal inflammation or pyelonephritis. (3) *Granular casts* (which are designated either coarsely or finely granular, depending on degree of degeneration) are derived from degenerating cells or cellular casts. They are probably the most common type of cast found in animals. (4) *Waxy casts* are wide and homogeneous, usually with distinctly square ends. They are the next stage of degeneration from granular casts and so indicate a more chronic tubular lesion. (5) *Fatty casts* contain fat globules from degenerating tubular epithelial cells and are most common in cats because of the high lipid content of feline tubular epithelium.

Crystals are another major component of urine sediment. Their precipitation and presence depend on the urine pH and

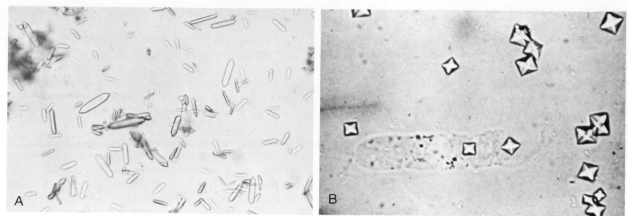

FIGURE 4–12. Canine urine sediment. Photomicrograph showing the two forms of calcium oxalate crystals. A, Monohydrate form. B, Dihydrate form. (Courtesy of Dr. Mary Anna Thrall.)

the solubility and concentration of the substance forming them. Crystals are common and usually are not indicative of disease. In carnivores, phosphates, urates, oxalates and cystine are normal; in herbivores, calcium carbonate crystals are the most common. Urine crystals that accompany pathological conditions include ammonium biurate, monohydrate calcium oxalate, bilirubin and cystine. Dihydrate calcium oxalate crystals can be found in normal urine. However, the monohydrate form of calcium oxalate is strongly associated with ethylene glycol (antifreeze) toxicity. Figure 4–12 illustrates these two types of calcium oxalate crystals. Bilirubin crystals may occur with the various problems that lead to bilirubinuria but probably are not abnormal in concentrated dog urine. Cystine crystals, though sometimes seen in normal dogs, are also found in a congenital defect of cystine metabolism that leads to cystinuria in dogs. Sulfonamide crystals may precipitate in the urine of animals on sulfa therapy.

Bacteria in unstained urine sediment may be difficult to detect. Rods may appear singly or in chains, but cocci may be lost in brownian movement. For this reason, any time bacteria are suspected, the sediment should be stained in order to examine it more thoroughly. Usually, the regular examination of the unstained sediment is completed and recorded first, and then the coverslip is removed and the underlying sediment on the slide is allowed to dry. Once dry, the slide can be stained with a Gram stain, and any bacteria present can be identified by shape and a Gram reaction. It may be helpful to also stain urine sediment with a Wright stain. The gram-negative rod-shaped bacteria can be difficult to see among all the pink-staining cellular debris present on a Gram stain. On a Wright stain, all bacteria stain a dark purple and are relatively easy to find.

Bacteria in a voided sample are often not significant, because they may be normal flora from the distal urogenital tract, especially from the prepuce or vagina. Bacteria are significant if they occur in catheterized or cystocentesis samples. Their presence should be correlated with leukocytes in urine; bacteria with no leukocyte response should raise suspicion of contamination of the sample. If bacteria are present in a urine sample, they can multiply as time passes, and so this should be taken into consideration when the sample is being analyzed.

Other miscellaneous and usually insignificant components of urine sediment include mucus, fat, sperm, parasites and fungi. Mucus appears as narrow, twisted, ribbon-like strands; it is normal in horse urine and can be seen in other species because of genital secretions or irritation of the urethra. Fat, as previously noted, takes the form of refractile, variably sized spheres in many planes of focus. Fat is rarely significant. Sperm are commonly seen in male dog urine. Parasites that can occur in urine include the ova of *Stephanurus dentatus, Dioctophyma renale,* and *Capillaria plica* and microfilaria of *Dirofilaria immitis.* Fungal elements in urine are almost always contaminants.

CLINICAL CHEMISTRY

Recently, several small relatively inexpensive clinical chemistry instruments have been developed. As with the electronic cell counters, a veterinary practice must have a significant demand for immediate availability of clinical laboratory data to justify the expense of these instruments. There are two general types of chemistry instrumentation: liquid reagent chemistry and dry chemistry. Instruments that use liquid reagents require more technical expertise and time in preparing reagents and monitoring their performance. The dry chemistry instruments are simpler to use and provide consistent performance. The principles of operation differ significantly between the two types of instruments, as does the extent to which specimen quality affects the measurements.

Clinical Chemistry Instrumentation

The liquid reagent–based instruments use the principle of photometry (the measurement of light transmittance by a solution). Beer's law, the basis for determination of concentration by measurement of light transmittance through a liquid, states that the concentration of a substance in a liquid is indirectly proportional to the amount of light that passes through the liquid. Most instruments have a spectrophotometer to measure the amount of light transmitted and convert the light into electrical energy. A spectrophotometer consists of a light source directed through a specific path and a photosensitive detector that converts light into electrical energy. Each substance will transmit light at a specific wavelength. To increase the specificity of the measurement, filters are placed between the light source and the sample to allow only a specific wavelength to pass through the sample. The magnitude of the electrical current produced by the detector corresponds to the concentration of the substance being measured. Solutions that contain a known concentration of specific substances are called standards and are used to calibrate the instrument. Each instrument has specific procedures for calibration, which should be carefully followed to ensure optimal performance.

The instruments that use dry reagents are becoming more popular for in-clinic use. The major advantage of these instruments is the elimination of liquid reagents, which must be reconstituted or diluted prior to use. Dry chemistry instruments use reagent strips (similar to the strips used for urinalysis) or reagent slides. A specific amount of the patient's sample is placed on the reagent strip, and the intensity of the color that develops is measured by the principle of reflectance. Light is transmitted to the analyte slide by fiber optics and the reflected light is conducted to a photodetector. The density of the color formed by the chemical reaction is determined and is proportional to the concentration of the substance being measured. Since this methodology does not depend on reading light transmitted through a liquid as with the spectrophotometer-based instruments, there is less interference due to lipemia or hemolysis.

Several dry chemistry instruments are available (such as the Abbot Serolyser, Refletron, Dupont Analyzer, Kodak DT 60 and the Vet Test 8008). The Vet Test 8008 is designed for use with veterinary samples (Fig. 4–13). Examples of chemistry tests available on this instrument are listed in Table 4–3. The primary advantage of using an instrument such as the Vet Test 8008 is the availability of predetermined reference ranges, which can be used until the laboratory can establish its own values. In many cases, especially with these instruments, little variation occurs from instrument to instrument or operator to operator. Veterinary samples can vary significantly from human samples in the concentration of particular substances. As with the thresholds on the hematology instruments, the limits of the chemistry test (the range of values which have a linear relationship within the methodology used) may have to be expanded to include values either above or below those seen in human samples. Good examples of this are the endocrine tests available on a few of the instruments. Thyroid hormone concentrations in dogs are much lower than in humans, and therefore assay procedures set up for humans will not be sensitive enough to detect normal dog values.

Quality Control Programs

A veterinary practice that decides to establish an in-clinic laboratory should make a commitment to quality control. Laboratory instruments will provide accurate answers only if the samples are handled correctly, a well-maintained instrument is used, and the tests are performed correctly. A quality control program consists of monitoring quality control results for identification of irregularities in reported values and following generally accepted laboratory procedures. Several textbooks on clinical chemistry and laboratory medicine provide excellent in-depth reviews of quality assurance programs. The following discussion will deal primarily with the basics in monitoring an instrument to ensure the accuracy of reported data.

Table 4–3 CHEMISTRY TESTS AVAILABLE ON THE VET TEST 8008	
Urea nitrogen	Creatinine
Albumin	Total protein
Alanine aminotransferase (ALT)	Aspartate aminotransferase (AST)
Serum alkaline phosphatase (SAP)	Cholesterol
Triglycerides	Glucose
Calcium	Creatine kinase (CK)
Gamma-glutamyltransferase (GGT)	Magnesium
Amylase	Lipase
Ammonia	Phosphorus

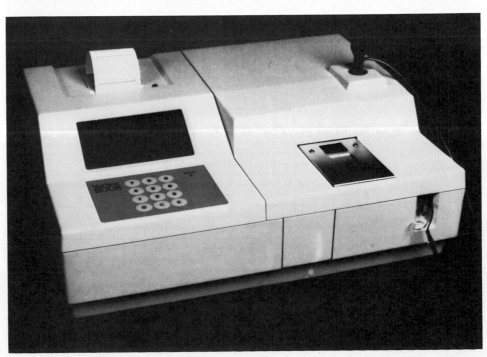

FIGURE 4–13. The Vet Test 8008 dry chemistry analyzer. (IDEXX Corp., Portland, ME.)

There are three levels of quality control: pre-analytical procedures, analytical procedures, and analytical quality monitoring procedures. The pre-analytical procedures deal with how the patient is prepared (fasting versus nonfasting samples), patient and specimen identification, specimen acquisition and specimen processing. Establishment of standard procedures for each of these steps will decrease the likelihood of samples being misidentified or of poor quality (hemolysed or lipemic). This aspect of quality control is important even in clinics that send their clinical pathology samples to a reference laboratory. Analytical variables include the analytical methodology, standardization and calibration procedures, documentation of analytical protocols and procedures and monitoring of equipment while in use. This aspect of quality control is usually well defined by the manufacturer of the instrument and should be followed closely. The final level, monitoring of analytical quality using statistical methods and control charts, is the aspect that involves the use of control products and record keeping. This aspect is the responsibility of the technician performing the tests.

Control products are solutions, usually serum-based, which have known concentrations of the different substances or analytes that can be assayed by the instrument. These products should be stable, available in aliquots to prevent alterations due to refreezing, and have little vial to vial variation. Control products can be purchased from an independent source or from the company that makes the test kit or instrument. Most control products are available as normal, high abnormal and low abnormal ranges. The control products are analyzed as patients' samples, and the values reported by the instrument are compared with the known values provided with the product.

Many control products are provided in a lyophilized form that requires rehydration with distilled water or a diluent provided by the manufacturer. It is essential that the solution be diluted properly to ensure that the concentration of the analytes will be correct. Imprecision in diluting the controls will be reflected by values that are not in concert with the known values of the product even though the instrument is working properly. It is highly recommended that volumetric or other precise pipettes be used to dilute the control products (a graduated cylinder is not acceptable).

The acceptable control values are within a specific range, which usually encompasses the mean ± two standard deviations. This range is established by the manufacturer of the product by repeated assay of the solution. When the instrument reports a control value above or below the established range, there is a problem with the procedure, and test results for that particular sample should not be reported until the problem is identified.

A useful visual display of the instruments' performance for quick inspection and review is the Levey-Jennings chart. Figure 4–14 illustrates the use of the Levey-Jennings chart to keep track of quality control data. By inspection of control data over a month, a technician may see the control values gently drift upward or downward, indicating possible deterioration of the control product or a change in the light source intensity. Wide scatter of values outside of the range on both the low and high end indicates imprecision on the part of the instrument or the technician. It is best to keep the chart close to the instrument, not hidden in a file drawer. Everyone who uses the instrument must be willing to run controls and chart the results. Other useful laboratory records include calibration logs, sample logs and maintenance logs.

Sample Handling

Sample handling is a critical step in obtaining accurate laboratory data. Several factors can interfere with analysis of a sample. The most common problems in veterinary medicine are hemolysis and lipemia. Difficulty in performing the venipuncture or excess pressure applied to the syringe during collection can cause significant hemolysis. The most common cause of lipemia is collection of a postprandial sample. There are times when both hemolysis and lipemia are unavoidable because they are the result of a disease process.

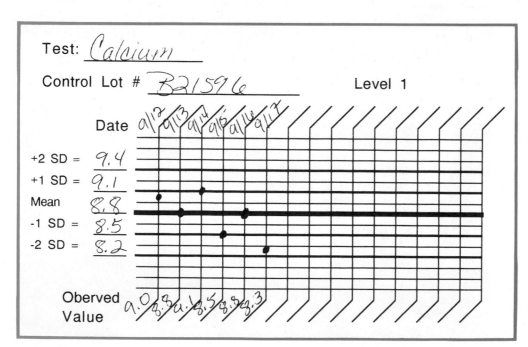

FIGURE 4–14. A Levey-Jennings chart illustrating the common procedure used for following the performance of an individual test control serum.

The effect hemolysis and lipemia will have on laboratory data is extremely method-dependent. There are no general rules to assist interpretation of changes due to sample quality. A good reference laboratory will provide information on how each of their tests is affected by these two changes. Manufacturers of the in-clinic instruments should provide information on how interfering substances such as hemolysis and lipemia affect the methods used in their instrument. Hemolysis will commonly change RBC indices, total protein determined on a refractometer, bilirubin, inorganic phosphorus and potassium in horses and some Akita dogs. Lipemia will interfere with any method that depends on optical density read on a spectrophotometer. Some chemistry instruments can compensate for this change. Again, the reference laboratory should be able to indicate which tests are affected. Lipemia can interfere with total protein determined on a refractometer. Often the lipemic samples have a very indistinct or unfocused line on the refractometer scale. Errors in processing the sample can also cause artifactual changes in laboratory data. It is important to use the appropriate collection tube for the test being performed. In general, EDTA is the preferred anticoagulant for hematology. Be sure to use a tube of appropriate size for the sample being drawn. It is often difficult to obtain large samples from small dogs and cats. The 2-ml pediatric collection tube is best for a patient this size. There are collection tubes made for smaller volumes (0.5 ml Microtainer tubes, Becton, Dickinson & Co., Parsippany, NJ). These tubes are excellent for samples from puppies, kittens and small exotic animal species. Excess anticoagulant in the collection tube can erroneously decrease the PCV and, in addition, can increase total protein determined on a refractometer.

Blood films should be made within 15 minutes of obtaining the sample to decrease *in vitro* morphological changes in the blood cells. If the practice uses a reference laboratory, unstained blood films should be sent with the EDTA sample. Slides sent through the mail should be packaged in a box or tube, not sent in a flat plastic or cardboard slide holder. The flat slide holders sent in an envelope often get processed through the automated canceling machine in the post office and arrive at the laboratory in numerous small pieces. If samples must be held overnight, refrigerate the whole blood but do not refrigerate the blood film. Water will condense on the surface of the blood film if it is placed in the refrigerator and cause lysis of the RBCs. In addition, the blood film should be protected from formalin vapors since they will interfere with staining.

Samples collected for chemistry profiles can be collected in clot tubes, which contain no anticoagulant, or in lithium heparin tubes. Blood collected in clot tubes (tubes without anticoagulant) must be allowed to completely clot before the sample can be centrifuged and the serum removed. Complete clot formation usually takes about 30 minutes. Clot tubes with activator gels will promote clotting, thus decreasing the time necessary for complete clot formation and facilitate separation of the serum from the RBCs. The sample should not be refrigerated before complete clot formation since this inhibits good serum separation. In addition, a fibrin clot forms above the RBCs if the blood is centrifuged before complete clot formation or at too fast a speed.

Blood collected in lithium heparin is excellent for emergency needs since it does not have to clot before it can be separated for analysis. Heparin may interfere with a few chemistry tests, so it is best to check with the reference laboratory before submitting heparinized plasma for chemistry panels. Lithium heparin is excellent for emergency electrolyte panels. EDTA is not suitable for most chemistry tests. Blood collected in EDTA will have markedly decreased calcium because EDTA binds the calcium to prevent clot formation. In addition, potassium EDTA will markedly increase the serum potassium levels. EDTA also interferes with many of the enzyme-based assays. Separation of the serum from the clot as soon as possible cannot be stressed enough. Prolonged exposure of serum to the clot will erroneously decrease the glucose, will increase the phosphorus, may increase potassium depending on species (especially in the horse) and may affect some enzyme activities. Do not depend on the reference laboratory courier service to get the sample to the laboratory in time to prevent these changes. It is best to take the time and responsibility to separate the serum and ensure the quality of the sample.

CYTOLOGY

Cytology is the study of cells; specifically it involves the microscopic examination of individual cells that have exfoliated from a tissue or structure. Unlike histopathology, cytology is not an evaluation of the architecture of a tissue; therefore, in some cases, it may not be diagnostically useful. In many instances, however, cytological appearance can be used to differentiate a noninflammatory lesion from an inflammatory one, or an inflammatory lesion from a neoplastic mass. Sometimes cytological appearance reveals a very specific diagnosis, and for certain samples, such as bone marrow or mast cell tumors, it may actually be more helpful than histopathology. It should be emphasized that cytology is an adjunct to, not a replacement for, histopathology.

One of the advantages of cytology is that it requires no special equipment or supplies other than those used in performing a CBC. A good microscope, some slides, and one or two stains will suffice for most cytological examinations. However, cytology does require a significant degree of expertise that can be acquired only by experience. This is especially true for cytology of solid masses. Most veterinary practices prefer to send cytology samples to a reference laboratory for evaluation. For this reason the discussion on cytology will be limited to fluid analysis and preparation of samples from solid tissues for submission to a reference laboratory. Veterinary technicians interested in becoming adept at cytology should obtain specific training through continuing education workshops.

For fluid analysis, a refractometer and a cell-counting method (such as Unopettes and a hemacytometer) are also needed. The two most helpful stains for cytological preparation are Wright's stain and Gram's stain. Diff-Quick stain, which can also be used for staining blood films, is suitable for almost all cytological samples. Once a sample for cytology has been obtained, slides should be made as soon as possible, before the cells degenerate. This is especially true of low-protein fluids, such as cerebrospinal fluid and tracheal washings. Most fluid samples can be prepared in the same manner as a blood film, leaving a feathered edge where the largest cells tend to migrate. If the fluid is thick or for some other reason the slide cannot be satisfactorily made, an alternative method is to place a drop of fluid on a slide, gently place another slide on top of it (do not press the two slides together, but allow the weight of the top slide to spread the drop of fluid) and then simply pull the two slides apart. This method works well for many types of sample, and it may result in fewer broken cells than the traditional technique.

If the fluid sample is not very cellular, as is the case with cerebrospinal fluid, a direct preparation may not provide enough cells for a thorough examination. It is always advisable to make one or two direct preparations in case the techniques used to concentrate the cells result in too many ruptured cells or other artifacts. There are "cytocentrifuges" that are especially designed to make cytological slides from hypocellular fluids. These cytocentrifuges are gentler to cells because they spin at a slow speed and have gradual acceleration and deceleration. They also may have a special apparatus that causes cells to be deposited directly on a slide, with filter paper taking away excess fluid. However, cytocentrifuges are probably impractical for all but the largest practices.

In many situations, an ordinary centrifuge can be used to prepare concentrated cells in the same way as urine sediment is prepared. If the centrifuge has adjustable speeds, a slow speed will be sufficient. The supernatant can be decanted or aspirated with a pipette, and a slide can be made from the material in the bottom of the tube. As previously mentioned, it is always wise to make one or two direct slides from a fluid sample prior to centrifuging, in case centrifugation creates too many artifacts (ruptured cells or poor staining). These preparations are then available if the sediment slides are unsatisfactory.

A routine fluid analysis of samples such as abdominal, thoracic or synovial fluid usually includes a WBC count, which actually should be referred to as a nucleated cell count (NCC), since some of the cells (mesothelial cells, synovial cells and so forth) may not be derived directly from blood. The NCC can be performed in the same manner as a CBC. Total protein is another helpful parameter in fluid analysis and can be done by refractometer, generally using the supernatant of a centrifuged portion of the fluid sample. Total erythrocyte (RBC) count is often included in the fluid analysis, but because of the frequency of peripheral blood contamination of samples, the RBC count alone is rarely helpful in evaluating fluid. It is more important to check for *erythrophagocytosis* (phagocytosis of RBCs by macrophages) during the cytological examination, since erythrophagocytosis generally implies that the RBCs were present in the fluid prior to sampling, rather than as contaminants.

The analysis of certain fluids includes specific tests that may add more information than routine tests. For instance, the *mucin clot test* is done on synovial fluid by mixing a dilute acetic acid solution (0.1 ml of 7 N acetic acid in 4 ml of distilled water) and then adding 1 ml of synovial fluid. Normal synovial fluid contains mucin, which forms a tight white clot in the acetic acid; if the mucin has been digested by bacterial or cellular enzymes, the clot will be less distinct or may not form at all, leaving only hazy or cloudy fluid. Therefore, good mucin clot formation usually accompanies normal or noninflamed joints, whereas a poor or absent mucin clot indicates inflammation, infection or both. The precipitation of mucin in joint fluid by acetic acid precludes the use of the WBC Unopette system because this system contains acetic acid as the diluent in the reservoir. NCCs on joint fluid should be done using the Unopette system for both WBCs and platelets. The reservoir in this system contains ammonium oxalate, which will not precipitate mucin.

Fluid samples that have neutrophils as the predominate cell type should be closely evaluated for the presence of bacteria. Bacteria should be present within cells (intracellular) to be considered significant (Color Plate IJ). If they are only extracellular, one should consider the possibility of contamination of the sample. If no bacteria are found, it should not be assumed that they are absent. They may be in very low numbers and difficult to find.

Cytological samples of solid masses can usually be aspirated with a syringe and needle (20 gauge or 22 gauge). It is not necessary to aspirate so strenuously that material appears in the barrel of the syringe; gentle aspiration will usually pull enough material into the needle, and it can then be expelled onto a glass slide. If the material is suspended in a fluid medium (as is the case with lymph node aspirates), the slide can be prepared as previously described. Excised solid masses should be blotted with absorbent paper to remove blood and tissue fluid and then gently touched to a slide to make an impression slide. Do not press too hard, or you will smear the material on the slide. If the mass is of a dense consistency that does not exfoliate cells easily, it may be necessary to scrape it with a scalpel blade and then spread the material thinly onto the slide. An alternative method is to cross-hatch cut the surface of the tissue with the scalpel blade and make an imprint preparation. The cross-hatching method is often gentler than the scraping method and preserves the cells better.

When handling excised pieces of tissue for cytological study, keep them wrapped in gauze and slightly moistened with saline, to prevent their drying out. Do not allow any contact with formalin or even with formalin fumes until after the cytological slides have been made and stained. Most reference laboratories prefer unstained slides, which can be stained at the laboratory by means of their standard stain protocol.

Recommended Reading

General

Benjamin MM: Outline of Veterinary Clinical Pathology. Ames, IA, Iowa State University Press, 1978.

Duncan JR and Prasse KW: Veterinary Laboratory Medicine/Clinical Pathology. Ames, IA, Iowa State University Press, 1986.

Laboratory Equipment

Hicks R, Schenken JR and Steinrauf MA: Laboratory Instrumentation. New York, Harper & Row, 1974.

Hematology

Jain NC: Schalm's Veterinary Hematology. 4th ed. Philadelphia, Lea and Febiger, 1986.

Rich LJ: The Morphology of Canine and Feline Blood Cells. St. Louis, Ralston Purina Co., 1974.

Urinalysis

Osborne CA and Stevens JB: Handbook of Canine and Feline Urinalysis. St. Louis, Ralston Purina Co., 1981.

Chemistry

Coffman JR: Equine Clinical Chemistry and Pathophysiology. Bonner Springs, KS, Veterinary Medicine Publishing Co., 1981.

Kaneko JJ (editor): Clinical Biochemistry of Domestic Animals. New York, Academic Press, 1987.

Quality Assurance Programs

land BE and Westgard JO: Quality Control: Theory and Practice. ı Henry JB (editor): Clinical Diagnosis and Management by Laboۀtory Methods. Philadelphia, WB Saunders Co., 1984.

؛tgard JO and Klee GG: Quality Assurance. *In* Tietz NW (editor): extbook of Clinical Chemistry. Philadelphia, WB Saunders Co., J86.

Cytology

nan V, Alsaker RD and Riis RC: Cytology of the Dog and Cat. ۈuth Bend, IN, American Animal Hospital Association, 1979.

Rebar AH: Handbook of Veterinary Cytology. St. Louis, Ralston Purina Co., 1978.

Avian and Reptilian Hematology

Campbell TW: Avian Hematology and Cytology. Ames, IA, Iowa State University Press, 1988.

Frye FL: Biomedical and Surgical Aspects of Captive Reptile Husbandry. Edwardsville, KS, Veterinary Medicine Publishing Co., 1981.

Jain NC: Schalm's Veterinary Hematology. 4th ed. Philadelphia, Lea and Febiger, 1986.

5

Parasitology and Public Health

JOHNNY D. HOSKINS and JOHN M. CHENEY

INTRODUCTION

Parasitism is responsible for significant disease and death in animals and humans. Ectoparasites (external parasites), including mites, ticks, lice, fleas, chiggers and myiasis-producing flies, and endoparasites (internal parasites), including protozoa, trematodes, tapeworms and nematodes, all have representative parasites on or in all animals and in every organ or tissue. Some parasites are host-specific, whereas other parasites are only capable of infesting or infecting a broad range of animal hosts. Modes of transmission vary considerably from simple, direct transmission to an extremely complex life cycle, involving the use of an intermediate host or transport host or specific environmental conditions. The nematode parasites have five stages in their development. Various nematodes, like the strongyle nematodes of ruminants and horses, produce an egg that passes into the environment. A first-stage larva develops within the egg. This free-living larva grows and molts (sheds the skin or cuticle) to a second-stage larva, which then grows and molts into a third-stage larva—the infective larva. The infective larva usually is ingested and develops into a fourth-stage larva and finally into a fifth-stage larva within the host.

Some nematodes have developed modifications from this life cycle. For example, hookworm larvae generally penetrate the skin and circulate in the host's tissue before completing their development in the small intestine. Others, such as the roundworms and whipworms, develop into the infective stage within the egg and do not hatch until ingested by the host. Other important nematodes, such as *Strongyloides,* have a first-stage larva in the egg when passed.

Most parasites are capable of causing significant damage to the host. This potential may be a function of the number of parasites present; for other parasites, location within the host, production of toxins or interference with normal physiological processes results from the parasitism.

Clinical signs of infection frequently are associated with parasitism, but not uncommonly the damage is more insidious, such as interference with normal weight gain or milk production.

Diagnosis is not difficult, but timing, choice of technique and interpretation of the results are often crucial for effective treatment and control. Treatment, including selection of the proper medication and appropriate control in the environment, always necessitates a thorough knowledge of the biology of the parasite.

The following sections discuss specific parasites as they relate to animal host and parasite class within each host. The veterinary technician should become familiar with both the common name and the scientific name (as an example, roundworm = *Toxocara canis*) of the common parasites. Each section contains information on the life cycle, tissue location, treatment and control for the specific parasite discussed. In addition, a section on diagnostic procedures and public health is presented.

ENDOPARASITES

Parasites of Dogs and Cats

Roundworms (Ascarids)

Toxocara canis, Toxocara cati and *Toxascaris leonina* are ascarids that are thick, white to cream-colored nematodes. Mature specimens measure about 3.5 to 5 cm for males and 10 to 15 cm for females. Eggs of the *Toxocara* spp. are large, oval and dark with a thick, rough shell. *Toxascaris leonina* is lighter in color and more egg-shaped and has a thick, smooth shell (Fig. 5–1). All three species are common in most geographical regions of the United States. The larval stage develops within the egg, and the second stage is the infective larva. Eggs are highly resistant to adverse conditions and, in ideal environmental conditions, become infective in about 2 weeks. Once ingested, *Toxocara* spp. hatch in the small intestine, penetrate the mucosa, migrate through the liver, pass through the heart and go into the lungs, in which they develop in a short time. Larvae are coughed, are swallowed and then mature in the small intestine in 4 to 6 weeks.

Toxascaris leonina eggs hatch in the small intestine, and the larvae penetrate the intestinal mucosa to develop for about 2 to 3 months and then return to the lumen as adults. In dogs older than 5 weeks of age, most of the larvae leave the circulation and are stored in the somatic organs until the dog becomes pregnant. Between the 42nd day and the 56th day of gestation, these larvae leave the somatic tissues, cross the placenta, enter the fetal lungs and remain there until birth. The larvae then complete the cycle already described. Consequently, a high percentage of dogs are infected by the *prenatal* or *transplacental* route. In the pregnant dog and cat, some of the activated larvae migrate to the mammary glands. These larvae are ingested by puppies and kittens when they first start to nurse. *Transmammary* infections are more common in cats than in dogs. The eggs of all three ascarids can be ingested by other animals (such as mice or chickens) and remain infective in their tissue until eaten by the appropriate host. All three species are readily diagnosed by a number of techniques, and they are amenable to treatment with a number of anthelmintics (Table 5–1). Control is difficult because the eggs are resistant, and control measures necessitate thorough cleansing of kennels, runs, yards, and so forth.

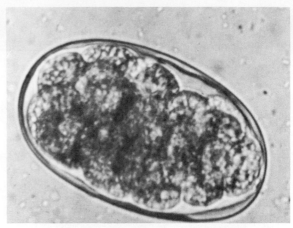

FIGURE 5–2. Strongyle-type egg, as seen in hookworms, measures approximately 62 μ × 40 μ.

Hookworm

Ancylostoma caninum occurs in dogs, foxes, coyotes, wolves, raccoons and badgers; *Ancylostoma braziliense* is found in dogs and cats; *Uncinaria stenocephala* occurs in dogs, cats, foxes, coyotes and wolves; *Ancylostoma tubaeforme* is found in cats and wild Felidae. Hookworms are all short, thick parasites, the adult males measuring 6 to 12 mm, the females measuring 6 to 20 mm. Hookworms produce a similar strongyle type of egg (Fig. 5–2). *Ancylostoma* spp. generally are found in coastal areas of high rainfall, whereas *Uncinaria stenocephala* are found in the northeastern United States. All hookworm species have a similar life cycle. Undeveloped eggs pass into the environment, develop and hatch, releasing a first-stage larva that undergoes a free-living existence until it develops to the third-stage infective larva. Hookworms are capable of establishing in the host following ingestion, but the normal mode of infection is *skin penetration*. After larvae penetrate, they enter the venous circulation, going ultimately to the lungs in which they develop for a short period. They are then coughed up and swallowed, and they enter the small intestine and mature. This generally occurs in 4 to 6 weeks.

Ancylostoma caninum has developed the added modes of infection—*transplacental* or *transmammary infection*. Third-stage larvae penetrate the skin and circulate in the pregnant female host, ultimately crossing the placenta. The larvae also are stored in somatic tissues until the female host becomes pregnant. Most of the somatic larvae activated at the time of pregnancy migrate to the mammary glands of the bitch and are passed on to nursing puppies. Diagnosis is readily performed by a number of techniques, and these species are amenable to treatment with a number of anthelmintics (see Table 5–1). Control is difficult, especially in warm, humid geographical regions, necessitating regular thorough cleansing of yards, kennels and so forth.

Intestinal Threadworm

Strongyloides stercoralis is a nematode that is a parasite of dogs, cats, foxes, humans, primates and possibly other wild carnivores. Only the female nematode is parasitic, and she reproduces parthenogenetically (without fertilization). Parasitic females live embedded in the mucosa of the small intestine. The

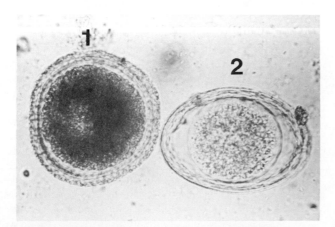

FIGURE 5–1. *Toxocara* egg (1) measures approximately 66 μ × 42 μ. *Toxascaris* egg (2) measures approximately 85 μ × 75 μ.

Table 5–1
PARASITICIDES USED FOR TREATMENT AND CONTROL OF INTERNAL PARASITES IN DOGS AND CATS

Drug	Toxocara-Toxascaris	Ancylostoma-Uncinaria	Strongyloides	Trichuris	Dirofilaria Adults	Dirofilaria Microfilariae	Taenia	Dipylidium	Giardia	Coccidia
Amprolium Corid	−	−	−	−	−	−	−	−	−	+
Butamisole hydrochloride Styquin	−	+	−	+	−	−	−	−	−	−
Dichlorophen/toluene Many trade names	+	+	−	−	−	−	+	+	−	−
Dichlorvos Many trade names	+	+	−	+	−	−	−	−	−	−
Diethylcarbamazine Many trade names	+	−	−	−	−	+	−	−	−	−
Disophenol sodium D.N.P.	−	+	−	−	−	−	−	−	−	−
Epsiprantel Cestex	−	−	−	−	−	−	+	+	−	−
Febantel Rintal Paste	+	+	−	+	−	−	+	−	−	−
Febantel/praziquantel Vercom Paste	+	+	−	+	−	−	+	+	−	−
Fenbendazole Panacur	+	+	−	+	−	−	+	−	−	−
Furazolidone Many trade names	−	−	−	−	−	−	−	−	+	−
Ivermectin Heartgard 30	−	−	−	−	−	+	−	−	−	−
Ivermectin Ivomec	+	+	−	+	−	+	−	−	−	−
Mebendazole Telmintic Powder	+	+	−	+	−	−	+	−	−	−
Metronidazole Flagyl	−	−	−	−	−	−	−	−	+	−
Milbemycin oxime Interceptor	+	+	−	+	−	+	−	−	−	−
N-butyl chloride Many trade names	+	+	−	−	−	−	−	−	−	−
Nitroscanate Lopatol	+	+	−	+	−	−	+	+	−	−
Oxibendazole/DEC Filaribits Plus	+	+	−	+	−	+	−	−	−	−
Piperazine Many trade names	+	−	−	−	−	−	−	−	−	−
Praziquantel Droncit	−	−	−	−	−	−	+	+	−	−
Pyrantel pamoate Nemex	+	+	−	−	−	−	−	−	−	−
Quinacrine hydrochloride Atabrine	−	−	−	−	−	−	−	−	+	−
Sulfadiazine/trimethoprim Many trade names	−	−	−	−	−	−	−	−	−	+
Sulfadimethoxine Many trade names	−	−	−	−	−	−	−	−	−	+
Thenium closylate Canopar	−	+	−	−	−	−	−	−	−	−
Thenium closylate/piperazine Thenatol	+	+	−	−	−	−	−	−	−	−
Thiabendazole Mintezol	−	−	+	−	−	−	−	−	−	−
Thiacetarsamide sodium Caparsolate	−	−	−	−	+	−	−	−	−	−
Tinidazole Available in England	−	−	−	−	−	−	−	−	−	−

+ = Indicated for use; − = not indicated for use.

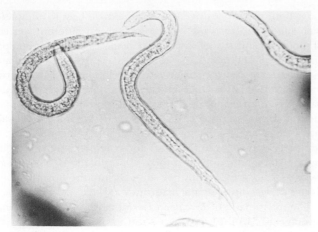

FIGURE 5–3. *Strongyloides* larvae from a dog. Note that the larvae are distorted in appearance because of the flotation solution.

eggs develop in utero, and the nematode gives birth to first-stage larvae (Fig. 5–3), whose chromosome number determines whether they will develop into a free-living generation before producing larvae destined to be parasitic or whether they will become a larval stage possessing a unique chromosome and be destined to develop into third-stage infective larvae. The infective larvae are capable of establishing infection by oral ingestion, after which they penetrate the small intestine and develop there. However, the primary mode of infection is by *skin penetration.* If the larvae use skin penetration, they then penetrate the venous circulation, going ultimately to the lungs to develop for a short time. Larvae are then coughed up and swallowed and penetrate the mucosa of the small intestine. In immunologically compromised animals, infections may be severe. *Strongyloides stercoralis* is widespread in tropical and subtropical regions, as well as in kennels, pet shops and so forth, in which environmental conditions are suitable. Diagnosis is not difficult. Frequently, a direct smear of fresh feces is suitable. Treatment is not always satisfactory, and alternate anthelmintics should be considered (see Table 5–1). Control necessitates thorough cleaning of facilities and allowing the facilities to dry.

Whipworm

Trichuris vulpis occurs in the cecum of the dog, fox and coyote. As with all whipworms, the anterior extremity is slender, and the posterior extremity is thickened, giving them a whip-like appearance. Males and females are about the same length, measuring 45 to 75 mm. The eggs are characteristic, possessing a thick, brown-yellow shell with a clear polar plug at each end (Fig. 5–4). *Trichuris vulpis* is widespread in temperate zones, and the incidence of infection is frequently high. The life cycle is simple and direct. The infective larva develops within the egg. When the egg is ingested, the larvae are released in the intestine, which they penetrate. Larvae develop in 8 to 10 days, return to the surface of the intestine, go to the cecum and attach and mature in an additional 60 to 80 days. Diagnosis can be effectively accomplished by a number of procedures, but eggs are quite heavy, and interpretation of the severity of infection based on the number of eggs present is not possible. A number of treatments are available (see Table 5–1). Control is difficult because eggs are highly resistant to

environmental conditions. Sanitation, as applied for ascarids, is the best approach.

Whipworm infection is uncommon in cats in the United States; however, *Capillaria campanula* has been reported to occur in the United States. Occasionally, *Capillaria aerophila,* a lungworm naturally occurring in the fox, has been found in both dogs and cats. The eggs are similar, but not as dark, and on the average, the eggs are somewhat smaller than those of whipworms.

Tapeworms

Dogs, cats, the wild Canidae and some of the wild Felidae are susceptible to infection by a number of tapeworms. The most commonly found tapeworm species are *Dipylidium caninum, Taenia hydatigena, Taenia pisiformis, Taenia ovis, Taenia krabbei, Multiceps serialis* and *Echinococcus granulosus* (the latter is mostly found in specific geographical locations such as Utah). Cats, as well as some of the wild Felidae, generally are infected with *Taenia taeniaeformis* and *Dipylidium caninum.* The species of tapeworms found in dogs and cats is dependent upon their geographical location and the amount of free-ranging activity the animals are given.

All tapeworms have an intermediate host in which the larval stage develops. *Dipylidium caninum* uses a flea, in which the larval (cysticercoid) stage develops. *Taenia hydatigena, Taenia ovis* and *Taenia krabbei* use ruminants—generally sheep, deer, elk, moose and so on, in which the larval stage (cysticercus) develops in the body cavity *(Taenia hydatigena)* or muscles *(Taenia ovis* and *Taenia krabbei). Taenia pisiformis* develops in the body cavity of rabbits, and *Taenia serialis* develops in subcutaneous areas or in the muscles (as a coenurus) of rabbits. The larval stage of *Taenia taeniaeformis* (strobilocercus) develops in the liver of mice, rats and other small rodents. *Echinococcus granulosus* uses ruminants, such as sheep, deer and elk, and humans as intermediate hosts. The larval stage is a rather large, fluid-filled bladder called a *hydatid cyst* that is easily recognized by its large size (25 to 100 mm in diameter), the presence of

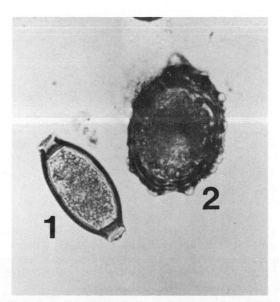

FIGURE 5–4. Trichurid egg (1), as seen in whipworms, measures approximately 80 μ × 36 μ. Ascarid egg (2) measures approximately 60 μ × 50 μ.

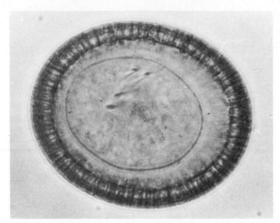

FIGURE 5–5. Typical *Taenia* egg measuring approximately 34 μ. *Dipylidium* eggs appear similar but are contained in packets of 1 to 20 eggs.

numerous small pieces of larval tapeworms (brood capsules) on the inner surface and the presence of compartments within the body of the cyst in which daughter cysts have grown and fused together.

Diagnosis of *Taenia* spp. and *Dipylidium caninum* infections is normally done by finding the proglottids (body segments), or chain of proglottids, around the host's anal region or on its hocks. Although the eggs will float, generally they are not released to mix with the feces (Fig. 5–5). *Taenia* spp. have one genital opening per proglottid, whereas *Dipylidium caninum* has two, one on either side. Further diagnosis of *Taenia* spp. beyond the genus designation is extremely difficult, requiring morphological study of the intact parasite.

Echinococcus granulosus eggs frequently mix with the feces (unlike *Taenia* spp.), but the eggs are typical Taenia-type eggs, possessing a thick, striated shell. *Dipylidium caninum* eggs, if seen in feces, occur in packets contained within a thin-walled membrane. A number of treatments are available (see Table 5–1), but the anthelmintics used for *Taenia* spp. frequently are not effective for *Dipylidium caninum*. Control is dependent upon the tapeworm species. *Dipylidium caninum* obviously necessitates vigorous control of fleas. For *Taenia* spp., the pet should not have access to the flesh or viscera of the intermediate host.

Heartworm and *Dipetalonema*

Dirofilaria immitis and *Dipetalonema reconditum* are the two filarial nematodes found commonly in dogs and the wild Canidae in the United States. *Dirofilaria immitis* infections may also occur in cats and the wild Felidae, but it is not as common as in dogs. The heartworm, *Dirofilaria immitis*, occurs primarily in the right ventricle and pulmonary arteries of the host, whereas *Dipetalonema reconditum* occurs in the subcutaneous tissues. Both nematodes produce a larval form called a microfilaria, which circulates in the blood (Fig. 5–6). These filarial nematodes are found commonly in areas of the United States where the intermediate hosts occur; however, heartworm is becoming more widespread as infected dogs and cats are brought into areas where the parasite is not normally found.

Dirofilaria immitis males measure 12 to 20 cm, and the females are 25 to 31 cm long, whereas *Dipetalonema reconditum* males are 9 to 17 mm long, and the females are 20 to 32 mm

long. Both nematodes need an intermediate host to complete their life cycle. *Dirofilaria immitis* uses several different species of mosquito and *Dipetalonema reconditum* uses the common dog and cat flea. Microfilariae, when ingested by the intermediate host, undergo reorganization and development to the third-stage infective larva. Once infective, they go into the mouthparts of the arthropod and remain there until the arthropod feeds upon a susceptible host. *Dirofilaria immitis* infective larvae enter the tissue for 85 to 120 days and develop into young adults. They then go to the heart and reach sexual maturity in another 60 to 70 days, for a total of 145 to 190 days. *Dipetalonema reconditum* apparently goes directly into the subcutaneous tissues to develop to sexual maturity.

The microfilaria of *Dirofilaria immitis* is 295 to 325 μm long (average = 313 μm) and 6 to 7 μm in diameter (average = 6.9 μm), whereas the microfilaria of *Dipetalonema reconditum* is somewhat shorter and more slender, measuring 250 to 288 μm long (average = 276 μm) and 4.5 to 5.5 μm in diameter (average = 4.6 μm). The microfilaria of *Dirofilaria immitis* shows a slight relative nocturnal periodicity and is more numerous in the peripheral circulation from late afternoon through the evening hours. *Dipetalonema reconditum* microfilaria, with the common dog and cat flea serving as its intermediate host, does not show any particular periodicity.

Diagnosis of heartworm disease in the dog is generally based on identifying microfilaria in the peripheral circulation. Various techniques have been used to detect microfilaria, including direct wet mount, capillary hematocrit tube and the Knott's or filtration concentration test. Wet mounts are helpful in the differential diagnosis of *Dirofilaria immitis* and *Dipetalonema reconditum* microfilariae. *Dirofilaria immitis* microfilariae move in place without directional motion, whereas *Dipetalonema reconditum* microfilariae have a directional movement across the viewing field. Concentration tests should always be used for the diagnosis of heartworm disease, as they are much more accurate than wet mounts or capillary hematocrit tube tests. Occult heartworm infections (adult heartworms without circulating microfilariae) occur in approximately 25 percent of dogs and 80 percent of cats. Several serological tests are available in commercial kits to test serum of dogs and cats for occult infection. Treatment of *Dipetalonema reconditum* is unimportant, because they are innocuous parasites. The treatment for *Dirofilaria immitis* necessitates the use of an agent effective for the

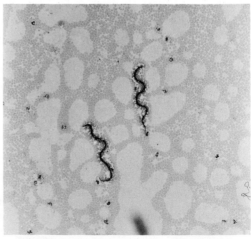

FIGURE 5–6. Microfilaria of *Dirofilaria immitis.*

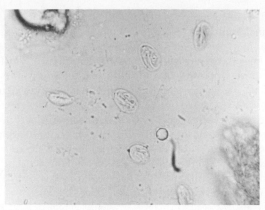

FIGURE 5–7. Cysts of *Giardia* sp. from a dog fecal flotation using ZnSO₄ at a specific gravity (SG) of 1.18.

adult heartworms followed by a microfilaricide (see Table 5–1). Control of *Dirofilaria immitis* necessitates daily or monthly heartworm preventive therapy and mosquito control in enzootic areas.

Giardia

Giardia spp. are common protozoan parasites of dogs and cats in the United States. A higher incidence of infection occurs among dogs, cats, humans and beavers than in other animals such as deer, sheep, moose and antelope. There are two forms of *Giardia*. The motile trophozoite, which is approximately 12 to 17 μm long and 7 to 10 μm wide, is found in the small intestine. The cyst form (the infective stage) is approximately 9 to 13 μm long (Fig. 5–7). When ingested, the cyst wall is digested away in the small intestine, releasing the trophozoite, which immediately divides into two organisms. These organisms attach to the epithelial cells lining the small intestine and continue to multiply by binary fission over the next 6 to 10 days until a large population exists. At that time, diarrhea develops and *Giardia* begins to produce cysts. Diagnosis can be accomplished by the direct, wet preparation or, more effectively, the zinc sulfate centrifugal flotation technique. Treatment is available (see Table 5–1), but reinfection frequently occurs. *Giardia* is more commonly found among dogs and cats crowded into kennels, animal shelters and so forth. The most effective control procedure is cleanliness and disinfection with soap or detergent.

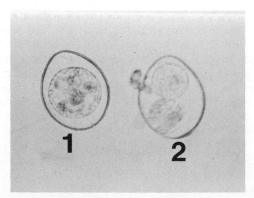

FIGURE 5–8. Unsporulated oocyst of *Isospora* (1) and sporulated oocyst of *Isospora* (2) measuring approximately 25 μ × 20 μ.

Coccidia

Dogs and cats are hosts for a number of species of *Isospora* (also called *Cystoisospora*) and *Sarcocystis,* and the cat is the definitive host for *Toxoplasma gondii.* The incidence and severity of coccidial infection is dependent on the host's age and immune status, conditions in which the hosts are housed or their diet *(Sarcocystis).*

The species of *Isospora* have a direct life cycle; however, recent studies have shown that some of *Isospora* spp. (*Isospora canis* and *Isospora felis*) can use an intermediate host, such as mice. The life cycle starts with an oocyst in the feces (Fig. 5–8). This oocyst must sporulate (develop into the infective form), which it does in less than a week, given optimum conditions of warmth and moisture. Once infective, the oocyst encloses two sporocysts, each of which encloses four small, spindle-shaped infective forms called *sporozoites* or a total of eight infective forms in each oocyst. When ingested, the oocyst and sporocyst walls are digested in the intestine, releasing sporozoites to penetrate the intestinal epithelium and enter a cell for subsequent development. Within the intestinal cell they become spherical and begin to grow to a large size. The nucleus replicates several times, and ultimately thousands of small, spindle-shaped organisms called *merozoites* develop. This asexual process of reproduction is called *schizogony,* and the large structure filled with the merozoites is called a *schizont.*

Once mature, the schizont ruptures, releasing merozoites. The next step in the life cycle is species-dependent, but usually they move further down the intestine, penetrate a cell and repeat the asexual process, but with smaller schizonts containing fewer merozoites. When released, the merozoites then penetrate a cell, and some of them become macrogametes (oval) and some become microgametes (sperm). Once fertilization occurs, the oocyst is produced and passes in the feces to begin the life cycle again. Although the life cycle is finite, for example, only a given number of oocysts can be produced from a single oocyst infection, the reproductive potential is great for some species.

Species of *Sarcocystis* have essentially the same type of life cycle, except that the carnivore is the host for the sexual stages (oocyst and sporocyst), and omnivores and herbivores act as hosts for the asexual (schizogony) stage. Infected carnivores pass a thin-walled oocyst, which will rupture, and which contains two small, thick-walled sporocysts in which four sporozoites have already developed and are immediately infective to the alternate host. Once ingested, the sporozoites are released and penetrate the epithelial tissue of the intestine. Generally, they enter the circulatory system and begin the first asexual (schizogony) phase in the kidney. The first schizont releases its small, spindle-shaped organisms, which then enter cardiac or smooth muscle, in which they develop into rather large schizonts called *sarcocysts.* When sarcocysts are ingested by a specific carnivore, and most species are specific for each carnivore-herbivore, the small, spindle-shaped organisms penetrate superficial epithelial cells of the intestine and immediately begin the sexual phase, terminating as a thin-walled oocyst about 11 to 14 days after ingestion of the infected flesh.

The life cycle of *Toxoplasma gondii* is similar to that of *Sarcocystis* except that most animals are suitable hosts for the development of the asexual (schizogony) stages, and only the cat is suitable as a host for the sexual stages. The typical life cycle occurs when a cat ingests the small sporulated oocyst. In the intestine, the parasite goes through two asexual stages and then into the sexual phase, producing oocysts. If, for example, a mouse should eat the oocyst, the first asexual phase occurs in this animal. When a cat eats these schizonts, the parasite goes into one asexual cycle, in the cat's intestine, followed by the sexual cycle. If the first mouse is eaten by another mouse, *Toxoplasma* goes into the second asexual cycle in this mouse. When then eaten by a cat, the parasites go directly into the sexual phase. The asexual cycle can go on indefinitely as animals eat the flesh of infected animals.

Diagnosis of *Isospora, Sarcocystis* and *Toxoplasma* is based upon recovery of the oocyst or sporocyst (for *Sarcocystis*) by a number of diagnostic procedures. Treatment is seldom administered for *Sarcocystis* or *Toxoplasma* infection, but when clinical coccidiosis occurs, treatment is recommended for *Isospora* spp. (see Table 5–1). Control of *Isospora* infections requires cleanliness, removal of the animal to clean premises or both; however, these oocysts are extremely resistant to environmental conditions. Control of *Sarcocystis* is generally not practiced for the carnivore host because *Sarcocystis* is considered nonpathogenic. If control is exercised, the best approach is to prevent consumption of raw flesh from any source, including ground beef and so forth. The best control for *Toxoplasma* in cats is to prevent consumption of raw flesh and contact with feces of infected cats.

Parasites of Horses

Roundworm

The ascarid of horses (*Parascaris equorum*) has a creamy white color. The males measure about 28 cm, whereas females are about 50 cm in length. They produce a dark brown, thick-shelled oval to spherical egg that is highly resistant to environmental conditions. The horse ascarid is common throughout the United States, and the incidence of infection, especially among younger horses, is frequently high. The larval stage develops within the egg, and the second stage is infective. Development to the infective stage requires about 2 weeks. When the egg is ingested, the larva is released in the intestine, penetrates the intestinal mucosa, enters the circulatory system and passes through to the liver, heart and, ultimately, the lungs, in which it develops for a period of time. Subsequently, larvae pass up the bronchial tree, enter the mouth and are swallowed. They are passed into the small intestine and mature. This entire life cycle requires 10 to 12 weeks. Diagnosis is readily performed using a number of techniques, and these parasites are amenable to treatment by a number of anthelmintics (Table 5–2). Control is difficult because eggs are extremely resistant to environmental conditions, and the coprophagous habits of foals tend to ensure infection.

Pinworm

The primary pinworm of horses, *Oxyuris equi*, is a white to slate grey–colored nematode with a slender, sharply pointed tail. Males are very small, measuring less than 12 mm, and females are 75 to 150 mm long. The eggs are slender and somewhat flattened along one side (Fig. 5–9). Frequently, they possess a first-stage larva when deposited. Pinworms are common in horses in the United States. The life cycle is simple and direct. Female parasites living in the cecum pass out though the anal sphincter and deposit masses of eggs on the perineum. Eggs are cemented into masses with a gelatinous material. Eggs drop off either singly or in masses, landing on ground or feed, and become infective in 3 to 5 days. Once ingested, the larva is released in the small intestine, penetrates the intestinal mucosa and develops for several days. Larva then returns to the mucosal surface, moves to the large intestine and reaches maturity about 50 days after the initial ingestion of the egg. Diagnosis can be performed effectively only by the adhesive tape technique. Pinworms are amenable to treatment by a number of anthelmintics (see Table 5–2). Control is difficult because of the coprophagous habits of foals.

Small and Large Strongyles

Strongylus vulgaris, Strongylus equinus and *Strongylus edentatus* are the three species of "large strongyles," along with 40 species of "small strongyles" of horses. The 40 or more species of small strongyles, of which there are several different genera, are bloodsucking nematodes. Strongyles vary in size from less than 12 mm (small strongyles) to lengths of 38 to 47 mm (large strongyles). However, some small strongyles, like *Tridontophorus*, are nearly as large as *Strongylus vulgaris*, the smallest of the large strongyles. All of the strongyles produce a similar thin-walled egg containing 4 to 16 brownish-colored cells when deposited and are referred to collectively as "strongyle eggs," a term that refers to the order of nematodes to which this group belongs (order *Strongyloidea*, the bursate nematodes).

All of the strongyles are common in horses throughout the United States, and the incidence of infection is generally high. The small strongyles that have been studied have a simple, direct life cycle. The eggs pass in feces, and a first-stage larva develops within the egg. Once developed, the larva hatches and undergoes a free-living existence, developing and molting to a second-stage free-living larva. It then develops to a third-stage larva that does not feed and awaits ingestion. In ideal environmental conditions, development from the egg stage to the infective larva will occur in less than a week. Once the small strongyle is ingested, the larva goes to the cecum, penetrates the cecal mucosa and develops for 1 to 2 weeks. The larva then returns to the mucosal surface and matures in an additional 1 to 2 weeks. The species in the genus *Strongylus* all have complex life cycles.

The development of the larval stages for large strongyles in the environment is the same as for the small strongyles, and once ingested they also penetrate the mucosa of the cecum and develop in a short period of time. *Strongylus vulgaris*, the most important of the large strongyles, leaves the mucosa and by some means (currently unknown) goes to the cranial mesenteric artery and its branches and develops in the lumen of the arteries over the next 6 months, becoming a young adult. It then returns to the cecum and matures, the entire prepatent period (the period of time after ingestion and before eggs pass in feces) requiring about 180 to 200 days. *Strongylus equinus* leaves the cecal mucosa and enters the peritoneal cavity. It then goes to the liver and develops into a young adult. The route taken back to the cecum is incompletely understood, but it may enter the pancreas. The entire prepatent period may be as long as 265 days.

Strongylus edentatus leaves the mucosa and enters the subperitoneal tissue, particularly in the right dorsal flank. Eventually,

Table 5–2
PARASITICIDES USED TO TREAT INTERNAL PARASITES IN HORSES

	Parasite						
Drug	*GASTEROPHILUS*	ASCARIDS	*STRONGYLUS VULGARIS*	*STRONGYLUS EDENTATUS*	SMALL STRONGYLES	PINWORMS	*STRONGYLOIDES*
Cambendazole Camvet	−	+	+	+	+	+	+
Dichlorvos Many trade names	+	+	+	+	+	+	−
Diethylcarbamazine Many trade names	+	−	−	−	−	+	−
Febantel Rintal	−	+	+	+	+	+	+
Fenbendazole Panacur	−	+	+	+	+	+	+
Ivermectin Equalan	+	+	+	+	+	+	+
Mebendazole Telmin		+	+	+	+	+	+
Oxibendazole Anthelcide EQ	−	+	+	+	+	+	+
Oxifendazole Benzelmin	−	+	+	+	+	+	+
Phenothiazine Pheno-Sweet	−	−	+	−	+	−	−
Piperazine Many trade names	−	+	−	−	+	+	−
Pyrantel Many trade names	−	+	+	+	+	−	−
Thiabendazole Many trade names	−	−	+	+	+	+	+
Thiabendazole/piperazine Equizole A	−	+	+	+	+	+	+
Thiabendazole/trichlorfon Many trade names	+	+	+	+	+	+	+
Trichlorfon Many trade names	+	+	−	−	−	+	−
Trichlorfon/phenothiazine/piperazine Dyrex	+	+	+	−	+	+	−

+ = Indicated for use; − = not indicated for use.

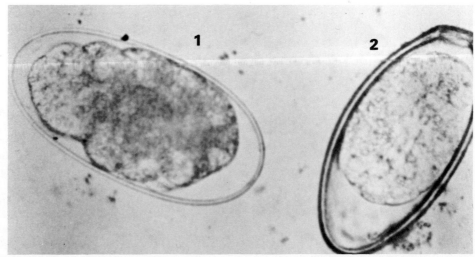

FIGURE 5–9. 1, Strongyle egg measuring 95 μ × 50 μ. 2, Egg of *Oxyuris equi* measuring 90 μ × 42 μ.

it enters the venous circulation and goes to the liver. Supposedly, it leaves the liver and about 2 months later migrates in the mesenteries to the perirenal fat for an additional 3 months. It again migrates in the mesenteries to the large intestine, which it penetrates, and develops to maturity in the lumen of the cecum. The entire prepatent period requires 300 to 322 days. Diagnosis of the strongyles can be accomplished by a number of techniques, and they are amenable to treatment by a number of anthelmintics (see Table 5–2). Control is difficult because the parasites are prolific egg producers and development of the larva occurs rapidly. Control is best applied by a treatment and management regimen based on environmental conditions and by limiting the number of horses on the pasture.

Intestinal Threadworm

Strongyloides westeri is a common parasite of horses, principally of foals (2 weeks to 6 months of age), and is widespread across the United States. The life cycle is essentially the same as *Strongyloides stercoralis* of the dog, with the exception that the parthenogenetic female produces a thin-walled egg containing a first-stage larva when deposited (Fig. 5–10). Diagnosis can be performed by a number of techniques; however, fresh feces must be used because the eggs will hatch in older feces. Treatments recommended are given in Table 5–2. Control necessitates good hygiene, together with treatment, because the parasite can be transmitted by the transmammary route.

Tapeworms

Anoplocephala perfoliata, Anoplocephala magna and *Paranoplocephala mamillana* are the tapeworms of horses. They are broad, thick and white and vary in length from about 2.5 cm *(Anoplocephala perfoliata)* to 75 cm *(Anoplocephala magna),* though most tapeworms are about 15 cm. The eggs of all species are similar and tend to have an amber color or almost no color. The eggs often have a peculiar shape, varying from almost round to somewhat square. The life cycles of all three tapeworms are similar in that the egg is ingested by a free-living mite for further development. In the mite, a small larval form, the

cysticercoid, develops to the infective stage in 2 to 4 months. Once ingested by the horse, the larval stage is released from the mite and develops into an adult tapeworm in 6 to 10 weeks. Diagnosis is readily performed by a number of techniques because the eggs mix with the feces. Treatment or control is seldom practiced.

Parasites of Ruminants

Strongyles

Cattle and sheep in the United States are commonly infected by a number of species of strongyle nematodes (order *Strongyloidea,* the bursate nematodes). Species in the genera *Haemonchus, Ostertagia, Trichostrongylus, Cooperia* and *Nematodirus* are the most common. These nematodes vary in size from about 6 mm *(Trichostrongylus)* to about 25 to 30 mm *(Haemonchus).* All except *Nematodirus* produce a similar "strongyle" egg, which is thin-walled and contains 4 to 16 brown cells when deposited (see Fig. 5–10). *Nematodirus* produces an extremely large egg (see Fig. 5–10). These parasites are widely distributed throughout the United States, but their incidence is dependent on their ability to develop in the external environment. Some, like *Haemonchus,* need considerable warmth and moisture, whereas others like *Ostertagia, Trichostrongylus* and *Nematodirus* will withstand colder, drier climates.

The life cycles, though somewhat variable among species, are similar. The first larval stage develops within the egg and hatches to undergo a free-living existence. The larval stage develops within the egg and grows and molts to the third-stage infective form in less than 2 weeks. Once ingested by the host, the larval stage generally penetrates the mucosa in the site it normally inhabits (stomach, small intestine, large intestine) and develops in a short time; it then returns to the surface of the mucosa and matures. Diagnosis can be effectively performed by most techniques. A number of treatments are available (Table 5–3). Control is best practiced by a combination of treatment and pasture management in areas where there is an abundance of warmth and moisture to promote survival of the larval stages on pastures.

Lungworms

The primary lungworms of cattle and sheep are *Dictyocaulus viviparus* (cattle) and *Dictyocaulus filaria* (sheep). They are slender, white nematodes, and males are 3 to 8 cm long, whereas females are 3 to 10 cm long. Females produce an egg containing a first-stage larva that hatches in the lungs. The first-stage larva passes up the bronchial tree and is swallowed, passing with the feces. Lungworms occur in animals throughout the United States, but their distribution is discontinuous because the larval stages require a certain amount of warmth and moisture to survive. The life cycle is simple and direct. The first-stage larvae live on stored food granules, developing to the third-stage infective form in less than a week in optimum environmental conditions. Once ingested, they enter the intestine, penetrate the intestinal mucosa, enter the lymphatic vessels and develop for a short period of time in lymph nodes. They then go to the heart, enter the circulatory system and then the lungs to mature in a total of 25 to 30 days. Diagnosis is best performed by use of the Baermann funnel technique. Only a few anthelmintics are considered acceptable (see Table 5–3).

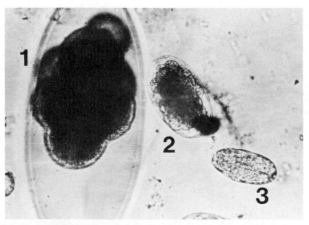

FIGURE 5–10. Egg of *Nematodirus* (1) measuring approximately 200 μ × 95 μ. Strongyle-type eggs (2) measuring approximately 86 μ × 40 μ. Egg of *Strongyloides* (3) measuring approximately 52 μ × 25 μ.

Table 5–3

PARASITICIDES USED TO TREAT INTERNAL PARASITES IN CATTLE, SHEEP AND GOATS

Drug	*HAEMONCHUS*	*OSTERTAGIA*	*TRICHOSTRONGYLUS*	*COOPERIA*	*NEMATODIRUS*	*STRONGYLOIDES*	*BUNOSTOMUM*	*TRICHURIS*	*OESOPHAGOSTOMUM*	*CHABERTIA*	*DICTYOCAULUS*	*MONIEZIA*	*FASCIOLA*	*COCCIDIA*
Albendazole Valbazen	+	+	+	+	+	+	+	−	+	+	+	+	+	−
Amprolium Corid	−	−	−	−	−	−	−	−	−	−	−	−	−	+
Chlorsulon Curatrem	−	−	−	−	−	−	−	−	−	−	−	−	+	−
Coumaphos Many trade names	+	−	+	+	−	−	−	−	−	−	−	−	−	−
Decoquinate Deccox	−	−	−	−	−	−	−	−	−	−	−	−	−	+
Fenbendazole Panacur	+	+	+	+	+	+	+	+	+	+	+	−	−	−
Haloxon Loxon	+	+	+	+	−	−	−	−	−	−	−	−	−	−
Ivermectin Ivomec	+	+	+	+	+	+	+	−	+	+	+	−	−	−
Levamisole Many trade names	+	+	+	+	+	+	+	+	+	+	+	−	−	−
Morantel tartrate Nematel	+	+	+	+	+	+	+	−	+	+	−	−	−	−
Phenothiazine Many trade names	+	+	+	−	−	−	−	−	+	−	−	−	−	−
Sulfonamides Many trade names	−	−	−	−	−	−	−	−	−	−	−	−	−	+
Thiabendazole Many trade names	+	+	+	+	+	+	+	−	+	+	−	−	−	−

+ = Indicated for use; − = not indicated for use.

Control is best exercised by proper management, ensuring that cattle and sheep do not occupy wet, swampy pastures.

Tapeworms

Tapeworms in cattle and sheep are *Moniezia expansa* and *Moniezia benedeni*. In addition, *Thysanosoma actinioides* occurs in sheep. The *Moniezia* spp. reach lengths of 4 m, whereas *Thysanosoma* is generally 25 to 30 cm long. *Moniezia* spp. are widespread across the United States, but *Thysanosoma actinioides* is found only in the western regions. The life cycle of *Moniezia* spp. is the same as for the *Anoplocephala* spp. found in horses, and they use similar free-living mites. The cycle of *Thysanosoma actinioides* is not known. Diagnosis of the *Moniezia* spp. is readily accomplished by a number of acceptable techniques because the eggs mix with the feces; however, diagnosis of *Thysanosoma actinioides* can be accomplished only by observation of the pearly white bell-shaped proglottid on the fecal mass. Treatment is seldom applied to *Moniezia* spp. or *Thysanosoma actinioides*. Control would be difficult, necessitating control of the mites.

Liver Flukes

The most common trematodes of cattle and sheep are *Fasciola hepatica* and *Fascioloides magna*. Both trematodes are green-ish, flat and leaf-like in shape. *Fasciola hepatica* is about 25 mm long and *Fascioloides magna* is about 50 to 75 mm long. The eggs of both trematodes are similar and are large and yellow-brown with an operculum, or "lid," at one end (Fig. 5–11). *Fasciola hepatica* and *Fascioloides magna* are widespread throughout the United States, but only in wet, swampy or subirrigated areas that will support substantial populations of the snail intermediate hosts. The normal hosts for *Fasciola hepatica* are cattle and sheep, but the natural hosts for *Fascioloides magna* are members of the deer family. *Fascioloides magna* cannot complete its life cycle (by passing eggs into the environment) in cattle and sheep.

The life cycles of both trematodes are similar and complex. Eggs passing in the feces must land in water to develop. Inside the egg, a small, ciliated miracidium develops, leaves the egg and penetrates the tissues of a specific snail, in which it undergoes asexual replication through larval stages called *sporocysts* and *rediae*, ultimately developing into a *cercaria*, which leaves the snail to encyst on vegetation and await ingestion. Once ingested, it goes into the intestine, penetrates through to the body cavity and penetrates the surface of the liver in which it wanders for several weeks. *Fasciola hepatica* eventually enters the bile ducts, whereas *Fascioloides magna* will form a cyst wall around itself with an opening into a bile duct if it infects members of the deer family. In cattle, a calcified cyst is found,

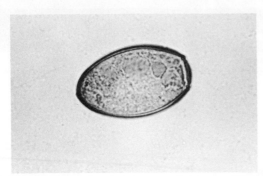

FIGURE 5–11. Egg of *Fasciola hepatica* measuring approximately 130 μ × 70 μ.

whereas in sheep the parasite continues to wander throughout the liver. The eggs are very heavy and will not float; consequently, a sedimentation procedure is used for diagnosis. Effective treatment is available (see Table 5–3). Control necessitates draining and drying wet, swampy pastures to prevent an overabundance of snails.

Coccidia

A number of species of coccidia infect cattle and sheep, and all belong to the genus *Eimeria*. Coccidia are common throughout the United States, and most animals are infected with at least one of the *Eimeria* species. The severity of the infection is dependent on the environmental condition (warmth, moisture), stocking intensity, age and previous exposure. Oocysts of the *Eimeria* species sporulate in the environment and reach the infective stage in the same manner as do *Isospora* spp. *Eimeria* spp., however, develop four sporocysts, each of which contains two sporozoites, for a total of eight infective forms per oocyst. The life cycle of *Eimeria* spp. is identical to that of *Isospora* spp., with the exception that an intermediate host is not required. Diagnosis may be accomplished effectively by several techniques. A number of treatments are available for the clinical disease (see Table 5–3). Control is difficult because oocysts are highly resistant. Proper management for coccidiosis includes prevention of overcrowding and contamination of feed and water and the use of dry bedding.

Trichomonads

Trichomonas foetus is a common protozoan parasite of cattle. This small, flagellated protozoan is equipped with three anterior flagella, an undulating membrane and a trailing flagellum. Generally, *Trichomonas foetus* is a slender, pear-shaped organism. The bull acts as a carrier, with the parasite living on the surface of the penis or in the prepuce. When transmitted by coitus to the cow, the organism develops in the vagina and uterus, causing abortion or fetal resorption. *Trichomonas* multiplies by binary fission; consequently, large populations can be generated in a short time. The cows, given a rest through two or three estrous cycles, will usually develop partial immunity. Diagnosis and treatment are performed on the bull. Diagnosis is difficult and complex (see Specialized Diagnostic Tests, further on). Control necessitates resting the cows and allowing immunity to develop, treatment or elimination of infected bulls and purchase of virgin bulls for breeding.

Parasites of Swine

Stomach Worms

Three stomach worms occur in swine: *Hyostrongylus rubidus, Ascarops strongylina* and *Physocephalus sexalatus. Hyostrongylus rubidus* is the most common and the most pathogenic of the three, usually occurring in adult pigs. Its parasitic development is similar to that of *Ostertagia* in ruminants. Diagnosis is based on finding strongyle eggs in the fecal sample, but the eggs can be confused with the eggs of *Oesophagostomum*, which also occurs in pigs. Treatment is given in Table 5–4. *Ascarops* and *Physocephalus* use beetles as their intermediate hosts and are rarely a problem in swine.

Ascarids

Ascaris suum is the large roundworm and is by far the most common parasite encountered in pigs. Its parasitic development is similar to that of *Parascaris* in the horse. *Ascaris suum* is usually more common in pigs younger than 1 year of age. Diagnosis is based on finding ascarid eggs in fecal samples. Treatment is given in Table 5–4.

Strongyloides

Strongyloides ransomi is found in the small intestine of young swine. Its parasitic development is similar to that of *Strongyloides* in the horse. Diagnosis is based on finding embryonated eggs in fresh fecal samples. Treatment is given in Table 5–4.

Oesophagostomum

Several species of *Oesophagostomum* occur in the large intestine of pigs. Their life cycle is similar to that of *Oesophagostomum* in ruminants. Diagnosis is based on finding typical strongyle eggs in fecal samples. Again, these eggs can be confused with the eggs of *Hyostrongylus* and *Trichostrongylus*. Treatment is given in Table 5–4.

Whipworm

The whipworm of swine is *Trichuris suis*. These worms usually occur in the cecum, and their parasitic development is similar to that of *Trichuris* in dogs. Diagnosis is based on finding typical *Trichuris* eggs in the feces. Treatment is given in Table 5–4.

Lungworm

There are three species of *Metastrongylus* that occur in the lungs of swine. Earthworms act as the intermediate host for the swine lungworm. Most commonly, the posteroventral part of the diaphragmatic lobe of the lung is involved. Diagnosis is made by finding rough-shelled, embryonated eggs in the feces. Treatment of lungworm infection in swine is given in Table 5–4.

Kidney Worms

Stephanurus dentatus is the kidney worm in swine. The adult worms live in the kidneys and perirenal tissues and pass eggs into the urinary bladder. Infection in pigs occurs by ingestion of third-stage larva, ingestion of earthworms containing the

Table 5–4
PARASITICIDES USED TO TREAT INTERNAL PARASITES IN SWINE

Drug	*Ascaris*	*Strongyloides*	*Oesophagostomum*	*Trichuris*	*Hyostrongylus*	*Metastrongylus*	*Stephanurus*	*Coccidia*
Dichlorvos Atgard	+	–	+	+	+	–	–	–
Hygromycin B Hygromix	+	–	+	+	–	–	–	–
Ivermectin Ivomec	+	+	+	–	+	+	+	–
Levamisole Many trade names	+	+	+	–	+	+	+	–
Piperazine Many trade names	+	–	–	–	–	–	–	–
Pyrantel tartrate Banminth	+	–	+	–	–	–	–	–
Sulfonamides Many trade names	–	–	–	–	–	–	–	+
Thiabendazole Many trade names	–	+	+	–	+	–	–	–

+ = Indicated for use; – = not indicated for use.

third-stage larva, skin penetration and in utero infection. Although eggs can be identified in urine, diagnosis is usually made at necropsy. Treatment is given in Table 5–4.

ECTOPARASITES

Parasites of Domesticated Animals

The ectoparasites of domesticated animals generally are members of the phylum Arthropoda. There are many different types of ectoparasites, including fleas, mites, lice, ticks, chiggers, bloodsucking flies and myiasis-inducing flies. Some are host-specific, whereas others infect any number of animals. Diagnosis generally is based upon the external morphological appearance, using taxonomic keys. A number of treatments are available (Tables 5–5 through 5–8). Control is often very difficult, sometimes necessitating treatment of the premises and prevention by prohibiting interaction with infected animals (such as fleas, ticks and lice on companion animals).

Fleas

Ctenocephalides canis (Fig. 5–12) and *Ctenocephalides felis* are the most common fleas of dogs and cats. Of these, *Ctenocephalides felis* is the most common. These fleas are not host-specific and will attack other animals and humans. They are widely distributed but are much more common in warm, humid environments. When environmental conditions are favorable, the flea has a great reproductive potential. Fleas thrive at low altitudes in temperature ranges of 65° to 80° F. Under these conditions, the flea life cycle can be completed, from hatching of an egg to the laying of the next generation of eggs, in as little as 16 days.

Adult fleas are long-lived insects and can survive several months without being fed. The female flea does need a meal of blood, however, in order to lay eggs and to feed her larvae. The female flea lays her eggs in the fur of a host. But the eggs are not sticky; they tend to fall out of the fur and survive in the protected places where the host sleeps or plays. The eggs will hatch into very small worm-like larvae. The larvae feed on organic debris, especially the dried blood droppings (flea dirt) left by adult fleas. Therefore, larvae depend on the host to return time after time to the places where the eggs dropped off. The larvae molt and form pupae, which spin cocoons, then emerge as young and hungry adults in about 3 weeks.

A complete flea control program must involve treatment of

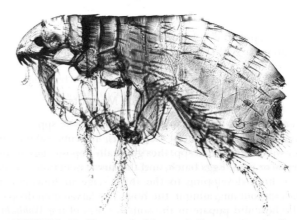

FIGURE 5–12. *Ctenocephalides canis,* the common dog flea.

Table 5–8
PARASITICIDES USED TO CONTROL EXTERNAL PARASITES ON SWINE

	Parasite			
Drug	LICE	FLIES	MITES	MAGGOTS
Coumaphos Many trade names	+	+	−	+
Crotoxphos Ciodrin	+	+	−	−
Dioxathion Del-Tox	+	−	−	−
Fenthion Tiguvon	+	−	−	−
Ivermectin Ivomec	+	−	+	−
Malathion Many trade names	+	−	+	−
Methoxychlor Marlate	+	−	−	−
Permethrin Many trade names	+	+	+	−
Pyrethrins Many trade names	−	+	−	−
Ronnel Korlan	+	−	−	+
Stirofos Rabon	+	−	−	−

+ = Indicated for use; − = not indicated for use.

Diagnosis is based on the morphological appearance of the larva, nymph or adult. Mallophaga have broad heads, and Anoplura have pointed heads. Treatment consists of dust, sprays, dips or shampoos, depending on the host and environmental conditions.

Mites

The mites commonly found on domesticated animals are given in Table 5–10. Most mites are host-specific, and even though morphologically similar, subspecies will not cross-infest other hosts. Mites live on the host continuously and infest other animals by contact. The life cycles of these mites are all slightly different because some burrow, whereas others live on the surface of the skin. *Sarcoptes* spp. and *Notoedres cati* females burrow in the skin and deposit eggs. The eggs hatch into six-

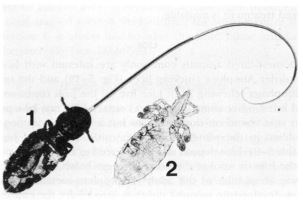

FIGURE 5–13. Chewing louse (1)′ of the order Mallophaga attached to a hair shaft. Sucking louse (2) of the order Anoplura.

Table 5–9
LICE ON DOMESTIC ANIMALS

Cattle
  Haematopinus eurysternus, sucking
  Linognathus vituli, sucking
  Solenopotes capillatus, sucking
  Haematopinus quadripertussis, sucking
  Damalinia bovis, chewing
Sheep
  Haematopinus tuberculatus, sucking
  Linognathus pedallis, sucking
  Linognathus ovillus, sucking
  Linognathus africanus, sucking
  Damalinia ovis, chewing
Horses
  Haematopinus asini, sucking
  Damalinia equi, chewing
Dogs
  Linognathus piliferus, sucking
  Trichodectes canis, chewing
Cats
  Felicola subrostratus, chewing

legged larvae, which develop and molt to eight-legged nymphs, which develop and molt into adults. The entire cycle requires 9 to 17 days.

Species of *Chorioptes, Psoroptes, Psorergates, Otodectes* and *Cheyletiella* have a similar life cycle except that they do not burrow to deposit eggs. *Demodex* spp. generally live in hair follicles. Their life cycle is probably direct, as in the preceding mites, but they can be found in many other tissues of the body.

Diagnosis of mites is based on the morphological appearance of the adult, and it generally requires a thorough skin scraping (Figs. 5–14 and 5–15). Sometimes mites, especially *Cheyletiella* and *Demodex,* can be diagnosed by fecal flotation in dog and cat feces. Treatment consists of dusts, sprays, dips or shampoos (see Tables 5–5 through 5–8).

Ticks

The ticks found on domesticated animals are not host-specific, though they do have host preferences, and their distri-

Table 5–10
MITES FOUND ON DOMESTIC ANIMALS

Sarcoptes scabiei
  Varieties are found on the body of cattle, sheep, horses, goats, swine and dogs
Psoroptes communis
  Varieties are found on the body of cattle, sheep, horses, goats and rabbits
***Chorioptes* spp.**
  Species occur on the body of cattle, sheep, goats and rabbits
***Psorergates* spp.**
  Species occur on the body of cattle and sheep
Otodectes cyanotis
  Occurs in the ears of dogs, cats and other related animals
Notoedres cati
  Occurs on the head of cats
***Cheyletiella* spp.**
  Occurs on the body of dogs, cats and rabbits
***Demodex* spp.**
  Occurs in hair follicles of dogs, cats, cattle, sheep, humans and horses

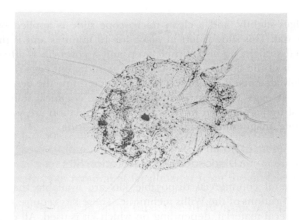

FIGURE 5–14. *Sarcoptes* sp. mite commonly found on dogs and swine.

bution is subject to environmental conditions. The species, and their host ranges, are given in Table 5–11. Ticks are identified as being soft or hard ticks. The most important soft tick is *Otobius megnini,* the spinose ear tick, which lives in the ear of its host. It attaches as a larva, enters the ear and develops through the larval, nymphal and adult stages. Adults mate and then drop off. The female deposits eggs and dies.

The hard ticks are generally classified into one-, two- or three-host ticks. Some, like *Dermacentor albipictus,* are one-host ticks, attaching as a larva and developing into an adult on that host. Adults drop off, lay eggs and then die. The three-host ticks attach as larvae, feed, drop off and molt in the environment to nymphs, reattach to a host, feed, drop off and molt to adults, which attach, feed, mate and drop off to lay eggs and die. *Rhipicephalus sanguineus,* a three-host tick, uses the same host (dog) for all three stages, whereas *Dermacentor venustus* uses small rodents for the larval stage, larger rodents and rabbits for the nymphal stage and dogs, horses, cattle and so on

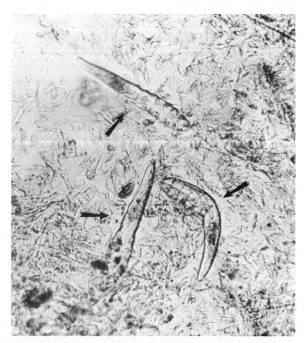

FIGURE 5–15. *Demodex* sp. mite commonly found on dogs.

Table 5–11
TICKS COMMONLY FOUND ON DOMESTIC ANIMALS

Otobius megnini: the spinose ear tick
  Most warm-blooded animals
Dermacentor albipictus: the winter tick
  One-host tick; cattle, sheep, horses, deer, elk, moose
Dermacentor venustus
  Three-host tick; cattle, sheep, horses, wild ruminants, dogs, humans; immature stages on rodents
Dermacentor variabilis: the American dog tick
  Three-host tick; dogs, primary host; immature stages on rodents
Dermacentor nitens: the tropical horse tick
  One-host tick; horses, donkeys, mules
Amblyomma americanum: the lone star tick
  Three-host tick; cattle, sheep, goats, horses, dogs, cats and wildlife; nymphs on rodents, larvae often found on birds
Amblyomma maculatum: the Gulf coast tick
  Three-host tick; cattle, sheep, goats, horses, dogs, cats and wildlife; nymphs on rodents, larvae often found on birds
Amblyomma cajennense: the Cayenne tick
  Three-host tick; mostly horses, but cattle, sheep, goats, wildlife
Ixodes dammini: the northern deer tick
  Three-host tick; adults feed on deer, dogs, horses, humans; immature stages found on small mammals, especially white-footed mice
Ixodes pacificus: the western black-legged tick
  Three-host tick; adults feed on deer, dogs, horses, humans; immature stages found on small mammals, especially white-footed mice
Ixodes scapularis: the black-legged tick
  Three-host tick; adults feed on deer, dogs, horses, humans; immature stages found on small mammals, especially white-footed mice
Rhipicephalus sanguineus: the brown dog or kennel tick
  Three-host tick; usually found on dogs

for the adult stage. Three-host ticks may complete the cycle in a short period *(Rhipicephalus),* whereas other ticks *(Dermacentor)* require 2 years—1 year for each stage—before reattaching to a host.

Treatment necessitates the use of dusts, sprays, dips or shampoos, depending on the host. Control of *Rhipicephalus sanguineus* requires treatment of the premises and, often, the house or kennel. Control of the other ticks is difficult at best, and the precaution of keeping animals away from infested areas can be practiced.

Myiasis-Producing Flies

Some of the myiasis-inducing flies (those developing in the tissue of animals), like *Hypoderma, Oestrus* and *Gasterophilus,* are host-specific and have been discussed under the appropriate host. Others, such as *Wohlfahrtia* spp. and *Cuterebra* spp., have a more limited host range and have been considered with the hosts generally infested. Blowflies in the genera *Lucilia, Calliphora* and *Phormia,* the flesh flies, species of *Sarcophaga,* and the screw worm fly, *Cochliomyia hominovorax,* are not host-specific and cause problems on a number of domesticated and wild animals. Blowflies and flesh flies generally deposit eggs (larvae for *Sarcophaga*) on the flesh of dead animals but can use traumatized or soiled areas. The eggs hatch, and the larvae develop through three larval stages and then drop out of the wound to pupate in the soil. Development of the larvae (maggots) is a function of temperature and varies from 2 to 19 days.

However, any 75-ml to 100-ml flask can be used to substitute for a Stoll flask. The method is as follows:

1. Fill the flask with decinormal caustic soda solution (0.1 N sodium hydroxide) or water to the first graduation.
2. Add feces until fluid goes to the top graduation (4-g displacement).
3. Add several glass beads, and stopper flask, and shake until the sample is mixed well. Samples can be stored and soaked overnight or longer in a refrigerator.
4. With a micropipette, transfer either 0.15 ml or 0.075 ml from the thoroughly mixed sample to a clean microscope slide. Cover the fluid with a coverslip and examine under the microscope, using low power (100×).
5. Examine the entire area under the coverslip, and count the eggs. Next, multiply by the proper dilution factor, either 100 (for 0.15 ml) or 200 (for 0.075 ml) for the eggs per gram of feces.

Stoll Centrifugation Technique

The greatest advantage to the centrifugation modification of the Stoll technique is that it is more sensitive and will detect parasitic eggs when other techniques do not. The method follows.

A regular Stoll flask or a plastic vial is prepared using 56 ml of water and 4 g of feces. Fill the flask or vial with 56 ml of water to the lower mark. Add feces until the vial is filled to the upper mark (approximately 4 g of fecal material). Mix feces with the water and, when possible, allow feces to soak 3 to 8 hours. (Mixture should be refrigerated if it stands more than 2 hours.) Mix the vial thoroughly and immediately remove 1.5 ml of mixture with a 3-ml syringe. Place the 1.5-ml sample in a 10-ml to 15-ml test tube and add flotation solution until a convex meniscus forms at the top of the tube. Place the tube in a swing head centrifuge and place a coverslip on top. Centrifuge at 1500 to 2000 rpm for 2 to 5 minutes. Remove the coverslip, and place on a clean microscope slide. Identify and count all the eggs under the coverslip. The count made multiplied by 10 gives eggs per gram. (If more than 50 eggs are seen on the first coverslip and highly accurate results are desirable, the test tube should be topped off with the chemical solution and a second coverslip added prior to centrifuging again.)

Interpretation of Quantitative Fecal Examination

There is no direct or positive correlation between the number of eggs or larvae found in the feces and the severity of parasitism in the animal. It must also be remembered that during the prepatent period, no eggs or cysts will be seen, although the animal may still be suffering from severe parasitism.

SPECIALIZED DIAGNOSTIC TESTS

Lungworm

The Baermann funnel technique is used primarily to recover larvae of lungworm, although it does have other uses. The funnel consists of a 12.5-cm to 22.5-cm diameter plastic or glass funnel, to which a short piece of rubber tubing is affixed and a centrifuge tube is attached. The funnel is filled with lukewarm tap water, and a screen, gauze or a single layer of facial tissue is lowered into the water. Feces, finely chopped tissues or culture material is carefully added, and the system is allowed to stand for 24 hours. Larvae filter into the centrifuge tube at the bottom, and the coarse material is held back. The system should not be left for more than 24 hours because eggs of some nematodes will hatch after this period and confuse the results. After 24 hours, the rubber hose is clamped, and the centrifuge tube is removed. The bottom 1 or 2 ml of fluid is examined microscopically for larvae.

Microfilaria

Filarial nematodes infect many different tissues of the body and produce an undifferentiated larva called a *microfilaria*. Depending on the species, microfilariae may be found in the blood or in the dermis of their host.

Species producing microfilariae that accumulate in the dermis are identified by the *skin maceration technique*. A biopsy of skin measuring at least 12 mm in diameter is finely macerated and is allowed to soak for at least 6 hours in physiologic saline solution at approximately 37° C or about 8 to 10 hours at room temperature (21° C). At the end of this time, the tissue is strained off, the liquid is centrifuged, and the bottom 1 or 2 ml are examined for microfilaria. Another method is histological sectioning of the skin, a procedure that is much more time-consuming and not as sensitive as maceration.

For microfilariae of filarial nematodes that occur in the blood, a number of procedures can be done.

Tests for Blood Microfilariae

Direct Smear. A thin film of blood is smeared on a slide and dried, and the film is stained with Wright's stain or Giemsa stain. This is a poor technique and will work only if microfilariae are numerous.

Saline Preparation. A few drops of freshly drawn blood are mixed with saline solution, and the resultant preparation is examined microscopically for motile microfilariae. It has the same disadvantages as the direct smear, but when used by technicians experienced in working with microfilariae, it can be effective.

Microhematocrit Technique. The microhematocrit tube is examined for microfilariae after centrifugation. Microfilariae will be found at the plasma-blood interface (buffy coat). This technique has the same disadvantages as the direct smear.

Knott Technique. Add 1 ml of blood to 9 ml of 2 percent formalin (or 2 ml blood in 18 ml formalin). The mixture is then shaken until the blood hemolyzes and is centrifuged at 1500 rpm for 5 minutes. The bottom 0.5 ml or 1 ml is then examined for microfilariae. Microfilariae are preserved, lay straight and are easily measured. Measurements often are necessary to distinguish species and must be done to separate *Dirofilaria* and *Dipetalonema*. This technique is the preferred technique for identification of microfilaria.

Filter Technique. Several filter techniques are available commercially for the recovery of microfilaria from the blood. These techniques require 1 ml of blood, which is then mixed with the lysing solution (usually 9 ml) to hemolyze the red blood cells. The mixture is then passed through a plastic chamber containing a filter membrane on which the microfilariae are collected. The membrane filter is then removed and is placed on a clean microscope slide. A drop of stain is placed on top of the membrane, which is covered with a coverslip for examining under the microscope.

The two simplest and most effective techniques described here are the filter and Knott procedures. Both have advantages, depending on the host and parasite.

Pinworms

Many animals and humans have pinworms (dogs and cats do not). Pinworm infection in horses and humans must be diagnosed by a special technique called the "adhesive tape" technique. With this technique, adhesive tape is folded over a test tube or a smooth, round rod with the adhesive side out. The perianal folds are spread, and the tape is applied to the skin in several places and then the tape is placed on a clean microscope slide with the sticky side down. A few drops of xylene are allowed to seep under the tape to clear the fecal debris, and the slide is then examined microscopically for typical pinworm eggs (always flat on one side).

Tapeworms

Most tapeworms occur in the small intestine of their host as adults or, as with *Thysanosoma*, have access to the intestine. All tapeworms use an intermediate host and since swine, domestic and wild ruminants or rabbits frequently serve in this capacity, diagnostic procedures for both adult and larval stages must be performed.

Adult Tapeworms

Some adult tapeworms such as *Moniezia* spp. in ruminants and the anoplocephalids in horses shed gravid proglottids that are destroyed in the intestine, releasing the eggs to mix with the feces. Any of the flotation procedures described under nematodes are satisfactory for diagnosis. However, *Thysanosoma* in ruminants and *Dipylidium caninum* and the *Taenia* spp. in carnivores produce a proglottid that does not break up in the intestine. The proglottid usually passes intact when the animal defecates. Thus, diagnosis necessitates *visual observation* of the proglottid (or chain) on the feces or around the anal region, which is frequently done by observant clients. *Echinococcus* spp. (taeniform tapeworm) in carnivores is an exception in that the eggs usually appear in the feces.

The fish tapeworms found in humans, bears and wild carnivores shed eggs from the proglottid. Thus, the eggs mix with the feces like *Moniezia* and the anoplocephalids, but this egg is heavy and will not float; therefore, the procedures used for diagnosis of trematodes must be applied (or the formalin–ethyl acetate technique).

Larval Tapeworms

Most species of tapeworms use arthropods, fish or mammals as intermediate hosts (an exception is *Hymenolepis diminuta*, which can use an intermediate host but does not need one). Some tapeworms using mammals have a larva that occurs as a large bladderworm (cysticercus) on the mesenteries or the liver; others produce a small bladderworm that occurs in the muscles. The heavily exercised muscles are the preferred sites for these larvae. Diagnosis may be performed by visual observation of the small bladderworms in the heart, diaphragm or jaw muscles, by pressing thin slices of tissue between two slides for microscopic examination, digestion with pepsin–hydrochloric acid or histological section. If the latter technique is used, remember that all tapeworms have small egg-shaped bodies called calcareous corpuscles that stain blue or purple with hematoxylin. This will identify the larva as a tapeworm, but it does not identify the species. For species identification, the specific host and the site within the host must be known.

Trematodes (Flukes)

Trematodes occur in the bile ducts of the liver, parenchyma of the liver, rumen, lungs, small intestine and other sites, such as skin and oviducts.

Fluke eggs (except *Troglotrema* and *Paragonimus* in the dog) are too heavy to float with the usual chemical solutions available for floating nematode and tapeworm eggs. *Troglotrema* and *Paragonimus* spp. are an exception in that they float with any of the chemical solutions listed earlier.

The diagnostic technique recommended for the recovery of fluke eggs, especially liver flukes and fish tapeworm eggs, is to add a small amount of material (one fecal pellet or equivalent amount) to a centrifuge tube and add 0.1 percent detergent. Macerate the feces, shake thoroughly and then fill with water. Allow to set 5 minutes, decant the supernatant and repeat the procedure. Continue this until the detergent solution is clear (usually two to five times). The detergent, acting as a wetting agent, separates eggs from fecal debris and allows them to settle. Examine the bottom 1 ml of fluid microscopically for the typical operculate eggs.

Protozoa

Single-celled parasites, like the helminths, occur in a variety of sites within the animal body. Various species occupy the circulatory system, especially the blood cells, gastrointestinal system (from mouth to anus) and reproductive system. Unfortunately, a variety of techniques must be employed for correct diagnosis.

Blood Parasites

Parasites occurring in the blood of an animal, such as *Plasmodium*, *Babesia*, *Theileria*, *Leucocytozoon* or *Trypanosoma*, can be identified by the direct smear technique. The slide is air-dried and is then stained with a Giemsa or Wright stain. *Trypanosoma* spp. may not be demonstrable by the direct smear technique; therefore, culture in blood agar slants overlaid with liver infusion tryptose medium is the best approach.

Gastrointestinal Protozoa

Trichomonas. *Trichomonas gallinae* from the oral cavity of birds, *Trichomonas equi* from the gastrointestinal tract of horses and *Trichomonas hominis* from dogs and humans are best demonstrated by direct smear of fresh samples. Lesions suspected of being caused by *Trichomonas gallinae* can be scraped (or swabbed), and this material can be mixed with some physiologic saline solution on a clean microscope slide and examined for these typical flagellates. The presence of an undulating membrane is diagnostic. For *Trichomonas equi* of horses, a drop or two of fluid expressed from the feces can be examined. If the feces are dry, add saline solution, mix and then examine a drop.

Hexamita meleagridis. This is the organism responsible for catarrhal enteritis of turkeys and is diagnosed by demonstration of the fast-moving flagellate in the upper part of the small intestine from freshly killed birds.

Coccidia. *Eimeria, Isospora* and *Toxoplasma* produce an oocyst, whereas *Sarcocystis* generally produces a sporulated sporocyst, all of which pass with the feces and may be easily demonstrated by either qualitative or quantitative concentration (flotation) techniques.

Sometimes, diagnosis of acute coccidiosis (in sheep or cattle) must be done at necropsy examination. In this situation, a scraping of the intestinal mucosa is mixed with physiologic saline solution on a clean microscope slide and is examined for schizonts, oocysts and the small, motile, teardrop-shaped merozoites.

Toxoplasma gondii and species of *Sarcocystis* have a typical coccidian life cycle. *Toxoplasma gondii* produces a very small oocyst in the cat (about the size of the cyst of *Giardia* spp.). *Sarcocystis* spp. produce a more normal-sized oocyst in dogs, cats and other carnivores, but they usually hatch so that only sporulated sporocysts are present in the feces.

Giardia Species. *Giardia* spp. found in domestic, wild and laboratory animals ostensibly can be diagnosed by the direct smear technique, but a more effective procedure is the zinc sulfate centrifugal flotation technique (see earlier description). The cysts are tinted with Lugol's solution, making the internal structures easily identifiable.

Entamoeba histolytica. The dog is sometimes a transient host for *Entamoeba histolytica* and, on occasion, will show clinical signs of infection. As with *Giardia*, the cyst form is best demonstrated by the zinc sulfate centrifugal flotation technique. Iodine will tint the cyst, facilitating identification. This is an extremely small cyst with four to eight nuclei.

Endamoeba Species. This commensal ameba often is found in primates, rodents, humans and other animals. The same techniques employed for *Entamoeba histolytica* are effective. The cyst has eight nuclei.

Balantidium Species. This large ciliate reportedly causes diarrhea in swine and humans, even though it is usually a commensal organism. Diagnosis is possible by direct smear, observing the large, motile trophozoite or by using zinc sulfate centrifugal flotation technique and recovering the large cyst. Iodine will stain the sausage-shaped macronucleus as an aid in identification.

Histomonas meleagridis. This ameba forms a cyst within the egg of the nematode parasite *Heterakis gallinae,* the cecal worm of poultry. In the event of an outbreak of "blackhead" in turkeys, recovery of the eggs of *Heterakis gallinae* from carrier birds and the presence of pathognomonic lesions in sick turkey poults is sufficient to delineate the cause of the infection as well as the source.

Trichomonas foetus. A positive diagnosis of trichomoniasis requires demonstrating the trichomonad from one or more infected animals. There is no serological test or other test based on immunological reactions that has yet proved practical or specific for trichomoniasis.

Diagnosis in the bull consists of checking the breeding records and finding which bulls are probably infected. After a few days of sexual rest, these bulls should be confined, the preputial hairs clipped and the preputial orifice washed with soap and water and dried and the bull examined. To collect the smegma sample, a dry plastic insemination pipette is attached to a 10-ml to 12-ml syringe. The pipette is introduced into the prepuce to its full length. A negative pressure is then created in the syringe, and the pipette is moved vigorously back and forth, scraping the glans penis and the preputial membrane. In most bulls, 0.5 to 1 ml of smegma can be collected in the pipette. This material is flushed into a vial containing 2 ml of lactated Ringer's solution or physiologic saline solution. The sample is then layered on Diamond's medium for culturing.

Trichomonas foetus may occur in small numbers; therefore, proper handling after collection to avoid extremes of temperature, contact with harmful chemicals and evaporation must be done. It is highly desirable to examine samples within a few hours after collection. Samples should be refrigerated but not frozen if they cannot be cultured immediately. The liquid transport medium (lactated Ringer's solution) is layered on the surface of Diamond's medium and is incubated at 37° C for 48 to 72 hours.

Diamond's medium is difficult to prepare and is not available commercially but is available from some diagnostic laboratories. Do not use other *Trichomonas* culture media, because the great majority will not grow *Trichomonas foetus.*

Arthropods

Infestations with ectoparasites means mites, lice, ticks, chiggers, fleas or the larval stages of *Diptera* such as screw worm flies, blowflies, *Hypoderma, Gasterophilus, Oestrus, Cuterebra, Cephenomyia* (wild ruminants) or *Wohlfahrtia*. Fortunately, except for mites, the arthropod parasites are sufficiently large that identification is not as difficult as with the other parasites. Generally, the host and the site on each host will be sufficient.

Mites and Chiggers

Some mites live on the surface of the skin (such as *Cheyletiella, Otodectes, Chorioptes, Psoroptes* and many bird mites), whereas others are burrowing types (such as *Demodex, Knemidokoptes* and *Sarcoptes*). Consequently, there is no uniform procedure for examination and recovery.

Mites and/or chiggers living under the skin, or even on the surface of the skin, are recovered by a deep scraping (deep enough to draw blood) at the periphery of the lesion. Suspected *Demodex* lesions, or even any suspected mite or chigger infestation, should be clipped of hair and "squeezed" at the time they are scraped to ensure adequate sample collections. This scraped material is then placed on a clean microscope slide, coverslipped and examined with a microscope.

Ticks, Fleas and Lice

Ticks, fleas and lice are all of a sufficient size to see with the unaided eye (though sometimes difficult to catch). Ticks and fleas are usually removed and identified. Sometimes lice are difficult to find (or catch); therefore, a careful examination for nits (louse eggs) attached to the hair may reveal their presence. Accurate louse identification often requires the service of a specialist.

Diptera

The species of *Diptera* that infest domestic and wild animals are often easily identifiable because they are host- or site-specific, or both, for example, *Hypoderma, Gasterophilus, Oestrus ovis* and *Cuterebra*. The larval stages of other dipterous insects are not as easily identified. *Screw worm larvae* can be identified by the presence of two black, pigmented tracheal trunks leading from the spiracular openings of the body. They can be clearly seen in the living third instar larva with the unaided eye. Preserved specimens often show this pigmentation, but if not, they can be mounted and cleared in polyvinyl alcohol for study. If a larva does not have pigmented tubules, it is one of myriad blowflies, which can be identified by the pattern of the spiracular openings at the caudal extremity of the body. Using a preserved specimen, cut off the caudal extremity with a sharp scalpel blade and mount upright in polyvinyl alcohol. With keys, identification to genus can be done using the third instar.

The larval stages of *Wohlfahrtia* spp. are parasitic in the very young, for skin must be tender for this parasite to penetrate. Identification of the larva is based on the morphological characteristics of the spiracular plates and cephalopharyngeal skeleton of the third instar larva.

Preserving, Mounting and Clearing Parasites

Ectoparasites and endoparasites may be adequately preserved in 10 percent formalin or 70 percent alcohol. Many of the helminths cannot be accurately identified until they have been cleared (nematodes) or stained (tapeworms and flukes). Nematodes may be cleared (made transparent or translucent) in glycerin, lactophenol or polyvinyl alcohol. When a nematode has been preserved in formalin, it can be transferred directly to lactophenol or mounted on a slide containing polyvinyl alcohol. If it is to be cleared with glycerin, a 10 percent solution of glycerin in water must be prepared. The preserved nematode is transferred to this solution, and the water is allowed to evaporate, leaving the parasite cleared in glycerin. This will require a few days at room temperature, but the dish can be placed in an incubator at 30° C to speed up the process. Specimens should be stored in a brown bottle to avoid yellowing by light. A short cut is to preserve the parasite in 70 percent alcohol containing 5 to 10 percent glycerin and allow the alcohol and water to evaporate.

Tapeworms and flukes are difficult to identify and often require staining. Preservation for morphological study is best accomplished by placing the specimen in a dish of water in the refrigerator until it relaxes (overnight) and then replacing this water with cold preservative (e.g., 10 percent cold formalin). This procedure ensures that the specimen does not contract, which makes study difficult. Special stains, such as acid carmine, are then used to stain and differentiate the internal structures for identification.

Nematodes, tapeworms, flukes, fleas, lice, mites, ticks, chiggers and the small larvae of *Diptera* can be preserved, mounted and cleared in polyvinyl alcohol, making a permanent preparation. Permount or Canada balsam can be used for this purpose, but the specimens must be passed through a graded alcohol series (including absolute alcohol) and then xylene before mounting. The graded alcohol series used is generally 10, 30, 50, 70, 90 and absolute. Depending on the size of the specimen, at least 1 minute is required in each. This is time-consuming and unnecessary if polyvinyl alcohol is available.

Preservation of feces can be done with 10 percent formalin, but this is satisfactory only for some eggs and larvae. Eggs of ascarids, as well as oocysts, will continue to develop. Refrigeration (or even freezing) of feces often is the best approach.

ZOONOSES AND PUBLIC HEALTH

Many infections and parasitic diseases are transmitted between animals and humans (zoonoses). These diseases are always of concern to occupational groups who come into daily contact with a variety of exotic, wild and domesticated animals. Consequently, the zoonoses selected here are those these personnel would possibly encounter. Some of the important diseases that have not been covered (i.e., anthrax, animal tuberculosis) are not as common in the United States because of control programs; however, they have not been eradicated and do occur sporadically from time to time.

Brucellosis is caused by *Brucella* spp. and is transmitted from animal to animal and to humans by direct contact, including fetuses and fetal membranes, and indirectly by ingestion of raw milk and fresh milk products.

Campylobacteriosis is caused by *Campylobacter* spp. The mode of infection is by direct contact with infected animals and consumption of fecal contaminated water or food. Dogs, cats and birds are considered probable sources of infection. Human-to-human transmission is also common, especially among young children.

Leptospirosis is caused by many different *Leptospira* spp. The disease is widespread and common among wild and domestic animal populations. Transmission generally occurs from the ingestion of water or food contaminated by urine of infected animals.

Plague is caused by *Yersinia pestis*. The disease occurs as the result of contact with wild rodents or rabbits, their fleas or both. Acquisition of the disease can be indirect such as through flea bites from rodent fleas on a dog or cat having access to infected rodents or through abrasions in the skin. Disease occurring as a result of direct contact with infected flesh can also occur.

Tularemia is caused by *Francisella tularensis*. The disease generally occurs from handling infected animals (rabbits, beaver, muskrat) or from a bite of an infected tick.

Salmonellosis is caused by *Salmonella* spp. A wide variety of the known serotypes from animals can infect humans. Transmission is by contaminated food and direct contact with domesticated and wild animals that are carriers or are clinically ill.

Dermatophytosis (ringworm) is transmitted by direct contact with infected dogs, cats, cattle and rodents or indirectly by the spores on the animal's hair.

Psittacosis or ornithosis infection occurs by inhalation of the airborne agent in contaminated environments (such as turkey-, duck- or goose-processing plants). Natural reservoirs for psittacosis or ornithosis are wild and domestic birds, especially the exotic psittacines.

Cat scratch disease is caused by a scratch or bite from an infected cat. After a lapse of 7 to 20 days, it manifests as regional lymphodermopathy, fever, malaise, generalized pains, vomiting and stomach cramps.

Contagious ecthyma is caused by direct contact with the lesions on infected sheep and goats.

Rabies is caused by a bite from infected dogs, cats, skunks, bats, foxes, raccoons and other warm-blooded animals. The highest incidence of dog and cat rabies in the United States generally occurs in areas where wildlife rabies is highest. The frequency of human rabies exposures attributed to rabid cats is now increasing at a greater rate than that associated with dogs. Rabid cats, which usually are reclusive, may attack humans and other animals when disturbed. Vaccination of both dogs and cats should be encouraged because it protects not only the community but also the veterinary technician.

Toxoplasmosis is caused by *Toxoplasma gondii*. Infection can be acquired from sporulated oocysts in cat feces or ingestion of raw or insufficiently cooked meat.

Hydatidosis is caused by infection with the hydatid cyst of the eggs of *Echinococcus granulosis* or *Echinococcus multilocularis*.

Tapeworms are acquired by ingestion of raw or poorly cooked beef (*Taenia saginata*) or pork (*Taenia solium*).

Creeping eruption is caused by penetration of the skin by larval stages of dog and cat hookworm of the genus *Ancylostoma*.

Visceral larva migrans is caused by ingestion of the infective larvae (within the egg) of *Toxocara canis*, especially by very young children.

Strongyloidosis is caused by infection, generally by *Strongyloides stercoralis*, which infects humans, dogs, cats and foxes.

Trichinosis is caused by infection with *Trichinella spiralis*, generally from consumption of raw or insufficiently cooked pork or bear.

Scabies is caused by the mites that are not strictly host-specific and can live for varying amounts of time on alternate hosts. Such mites include *Sarcoptes*, *Notoedres* or *Cheyletiella*.

APPENDIX

Pepsin Digest

Add 10 g of pepsin to 100 ml of distilled water and then add 10 ml of concentrated hydrochloric acid. Tissues should be finely minced (cut) and added to the digest, 1 part tissue to 10 parts digest (volume/volume). The digesting material must be incubated at 37° C and stirred frequently until digestion is complete. Digestion time is variable, depending on the density of the tissue; for example, brain or lung will digest sooner than muscle. After digestion, decant most of the supernatant and examine the sediment for parasites.

Lugol's Solution

Add 10 g of potassium iodide and 5 g of iodine crystals to 1 liter of distilled water and place in a brown (amber) bottle (otherwise it will lose strength). These chemicals do not go into solution readily; heating or preparing several weeks in advance of use is necessary.

Zinc Sulfate

Zinc sulfate at a specific gravity of 1.18 is made by adding 331 g of zinc sulfate to 1 liter of distilled water (tap water will do). However, since zinc sulfate is hygroscopic, 331 g seldom is adequate, and a hydrometer *must* be used to adjust the specific gravity. To make a solution of specific gravity 1.20, keep adding zinc sulfate until the proper density is obtained.

Lactophenol

Lactophenol is an excellent medium for clearing nematodes to facilitate study of their morphological characteristics, which is often a necessity to identify nematodes to genus and species. The recipe is one part lactic acid, one part carbolic acid, one part distilled water and two parts glycerin. Nematodes preserved in 70 percent alcohol or 10 percent formalin can be placed directly into this clearing agent and can be ready to examine within 12 to 24 hours, depending on the size of the nematode. Lactophenol has the additional advantage that the nematode can be returned to the solution and kept permanently.

Glycerin

Glycerin also is an excellent clearing agent, and once cleared in glycerin, preserved nematodes can be permanently maintained; however, sunlight will soon cause the nematode to become yellow. Specimens must be kept in an amber bottle. If nematodes are preserved in 70 percent alcohol, they are transferred to a dish containing 70 percent alcohol and 5 to 10 percent glycerin, and the alcohol and glycerin are allowed to evaporate. If they are preserved in 10 percent formalin, they must be transferred to 5 to 10 percent glycerin in water, and the water is allowed to evaporate. This process will require several days but can be hastened by introducing the dish into an incubator at 37° C.

Ingredients for Willis Technique

General. As indicated in the text, the simple flotation (Willis technique) of nematode eggs, tapeworm eggs, coccidia and so forth, which is often used to detect gastrointestinal parasitism in animals and humans, uses concentrated sodium chloride, magnesium sulfate, sodium nitrate or sugar solutions. All solutions are essentially equally effective, but some (sodium chloride) are more readily available and are less expensive than others (sugar). The recipes for each are given below.

Sodium Chloride. Saturated sodium chloride has a specific gravity of 1.20. A saturated solution is made by adding 311 g of sodium chloride to 1 liter of water. A simple procedure is to keep adding salt to warm or hot water until no more goes into solution. Cool to room temperature. Do not decant the excess salt for this will ensure that a saturated solution is maintained.

Sodium Nitrate. This is used as a saturated solution at a specific gravity of 1.36. It is made by adding 616 g of sodium nitrate to 1 liter of water. As with sodium chloride, a simple procedure is to add sodium nitrate to warm or hot water until no more goes into solution.

Magnesium Sulfate. A saturated solution of magnesium sulfate has a specific gravity of 1.30 and is made by adding 337 g of magnesium sulfate to 1 liter of water. As with sodium chloride and sodium nitrate, it can be added to warm or hot water until no more goes into solution.

Sugar. Table sugar (cane or beet source) is used at a specific gravity of 1.2 to 1.3 and is made by adding approximately 1500 g of sugar to 1 liter of water. As in the preceding recipes, heating the water will make the sugar go into solution more easily. Between 18 ml and 20 ml of phenol or formaldehyde must be added as a preservative.

The Baermann Funnel

The Baermann apparatus may be used for the recovery of larvae from the feces, soil or minced tissues of an animal (Fig. 5–16). Although variable results are frequently obtained with this technique, semiquantitative results may be expected from its careful use. It depends on the migration of the larvae from the feces, tissues or soil into water of a warmer temperature, which is brought into contact with the bottom of the material to be examined. The equipment used consists of a glass funnel about 25 cm in diameter in which a wire gauze of 1-mm mesh (about 22.5 cm in diameter) is placed. The funnel is joined to a centrifuge tube by means of a rubber tube, the latter being provided with a pinchcock. In use, the assembled funnel is placed in a ringstand. Before use, the funnel is filled with lukewarm water to the level of the wire gauze. The material to be examined is thoroughly broken up and is placed on the gauze. Usually within 10 to 15 minutes, larvae may be observed migrating into the water, and a large number may be recovered by drawing the material into the centrifuge tube by means of the pinchcock. The largest yield will be obtained by allowing the material to remain in the funnel for 24 hours before drawing off the larvae.

Polyvinyl Alcohol Mounting Medium

Several methods of handling and mounting nematodes are available, but most methods have undesirable features. Most permanent preparations are made only after long and tedious effort. Those methods that are more rapid usually produce preparations of a temporary or, at best, semipermanent nature, and extreme care is necessary in handling the mounting medium.

There is one method that is short, gives consistently good results, is considered equal to or better than the methods now employed for handling nematodes and produces permanent mounts. It is the polyvinyl alcohol method. This method also has been described and employed for mounting other biological specimens. By using this method, permanent mounts of the small and large nematodes have been made. Large nematodes ordinarily cannot be cleared and mounted successfully by any other technique. The method is equally useful for making permanent mounts of certain parasite eggs.

Lactic acid, phenol and a stock solution of polyvinyl alcohol constitute the mounting medium used and the basis of this

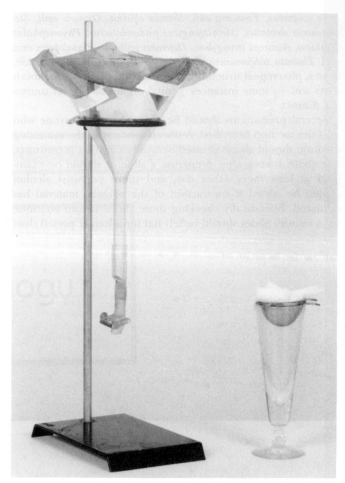

FIGURE 5–16. Baermann apparatus used for recovery of larvae from feces, soil or minced tissues of an animal.

method. The stock solution of polyvinyl alcohol is prepared by dissolving the powdered polyvinyl alcohol (Elvanol 71–24) in distilled water in the ratio of 15 g polyvinyl alcohol to 100 ml water. The process is hastened by the use of an 80° C water bath. The polyvinyl alcohol goes into solution in water gradually, and the end product has a molasses-like consistency.

The stock solution of polyvinyl alcohol is mixed with lactic acid and phenol in the following proportions:

Stock solution	56 parts
Lactic acid	22 parts
Phenol	22 parts

The resulting mixture is used as the mounting medium in preparation of slides and should be stored in a dark or amber bottle.

Specimens may be mounted directly in the mounting medium from reagents, such as formalin, alcohol-glycerin, any concentration of alcohol and even directly from water, if the specimens have previously been killed. Mounts are made in the usual way except that this polyvinyl alcohol mixture is used for the medium. Since it is just that simple and no collapsing or inflation occurs, it has many advantages.

This method has been used on *Ancylostoma caninum, Gongylonema pulchrum, Strongylus* spp., *Tridontophorus* spp., *Haemon-*

edge and skills. The decision to equip and operate a local laboratory must be based in part upon services available through referral laboratories. When comparing the cost of services obtained from these laboratories, the packaging and shipping costs, as well as the direct charge, must be considered. The turnaround time from collection of the specimen until results are received may be unacceptable. Specimens can be submitted only on laboratory work days, whereas the specimens can be processed in a local laboratory when they are obtained, including weekends and holidays. Shipping delays are avoided, and preliminary and final results are immediately available in the practice with its own laboratory so that waiting for communication of results from an outside laboratory is unnecessary. The overhead costs of equipment and stocking supplies are modest and acceptable to most practices. As a technician gains proficiency in the microbiology laboratory, the time commitment will be reduced. If specimens are sent out, considerable time can be spent packaging them, delivering them to shipping terminals and calling for results. Many practices find it cost-effective to operate a microbiology laboratory that is capable of processing routine bacterial cultures.

DIAGNOSTIC METHODS

The choice of methods for examining a specimen in the microbiology laboratory is dependent on the type of specimen and the pathogen sought. Traditionally, microbiologists have attempted to *isolate agents* in various types of culture systems and then use various identification schemes to characterize them. This is still the most frequently used method in bacteriology. However, there are times when the organism may be difficult to cultivate or may not be viable in the specimen presented to the laboratory. In these cases, demonstration of *specific microbial antigens* in the specimen may be more rapid and cost-effective. Immunofluorescence stains have been the most commonly used method of antigen detection. Other immunological assays (e.g., enzyme immunoassays, latex particle agglutination and protein A coagglutination procedures) are now being introduced into veterinary diagnostics. In some diseases, such as botulism and mycotoxicoses, establishing the presence of a *microbial toxin* is necessary, rather than identifying the organism that produces it. Sometimes, a specific *immunological response* by the patient to an infectious agent can estab-

lish the diagnosis. Serum can be tested for the presence of specific antibodies, or skin tests can be performed. Another diagnostic method is *direct examination* of exudates and tissue biopsies. Some microorganisms present such unique morphological characteristics, host inflammatory responses and lesions that a definitive diagnosis can be established without the need for further laboratory testing. Therefore, a direct examination is one of the most important procedures that can be performed in the clinical laboratory.

COLLECTION OF SPECIMENS

There is no other area in the clinical laboratory in which specimen sources and types are so diverse as in the microbiology laboratory. To compound this diversity, specimen selection, collection and transport to the laboratory will have a major impact on results. Therefore, it is important that close communication between the technician and veterinarian be established.

Proper Specimen Collection

The goal of specimen collection is to obtain a sample from the patient that is representative of the disease process. Therefore, the culture specimen must be from the actual *infection site* (Fig. 6–1). It must be collected with a minimum of contamination from adjacent tissues or secretions. Material swabbed from superficial body surfaces (skin or mucous membranes) will usually yield a mixed growth of bacteria, often making it difficult to identify a significant pathogen. Culture specimens recovered from body orifices and draining tracts are frequently contaminated with normal flora. The most satisfactory specimens are those aspirated from normally sterile, closed body compartments after the surface has been aseptically prepared.

Optimal times and *sites* for specimen collection must be observed. Knowledge of the pathophysiology of infectious disease processes is important for determining the optimal specimens that will provide the best chance of recovering the agent. Infections by some viruses and mycoplasma are acute processes that are followed by secondary invasion by opportunistic bacteria. Therefore, sampling must be performed early in the course of disease. Most viruses and some bacteria localize in specific

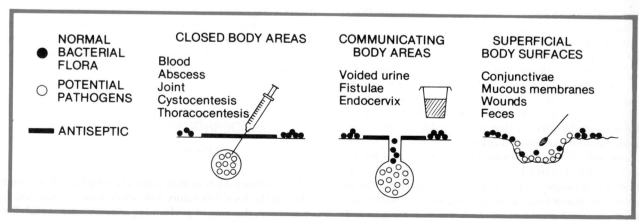

FIGURE 6–1. Methods used to collect bacterial culture specimens and probable sources of contamination.

tissues. Knowledge of these characteristics can be used to improve specimen selection.

Specimens obtained at necropsy for culture should be collected as soon as possible after the death of the animal (see Chapter 23). Whenever possible, culture specimens should be obtained prior to the administration of antimicrobials, especially if the suspected pathogen may be susceptible to the antimicrobial or the antimicrobial may be concentrated at the site of infection. However, the administration of antimicrobials does not necessarily preclude the usefulness of cultures. The antimicrobial drug may be diluted to an ineffective level in culture medium, thereby allowing the pathogen to grow. Antimicrobial-resistant or superinfecting bacteria may still be recovered. In addition, the effectiveness of therapy can be evaluated by determining the relative numbers of bacteria present.

An *adequate quantity* of material should be obtained for complete examination. All too frequently, a good specimen is collected, but only a minute amount is submitted to the laboratory on a swab for examination. Aliquots of body fluids, exudates or pieces of tissue are always more useful than a swab. Smears can be prepared for direct examination, and multiple culture media can be inoculated when adequate material is submitted. Quantitative results can also be obtained, if needed.

Appropriate collection devices and specimen handling must be used to ensure optimal survival and recovery of significant microorganisms (Fig. 6–2). Sterile swabs are acceptable for transferring most samples from the patient to culture media. If the culture medium is not immediately inoculated, the swab must be placed in a humidified transport chamber such as the Culturette (Baxter Scientific Products), or into a transport medium. *Transport media* are designed to maintain optimal conditions for survival of the suspected pathogen without allowing overgrowth by contaminating saprophytes. Semisolid transport

media, such as Amies transport medium with charcoal for *aerobic bacteria* (growth in the presence of oxygen) or Port-A-Cul tubes (Becton Dickinson Microbiology Systems) for *anaerobic bacteria* (requires absence of oxygen) can preserve specimens on swabs for several days. Swabs should not be placed in nutritive broths before inoculating isolation media, because an insignificant nonpathogen may overgrow and prevent recovery of the pathogen. Specimens can be collected in various sterile containers that do not contain preservatives or anticoagulants for transport. If tissues are collected for culture, each piece must be packaged separately in a leak-proof, sterile container.

Each culture specimen container must be *properly labeled.* Identification of the patient by name, species, case number or owner, as appropriate, should be legibly indicated. If more than one veterinarian works in the practice, the one in charge of the case should be identified so that questions about history and preliminary reports can be communicated efficiently. The source of the specimen should also be included on the label. Nothing can be more frustrating in the laboratory than to be presented with a swab for culture and wonder if it represents conjunctiva, ear canal, skin or endometrium. As will be discussed later, the source of the specimen will be a significant factor in deciding how to set up the culture, which bacteria to identify and how to interpret the results. If the culture specimen is to be sent to a referral laboratory, additional clinical history should be included. Results of previous culture attempts, other laboratory tests and antimicrobial treatments should be reported, as well as the major clinical manifestations and duration of illness, so that laboratory personnel will be able to recognize and identify significant findings.

Special Collection and Handling Procedures

Some groups of microorganisms require special collection and handling for optimal isolation. Anaerobic bacteria must be protected from oxygen. Often a sterile syringe with a fine-gauge needle (22- to 23-gauge) is the best collection device for aspirating exudates from an infected site. Any air in the syringe is expelled, the needle is plugged by inserting it into a rubber stopper and the plunger is taped to the body of the syringe. The syringe can then be transported to the laboratory. Survival and subsequent isolation of anaerobes is enhanced by keeping them in the reduced microenvironment in which they are found. Therefore, as stated previously, exudate and pieces of tissue are better specimens than swabs. If a swab is collected, it must be placed in an appropriate anaerobic transport device. Handling a specimen as if it contains anaerobes will not jeopardize the viability of aerobic bacteria.

In attempts to isolate fungi and mycobacteria, swabs generally are not the best specimens. These agents tend to cause chronic infections, often with small numbers of organisms present. Too few organisms may be present on a swab, or in the case of mycobacteria, they may adhere to the swab, and culture results will be negative. Exudates, biopsy material and tissue should be submitted as quickly as possible to the microbiology laboratory.

The more fastidious groups of microorganisms, for example, *Mycoplasma, Chlamydia, Rickettsia* and viruses, require special selective transport media. These media are usually formulated to contain antimicrobials that will inhibit the growth of other

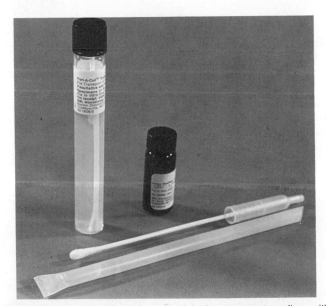

FIGURE 6–2. Culturette swab, tube of Amies transport medium with charcoal and Port-A-Cul anaerobic transport tube. The Culturette swab is replaced in the plastic tube after it is inoculated, and the ampule at the bottom is crushed in order to provide moisture for the swab. The transport tubes are used by inserting the swab deeply into the medium and breaking off the end of the swab that has been handled. The Port-A-Cul tube contains an indicator that changes color when exposed to oxygen and shows how far oxygen has diffused into the agar.

microorganisms, while preserving the viability of the desired agent. Specific transport media and instructions for proper use should be obtained from a referral laboratory that is capable of providing the desired culture service.

PROCESSING SPECIMENS

Each specimen received in the microbiology laboratory should be carefully and individually evaluated, just as each patient is individually examined, rather than being subjected to an inflexible processing scheme. Variables to be considered include anatomical source and condition of the specimen, animal family of the patient, clinical history, special requests from the veterinarian and results of direct examination of the specimen which will collectively focus on the most likely agents.

Condition of the Specimen

Each specimen received in the microbiology laboratory should be examined to see if it is suitable for further processing. If there is evidence that the specimen has become grossly contaminated or dried out, if it is of insufficient quantity, if there has been excessive delay in receipt or any other evidence of mishandling is present, an attempt should be made to obtain a second sample. Specimens should be processed the same day they are collected, or they should be held at refrigeration temperatures if a delay is anticipated.

Clinical Information

When the microbiology laboratory receives information about the clinical history of the suspected infectious disease and the source of the specimen, the pathogen can be identified much more efficiently. Each pathogen has a preferred habitat where it will grow and specific mechanisms for causing disease. Therefore, for a particular manifestation of disease, there will be a limited number of agents that should be considered as likely pathogens. Comparison of the clinical description of disease with the biology and pathogenicity of microorganisms will usually identify a limited number of agents that typically are involved in each type of disease process.

If the veterinarian has carefully examined the patient, the differential list of infectious agents can usually be limited to two to five microorganisms. Table 6–1 lists the most common bacterial species associated with infections of various sites in animals. If the technician can focus the search for pathogens on these most likely agents, results will often be obtained much more rapidly and with less expense.

Direct Microscopic Examination

Direct microscopic examination of exudates, impression smears from tissues or infected body fluids is the most important laboratory procedure that can be used for microbiological diagnosis. It provides immediate information on the types and numbers of microorganisms present as well as the type of host cellular inflammatory response. The likelihood of infection can be determined as can the probable type of agent (i.e.,

virus, bacteria or fungus), which, in turn, determines the nature of the diagnostic assays needed. Suitability of the specimen for culture can also be evaluated. The most likely pathogen (or predominant organism) may tentatively be identified. This information may be used as the basis for the interpretation of the significance of subsequent culture results.

In many situations, Gram's stain is the procedure of choice because it provides differentiation of gram-positive and gram-negative bacteria. However, some bacteria do not stain well with Gram's stain. Gram-negative bacteria may not be well differentiated from the background in exudates and tissue impression smears.

Other tissue stains (i.e., Giemsa's and Wright's stains or methylene blue wet mounts) may be more useful for detecting all microorganisms present in the smear. Although these stains are more efficient in demonstrating the presence and morphology of bacteria, they do not provide differentiation of gram-positive and gram-negative bacteria. Careful direct examination may be sufficient for diagnosis without cultures, or it can narrow the diagnostic likelihood to a few bacterial species. This information helps in the selection of optimal culture conditions for identification of suspected pathogens.

Gram's Stain Procedure

The technique for preparing a Gram-stained smear is as follows:

1. Prepare a thin smear from tissue exudates or bacterial suspension on a clean slide and allow smear to air dry.
2. Fix material to the slide so that it does not wash off during the staining procedure by passing the slide, right side up, through a flame three or four times.
3. Flood smear with crystal violet solution, and let stand for 1 minute.
4. Wash smear briefly with tap water.
5. Flood smear with Gram's iodine solution, and let stand for 1 minute.
6. Wash with tap water, and decolorize until solvent flows colorlessly from the slide. This usually requires 5 to 10 seconds.
7. Wash briefly with tap water, and flood the slide with safranin counterstain for 30 to 60 seconds.
8. Wash briefly with tap water, blot dry and examine the stained smear under the 100 × (oil immersion) objective of the microscope. *Gram-positive bacteria* stain dark blue to purple; *gram-negative bacteria* appear pink to red.

BACTERIAL ISOLATION AND IDENTIFICATION PROCEDURES

Equipment

The following is a list of equipment and supplies required for the performance of basic diagnostic bacteriology tests.

1. Binocular microscope
2. Incubator
3. Anaerobic culture system
4. Stains: Gram's stain kit, acid-fast stain kit, lactophenol cotton blue
5. Bacteriological loops, inoculating needles and calibrated loops

Table 6–1
COMMON BACTERIAL SPECIES ASSOCIATED WITH INFECTIONS

Type of Infection	Canine	Feline	Equine	Porcine	Ruminants
Conjunctivitis	Staphylococcus Streptococcus Pseudomonas	Staphylococcus Pasteurella Chlamydia	Streptococcus Staphylococcus	Streptococcus Staphylococcus	Moraxella bovis Branhamella Streptococcus Staphylococcus Escherichia coli
Central Nervous System	Rare	Rare	Streptococcus Actinobacillus Escherichia coli	Streptococcus Escherichia coli	Haemophilus somnus Listeria Escherichia coli Pasteurella haemolytica
Gastroenteritis	Salmonella Clostridium perfringens Campylobacter	Salmonella	Salmonella Escherichia coli Actinobacillus Rhodococcus equi	Salmonella Escherichia coli Treponema Clostridium perfringens	Salmonella Escherichia coli Clostridium perfringens Mycobacterium paratuberculosis
Genital tract	Brucella canis Escherichia coli Streptococcus Staphylococcus Mycoplasma	Streptococcus Pasteurella Escherichia coli	Streptococcus Escherichia coli Klebsiella Pseudomonas	Brucella suis Streptococcus Leptospira	Brucella Listeria Actinomyces pyogenes Campylobacter Mycoplasma
Mastitis	Staphylococcus	Staphylococcus	Streptococcus	Streptococcus Staphylococcus Escherichia coli Actinobacillus Actinomyces pyogenes	Streptococcus Staphylococcus Actinomyces pyogenes Nocardia Mycobacterium Escherichia coli Klebsiella
Musculoskeletal	Staphylococcus Escherichia coli Pseudomonas Brucella canis Anaerobes	Rare	Streptococcus Actinobacillus Escherichia coli Rhodococcus equi Staphylococcus	Streptococcus Mycoplasma Escherichia coli Erysipelothrix Actinomyces pyogenes	Clostridium Actinomyces pyogenes Escherichia coli Streptococcus Erysipelothrix Haemophilus somnus Mycoplasma Chlamydia
Otitis	Staphylococcus Pseudomonas Streptococcus Clostridium perfringens	Rare	Rare	Rare Streptococcus	Rare Streptococcus Pasteurella Actinomyces pyogenes
Respiratory Upper	Bordetella bronchiseptica	Pasteurella multocida	Streptococcus equi	Bordetella bronchiseptica Pasteurella multocida	Haemophilus somnus Actinomyces pyogenes Fusobacterium
Pneumonia	Bordetella bronchiseptica Pasteurella Klebsiella Escherichia coli Mycoplasma Streptococcus Staphylococcus	Rare Pasteurella Chlamydia	Streptococcus Actinobacillus Rhodococcus equi Pasteurella Staphylococcus Klebsiella Pseudomonas Bordetella bronchiseptica	Mycoplasma Haemophilus Pasteurella Streptococcus Actinobacillus	Pasteurella Actinomyces pyogenes Haemophilus somnus Mycoplasma
Pleuritis	Fusobacterium Bacteroides Actinomyces	Bacteroides Fusobacterium Pasteurella Nocardia	Streptococcus	Actinobacillus	Pasteurella Actinomyces pyogenes
Skin wounds abscesses	Staphylococcus Streptococcus Pseudomonas Nocardia Actinomyces Fusobacterium	Pasteurella multocida Streptococcus Staphylococcus Anaerobes	Streptococcus Corynebacterium pseudotuberculosis Pseudomonas Dermatophilus Staphylococcus	Streptococcus Staphylococcus Actinomyces pyogenes	Actinomyces pyogenes Dermatophilus Actinomyces Actinobacillus Staphylococcus
Urinary tract	Escherichia coli Proteus Staphylococcus Streptococcus Klebsiella Pseudomonas Pasteurella	Staphylococcus Escherichia coli	Streptococcus Escherichia coli	Eubacterium suis Streptococcus	Corynebacterium renale Actinomyces pyogenes

6. Alcohol wick burner, Bunsen burner or sterno burner
7. Glass slides and coverslips
8. Forceps, spatulas and scalpels
9. Specimen-collection devices: swabs, tubes, cups, and so forth
10. Transport media: Amies, Port-A-Cul
11. Culture media (Table 6–2)
12. Antibiotic disk dispenser and disks
13. 3 percent hydrogen peroxide
14. 3 percent potassium hydroxide

15. Oxidase test reagent
16. Coagulase plasma
17. *Salmonella* polyvalent antiserum
18. Packaged identification system for Enterobacteriaceae (Table 6–3)
19. Kovac's reagent

The most expensive item is a good-quality binocular light microscope with a 100 × oil immersion objective. Dark-field and phase-contrast options are useful but not essential. Small coun-

Table 6–2
BACTERIOLOGICAL PLATE AND TUBE MEDIA FOR THE PRACTITIONER'S LABORATORY

Media	Purpose and Inoculation	Reactions and Interpretations
Blood agar plate (trypticase soy agar with 5% sheep blood)	Primary isolation medium for all specimens in which pathogenic bacteria are suspected. Always streak for colony isolation.	Observe growth rates, colony morphological characteristics, hemolysis. Test selected colonies for Gram reaction, catalase and oxidase. Inoculate differential tests and antimicrobial susceptibility tests from well-isolated colonies.
MacConkey agar	A primary isolation and differential plating medium for selection and recovery of Enterobacteriaceae and related gram-negative bacteria. Inoculate by streaking for isolated colonies.	Growth is usually gram-negative. Pink to red colonies (with increased redness of the medium) are lactose fermenters, e.g., species of *Escherichia, Klebsiella* and *Enterobacter*. Colorless colonies (often with a slight change of the medium to yellow) are nonlactose fermenters.
Hektoen enteric agar	A direct plating medium for fecal specimens that is highly selective for *Salmonella*. Inoculate by streaking for isolated colonies.	Disaccharide fermenters are moderately inhibited and produce bright orange to yellow to salmon to pink colonies. *Salmonella* colonies are blue-green typically with black centers from hydrogen sulfide. *Proteus* colonies may resemble *Salmonella*.
Selenite broth or Tetrathionate broth	Enrichment broth for the selective enhancement of growth by *Salmonella* from specimens containing heavy concentrations of mixed bacteria, such as feces. Inoculate relatively heavily and incubate for 8 to 12 hr.	Subculture to MacConkey agar and Hektoen enteric agar for isolation of *Salmonella*.
Triple sugar iron (TSI) agar slant	A differential medium for detection of carbohydrate (glucose, lactose, sucrose) fermentation and production of hydrogen sulfide. Inoculate by stabbing the butt once with an inoculating needle and by streaking the slant. Incubate with a loose cap.	Yellow color change indicates acidification caused by carbohydrate fermentation. In the butt, glucose fermentation is detected; in the slant, lactose and sucrose fermentation is detected (includes glucose fermentation as an intermediate product). Red color change indicates alkalinization caused by lack of carbohydrate fermentation. Black color indicates hydrogen sulfide production. Results are recorded as slant/butt; A = acid (yellow), K = alkaline (red) or NC = no change.
Christensen's urea agar slant	A differential medium for detection of urease production by an organism. Inoculate by streaking heavily over the slant.	Urease-positive bacteria produce a pink-red color change in the slant and sometimes throughout the butt. Urease-negative bacteria allow the medium to remain the original yellow color.
Motility media*	A test medium for determining if an organism is motile or nonmotile. Inoculate by stabbing the center of the tube with an inoculating needle. Incubate at 35°C for most organisms; incubate at room temperature if *Listeria* is suspected.	Motile organisms migrate from the stab line, flaring out to cause turbidity in the medium. Nonmotile organisms grow only along the stab line; the surrounding medium remains clear.
Indole test media*	A test medium for detecting the ability of bacteria to produce indole as one of the degradation products of tryptophan metabolism. Inoculate, incubate 24 to 48 hr, then add Kovac's reagent to detect indole.	Development of a red color at the interface of the reagent and the broth within seconds after adding the reagent is indicative of a positive test.

*Combination media can be purchased that provide for several tests in the same tube, such as SIM (sulfide-indole-motility), MIO or MIL (motility-indole-ornithine or motility-indole-lysine).

Table 6–3
COMMERCIAL KIT SYSTEMS FOR IDENTIFICATION OF MICROORGANISMS

Enterobacteriacea
API 20E
 bioMérieux Vitek, Inc.
Enterotube II
 Roche Diagnostics
Minitek Enterobacteriaceae Set
 Becton Dickinson
 Microbiology Systems
Micro-ID
 Organon Teknika Corp.
Rapid E
 bioMérieux Vitek, Inc.
Staphylococcus
Minitek Gram-positive Set
 Becton Dickinson
 Microbiology Systems
STAPH-IDENT
 bioMérieux Vitek, Inc.
STAPH-Trac
 bioMérieux Vitek, Inc.
Streptococcus
API 20S
 bioMérieux Vitek, Inc.
Minitek Gram-positive Set
 Becton Dickinson
 Microbiology Systems
Rapid STREP
 bioMérieux Vitek, Inc.
Small Gram-positive Bacilli
API Coryne
 bioMérieux Vitek, Inc.

Other Gram-negative Bacteria
API 20E
 bioMérieux Vitek, Inc.
Minitek Nonfermenter Set
 Becton Dickinson
 Microbiology Systems
OXI/FERM
 Roche Diagnostics
Rapid NFT
 bioMérieux Vitek, Inc.
Yeast
API 20C
 bioMérieux Vitek, Inc.
Minitek Yeast Set
 Becton Dickinson
 Microbiology Systems
Yeast-Ident
 bioMérieux Vitek, Inc.
Anaerobic Bacteria
An-Ident
 bioMérieux Vitek, Inc.
API 20A
 bioMérieux Vitek, Inc.
Minitek Anaerobe II
 Becton Dickinson
 Microbiology Systems
RapID-ANA II
 Innovative Diagnostic
 Systems, Inc.

See Table 6–4 for addresses of product manufacturers and distributors.

tertop incubators are available. Important characteristics of a quality incubator include (1) insulated walls to maintain a constant temperature; (2) an adequate seal to maintain a humid atmosphere; (3) a capacity for plates, tubes and candle jars; (4) a thermometer to check the temperature, which should not fluctuate more than $\pm 2°C$; and (5) an adjustable, thermostatically controlled heating element. Storage space for media in a refrigerator is needed, as well as a convenient, clean laboratory workbench with a sink.

Culture Media

A number of different media are needed in the bacteriology laboratory for isolation of various microbial agents and for identification of these microorganisms. Both dehydrated and prepared media are readily available today. It is usually much more convenient for small laboratories to purchase prepared media than to prepare their own. In addition, the quality of purchased media will be much more consistent and usually will be quality-tested before it is distributed. There are numerous distributors of prepared media throughout the United States. A few national and regional distributors are listed in Table 6–4. Names and addresses of other suppliers can be obtained from local hospitals. These microbiology supply distributors usually have a full line of prepared plates and tubes of media available, as well as the ancillary biochemical reagents, stains and miscellaneous supplies that are necessary in the laboratory (see preceding list).

Table 6–4
COMMERCIAL SOURCES OF MICROBIOLOGY LABORATORY SUPPLIES

This table presents a partial listing of manufacturers and distributors of various microbiology laboratory supplies such as prepared plate and tube media, stains and reagents, susceptibility test supplies, loops, slides, swabs, incubators, microscopes, anaerobic systems and diagnostic kits. Through consultation with other local microbiology laboratories (e.g., hospitals) other local or regional suppliers may be discovered.

Abbott Laboratories, Diagnostics Division, North Chicago, IL 60064, (800) 323-9100
Anaerobe Systems, 2200 Zanker Road, Suite C, San Jose, CA 95131, (800) 443-3108
Baxter Scientific Products, 1430 Waukegan Road, McGraw Park, IL 60085, (708) 689-8410
Becton Dickinson Microbiology Systems, PO Box 243, Cockeysville, MD 21030, (410) 771-0100
Becton Dickinson Vacutainer Systems, Rutherford, NJ 07070, (201) 847-6800
Bethyl Laboratories, Inc., PO Box 850, Montgomery, TX 77356, (800) 338-9579
bioMérieux Vitek, Inc., 200 Express Street, Plainview, NY 11803, (800) 645-7034
Carr-Scarborough Microbiologicals, Inc., PO Box 1328, Stone Mountain, GA 30086, (800) 241-0998
Curtin Matheson Scientific, Inc., PO Box 1546, Houston, TX 77251, (713) 878-2349
Difco Laboratories, PO Box 331058, Detroit, MI 48232, (800) 521-0851
Fisher Scientific, 711 Forbes Avenue, Pittsburgh, PA 15219, (412) 562-8300
ICN Biomedicals, Inc., 3300 Hyland Avenue, Costa Mesa, CA 92626, (714) 545-0113
IDEXX Corp., 100 Fore Street, Portland, ME 04101, (800) 248-2483
ImmuCell Corp., 966 Riverside Street, Portland, ME 04103, (207) 797-8386
Innovative Diagnostic Systems, Inc., 3404 Oakcliff Road, Suite C-1, Atlanta, GA 30340, (800) 225-5443
Marion Scientific Corp., 9233 Ward Parkway, Kansas City, MO 64114, (816) 966-4000
Meridian Diagnostics, Inc., 3471 River Hills Drive, Cincinnati, OH 45244, (800) 543-1980
Microbio Products, Inc., 3901 Nome Street, Unit 1, Denver, CO 80239, (303) 371-4166
Miles Scientific, Mobay Corp., Shawnee, KS 66201, (800) 422-9874
Organon Teknika Corp., 100 Akzu Avenue, Durham, NC 27704, (919) 620-2000
Oxoid USA, Inc., PO Box 691, Ogdensburg, NY 13669, (800) 567-8378
Pitman-Moore, Inc., 421 E. Hawley Street, Mundelein, IL 60060, (800) 525-9480
Remel, 12076 Sante Fe Drive, Lenexa, KS 66215, (800) 255-6730
Roche Diagnostic Systems, 340 Kingsland Street, Nutley, NJ 07110, (908) 235-7200
Synbiotics Corp., 11011 Via Frontera, San Diego, CA 92127, (800) 228-4305
TechAmerica Veterinary Products, PO Box 901350, Kansas City, MO 64190, (816) 891-5500
Veterinary Medical Research & Development, Inc., PO Box 502, Pullman, WA 99163, (800) 222-8673
VWR Scientific, PO Box 13645, Philadelphia, PA 19101, (215) 431-1700

Purpose of Specific Media

Solid media in plates are used for primary isolation of bacteria from clinical specimens. This type of medium allows distribution of the specimen in such a way that *isolated colonies*

colonized by microflora (e.g., intestinal tract) interpretation becomes much more difficult. In general, if there is scant aerobic growth of three or more bacteria, the result probably reflects normal flora. Most bacterial infections, other than mixed anaerobic infections, are usually caused by only one or two agents. When a specimen from an infectious process is carefully collected, growth of a single organism in nearly pure culture will often be observed. Therefore, the most abundant colony type is usually the most important.

Some general guidelines for selection of significant isolates can be derived from colony morphological characteristics, though exceptions will always occur. Usually circular, smooth, raised or convex opaque to gray colonies with an entire edge are more likely to be significant. Large, rough, granular, irregular, spreading or heavily pigmented colonies are likely to be insignificant unless large numbers are recovered in nearly pure culture.

Changes in the media should be carefully noted. Hemolysis in blood agar is often a good indication of a possible pathogen. Sometimes the hemolytic pattern provides adequate identification, such as the double zone of hemolysis produced by many coagulase-positive isolates of *Staphylococcus*. Pigment production can be an important characteristic to note on primary cultures. The differential features of MacConkey agar (i.e., ability to grow and lactose fermentation) are important bits of information that can aid in the identification of an isolate. Odors produced by bacteria are difficult to describe adequately, but after experience is gained, they can be another useful identifying characteristic.

The novice microbiologist may be required to rely on several differential tests for the identification of isolates. As experience is gained and confidence develops, more isolates will be recognized on the primary plates. Knowledge of the more common bacterial species to expect from a specimen (see Table 6–1) will provide a differential list of bacteria to consider so that it is not necessary to face each culture as a complete unknown.

Recording, Interpreting and Reporting Results

Although it is impossible to devise rigid rules that provide for adequate processing of all specimens, some rigid routines are necessary for observing and recording results of cultures. A laboratory worksheet should be developed for recording all observations. It is essential that these records contain sufficient detail so that anyone who works in the laboratory can take over and complete the culture without a special briefing. A worksheet that provides adequate room for a flow chart type of illustration of culture processing and observation is easy to follow (Fig. 6–5). These work records may become part of the medical record, so care should be taken to ensure that they are complete and accurate (see Chapter 3).

As an aid to interpreting culture results, the relative abundance of growth of each type of colony should be recorded. A convenient system of recording is a scale of 1+ to 4+, in which each step on the scale represents the number of quadrants of the primary culture plate in which the colony is growing. For example, if the only colonies are in the initial streak lines in which the specimen was inoculated on the plate,

FIGURE 6–5. Example of a laboratory worksheet for recording results of various laboratory procedures, including microbial identification and susceptibility tests.

growth would be rated 1+. If growth is so abundant that colonies are found in the fourth quadrant (the final streak lines), growth is rated 4+. Any bacterium isolated from broth subculture, but not on primary inoculated plates, is rated 1+, regardless of the abundance of growth on the subculture plate. Because bacterial cultures should not be evaluated empirically as positive or negative, this semiquantitative method helps the clinician to interpret the significance of the results. Specimens from most acute bacterial infections that have not been treated with antimicrobials will yield 3+ to 4+ growth. However, because of poor collection technique, mishandling the specimen, presampling antimicrobial therapy or chronic infections, a smaller number of bacteria may be recovered. The clinician must decide whether these smaller numbers of bacteria are significant. If the culture is from a normally sterile body site, these culture results are often significant.

Normal Flora

Specimens cultured from sites with a normal flora are more difficult to interpret. Usually these cultures are insignificant if they result in scant growth, especially if it is a mixture of bacteria. To avoid wasting undue time precisely identifying the microflora, the technician should become familiar with flora normally found at various sites of the body (Table 6–5). Many of these bacteria are potential pathogens. If they are identified because of common recognition and are specifically reported while other, less familiar bacteria are overlooked, the report may mislead the clinician by implying undue significance.

Therefore, reporting results of cultures from sites with normal flora can be a perplexing problem. Often it is better to specify which specific pathogens have been *excluded* by careful cultural examination, such as "no *Salmonella* isolated." Be-

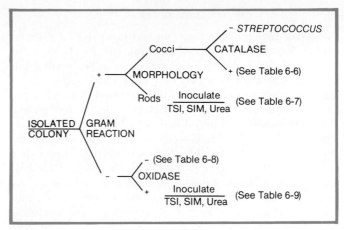

FIGURE 6–6. General flow chart for identification of common aerobic veterinary bacterial pathogens.

tween the extremes of trying to identify everything and reporting "normal flora," the technician and clinician must communicate the specific needs and most useful information expected from a given specimen. Perhaps certain potential pathogens that may be considered significant for the specimen should be carefully looked for. In other situations, a predominant bacterium can be identified or groups of organisms reported (e.g., coliforms, diphtheroids, and so forth).

Identification Procedures

Rapid identification of clinically significant bacteria is best accomplished by means of a few rapid tests that can presumptively differentiate organisms. To one who is experienced, such characteristics as colonial morphology, hemolysis, growth on MacConkey agar and odor may be adequate for presumptive identification. Often, additional differential tests are needed for more precise identification. Figure 6–6 presents a useful approach to identification of unknown isolates.

Gram's Reaction

The first differential characteristic that must be determined is the *Gram stain reaction*. Gram's stain can be performed on thin smears of bacteria from a single colony (see instructions for Gram's stain preparation in the section on Direct Microscopic Examination). Potassium hydroxide, 3 percent, may be used as an alternate and more rapid test for the Gram reaction of isolated colonies. A small drop of 3 percent potassium hydroxide (no larger than a colony) is dispensed on a slide, and a colony of bacteria is picked from the blood agar plate with a bacteriological loop and is mixed into the 3 percent potassium hydroxide. The loop is slowly and gently lifted at 5-second intervals to see whether a viscous gel is sticking to the loop. The formation of any sticky strand that can be lifted with the loop is indicative of a gram-negative bacterium. The reaction should appear within 20 to 30 seconds. Gram-positive organisms will diffusely mix in the 3 percent potassium hydroxide. Luxuriant growth on the MacConkey plate is presumptive evidence of a gram-negative organism and usually does not need to be confirmed. Cellular morphological characteristics of the gram-positive bacteria are important differential characteristics that require careful examination of a stained smear.

Table 6–5
NORMAL FLORA

Site	Aerobes	Anaerobes
Skin, ear	*Staphylococcus, Micrococcus,* diphtheroids, transient environmental and fecal contaminants	
Mouth, nasopharynx	*Micrococcus, Staphylococcus, Streptococcus* (alpha and beta), *Bacillus,* coliforms, *Proteus, Pasteurella, Actinobacillus, Haemophilus, Mycoplasma*	*Bacteroides, Fusobacterium, Actinomyces,* spirochetes and others
Trachea, bronchi, lungs	No residents, only transient contaminants	
Stomach, small intestine	Small numbers of alpha-*Streptococcus*	*Lactobacillus*
Large intestine	*Streptococcus, Escherichia coli, Klebsiella, Enterobacter, Proteus* and others	*Clostridium, Fusobacterium, Bacteroides,* spirochetes, *Lactobacillus*
Vulva, prepuce	Diphtheroids, *Micrococcus, Staphylococcus* and fecal organisms	
Conjunctiva, uterus, mammary glands	These areas may occasionally contain small numbers of insignificant bacteria	

Catalase Test

Catalase activity is an important and rapid test for differentiating *Staphylococcus* from *Streptococcus,* and *Erysipelothrix* and *Actinomyces (Corynebacterium) pyogenes* from other small gram-positive rods. Hydrogen peroxide (3 percent) is the only reagent needed and can readily be purchased from any drugstore. It should be stored in a dark bottle in the refrigerator. The *slide catalase test* is performed by picking bacteria from the center of a colony with a needle or loop and smearing the bacteria on a clean, dry slide. A drop of hydrogen peroxide is added over the bacteria and immediately observed for bubbling. Lack of bubbling is a negative test. The order of the test procedure must not be reversed or false-positive results can be obtained. If any blood agar is introduced into the test, it can also cause a false-positive result.

Oxidase Test

Cytochrome oxidase activity should be determined for all gram-negative bacteria except strong lactose fermenters, which will be negative. Commercial cytochrome oxidase test reagents are readily available and conveniently packaged for use in small laboratories. The reaction is supposed to be clearly visible within a few seconds, but with some of the reagents the reaction may be delayed for up to 2 minutes for *Pasteurella* and *Actinobacillus.* A heavy inoculum must be used for accurate testing. A wooden stick or platinum loop should be used to pick colonies for testing, because trace amounts of iron from other loops can cause false-positive results.

Presumptive Identification

When the Gram reaction, cellular morphological characteristics, catalase and oxidase results have been determined, the bacteria can be tentatively grouped, and differential tests can be selected as indicated in Figure 6–6 for identification.

Isolates of *Streptococcus* are usually characterized by the type of hemolysis they produce. Beta-hemolytic *Streptococcus* is usually considered to be a potential pathogen. Alpha- and nonhemolytic *Streptococcus* usually originate from normal flora of skin and mucous membranes and are not considered significant unless they are isolated from normally sterile sites.

Isolates of *Staphylococcus* should be differentiated from *Micrococcus* (Table 6–6), which are considered to be nonpathogenic.

Table 6–6
DIFFERENTIATION OF GRAM-POSITIVE, CATALASE-POSITIVE COCCI

Organism	Hemolysis	Hyaluronidase	Glucose Fermentation	Coagulase
Staphylococcus aureus	+ *	+	+	+
Staphylococcus intermedius	+ *	−	+	+
Staphylococcus epidermidis	±		+	−
Micrococcus	−		−	−

*Double zones of complete and incomplete hemolysis are frequently observed.

Glucose-fermenting ability, determined in TSI agar slants, can be used for differentiation of these genera. If a double zone of hemolysis is observed on the blood agar plate, the bacterium can be identified as a coagulase-positive *Staphylococcus* without need for further testing. All other *Staphylococcus* isolates should be tested for coagulase activity because coagulase activity correlates with pathogenicity. Speciation of coagulase-positive and coagulase-negative *Staphylococcus* spp. may be attempted in special cases.

The small gram-positive rods can be differentiated by inoculating TSI, urea and sulfide-indole-motility (SIM) media. The results of these tests, as well as colonial morphology and catalase activity, can identify the isolate (Table 6–7). Individual characteristics of the important pathogens in this group will be discussed later.

Most gram-negative, oxidase-negative bacteria are members of the Enterobacteriaceae family. These bacteria are reactive in biochemical tests and can be identified by one of several different systems. The most rapid and economical methods for differentiating the Enterobacteriaceae family members are the commercially available packaged multitest systems. These systems are discussed further on. There are a few other organisms that may be isolated infrequently that are oxidase-negative. The most common reason for nonenteric oxidase-negative results is a false-negative oxidase test result. When such results are suspected, further differentiation of oxidase-negative bacteria, as shown in Table 6–8, is necessary.

Table 6–7
DIFFERENTIATION OF SMALL, NONSPORE-FORMING GRAM-POSITIVE RODS

Organism	Motility (22°)	Catalase	Hydrogen Sulfide in TSI	Urease	Hemolysis	Colony Morphological Characteristics
Listeria monocytogenes	+	+	−	−	Complete	Very small
Erysipelothrix rhusiopathiae	−	−	+	−	Slow, greenish	Very small
Actinomyces pyogenes	−	−	−	−	Complete	Very small
Corynebacterium renale	−	+	−	+	V	Medium size, entire
Corynebacterium pseudotuberculosis	−	+	−	+ (w)	V	Dry, grainy white
Rhodococcus equi	−	+	−	+ (d)	−	Large, mucoid, pink
Other diphtheroids	−	+	−	V	V	V

d = delayed, may require up to 2 weeks
V = variable results
w = weak

Table 6–8
DIFFERENTIATION OF GRAM-NEGATIVE, OXIDASE-NEGATIVE BACTERIA

	Growth on MacConkey	TSI	Motility	Identification Method
Enterobacteriaceae	+	A/A, K/A	+*	Micro-ID or API 20E
Pasteurella, Actinobacillus	–	A/A, A/NC	–	See Table 6–9†
Pseudomonas	+	K/NC	+	
Acinetobacter	+ (w)	K/NC	–	

*Klebsiella is nonmotile.
†Negative oxidase results are caused by very weak reactions.
w = weak
A = acid
K = alkaline
NC = no change

The most frequently isolated oxidase-positive, gram-negative bacteria of veterinary importance can be differentiated by using three tubes of media (TSI, urea and SIM) as shown in Table 6–9.

Definitive Identification

The identification procedures discussed in this chapter are presumptive methods. Definitive identification of some isolates may require extensive testing. The cost of such identification in time, media and specialized techniques is usually not justifiable in a small practice laboratory. Unusual isolates should be forwarded to a referral laboratory for further identification. The isolate should be subcultured to an agar slant medium that does not contain a fermentable carbohydrate, or it should be heavily inoculated onto a swab. The swab can be transported in a transport medium such as Amies transport medium. Do not attempt to ship agar plates. Invariably, they become contaminated and overgrown, dehydrated or broken.

Commercial Identification Kits

Commercial development of kit systems for identification of bacteria has been one of the most important advances in clinical bacteriology. These systems provide a cost-effective method for identification of bacteria in low-volume laboratories. Most kits consist of a number of test compartments arranged in a compact unit. The systems generally utilize microtechnique tests in various types of media systems. They may include compartments of solid agar, dehydrated broth, substrate or reagent disks and supplementary conventional tests. All compartments are inoculated with organisms from an isolated colony or colonies. After the specified period of incubation and the addition of required reagents, the results are recorded as positive or negative for each test. For many of the systems, these reactions have variously weighted values so that the positive results will produce a unique profile number for each combination of positive and negative results. Most systems provide profile directories or registers for identification of the isolate most likely to produce the set of observed reactions.

It is advantageous for the low-volume laboratory to use these systems because they are usually more cost-effective than attempting to maintain a large inventory of conventional media. They have a reasonable shelf life (6 to 18 months) and require minimum storage space because of the compact construction. Accuracy is better than conventional media in most small laboratories, as most reactions are easy to interpret and results can be decoded more rapidly than sorting through conventional identification tables. Finally, depending upon the spe-

Table 6–9
DIFFERENTIATION OF GRAM-NEGATIVE, OXIDASE-POSITIVE BACTERIA

Organism	Glucose Fermentation in TSI Agar	Growth on MacConkey Agar	Motility	Hemolysis	Urease	Indole
Aeromonas spp.	+	+	+	+	–	+
Actinobacillus spp.	+	±	–	+ (V)	+	–
Pasteurella haemolytica	+	±	–	+*	–	–
Pasteurella multocida	+	–	–	–	–	+
Pasteurella pneumotropica	+	–	–	–	+	+
Pasteurella spp.	+	–	–	–	±	+
Pseudomonas aeruginosa	–	+	+	+	±	–
Pseudomonas spp.	–	+	+	V	V	–
Bordetella bronchiseptica	–	+ (w)	+	–	+	–
Moraxella bovis	–	–	–	±	–	–
Moraxella spp.	–	–	–	–	–	–
Brucella canis	–	–	–	–	+	–

*Hemolysis under the colony
V = variable
w = weak

cific system, most bacteria can be identified within 4 to 24 hours after isolation.

It is absolutely essential that the manufacturer's directions and precautions be followed implicitly or misidentification will occur. If the system is limited to oxidase-negative enteric bacteria, only those organisms should be inoculated. Other organisms can still yield a profile number, which will result in an incorrect identification. Therefore, these systems still require evaluation by a competent microbiologist who can determine whether the results correlate with other laboratory findings and the clinical history. Problems can also arise from inoculation with an older culture, improper concentration of inoculum or mixed cultures. For the proper use of these systems, some personnel retraining may be necessary. As experience is gained, accuracy will be increased.

When selecting one of these systems, factors to consider include (1) the ease of inoculation, (2) manipulations required to add reagents, (3) the availability of interpretive charts or numerical coding devices and (4) the data base used in development of profile registers. Often it is difficult to discover whether significant numbers of veterinary pathogens are included in the data bases in order for there to be a reasonable probability of correct identification of unique veterinary pathogens.

The most beneficial use of these systems is the identification of members of the Enterobacteriaceae family (see Table 6–3). All enteric identification systems give essentially the same degree of accuracy and reliability of performance if strict attention is paid to the manufacturer's instructions. The systems that seem to have gained widest acceptance in veterinary bacteriology include API 20E, Micro-ID and Enterotube II. The data base and accuracy of the identifications provide excellent results.

Several packaged kit systems are marketed for identification of gram-negative bacteria other than Enterobacteriaceae (see Table 6–3). These systems have limited usefulness in small veterinary laboratories. Present data bases are largely based on human pathogens rather than unique gram-negative bacteria that are host-specific to various animals (*Pasteurella, Actinobacillus, Haemophilus, Moraxella,* and so forth). Presumptive identification methods outlined in this chapter are frequently more accurate and less expensive.

Identification kits are available for gram-positive cocci (see Table 6–3). Although these systems may provide more definitive identifications of some organisms, the clinical relevance and cost-effectiveness of their use has not been adequately evaluated in veterinary microbiology.

The identification kits for yeast and anaerobes are useful for large-volume laboratories, but usually the need for them in the small laboratory is not adequate to be cost-effective.

Special Culture Procedures

Blood Cultures

The detection of viable bacteria in an animal's blood has considerable diagnostic and prognostic importance. Blood cultures are indicated for fever of unknown origin, suspected bacteremia associated with endocarditis, arthritis, meningitis and neonatal septicemias. Blood cultures should be obtained from dogs that have antibodies to *Brucella canis* to aid in confirmation of the diagnosis.

Special care must be taken to avoid contaminating blood cultures with skin microflora. The venipuncture site should be decontaminated using surgical scrubbing procedures (see Chapter 12) and should not be palpated after preparation unless a sterile glove is used. Blood can be obtained by using a syringe and needle or a closed-vacuum bottle system. Often the concentration of bacteria in blood is too low to detect by direct inoculation of plate media. Therefore, inoculation of broth media is a more sensitive culture system. Ideally, a sample of 5 to 10 ml of blood should be obtained for culture. The blood should be inoculated into an approved blood culture bottle immediately. Blood samples in anticoagulants, such as heparin and ethylenediamine-tetraacetic acid (EDTA), are not acceptable for culture because of the poor survival of some bacteria in the presence of these anticoagulants. Commercially available blood culture media bottles are recommended.

Blood culture samples should not be obtained more frequently than once per hour. If a patient in critical condition is to be started immediately on antibiotics, multiple samples should be collected from different venipuncture sites. Usually, arterial blood provides a yield that is no better than that provided by venous blood. For fever of unknown origin and subacute endocarditis, obtain two separate blood cultures on the first day and again on the second day if bacterial growth is not present in the first set of cultures.

Blood culture bottles should be incubated at 35°C to 37°C for at least 7 days and examined daily for macroscopic evidence of growth. Positive cultures can be recognized by one or more of the following characteristics: turbidity, gas bubbles, fluffy or compact colonies and hemolysis of the blood. When growth is observed, gram-stained smears and subcultures on plate media should be prepared for examination and identification of the organism. Negative-appearing blood culture broths should be blindly subcultured before being discarded and reported as negative.

Brucella isolation from blood can be enhanced by using a Castaneda culture bottle. The biphasic system provides an agar surface for more efficient isolation of *Brucella*. Cultures for this agent should be held for 2 to 4 weeks before being discarded as negative.

Urine Cultures

Urine is an excellent growth medium for many bacteria because it contains electrolytes, water-soluble vitamins, residual amounts of glucose and various nitrogenous compounds. Therefore, it is imperative that careful attention be given to proper collection and handling of urine for culture, or a small and insignificant number of bacteria can rapidly multiply to significant numbers. Urine specimens for culturing can be collected in three ways: (1) free catch, (2) catheterization or (3) cystocentesis (see Chapter 8). The distal urethra and genitalia are colonized with microflora that contaminate free-catch and catheterization specimens. If the skin has been adequately prepared for cystocentesis specimens, and the needle does not contact any abdominal organ other than the bladder, any bacteria isolated from the specimen should be significant. To reduce overgrowth with insignificant bacteria that may contaminate urine specimens, cultures should be set up within 2 hours of collection. If cultures cannot be established within 2 hours, the sample must be refrigerated to slow the bacterial growth. Refrigeration begins to fail after 18 to 24 hours. Therefore, the best method for identifying urinary tract infections is to establish cultures as soon as possible.

The bacteriological examination of urine specimens collected by methods other than cystocentesis should provide an estimate of the number of microorganisms per milliliter of urine as an aid in evaluating the significance of culture results. Direct microscopic examination of a gram-stained smear of uncentrifuged urine is recommended. If one or more bacteria per oil immersion field are observed, usually greater than 10^5 per ml are present, and this is indicative of significant bacteruria. If the specimen is contaminated with normal urogenital flora, bacteria will usually be found at concentrations of less than 10^4 per ml and will not be observed by direct microscopic examination. Between 10^4 and 10^5 bacteria per ml in a specimen may be an indication of urinary tract infection and should be correlated with clinical signs for determination of the significance. Bacterial counts can be low because of improper handling of the specimen, dilution from forced fluid therapy or cystocentesis samples from patients with urethritis that has not become established as a concomitant cystitis.

The use of blood agar and MacConkey agar as selective and differential isolation media is recommended for the culture of all urine specimens. There is no need for broth medium for enrichment culturing. A blood agar plate should be inoculated with a standard dilution loop calibrated to deliver approximately 0.001 ml as illustrated in Figure 6–7. Each colony represents 10^3 organisms per ml in the specimen; therefore, the number of colonies is multiplied by 1000 to obtain the concentration of organisms in the specimen. Bacteria are identified as described in this chapter. If more than two types of bacteria are isolated, a second specimen should be collected and cultured to distinguish a mixed infection from contamination or mishandling of the specimen.

COMMON BACTERIAL SPECIES

The bacterial pathogens frequently associated with many infectious processes are listed in Table 6–1. Some of the colony morphological characteristics, growth and identifying characteristics of these bacteria are listed in Table 6–10. Additional details are given in the following discussion for special isolation and identification techniques. Clinically important characteristics are noted.

Gram-Positive Cocci

Staphylococcus

Staphylococcus spp. are catalase-positive cocci that occur in grape-like clusters. They are frequently isolated from pyogenic lesions, such as wounds, dermatitis, otitis, mastitis, cystitis and osteomyelitis. As stated previously, they are usually divided into coagulase-positive and coagulase-negative strains. The coagulase-positive species, *S. aureus* and *S. intermedius*, are more important pathogens, and the others are usually considered to be less pathogenic. One of the most important identifying characteristics that should be noted is the development of a double zone of hemolysis (an inner zone of complete hemolysis and a second zone of incomplete hemolysis). This is a common identifying characteristic of most coagulase-positive isolates from

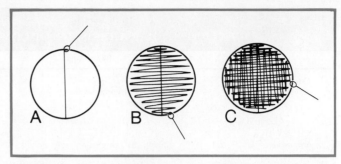

FIGURE 6–7. Procedure for inoculating media for semiquantitative bacterial colony counts when culturing urine. A, Primary inoculation with calibrated loop. B, Streak at right angles to primary inoculation. C, Streak at right angles to previous streak.

animals. Mannitol fermentation is not a reliable correlate of coagulase activity in staphylococcal isolates from animals. Because of a high incidence of acquired antimicrobial resistance, these organisms should be tested for antimicrobial susceptibility.

Streptococcus

Streptococcus spp. are catalase-negative cocci that occur singly, in pairs or in short chains. Chain formation is more easily demonstrated in broth cultures. *Streptococcus* is the most common bacterial pathogen of the horse and can be found to cause pyogenic infections and mastitis in all species of animals. However, the species tend to be rather host-specific. Therefore, the streptococcal pathogens of humans rarely cause infections in animals, and animals are usually not reservoirs of human pathogens. Some species cause specific diseases. *Streptococcus equi* is the cause of strangles in horses. *Streptococcus agalactiae* is an important cause of bovine mastitis. It can be identified by the CAMP test. Definitive biochemical and serological (Lancefield typing) testing is usually not clinically important. It is important to evaluate the hemolysis produced on blood agar. Beta-hemolysis (complete clearing) usually correlates well with potential pathogenicity; alpha-hemolysis (incomplete greenish discoloring) and gamma-hemolysis (nonhemolytic) are usually indications of normal flora of skin and mucous membranes. However, when isolated in nearly pure culture from normally sterile body sites, these organisms can be considered to be clinically significant. Susceptibility to antimicrobials is usually predictable, which means that antimicrobial susceptibility testing may be an unnecessary expense.

Anaerobic Cocci

Anaerobic cocci belong to the genera *Peptococcus* and *Peptostreptococcus*. When isolated, these agents are usually associated with mixed anaerobic infections.

Gram-Positive Rods

Spore Formers

Bacillus spp. are the most common contaminants isolated in the laboratory. They are ubiquitous in soil, water, air and dust. They are large spore-forming rods that usually grow as large,

Table 6–10
IDENTIFYING CHARACTERISTICS OF COMMON VETERINARY BACTERIAL PATHOGENS

	Blood Agar	MacConkey Agar	Other Characteristics
Gram-positive			
Staphylococcus	Smooth, glistening white to yellow pigmented colonies.	No growth.	Catalase-positive glucose fermenter. Double-zone hemolysis usually indicates coagulase-positive. Coagulase activity is a useful differential test.
Streptococcus	Small, glistening colonies; hemolysis.	No growth except some enterococci.	Catalase-negative, usually identified by type of hemolysis. Beta-hemolytic strains more likely to be pathogens, others are often part of flora; Streptococcus agalactiae CAMP-positive.
Actinomyces pyogenes	Small, hemolytic strep-like colonies.	No growth.	Catalase-negative; slow growth, often requiring 48 hr for distinct colonies, growth enhanced in candle jar.
Corynebacterium pseudotuberculosis	Slow-growing, opaque, dry crumbly colonies; usually hemolytic.	No growth.	Catalase-positive; weak urease-positive.
Corynebacterium renale	Small, smooth, glistening colonies (24 hr); become opaque and dry later.	No growth.	Catalase-positive, urease-positive.
Rhodococcus equi	Small, moist, white (24 hr) become large, pink colonies, no hemolysis.	No growth.	Catalase-positive, delayed urease-positive.
Listeria monocytogenes	Small, hemolytic, glistening colonies.	No growth.	Catalase-positive, motile at room temperature.
Erysipelothrix rhusiopathiae	Small colonies after 48 hr; greenish (alpha) hemolysis.	No growth.	Catalase-negative, hydrogen sulfide-positive.
Nocardia	Slow-growing, small, dry, granular, white to orange colonies.	No growth.	Partially acid-fast, colonies tenaciously adhere to media.
Actinomyces	Slow-growing, small, rough, nodular white colonies.	No growth.	Require increased carbon dioxide or anaerobic incubation, not acid-fast.
Clostridium	Variable, round, ill-defined, irregular colonies usually hemolytic.	No growth.	Obligate anaerobes.
Bacillus	Variable, large, rough, dry or mucoid colonies.	No growth.	Usually hemolytic, large rods with endospores.
Gram-negative			
Escherichia coli	Large, gray, smooth, mucoid colonies, hemolysis variable.	Hot-pink to red colonies; red cloudiness in media.	Hemolysis frequently associated with virulence.
Klebsiella pneumoniae	Large, mucoid, sticky, whitish colonies, not hemolytic.	Large, mucoid, pink colonies.	Nonmotile, require biochemical tests to differentiate from Enterobacter.
Proteus	Frequently swarming without distinct colonies.	Colorless, limited swarming.	
Other enterics	Gray to white smooth, mucoid colonies.	Colorless colonies.	Biochemical tests for identification, serotyping indicated for Salmonella.
Pseudomonas	Irregular, spreading, grayish colonies, variable hemolysis, may show a metallic sheen.	Colorless, irregular colonies.	Oxidase-positive, fruity odor, may produce yellow-greenish soluble pigment in clear media.
Bordetella bronchiseptica	Very small, circular dewdrop colonies, variable hemolysis.	Small, colorless colonies.	May require 48 hr for distinct colonies, oxidase-positive, rapid urease-positive, citrate-positive.
Brucella canis	Very small, circular, pinpoint colonies after 48–72 hr, not hemolytic.	No growth.	Oxidase-positive, catalase-positive, urease-positive.
Moraxella	Round, translucent, grayish-white colonies, variable hemolysis.	No growth.	Oxidase- and catalase-positive, often nonreactive in routine biochemical tests. Colonies may pit media.
Actinobacillus	Round, translucent colonies, variable hemolysis.	Variable growth, colorless colonies.	Glucose fermenter, nonmotile, urease-positive. Sticky colonies.
Pasteurella haemolytica	Round, gray, smooth colonies; hemolysis under the colony.	Variable growth, colorless colonies.	Glucose fermenter in TSI, weak oxidase-positive.
Pasteurella multocida	Gray, mucoid, round to coalescing colonies, no hemolysis.	No growth.	Glucose fermenter in TSI, weak oxidase- and indole-positives.

rough, granular or spreading colonies. They are usually hemolytic. Occasionally strains of *Bacillus* will be isolated that react as if they are gram-negative and oxidase-positive. However, they can be identified by the presence of spores in stained smears. *Bacillus anthracis* (the agent that causes anthrax) is the only important pathogenic species. It is extremely virulent for humans. *Do not attempt to culture it.*

Clostridium spp. are large, spore-forming anaerobic rods. There are many nonpathogenic species of soil origin. The pathogenic species are noted for their potent toxins and extensive destruction of tissue. Infections may be accompanied by an accumulation of gas (emphysema) in the tissues. Laboratory diagnosis of the toxic diseases (tetanus, botulism and enterotoxemia) and differentiation of the infectious diseases (black-

leg, malignant edema, bacillary hemoglobinuria, and so forth) require the assistance of reference diagnostic laboratories. Often a Gram-stained smear is a useful technique for ruling out clostridial disease or indicating it as a possibility. *Clostridium perfringens* is occasionally isolated from deep wounds with extensive tissue necrosis, such as compound fractures. The bacterium requires an anaerobic atmosphere for growth and frequently produces a double zone of hemolysis.

Small Rods

Corynebacterium spp. are small, club-shaped rods that tend to occur in palisades or in an angular arrangement because of their "snapping" division. Colonies are usually quite small at

24 hours but continue to enlarge and vary markedly by species. Most species are catalase-positive. *Actinomyces pyogenes* (previously called *C. pyogenes*) produces a small pinpoint colony, hemolysis and negative catalase reaction. Cellular morphological characteristics must be evaluated carefully to differentiate it from *Streptococcus*. It is the most common pyogenic agent in ruminants. *Rhodococcus equi* (also known as *Corynebacterium equi*) is a cause of pneumonia and abscesses in foals. Morphologically, individual cells are coccobacillary and larger than other *Corynebacterium* organisms. *Corynebacterium pseudotuberculosis* (formerly known as *C. ovis*) causes chronic abscesses in goats and sheep. *Corynebacterium renale* is a cause of pyelonephritis and cystitis in cows. There are many other *Corynebacterium* spp. that are nonpathogenic commensals of the skin. They are frequently referred to collectively as diphtheroids.

Listeria monocytogenes is a small, non-spore-forming rod that is catalase-positive. It is the only small gram-positive rod that is motile at room temperature. It is an infrequent cause of abortion in large animals and septicemia in young animals. In ruminants, it causes an encephalitis known as circling disease. The bacteria localize in the pons and medulla (brain stem). Cultures from other parts of the brain may be negative. Isolation may require a cold enrichment technique. The brain is stored in a refrigerator and cultured weekly for up to 12 weeks before the results are considered negative.

Erysipelothrix rhusiopathiae is a pleomorphic rod, which is usually slender and small. The colony is small, and an incomplete, greenish hemolysis (alpha-like) is produced. The cellular morphological characteristics must be carefully evaluated to differentiate it from *Streptococcus* because both are catalase-negative. A definitive characteristic that differentiates it from other gram-positive rods is the production of hydrogen sulfide. *Erysipelothrix* is most commonly encountered as a cause of septicemic or arthritic disease of pigs, but it is occasionally a cause of endocarditis in dogs.

Filamentous Rods

The Actinomycetaceae family contains several clinically important bacteria. Most *Actinomyces* spp. are anaerobic bacteria that may tolerate low levels of oxygen. Therefore, some species can be isolated in a candle jar, but the most efficient isolation can be achieved with an anaerobic system. *Actinomyces* spp. are usually branching, filamentous gram-positive rods. Colonies are slow to develop, requiring up to 5 days, and are usually raised and irregular in shape. When isolated, they are usually recovered from pyogranulomatous lesions of soft tissue, pyothoraces or osteomyelitis. *Nocardia* spp. have cellular morphological characteristics similar to those of *Actinomyces*. They are partially acid-fast, which means a modified staining procedure must be used. In place of the acid-alcohol decolorizer, only an acid decolorizer is used to demonstrate acid-fastness. *Nocardia* spp. are aerobic bacteria with colonies usually appearing after 2 to 5 days of incubation. The colonies are rough and have a dry, granular texture. They adhere tenaciously to the media. *Nocardia* is occasionally isolated from pyothoraces and wounds. It may be a serious mastitis pathogen in some dairy herds. *Dermatophilus congolensis* is another branching, filamentous bacterium. It often has a beaded appearance with transverse and longitudinal divisions. It is an uncommon cause of skin infections of horses and ruminants. The organism can be demonstrated in smears of pus from under the elevated scabs containing tufts of hair. *Streptomyces* spp. are aerobic, filamentous bacteria that are not acid-fast. They are abundant in soil and may be isolated as contaminants.

Anaerobes

Anaerobic gram-positive non-spore-forming rods belong to the genera *Bifidobacterium*, *Eubacterium* and *Propionibacterium*. If definitive identification of these organisms is needed, they should be sent to a reference diagnostic laboratory. They are usually isolated in mixed cultures from pyogenic lesions.

Acid-Fast Bacteria

Mycobacteria are mostly small, short rods but are occasionally pleomorphic. They stain poorly with Gram's stain but are acid-fast. These bacteria are rarely isolated in veterinary practice laboratories, because special procedures and media are usually required. However, preparation of an acid-fast stained impression smear can be a useful diagnostic procedure for making a presumptive diagnosis of mycobacterial infection. Positive findings are significant; however, negative findings have limited predictive value. *Mycobacterium paratuberculosis* may be demonstrated in acid-fast stained smears prepared from intestinal mucosa or mesenteric lymph nodes of ruminants. *Mycobacterium avium* infection of birds can frequently be confirmed by examination of acid-fast smears prepared from the liver or intestinal mucosa. Occasionally, abundant acid-fast organisms can be demonstrated in the feces.

Isolation of the agents of tuberculosis, *Mycobacterium bovis* and *Mycobacterium tuberculosis*, should not be attempted in a clinic laboratory. Infrequently, a rapid-growing *Mycobacterium* may be isolated from cases of bovine mastitis. The colonies will usually appear at 3 to 5 days of incubation. These organisms should be forwarded to a reference laboratory for definitive identification.

Gram-Negative Bacteria

The Enterobacteriaceae family of bacteria is the largest group of potential pathogens and the most frequently isolated bacteria. The normal habitat of these organisms is the digestive tract and soil; therefore, they will usually grow on MacConkey agar and are frequently insignificant contaminants of specimens. They are small gram-negative rods, with some pleomorphism. Some of the common identifying characteristics include oxidase negativity, glucose fermentation and motility (except *Klebsiella*). Genus and species identification requires numerous biochemical tests, and serotyping is frequently needed to identify pathogenic strains. Acquired antimicrobial resistance from R-factors (plasmids) is common in this family of bacteria, making antimicrobial susceptibility testing a necessary clinical evaluation of isolates.

Most non-Enterobacteriaceae gram-negative bacteria are oxidase-positive, and growth on MacConkey agar is variable.

Coliforms

Escherichia coli can frequently be presumptively identified by the strong lactose fermentation reaction it produces on MacConkey agar. Strains causing tissue infections and cystitis are frequently hemolytic. *Escherichia coli* is frequently associated with diarrhea in neonates (especially pigs, calves and lambs). The pathogenic strains causing diarrhea have special surface antigens (pili) and produce enterotoxins. Identification of these characteristics requires specialized laboratory testing, such as use of the K-99 *E. coli* antigen test kit (Kolichek, Synbiotics Corp.). However, presumptive evidence of *Escherichia coli* involvement in diarrhea (scours) can be obtained by Gram-staining a smear taken from small intestinal mucosa shortly after the death of the animal. If a large number (>25) of gram-negative rods are observed in each oil immersion field, it is a strong indication that *Escherichia coli* is a cause of diarrhea.

Klebsiella spp. and *Enterobacter* spp. are occasionally involved in infections of the respiratory and urinary tracts and in mastitis. They are becoming more important in veterinary medicine as superinfecting agents following antimicrobial therapy.

Salmonella

Salmonella spp. can cause diarrhea and septicemia in all animals and in humans. When culturing feces, selective and enrichment media should be used to increase the probability of successful isolation of *Salmonella*. Hektoen enteric agar and selenite enrichment broth (see Table 6–2) are recommended. The enrichment broth should be subcultured to both MacConkey and Hektoen enteric agar. Non-lactose-fermenting colonies can rapidly be screened with *Salmonella* polyvalent O antiserum to identify them. In order to be able to define the epidemiology of salmonellosis outbreaks, the isolates should be forwarded to a reference laboratory for serotyping.

Proteus

Proteus spp. are frequently isolated as specimen contaminants or secondary invaders. They are important pathogens of the urinary tract. Related genera of bacteria that do not swarm on blood agar are *Morganella* and *Providencia*. The swarming *Proteus* spp. sometimes interfere with isolation of other organisms. This problem can be solved by using phenylethyl alcohol (PEA) blood agar plates. *Proteus* and other gram-negative organisms will be inhibited, providing easier isolation of gram-positive organisms.

Other Enterics

There are many other members of the Enterobacteriaceae family, including *Serratia*, *Citrobacter*, *Edwardsiella* and *Hafnia*, that are infrequently isolated. Careful clinical evaluation is necessary to determine their significance. Often, a repeated culture helps confirm the significance of isolation.

Aeromonas

Aeromonas spp. are oxidase-positive rods that grow on MacConkey agar. They are commonly found in soil, water and sewage and frequently infect aquatic animals. They are infrequently a cause of septicemia in terrestrial animals. Some strains grow best at room temperature.

Actinobacillus

Actinobacillus spp. are oxidase-positive, small rods that usually grow on MacConkey agar. The colony morphological characteristics are similar to those of *Pasteurella*. *Actinobacillus equuli* is the most frequently isolated species. It produces a very sticky colony. It is frequently the cause of septicemic infections in foals. It can be isolated from most horses as part of the naso-oropharyngeal flora but is generally only an opportunistic pathogen in older horses.

Pasteurella

Pasteurella spp. are usually associated with respiratory infections in most animals. In cats, they are frequently recovered from abscesses. They are small, oxidase-positive coccobacilli. Identification can be aided by noting the typically weak glucose fermentation reaction in a TSI tube. *Pasteurella* spp. tend to be nonreactive in most commercial identification kit systems and may be misidentified. All *Pasteurella* spp. are nonhemolytic except *Pasteurella haemolytica*. Its colony must be removed in order to observe the hemolysis that occurs directly under the colony. *Pasteurella multocida* produces a characteristic "musty" odor.

Haemophilus

Haemophilus spp. are often part of the normal flora of mucous membranes. A few species are important pathogens, usually of the respiratory system. They are small coccobacilli that require specially enriched media for growth. They may grow as satellite colonies around *Staphylococcus* on blood agar. In addition to the nutritional growth requirements, an increased concentration of carbon dioxide is necessary. These bacteria are very susceptible to antibiotics and environmental stress factors, such as drying; therefore, specimens must be collected and handled carefully or isolation will be unsuccessful.

Pseudomonas

Pseudomonas spp. are common soil and water bacteria. They are usually considered to be opportunistic pathogens of wounds and otitis. Infrequently, they are isolated from the respiratory and urinary tracts. There are many species, but *Pseudomonas aeruginosa* is the most common pathogen. It produces water-soluble yellow-green pigments that diffuse into the media, and it has a distinctive odor that aids in recognition.

Bordetella

Bordetella bronchiseptica is a small coccobacillus that is frequently recovered from respiratory infections of dogs. It is associated with atrophic rhinitis in pigs and is infrequently isolated from respiratory infections of other animals. Colonies are slow to develop and may only be pinpointed after 48 hours. Growth occurs on MacConkey agar. It is oxidase-positive, urease-positive (often within 4 hours) and citrate-positive.

Brucella

Brucella spp. are very small coccobacilli that are usually associated with reproductive failure—abortion and infertility. Some species require increased carbon dioxide for growth; however, *Brucella canis* can be isolated in an aerobic atmosphere. Growth is slow, often requiring from 3 to 7 days for colonies to be detectable. Suspected *Brucella* isolates should be sent to a reference laboratory for definitive identification because of the economic and zoonotic importance of these agents.

Other Gram-Negative Rods

There are a large number of gram-negative bacteria that have little or undetermined clinical importance. Included are bacteria such as *Moraxella, Acinetobacter, Neisseria, Branhamella* and related pleomorphic coccobacilli. These organisms are commonly found as part of the flora of mucous membranes and are usually secondary, opportunistic pathogens. They are relatively nonreactive in most conventional biochemical tests. Thus, identification is usually difficult, even for reference diagnostic laboratories.

Anaerobes

The gram-negative anaerobes, *Bacteroides* and *Fusobacterium*, are frequently involved in mixed infections in abscesses and necrotic tissue. They are normally found in the digestive tract, so infections resulting from contamination of tissues with mucous membrane flora or intestinal contents frequently contain these organisms. Usually Gram's stain of the exudate will indicate that bacteria that do not grow aerobically are present. If obligate anaerobes are isolated, evaluation of the cellular morphological characteristics provides adequate clinical information. Species identification is rarely important. Recent taxonomic advances have resulted in the reclassification of some former *Bacteroides* spp. into the genera *Dichelobacter, Porphyromonas* and *Prevotella*.

Spirochetes and Curved Bacteria

Leptospira spp. cause febrile infections often followed by abortion and infertility. These spirochetes are difficult to isolate and usually die within a few hours while being transported to a laboratory. Darkfield examination of urine may aid in establishing a diagnosis. Most diagnoses are made by serological testing.

Borrelia burgdorferi is a tick-transmitted spirochete that causes Lyme disease in humans and arthritis and lameness in dogs. Canine borreliosis may be accompanied by high rectal temperature and lymphadenopathy. Detection of serum antibodies to *B. burgdorferi* by indirect fluorescent antibody tests currently is the diagnostic test of choice in dogs. Isolation of *Borrelia* by culture is difficult and often nonproductive. Borreliosis appears to be a disease of emerging importance in the United States in dogs and other animals within areas infested by ticks carrying this agent.

Treponema (Serpulina) hyodysenteriae is a spirochete that causes dysentery in pigs. Cultural isolation is beyond the capability of most laboratories. Diagnosis of this infection may be made by examining smears of colonic mucosa for numerous large spirochetes.

Campylobacter spp. cause two different types of disease conditions. One group contains important reproductive pathogens, causing abortion and infertility. Because of special needs for enrichment and selective media and a microaerophilic atmosphere, specimens for isolation of *Campylobacter* should be sent to veterinary diagnostic laboratories specially equipped for *Campylobacter* culture. The second group is emerging as important zoonotic enteric pathogens. Most public health and hospital laboratories are equipped to isolate this group. *Campylobacter* spp. are curved gram-negative rods. They can be recognized by darkfield or phase-contrast microscopy by their darting motility.

Mycoplasma

Mycoplasma spp. are small bacteria that lack a cell wall and, as a result, are not easily stained and observed in exudates. Arthritis and pneumonia are the most common mycoplasmal diseases. The role of *Mycoplasma* in urogenital infections is not well characterized. Special media and techniques are required for isolation and identification of *Mycoplasma*. Therefore, arrangements should be made with a reference laboratory for *Mycoplasma* transport media and specimen shipping instructions.

ANTIMICROBIAL SUSCEPTIBILITY TESTING

One of the purposes of the clinical microbiology laboratory is to provide information that can assist in the selection of appropriate therapy for infectious diseases. All antimicrobial agents have limitations in their spectra of activity. Therefore, a universal antimicrobial for all infections is not available. Some organisms are intrinsically resistant to an antimicrobial, whereas others acquire resistance. The most common mechanism for acquired resistance is the acquisition of extrachromosomal pieces of DNA (deoxyribonucleic acid) such as plasmids (R-factors) and bacteriophages. As a result, the bacteria are able to produce enzymes that modify or inactivate the antimicrobial, enable the cell to resist penetration of the drug or alter target sites and reduce the activity of the drug. Because the acquired resistance traits are not static, the antimicrobial susceptibility pattern *(antibiogram)* is not predictable for many organisms. Therefore, susceptibility tests are necessary.

Indications for Susceptibility Testing

Susceptibility testing is indicated for most rapidly growing, aerobic and facultative anaerobic, clinically significant bacteria. Testing should be avoided for isolates representing normal flora and for those bacteria with predictable susceptibility to the antimicrobial of choice. Gram-positive bacteria other than *Staphylococcus* have rather predictable antibiograms; therefore, routine testing is not needed. However, susceptibility testing may be indicated if the antimicrobial of choice cannot be safely and economically administered to the patient. *Unpredictable resistance patterns are frequently observed with the gram-negative bacteria,* thus requiring testing. Most slow-growing and anaerobic bacteria have rather predictable antibiograms, so testing is not necessary. If acquired resistance is found to be a problem in these organisms, special test methods will be necessary for testing them.

In most cases, the veterinarian will have started antimicrobial therapy before the laboratory results are available. When the test results become available, therapy can be altered or modified to provide safe, effective, least-cost therapy. In some situations, the culture specimen will be from a moribund or dead animal. Susceptibility testing may still be important because it

A grid's purpose is to allow only the primary x-ray beam to pass through and prevent scattered radiations from reaching the film. The grid is constructed in such a way as to absorb all radiations that do not pass between the lead strips. This arrangement may absorb most scattered radiations if grids of high ratios are used. However, it has the disadvantage of absorbing part of the primary x-ray beam and therefore requires greater exposure time to obtain a given film density. Figure 7–24 illustrates how a grid absorbs scattered and secondary radiation and prevents it from reaching the film.

Grids are made of different ratios and number of strips per 2.5 cm. The ratio varies from 5:1 to 16:1 and from 60 lines (strips) per 2.5 cm to 120 lines per 2.5 cm. The higher the ratio and the number of lines per 2.5 cm, the more expensive the grid. The ratio of a grid refers to the relation between the depth of the lead strips to the width of the radiolucent spaces. For example, if the depth of the lead strip is 12 times greater than the space's thickness, the grid ratio will be 12:1, and if it is 10 times greater, the ratio will be 10:1 and so on. The greater the ratio, the more efficiently the grid absorbs scattered radiations. Figure 7–24A illustrates the ratio of a 5:1 grid.

The grid is most useful in radiographing parts of the body in which scattering is considerable, which in practice includes all thick parts of the body (e.g., thorax, abdomen, skull) and those joints and bones in excess of 10-cm thickness. It is true that the film will show lines of the lead strips in the grid, but there will be a much improved quality of film of the part radiographed, with good detail because of the decreased scattered radiations.

Grids may be *parallel* or *focused*. A parallel grid is one constructed with strips parallel to each other. A focused grid is one in which the lead strips and spacers are gradually angulated from the center to the periphery of the grid. The distance from the point of convergence, or focal point, is referred to as its focal distance, or radius. The advantage of a focused grid is that it allows unobstructed amounts of radiation to pass through it at the center and at the edge of the grid as long as the radiations are parallel to the axis of the lead strips. Such grids can be used only at a specific focal-film distance specified by the manufacturer. If distances above or below the focal distance are used, grid cutoff will occur, which means that part of the primary beam will be absorbed by the grid.

For veterinary work, a grid with a ratio of 8:1 at 103 lines per 2.5 cm is recommended. With some minor work, a grid can be used with all sizes of cassettes if a wooden insert is constructed to fit around the smaller cassettes, always holding them at the center of the grid in a grid holder.

Cross-hatched grids are among other types of grids that are used. These are stationary grids in which the lead strips crosscut others in a honeycomb pattern. The usual grid ratio of cross-hatched grids is 8:1, though a grid of 16:1 may be used with a very high kilovoltage technique. Cross-hatched grids can be obtained when necessary by placing two parallel grids at right angles to each other. There is very little need for such grids in veterinary practice.

Potter-Bucky Diaphragm

One other type of grid encountered in veterinary hospitals is the *Potter-Bucky diaphragm*. This is simply a movable grid. The movement of the diaphragm is timed to suit a particular exposure, and the grid moves across the film during the exposure

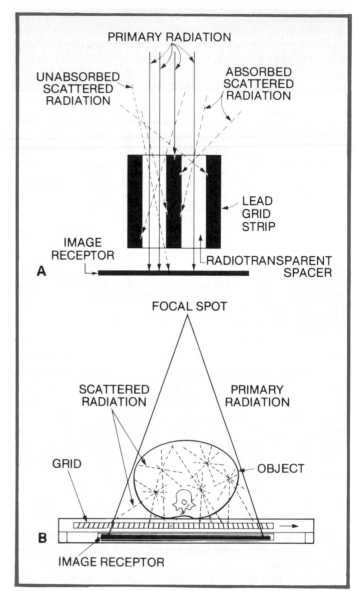

FIGURE 7–24. Cross-section of a grid. A, Diagram of a small section of a grid showing how a large proportion of the scattered radiation is absorbed and image-forming primary radiation passes through to the image detector. B, Diagram of focused Potter-Bucky diaphragm being moved toward the right. (From Eastman Kodak Co.: The Fundamentals of Radiography, 12th ed., 1980. Rochester, NY, Eastman Kodak Co., Radiographic Markets Division.)

so that the lead lines are not shown on the resulting film. When using a movable grid, the exposure time must be increased by a factor of four or the kilovoltage increased by about 20 percent. Usually, Potter-Bucky diaphragms are positioned under the table and are electronically linked to the timer of the x-ray machine (Fig. 7–24B).

Another method to reduce scattered radiation is the *air gap technique*. It is a simple technique that consists of increasing the distance between the patient and the surface of the cassette. With this technique, the amount of scattered radiations produced is not reduced, but less scattered radiations reach the film because of the increased distance between patient and film.

With the air gap technique, it is not necessary to increase the exposure factors as must be done with a grid. However, this technique will decrease the sharpness of the image because of increased subject-to-film distance. It is also less effective at high kilovoltage settings, because more scatter occurs in a forward direction. This technique is used most commonly in veterinary radiology for magnification purposes and for equine thoracic radiography.

THE DARKROOM

The importance of the darkroom in radiography cannot be overemphasized. Radiography unquestionably begins and ends in the darkroom, where films are loaded into cassettes ready for exposure and returned for processing into a finished radiograph. Most mistakes made in veterinary radiography are related to the processing of radiographs. It is necessary to keep the darkroom very clean and light-proof. It is also essential for the technician to have a thorough knowledge of x-ray darkroom technique and of conventional or automatic processing. The chemicals should be changed, replenished, maintained and mixed according to the strict directions of the manufacturer.

Equipment

A darkroom need not be spacious. For most veterinary practices, a small room of about 120 cm × 240 cm is adequate. However, it is essential that this room be made totally dark. If there is a window in the room, there is no reason not to open it for ventilation when the room is not in use; however, the window should be light-proof when closed. It is important also that a lock be placed on the door to avoid its being opened while films are being processed. A darkroom need not be completely dark, since a safelight (a special light for darkroom use that will not expose film) can be used during film processing. It is important, however, that the safelight does not exceed the wattage recommended for the type of filter used; otherwise the exposed films will be "fogged" and the quality of the radiographs compromised. The proper type of filter must be used in the darkroom. Orange, red or yellow filters may be used with most x-ray films, but with the rare earth type of x-ray film, a special red filter must be used (Fig. 7–25). As a princi-

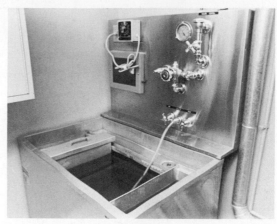

FIGURE 7–26. Processing tanks. The developer is in the right tank. The middle tank holds screening water to wash the films, and the left tank contains the fixer. There is a mixing valve that maintains the solutions at a constant temperature.

ple, it is important to keep in mind that no films should be exposed to the safelight any longer than necessary. It is important to work rapidly but carefully when processing x-ray films and loading and unloading films in the cassettes.

There must be a workbench in the darkroom located as far away from the processing tanks as possible so that liquid or dry chemicals will not be spilled on it. Above or below the bench there should be shelves to store film hangers and unexposed films and cassettes. It is necessary to keep x-ray film in a cool, dry place protected from extraneous x-rays.

Hand Processing Equipment

The processing equipment should include a developing tank, a rinsing tank and a fixer tank. The tanks should be big enough to accommodate several 35 cm × 42.5 cm films at the same time. Running water in the rinsing tank is ideal. If it is not available, the water should be changed frequently. Development and fixer solutions should be changed every 90 days regardless of use and more frequently if radiograph volume is high. The tanks should be made of stainless steel for ease of cleaning (Fig. 7–26).

In certain areas of the country, it will be necessary to heat up or cool down the solutions during certain times of the year. This may be accomplished with an electric heater or a cooling device. During the heat of the summer, it may be necessary to add ice to the washing water in order to keep the solutions at the proper temperature. It is also essential to have stirring rods made of stainless steel, plastic or rubber to mix the solution every day before starting the processing of films. An inexpensive way to keep the solution temperature constant in processing tanks is by installing a good quality shower-bath mixer valve. This type of valve is sufficient and economical enough to maintain the solution at a constant temperature in a low-volume practice. Good ventilation is necessary to keep the room dry and avoid accumulation of volatile chemicals.

Automatic Film Processors

There are several makes and sizes of automatic processors on the market. In recent years, some larger veterinary hospitals

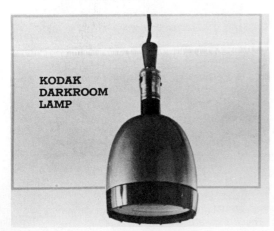

FIGURE 7–25. Darkroom lamp with a special filter to avoid fogging of x-ray films during loading and unloading of cassette.

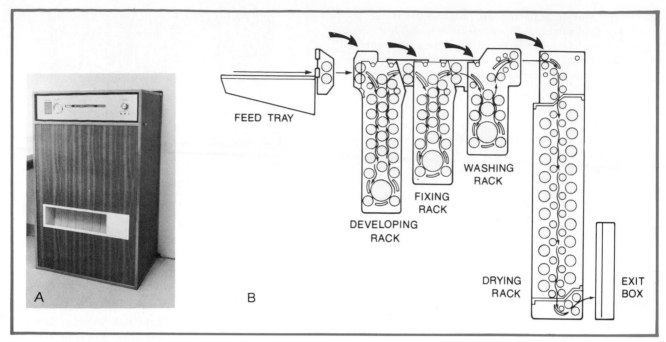

FIGURE 7–27. Automatic processor. A, Kodak X-OMAT processor used in some veterinary hospitals. It is a 90-second processor. B, Diagram of a typical automatic x-ray processor.

have invested in automatic processing systems. There are small-capacity, 90-second processor units that can be installed in most darkrooms without remodeling. The larger processor units necessitate some remodeling, because the input tray must be in the darkroom and the output side must be out of the darkroom. This usually necessitates some structural and plumbing modifications (Fig. 7–27).

As with manual processing tanks, it is necessary to maintain fresh solution and assure that the solutions are flowing properly within the processor. It is important to provide ventilation in the darkroom when automatic processors are used. Usually, a good quality exhaust fan installed in the ceiling is adequate.

Film Storage

X-ray films must be handled and stored properly for maximum usefulness. The film must be protected from light, x-radiations and gamma radiations, heat, moisture and pressure. Therefore, they must be stored away from these hazards. As previously mentioned, the darkroom can fulfill this function if the room is kept clean and free of moisture. It may be helpful if the x-ray films are kept in their original boxes and placed in a cabinet. Special bins to store x-ray films can be purchased, but they are expensive for most veterinary practices (Fig. 7–28).

Cassette Loading and Unloading

Care must be taken when transferring x-ray film from its box to the x-ray cassette to avoid static electricity. The film should be handled carefully, held only by the corners and pulled from the box in a continuous and slow motion (Fig. 7–29). The film should be carefully placed in the cassette. Great care should

also be taken in removing x-ray film from the cassette to prevent damage to the intensifying screen.

Hanging X-ray Film

When exposed films are placed on a film hanger after exposure, they must be handled carefully. The films should be handled *only* by the corners and clipped to the stationary bottom clip first and then to the flexible top clip. It is most important to have dry hands when handling exposed, nonpro-

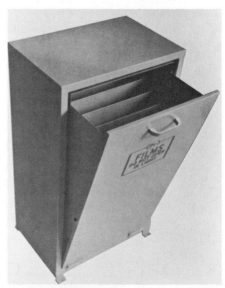

FIGURE 7–28. Film bin. Film storage bin commonly used in darkrooms. These bins are designed to store open x-ray box films for loading x-ray cassettes.

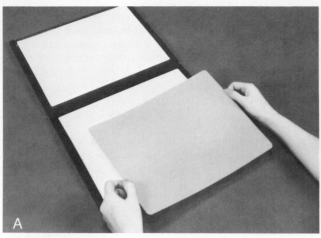
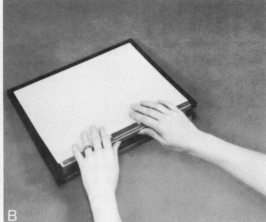

FIGURE 7–29. Loading a cassette. A, Using both hands to avoid kink marks, place the film carefully into the cassette. B, The cassette must be closed and latched gently. (From Eastman Kodak Co.: The Fundamentals of Radiography, 12th ed., 1980. Rochester, NY, Eastman Kodak Co., Radiographic Markets Division.)

cessed films. Any developer or fixer solution touching the film will create an artifact on the processed film (Fig. 7–30).

Developing X-ray Film

As previously mentioned, processing solutions should be stirred before developing the film. When the film is placed in the developer, it should be agitated up and down a few times to remove air bubbles from the surface of the film. The film should be developed for 5 minutes at 20°C. If the temperature is above or below 20°C, the developing time should be adjusted according to the directions of the manufacturer.

In the developing solution, the chemicals reduce the exposed silver halides from the exposed x-ray film to metallic silver, which is black. Gradually through the developing process, the latent image is revealed. The film is then removed from the developer tank and quickly rinsed in the central water bath. It is then placed in the fixer solution, which stops the development process and preserves the film. The film should remain in the fixer for approximately twice the development time. The film is then placed in the central rinse tank

for about 15 to 20 minutes. Films can be dried in a special air-circulated film dryer box or allowed to hang until dry in a well-ventilated dust-free area. For a more complete discussion of the chemistry of x-ray processing, please refer to the Kodak publication, *The Fundamentals of Radiography*, 1980.

Silver Recovery

In larger veterinary practices, the silver contained within the x-ray film emulsion may be removed and recovered. Most of the silver that is not exposed to x-rays is not converted to metallic silver and accumulates within the fixer solution. Silver recovery units can be attached to the fixer solution to remove the silver by an electrolytic process. This, however, is only economical for the larger-volume veterinary hospital. The silver can also be recovered from exposed and nonexposed x-ray film. There are a few companies that specialize in recycling x-ray film for silver recovery. This could be the source of a small "bonus" at the time an x-ray file is "purged" of the old cases on file.

RADIOGRAPHIC FILM QUALITY

It is of utmost importance to produce radiographs of excellent quality in order to arrive at a radiographic diagnosis. A film of good diagnostic quality should have excellent detail, correct scale of contrast and optimal density. Each of these film characteristics will be briefly discussed.

Detail

Radiographic detail refers to the degree of sharpness that defines the edge of an anatomical structure. It is the best possible reproduction of an organ. Detail is influenced by every possible factor, but some are more influential than others.

The focal-film distance is one important factor in the loss of detail. If the focal spot is too close to the part radiographed,

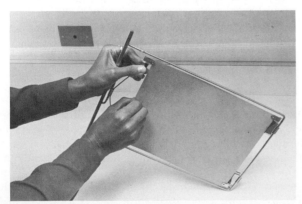

FIGURE 7–30. Hanging x-ray films. Films should be handled by the corners only and should be clipped to the stationary bottom clip first then to the flexible top clip.

there will be magnification and lack of distinction at the margins of the structures radiographed. Therefore, it is important to keep the focal-film distance as long as possible without increasing the time of exposure to avoid movement. Most veterinary hospitals have radiographic technique charts that use a focal-film distance between 36 and 48 inches or 80 and 110 cm.

Movement in veterinary radiology is a constant problem, especially with older units that have a minimum exposure time of 1/10 second. It is difficult to produce diagnostic films of the thorax with a unit that does not have a minimum time of exposure of at least 1/30 second and ideally 1/120 second. With large animals, movement is a constant problem with a small, portable unit. This is why rare earth screens are becoming so popular in veterinary medicine, because they have the advantage of providing a much shorter exposure time.

The size of the focal spot is another important factor that regulates detail. The larger the focal spot, the poorer the detail. Since most equipment in veterinary medicine has a rather large focal spot of 0.8 mm or more, loss of detail may be significant, especially with older units that have focal spots of 1.2 to 2 mm. Therefore, it is important to place the part to be radiographed as close as possible to the x-ray film. If the part is too far from the film, there will be magnification, resulting in a loss of detail. This is especially important in large-animal radiology.

Other factors that affect detail are poor film-screen contact and over- or underexposed radiographs that often result from an improper technique chart or carelessness. Poor radiographic processing causes more ruined radiographs than all other factors combined. All processing errors affect detail. It is therefore important to standardize the developing process by following to the letter instructions of the manufacturer. Any conditions, such as light leakage, excessive heat, backscatter or secondary radiations, result in film fogging.

Radiographic Contrast

Radiographic contrast refers to the density or opacity difference between two areas on a radiograph. High contrast means the opacity differences are large and there are fewer shades of gray. High-contrast radiographs are very black and white. Latitude refers to the range of different opacities on the radiograph. Long-latitude radiographs have a much larger number of shades of gray, but the difference or contrast between each shade is small. High-contrast radiographs are preferred for spine and extremity films. Long-latitude, low-contrast radiographs are preferred for thoracic films.

Kilovoltage is the factor that has the greatest influence on radiographic contrast. The higher the kilovoltage, the greater the latitude and, therefore, the greater the number of shades of black, gray and white. The absorption of the x-ray beam at high kilovoltage is more uniform among the various tissues in the body, resulting in less contrast. This is most important with thoracic radiographs, because the ribs are more closely penetrated to the soft tissue of the lungs. At a lower kilovoltage, the difference in density between the various tissues in the body is much greater. The bone stands out against the surrounding soft tissue because there is a much shorter scale of contrast. Therefore, for thoracic examinations, a high kilovoltage technique is recommended. For skeletal studies, a lower kilovoltage technique is recommended.

Other factors influencing contrast are secondary and scattered radiations (which can be markedly improved by the use of a grid), light leakage and poor processing technique, especially with short developing times resulting from warm solutions.

Radiographic Density

Radiographic density refers to the degree of blackness of the film. It is the result of the amount of light that was transmitted to the x-ray film following interaction of the crystals in the intensifying screens with the x-ray beam. When a film is properly exposed, the anatomical part radiographed will have good contrast with good differential absorption of the x-ray beam by the various tissue densities. Therefore, the part radiographed should be clearly seen but should not be so dark as to overexpose the anatomical structures to the degree that they are difficult to differentiate from the background film density. The thickness and density of the anatomical part radiographed do affect density. The thickest part will absorb more radiation, sometimes as much as denser tissues if of lesser thickness.

The primary factor affecting density is the milliampere-seconds setting. As you remember, the milliampere-seconds factor is a quantity factor that regulates the amount of x-ray produced that reaches the film. If more x-rays reach the film, more light will be emitted by the screens, and the film will be darker. Therefore, it can be stated that *high milliampere-seconds settings will increase film density and low milliampere-seconds settings will reduce film density.*

Another factor that affects film density is the kilovoltage setting. At a higher kilovoltage, the x-ray tube is more efficient in producing x-rays and therefore increases the energy level of x-rays produced. If all other exposure and development factors are kept constant, increasing the kilovoltage will increase the radiographic density. This effect is more apparent at lower kilovoltage settings for a given part than at higher kilovoltage settings.

The distance from the focal spot to the surface of the film is another important factor in film density. If everything remains constant but the distance, a given examination could be markedly overexposed if the distance is reduced, or it could be underexposed if the distance is increased. This effect can be dramatic because the intensity of the radiation is reduced or increased as the square of the distance is changed. This effect was discussed earlier under the section that discussed the inverse square law. It does emphasize the need for consistency and for accurate measurement of the focal-film distance.

Magnification

Magnification is a technique rarely used in veterinary practices, but it is becoming more and more popular in most veterinary teaching hospitals. Magnification is based on the principle that a larger image of an anatomical structure can be obtained if the distance between the object and the film is increased. However, in order to obtain diagnostic films, it is necessary to have a very small focal spot. A focal spot of 0.3 mm or smaller is needed for radiographic magnification. If larger focal spots are used, the advantage of direct magnification is lost because of the blurring at the margin of an organ produced by the larger focal spot. Excellent magnification studies up to four and five times in size have been obtained of small objects with focal spots as small as 0.1 mm. This technique would be useful to veterinarians, especially for studies of extremities in small dogs and for studies of the skull. It is anticipated that the price of small focal-spot tubes will come down enough to make their use a worthwhile consideration for some practices.

Technical Errors and Artifacts

Several errors in handling x-ray films or in setting up a technique for an examination can be made. In general, these errors will reduce the quality of the x-ray film and in certain cases may nullify its diagnostic value. Tables 7–4, 7–5 and 7–6 are intended to help the technician identify the cause of errors and take corrective measures. Table 7–4 deals with technical errors other than those occurring as a result of film processing. Tables 7–5 and 7–6 deal with errors originating from film processing.

The advent of automatic processing equipment has helped tremendously in eliminating many errors made in wet processing techniques. It has standardized film processing and has made it easier to trace the cause of processing mistakes, which are usually mechanically related. Even with automatic processors, many mistakes can be made and must be recognized and corrected to obtain the best possible radiographs.

Several other mechanical failures may occur with automatic processors. It is important to keep the processor clean at all times. It is especially important to wash the roller thoroughly at least once a month. Processors are sophisticated machines that must be serviced regularly by professionals. It is unreasonable and cost-ineffective for a veterinarian to expect the technician to service the processor. However, it is the responsibility of the technician to be able to recognize processor problems and correct them when possible. It is also the technician's responsibility to keep the processor clean at all times.

RADIATION SAFETY

Since 1970, there has been a tremendous growth in the use of x-ray equipment by veterinarians. There are few diagnoses in medicine or surgery that cannot be aided by the use of diagnostic radiology. It therefore behooves one to be aware of the hazard of using x-rays or any other type of ionizing radiation.

It is the responsibility of the veterinarian to ensure that proper radiation safety measures are observed in the hospital. It is also the veterinarian's responsibility to instruct the technician in the proper use of the equipment and to ensure that the design of the x-ray room meets state regulations.

All animal tissues are sensitive to radiation, that is, absorption of radiation doses above a certain minimum roentgen value will change or alter the tissue. The following tissues (not in order of sensitivity) are most readily affected by ionizing radiation: dermis, lymphatics, hemopoietic and leukopoietic (blood-forming) tissues, breast, thyroid, bone (especially the epiphysis or growing centers) and the germinal epithelium or gonads. These tissues are sensitive to alpha, beta or any other kind of ionizing radiations. All animal species are affected, including humans, even though there are different degrees of

Table 7–4
TECHNICAL ERRORS

Increased Film Density
Too high mAs or kV settings
Too short focal-film distance
Wrong measurement of anatomical part
Equipment malfunction
Speed of intensifying screen too fast
Decreased Film Density
Too low mAs or kV settings
Too long focal-film distance
Wrong measurement of anatomical part
Speed of intensifying screen too slow
Black Marks or Artifacts
Film scratches
Crescent mark due to rough handling
Static electricity (linear dots or tree pattern)
Top of film black, resulting from exposure to light while still in box
Defective cassette that does not close properly, exposing margins of film to light
White Marks (Artifacts)
Dirt or debris between the film and screen
Defect or crack in screen
Contrast medium on tabletop, skin or cassette
Gray Film
Film accidentally exposed to radiation—scattered, secondary or direct
Lack of grid for examination of a thick part
Outdated film
Film stored in too hot or too humid place
Distorted or Blurred Radiograph
Motion—patient, cassette or machine
Too great focal-film distance, causing magnification and distortion
Poor film-screen contact
Poor centering of primary x-ray beam
Linear Artifacts
Gridlines
Grid out of focal range
Primary beam not centered
Grid upside down
Grid damage, causing distorted gridlines
Miscellaneous Artifacts
Cone cut, causing underexposed margins
Target damage, resulting in inconsistent film density— requires tube replacement
Double exposure
Blank film—faulty equipment, nonexposed film processed

sensitivity among species. The more rapidly dividing tissues are affected most by radiation.

Technicians should remember that one of the best protective devices at their disposal is the ability to avoid retakes. It is, in addition, cost-effective and saves time and resources.

Radiation Filtration

Aluminum has a marked effect on filtration of softer (lower energy level) x-rays. Insertion of 1 mm or even 2 mm of an aluminum filter into the path of the primary beam at the portal of the x-ray tube is essential to filter out or absorb the soft x-rays that are a component of all x-ray beams in the diagnostic range. By absorbing these soft radiations, the filter reduces the amount of radiation absorbed by the patient and, therefore, the amount of scattered and secondary radiations

Table 7–5
FILM PROCESSING MISTAKES IN WET TANKS

Increased Film Density
Film overdeveloped
Temperature of solution too high
Wrong concentration of developer
Defective thermometer
Decreased Film Density
Film underdeveloped
Temperature of solution too low
Exhausted developer
Contamination of developer
Developer too diluted or improperly mixed
Failure to add replenisher solution as needed
Defective thermometer
Fogged Films
Light leakage in darkroom from defective safelight, door,
windows, around processor pipes, turning lights on in
darkroom before film is cleared
Film exposed to radiation from any source—through wall
if storage room adjacent to x-ray room, cassette left in
x-ray room while exposure made
Overdeveloped film
Contaminated developer
Yellow Radiograph
Fixation time too short
Exhausted fixer solution
White Spots
Defective screens—pitted, scratched
Dust or grit on surface of film
Fixer on film before processing
Black Spots
Drops of developer solution on film before processing
Films stacked together in fixer
Air Bells
Film not agitated when placed in developer; air bubbles
form on surface of film
Reticulation
Solutions have uneven temperature from bottom to top of
tanks
Need to stir up solution to even up temperature in tanks
Weak fixer or lack of hardening solution
Brittle Radiographs
Drying temperature too high
Drying time too long
Miscellaneous Mistakes
Film wet—too short drying time
Grit on films—dirty tanks and solutions
Corner marks—wet or dirty fingers on hangers
Sticky film—film washed or dried improperly
Static electricity—low humidity and rough or too fast
handling of films
Scratches—careless handling

that may affect the technician. Increased aluminum filtration also generally improves latitude and detail by improving the quality of the x-ray beam.

Radiation Measurement

To understand radiation safety and radiation dose units of measurement, it is necessary to define a few terms commonly used in the measurement of radiation exposure.

Roentgen. The roentgen (R) is defined as a unit of radiation exposure that will liberate a charge of 2.58×10^{-4} coulombs per kilogram of air. As an example, a roentgen is the approximate exposure to the body surface for an anterior-posterior radiograph of the abdomen for an average adult human.

Rad. The unit of absorbed dose of ionizing radiations is called rad. It is the energy imparted by ionizing radiations to unit mass of irradiated material and is equal to 100 erg/g. The number of rads deposited in tissue per roentgen of radiation exposure varies with the energy of the beam and with the composition of the absorber.

Rem. Short for rad equivalent man, rem is the product of the dose in rads and the relative biological effectiveness of the radiation used. This unit of measurement makes allowance for the fact that the effect of radiations on different tissue varies with the type of radiation or relative biological effectiveness. A rem is equal to the absorbed radiation dose in rads multiplied by a quality factor.

$$Rem = rads \times quality\ factor$$

Because the quality factor for diagnostic radiation is 1, for all practical purposes in veterinary practice a rem = rad. For larger particles of radiation such as neutrons, protons and alpha particles, the quality factor increases from 3 to 20. These larger, more dangerous particles of radiation are not emitted from diagnostic x-ray machines.

Maximum Permissible Dose. This dose should be of great interest to the veterinary technician, as it is the maximum dose of radiation a person is allowed to receive during occupational exposure over a certain time. This dose is 0.1 rem average weekly dose, 3 rem over 13 weeks, 5 rem per year and a maximum accumulated dose of 5 (N − 18) rem, where N is age in years. The technician should remember also that a permissible dose is the dose that will not harm the person receiving it during her or his lifetime. All radiations can be said to be harmful; therefore, in working out an arbitrary permissible level of exposure, one must take into consideration the effect of the cumulative dose over a person's whole lifetime.

Table 7–6
COMMON TECHNICAL ERRORS WITH AUTOMATIC PROCESSORS

Increased Density
Temperature of developer too high
Over-replenishment
Light leak from cover or in darkroom
Speed too slow
Faulty thermostat
Decreased Density
Temperature of developer too low
Under-replenishment
Exhausted developer, necessitating thorough
cleaning of tanks every 6 months
Faulty thermostat
Processing Streaks
Cross-over rollers dirty
Dirty wash water
Air tubes need cleaning
Scratches on Film
Guide shoes malaligned or dirty
Dryer air tubes malpositioned
Wet or Damp Film
Thermostat malfunction
Dryer temperatures too low
Insufficient air venting
Film not hardened sufficiently
Film Overlap
Film fed too rapidly into processor
Tension on rollers too high

Personnel Monitoring. In order to protect the staff from over-dose, the radiation that each person receives can be measured on a *film badge*. A film badge is a container that holds a special film designed to record a wide range of exposures. The film holder incorporates several different types of metal filters that permit differentiation of the type of ionizing radiation exposures. This badge should be worn outside the apron on the collar at the level of the thyroid gland. Film badges can be exposed by heat, pressure and chemical fumes. The film badge should be taken care of and stored outside the radiology area so that the amount of radiation it detects is actually the amount to which the person was exposed.

Radiation monitoring badges come in several forms: rings, clips and wrist badges. Several companies offer a badge service. These badges are analyzed on a monthly or quarterly basis.

Another device used to detect radiation exposure is the pocket dosimeter, which is a simple ionizing chamber. Thermoluminescent dosimeters can also be used for personal monitoring. However, badges are the most common and practical means of measuring radiation exposure. Film badge readings are reported in millirems or 1/1000 rem. Technicians should insist that the veterinarian for whom they work provide them with a radiation monitoring device.

Protection Practices

1. Always use a collimator and always use the smallest possible aperture that will cover the anatomical areas of interest (Fig. 7–31).

2. Make sure there is an aluminum filter at the portal of the x-ray tube.

3. Make sure the proper exposure factors are used to avoid retake.

4. Make sure the animal is positioned properly the first time—again to avoid retakes.

5. Never stand in the direct x-ray beam when holding the part to be radiographed.

6. Always wear an apron and gloves when holding an animal or an apron alone if one has to be in the room when an exposure is made. The apron should have 0.5-mm lead equiv-

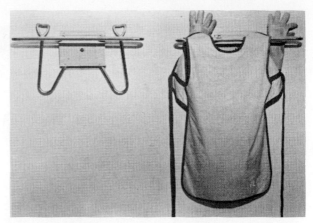

FIGURE 7–32. Apron and gloves on a stand. It is important to keep the apron on a stand and the gloves well aerated when not in use in order to increase the useful "life" of the apron and gloves. The apron should have a minimum of 0.5 mm of lead equivalent.

alent minimum to assure good protection from secondary and scattered radiations (Figs. 7–32 and 7–33).

7. Use accessory equipment designed to reduce radiation exposure, such as cassette holders, restraining devices and positioning devices (Fig. 7–34).

8. Anesthesia and tranquilization of the patient should be used every time an animal cannot be controlled easily and adequately for a given examination.

9. Only required personnel should be in the examining room at the time of exposure. A pregnant woman should not be in the room nor should anyone less than 18 years of age.

10. Use good, fast screens to reduce the mAs settings as much as possible.

11. Higher kilovoltage techniques allow reduction of the milliampere-seconds setting and should be used whenever possible.

Radiation safety is a frame of mind. It is a habit, and it requires awareness of the danger of radiation. It is easy to become careless with radiation because it is invisible, tasteless, odorless, and produces no external stimulation at diagnostic levels. Technicians should always remember that though invis-

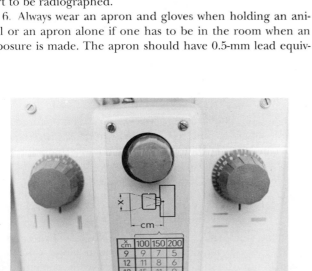

FIGURE 7–31. Collimator, which is used to limit the size of the x-ray beam to the part to be examined. By coning down on an area, the amount of scattered and secondary radiation can be drastically reduced.

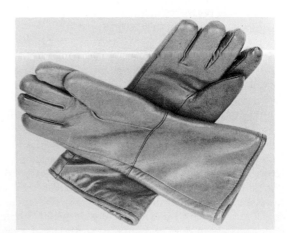

FIGURE 7–33. Lead gloves should have a minimum of 0.5 mm of lead equivalent; they ideally should have 1 mm of lead equivalent. They should always be worn when restraint is needed for an examination.

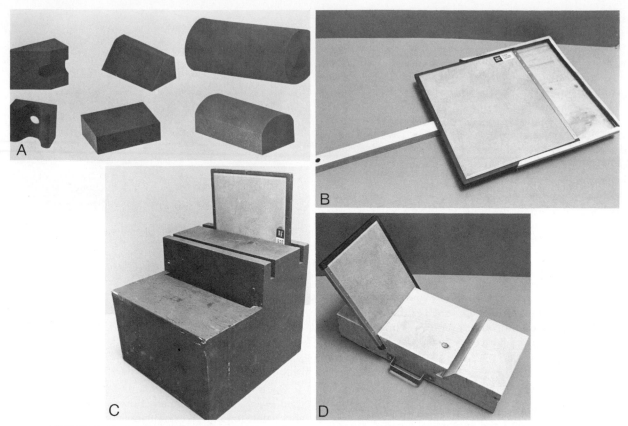

FIGURE 7–34. Positioning devices. A number of commercially available devices can be used to help position animals in order to reduce the time needed to perform the examination. A, Various foam devices used to position small animals; B, cassette holder for large animal examinations; C, block for examination of large animal foot; D, block for examination of large animal fetlock and pastern joints.

ible, radiations are dangerous to one's health. X-ray effects are cumulative. The ionization that results from continued exposure to x-rays and other high-energy rays constitutes the cumulative effect. They can destroy all living tissue if the absorbed doses are high enough. Secondary radiations are less harmful than primary radiations but are still extremely harmful. Therefore, carelessness has no place in radiology. Remember "the big three" methods of radiation protection: *time, distance* and *shielding.* "Time"—avoid retakes, do it right the first time. "Distance"—stay as far away as possible from the patient and x-ray beam. "Shielding"—always wear your apron and gloves.

RADIOGRAPHIC CONTRAST AGENTS

A number of radiographic examinations involve the addition of a contrast medium to the body system for better visualization of that system. Contrast media are classified largely as pharmaceuticals by the Federal Food and Drug Administration (FDA). Therefore, one must have at least a fundamental knowledge of the dosage of these agents in order to anticipate their effect on the patient. The literature contains many references concerning contrast media, but the scope of this text is to present the basic facts about common contrast materials in a concise form. More extensive treatment of this topic is found in Kleine and Warren (1983) and Morgan and Silverman (1987).

In radiology, "contrast" means density difference. Contrast materials are "contrast" materials in the true sense of the word. Two classes of contrast materials are used in radiology: *radiopaques* (positive contrast agents) and radiolucents (negative contrast agents). Air, nitrous oxide and carbon dioxide do not absorb or emit appreciable amounts of radiation and are used as negative contrast agents to produce a decreased radiographic density.

Radiopaque media are divided into soluble and insoluble materials. About the only insoluble material used in radiology is *barium sulfate.* All the other contrast materials are soluble and contain iodine in either an ionized or a non-ionized form. Barium sulfate is used almost exclusively for gastrointestinal studies, whereas the iodine compounds are used for renal, articular, vascular and myelographic studies. Two forms of iodine compounds are used for gastrointestinal study: oral meglumine diatrizoate (Gastrografin made by Squibb) and oral sodium diatrizoate (Oral Hypaque made by Winthrop Laboratories).

Soluble iodinated contrast materials are hyperosmotic, which causes an increase in intravascular blood volume followed by an osmotic diuresis. This is usually not much of a clinical problem and is mostly asymptomatic; however, care should be taken with dehydrated older and debilitated animals. Very few adverse reactions occur with contrast media in veterinary medicine. However, adverse reactions have occurred, and one should always be on guard to take emergency measures if needed.

Common Contrast Media and Applications

Esophagus

Contrast Agents. Barium sulfate, which comes in various forms from a pulverized powder to a micronized form and from a suspension to a colloidal form in various concentrations, is used alone and diluted to evaluate an enlarged esophagus or is used as a thick paste if the esophagus is not enlarged. Barium mixed with food is more appropriate for diagnosis of esophageal strictures. Gastrografin or Oral Hypaque is used when a perforation of the esophagus is suspected.

Procedure. No special preparation is needed. Ideally, the study is done under fluoroscopy. If not available, the exposure must be made when the animal swallows. The barium is administered with a syringe in the buccal pouch.

Stomach and Small Bowel (Upper Gastrointestinal Studies)

Contrast Agents. Three kinds of contrast agents are used for upper gastrointestinal studies: barium sulfate 25 to 30 percent w/v, oral iodines such as Gastrografin, and negative contrast, including air, carbon dioxide and nitrous oxide. Barium sulfate is the most commonly used agent for upper gastrointestinal studies when perforation is not suspected. Negative contrast media are used in combination with barium sulfate for double-contrast study. Oral-iodinated products are given when perforation is suspected because barium sulfate is inert and will not be resorbed once it leaks into a body cavity.

Procedure. Food should be withheld for 24 hours, and warm water enemas should be administered about 2 to 3 hours before the gastrointestinal study. Acepromazine (Ayerst Laboratories) can be used without adverse effects on the gastrointestinal study.

Dosage. Barium sulfate, 10 ml/kg; Oral Hypaque or Gastrografin, 3 ml/kg.

Film Sequence. The survey film consists of a ventrodorsal (VD) and a lateral (L) view. Immediately after administration of contrast medium four films should be taken to completely evaluate the stomach: a VD, a dorsoventral (DV) and both a right and left lateral. At 15 minutes and 30 minutes and 1 hour, the film sequence consists of VD and L right. These same views are taken at various intervals until contrast reaches the large bowel. The timing sequence will vary with the patient and the suspected disease process.

Large Bowel (Lower Gastrointestinal Study, Barium Enema)

Contrast Agents. Barium sulfate, 10 to 15 percent, w/v or iodinated preparations, such as Gastrografin or Oral Hypaque, are used for the lower gastrointestinal studies.

Precautions. Barium sulfate should not be used when a perforation is suspected. A barium enema should not be performed for 48 hours after taking a biopsy of the colon or rectum.

Preparation. The preparation is similar to that for upper gastrointestinal studies. Warm water enemas must be given before the examination because it is essential that the entire large bowel be cleansed before a barium enema is performed. A Bardex (French, Bard Hospital Division, C. R. Bard, Inc.) catheter and barium container are needed for the study.

Procedure. The animal should be anesthetized. A 15 percent w/v barium sulfate solution is used for barium enemas. The dose is 5 to 10 ml per 0.45 kg of body weight. Ideally, the study is done under fluoroscopy. Radiographic views needed are L, VD and right and left oblique views. After completion, the barium is evacuated and air is injected to obtain a double-contrast study of the large bowel.

Urinary Tract

Contrast Agents. Several kinds of contrast studies are available for study of the kidneys. However, since the *intravenous pyelogram* (IVP) is the one most used in practice, our discussion will be limited to it.

An IVP or excretory urogram is performed by injecting contrast medium intravenously. Tri-iodinated products are most commonly used. A meglumine diatrizoate and sodium diatrizoate preparation (Renografin, Squibb) is probably the most popular contrast product used in medicine for IVP examinations.

Complications. The most common complications encountered with an IVP are vomiting, anaphylactoid reactions and hypotension. Vomiting is a transient reaction of short duration and is not serious in nature. The anaphylactoid reactions are rare but must be attended to immediately. It is necessary to have epinephrine available for immediate administration whenever an IVP is done. Hypotension is rare, but when it occurs, it can be life threatening and may lead to renal failure.

Contraindications. The only serious contraindication is dehydration.

Procedure. The animal should fast for 24 hours, but water should be available to avoid dehydration. Enemas should be given when needed, at least 2 to 3 hours before the IVP. VD and L films should be taken before the examinations. Films should be taken in the VD and L positions immediately after injection of the contrast medium at 5 minutes and 15 minutes after injection. When needed, follow-up studies at 20 minutes or 25 minutes after injection may be indicated.

Urinary Bladder

Contrast Agents. Tri-iodinated contrast materials are most desirable for retrograde cystography. Non-opaque contrast materials, such as air, carbon dioxide and nitrous oxide, are popular with some veterinarians. Do not use barium sulfate or sodium iodide.

Procedure. The colon should be cleansed. Depending on the breed and size of the animal, different catheters may be used. A Foley catheter, a tomcat catheter and a soft flexible male catheter may be needed. In addition, a syringe and three-way valve are needed. Two types of cystography are commonly performed in veterinary practice: positive-contrast cystography and double-contrast cystography. Positive-contrast cystography is used to detect leaks or rupture of the lower urinary tract following trauma. Tri-iodinated contrast at concentrations of 10 to 15 percent is injected retrograde into the urinary bladder at 5 to 15 ml per kg body weight. Double-contrast cystography is used to detect all other forms of urinary bladder disease. A catheter is placed into the urinary bladder and all urine is removed. Next, 3 to 10 ml of tri-iodinated contrast is injected, followed by carbon dioxide or room air at 5 to 15 ml per kg body weight. Because of the variability of urinary bladder volume, it is best to fill the bladder to palpable turgidity. Lateral and oblique VD radiographic views are most helpful.

Urethrography

Contrast Agents. Tri-iodinated compounds at 30 percent concentration are best for urethrography.

Procedure. A male catheter is placed in the urethra, and 10 to 20 ml are injected while pressure is applied at the end of the urethra. A Foley catheter can be used also. The x-ray is taken while injecting the last few milliliters. An L view and two oblique (O) views should be taken during the injection of the contrast material.

Spinal Cord

Myelography is the contrast examination most frequently performed to localize and characterize spinal cord lesions. Myelograms are always performed with the animal under general anesthesia. Non-ionic iodinated contrast medium is injected into the subarachnoid space (CSF space) at the cisterna magna (skull–C1 space) or in the caudal lumbar spine area (L4–L6). Myelography is most commonly performed prior to surgical intervention.

Contrast Agents. Two non-ionic contrast agents are currently in wide use in veterinary medicine, iopamidol (Isovue, Squibb and Sons, Princeton, NJ) and iohexol (Omnipaque, Sanofi Winthrop, New York, NY). Both of these contrast agents are superior to older myelographic contrast agents such as metrizamide (Amipaque, Winthrop, New York, NY) because they are available in sterile solution and have a decreased incidence of nausea, vomiting and seizures. The dose of contrast medium ranges from 0.25 ml/kg for cervical evaluation with a cisternal injection to 0.45 ml/kg for cervical evaluation from a lumbar injection. The concentration of iodine should not exceed 300 mg/ml, and injection volume should not exceed 15 ml.

Contraindications. Infection of the spinal cord and meninges or when the disease is to be treated medically only are included.

Procedure. Survey films should be taken first. The site of injection should be aseptically prepared. Spinal needles, in size of 20-gauge to 22-gauge and 3.75 to 8.75 cm should be available, because the size of the animal may vary considerably, and some dogs may be so obese that even an 8.75 cm needle may be short! Films are taken in the VD and L positions immediately after administration of the contrast medium.

POSITIONING

Proper positioning is essential to obtain diagnostic radiographic examinations. It is again the responsibility of the veterinary technician to position the animal properly. It is not the intent of this chapter to discuss positioning at length. Please refer to the excellent treatment of this topic by Kleine and Warren (1983) and Ticer (1984) for small animals and Morgan and Silverman (1987) for both large- and small-animal positioning.

Principles of Positioning

In order to achieve proper positioning, it is useful for the technician to remember that two views at right angles are necessary to obtain a diagnostic study. This principle applies to all examinations in small animals and to extremities in large animals. The exceptions to this rule are thoracic examinations and spinal examinations in the horse and, additionally, in cases of trauma or in debilitated animals when only L views can be taken without causing undue stress to the animals.

Another principle to remember is the importance of centering the primary beam on the lesion itself, when known. This is especially important in orthopedic cases in both small and large animals. For example, fracture healing may look very different when the x-ray beam is centered over the fracture line as opposed to a short distance away from it. Costly errors have been made by veterinarians who removed supporting devices before the correct time. These errors occurred because fractures may have appeared healed when the primary beam was centered away from the fracture line itself.

It is also important, when performing a radiographic examination, to use an x-ray film that is large enough to completely cover the system to be examined. For example, the thorax should be included in its entirety on one film; the same applies for the abdomen. For extremities, the primary beam should be directed at the lesion. It is good to have a radiograph large enough to include the proximal and distal joint in order to obtain a good spatial anatomical relationship of the lesion.

These principles are basic but essential. Proper positioning is obtained by practice. These topics are well illustrated and discussed in the references mentioned.

RESTRAINT

The importance of restraint in order to achieve proper positioning cannot be emphasized enough. It is part of radiation safety. Without proper restraint, many examinations should not be undertaken. In some cases, attempting to make examinations without restraint would be life threatening with large animals and dangerous with certain small animals.

There are many types of restraint; some are mechanical or manual, and some are chemical. For the purpose of radiation safety, manual restraint should be avoided as a routine procedure. When it is essential to be in the room with the animal, one should wear a protective lead apron and gloves, and the x-ray beam should be limited to the system to be examined by coning devices or by adjusting the collimator.

Mechanical restraint comes in various forms. A number of commercial devices designed for animal positioning are available, varying in price from a few dollars to several hundreds of dollars (Fig. 7–34). One of the most useful and inexpensive devices to use in the dog is a simple muzzle, which often has a calming effect on an animal (see Chapter 1). Sandbags and sponges can also be used to obtain excellent positioning. When the animal is positioned properly, it is most important to take the radiograph as rapidly as possible, as one can hope for only a few seconds of restraint before the animal moves.

Chemical restraint can be achieved with tranquilizers, analgesics or anesthesia (see Chapter 11). Chemical restraint has contributed greatly to the progress made in radiology by devising a position that would otherwise be impossible to achieve. For example, complete examination of the skull should not be attempted without anesthesia. Every time total immobility or relaxation is required for proper positioning, anesthesia should be used. Most spinal examinations will prove nondiagnostic unless the examination is done under anesthesia. In several circumstances, tranquilization is adequate to control most animals. Tranquilizers are excellent to control frightened or aggressive dogs and cats. They are also most useful for controlling large animals.

Again, good positioning is essential in producing diagnostic x-ray films. It takes time to learn and become proficient at achieving every position needed for a variety of examinations in large and small animals. However, most organs can be radiographed with proper techniques, equipment, accessory devices and the use of mechanical or chemical restraint, or both.

DIAGNOSTIC ULTRASOUND

Ultrasound should be the next new major diagnostic modality to enter veterinary practice. It is portable, does not require the use of ionizing radiation and is non-invasive, well tolerated by patients and accepted by clients. As ultrasound equipment becomes affordable, the only problem with its introduction into practice is the long learning curve associated with its use. Newer veterinary graduates are more familiar with the uses and indications for ultrasound, but few veterinary schools have fully integrated ultrasound into the curriculum. I encourage all new veterinary technicians to familiarize themselves with the basics of diagnostic ultrasound. But remember, ultrasound is user-dependent. The image and the interpretation are only as good as the person doing the examination.

Ultrasound Basics

Sound is a mechanical pressure wave made up of a series of compressions and rarefactions transmitted through a medium. Sound waves are characterized by their wavelength or distance between compressions, their frequency in cycles per second and their velocity or speed of transmission (Fig. 7–35). These characteristics are integrated by the following formula:

$$\text{Velocity} = \text{wavelength} \times \text{frequency}$$

For simplicity we can assume the speed of sound in the body is 1540 meters per second. Therefore, as the frequency of sound increases, the wavelength decreases. Shorter sound waves produce increased image resolution but decreased patient penetration. The frequencies used in veterinary diagnostic ultrasound generally range from 2.5 to 10 megahertz (MHz). A hertz (Hz) is 1 cycle per second. Therefore typical ultrasound frequencies will range from 2 to 10 million cycles per second or 2.5 to 10 MHz. Audible sound will range from 20 to 20,000 Hz.

Real-time gray-scale ultrasound is based on the *pulse-echo principle*. A short pulse of sound usually 2 to 3 cycles long is produced from the transducer and transmitted into the patient. The sound wave strikes an echogenic surface and returns some of the sound to the transducer. The strength of the returning sound wave determines the brightness of the image, and the time it takes for the sound to travel into the patient and back to the transducer determines where the echo will be seen on the screen. Remember, the time it takes for a sound wave to

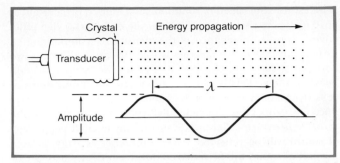

FIGURE 7–35. Sound wave with a wavelength = λ. Closely spaced dots are compressions. Widely spaced dots are rarefactions. The amplitude is proportional to the loudness.

traverse a distance and be reflected back is a function of the distance between the sender and reflector and the speed of the sound wave in that medium. For all practical purposes, the speed of sound in small animal tissues is constant at 1540 meters per second.

Ultrasound production and reception is based on the *piezoelectric effect*. A piezoelectric crystal will change shape or thickness when subjected to a voltage pulse. Rapid pulses of electrical energy are transformed into mechanical energy or sound waves by the vibrating crystal. Returning sound waves cause the crystal to vibrate, and that mechanical energy is transmitted into electrical energy by the transducer. This electrical signal is transformed into the gray-scale image on the screen. The transducer acts as both the sound transmitter and the receiver. The operating frequency of the transducer is partially determined by the thickness of the piezoelectric crystal. The thinner the crystal, the higher the transducer frequency. The transducer transmits sound 0.01 percent of the time. It receives returning sound waves 99.9 percent of the time.

Ultrasound Tissue Interaction

In order to better understand the ultrasound image it is important to understand the interaction of ultrasound within tissue. As the sound wave proceeds through the body it is progressively attenuated or weakened. This *attenuation* limits the depth of penetration of the sound wave and therefore limits the depth of structures that can be effectively imaged. The ultrasound beam is attenuated or weakened by absorption, reflection, scattering, refraction and diffraction. Reflection is a redirection of the sound beam back to the transducer and is the basis of the diagnostic image. Absorption is sound energy converted to heat within the tissues. Scattering is the intertissue microreflection of sound which is responsible for much of the echo texture of various organs. Refraction and diffraction are the bending of the sound beam as it crosses areas of differing tissue densities. Refraction attenuation is important in the generation of several ultrasound artifacts.

Sound reflection or echo production forms the basis of the ultrasound image. An echo is produced whenever the ultrasound beam crosses an acoustic interface. An acoustic interface is the boundary between two tissues of differing acoustic impedances or Z. See equation below.

$$\text{Acoustic impedance (Z)} = \text{density (P)} \times \text{speed of sound transmission (C)}$$
$$Z = P \times C$$

If we assume the speed of sound in soft tissue to be constant at 1540 meters per second (m/s), then the main factor that influences acoustic impedance is the density or composition of tissue. The take-home message is that the more different two adjacent tissues are, the greater will be the echo reflection between them. This is why very homogeneous populations of cells (lymphoma lymph nodes, regenerative liver nodules) produce few echoes and are generally hypoechoic (darker). If the acoustic interface difference is small, only a small percentage of sound will be reflected. If the difference is .large, a large portion of sound will be reflected. Most soft tissues have a Z or acoustic impedance within 1 to 2 percent of liver.

Interface	% Reflection
Fat-muscle	0.94
Fat-bone	49.00
Tissue-air	100.00

Patient Preparation

Patient preparation is important because 100 percent of the sound is reflected when the ultrasound beam intersects air. Hair traps air, which is how it insulates the animal, but if one tries to pass ultrasound through hair the majority of the ultrasound beam is reflected before it ever enters the animal. A careful close clip of the area to be examined, as well as removal of dirt and scales, will improve the ultrasound image. A generous volume of ultrasound gel is also beneficial to displace air and couple the transducer to the skin. Small animals are placed in a padded V-trough table on their backs for abdominal examination, and in lateral or sternal recumbency for cardiac examination. Most small animals tolerate abdominal and cardiac examinations well and rarely require tranquilization. A special table with a large hole cut in it may help with cardiac examinations. The animal is placed in lateral recumbency with the chest area over the hole, which allows for better ultrasound transducer access. Large animal examinations are done in the standing tranquilized animal. Again, close clipping, especially for tendon examinations, is critical for an optimal examination.

Ultrasound Display Modes

The returning echo can be displayed in several ways. *"A"-mode* or *amplitude mode* displays the returning echoes as spikes from a baseline. The echo depth is determined by its location along the baseline. The echo intensity is displayed by the height of the spike. A-mode ultrasound machines are used predominantly in ophthalmology and would have little value in veterinary practice.

"B"-mode or *brightness mode* forms the basis for two-dimensional imaging. The returning echoes are displayed as dots. The brightness of the dot is a function of the strength of the returning echo. The placement of the dot is a function of the time it took for the echo to return to the transducer. The cross-sectional image is formed through data storage. There are two basic types of B scanners, *static* and *real-time*. With static scanners the transducer is manually moved across the patient and the image is held on the screen during the transducer sweep. These machines are large and cumbersome, require skill to produce an adequate image, increase the time required for an examination and do not allow visualization of motion.

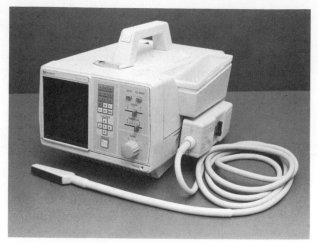

FIGURE 7–36. Portable real-time ultrasound unit with a linear array transducer—most popular for large animal ultrasound.

These machines are readily available, generally free from hospital surplus, but are not as valuable as real-time equipment in veterinary practice. With real-time equipment, the sound beam is automatically swept across the patient while the transducer is held steady (Fig. 7–36). New images are produced rapidly, permitting direct observation of moving structures. With B-mode real-time equipment, images are displayed in gray scale. Gray scale is a technique in which the various echo strengths are displayed in numerous shades of gray from black to white.

M-mode or *time-motion (TM) mode* is produced by passing a narrow sound beam across a body part. Each echo interface is presented as a dot. The motion of the body part is displayed by sweeping the image across the screen or image recorder. M-mode can be thought of as a very thin sector of B-mode displayed as a function of time. M-mode is primarily used for echocardiography. Ideal ultrasound equipment for veterinary practice would be a real-time B-mode scanner with M-mode capabilities (Fig. 7–37).

The selection of appropriate transducers is critical when purchasing ultrasound equipment. Transducers will vary in type, size, style, shape and frequency. Linear array transducers are made with several piezoelectric crystals stacked side by side. The crystals are fired in rapid sequence to produce a rectangular cross-sectional image. The major drawback for linear array transducers is their large footprint or contact area. It is difficult to use these transducers for intercostal cardiac studies and for subcostal studies in the cranial–abdominal area in small animals. Linear array transducers are primarily used for transrectal reproductive examinations in cattle and horses.

Sector scanners produce a triangular field (Fig. 7–38). The crystal is swept across the area by mechanical or electronic means, and the transducer generally has a small contact area. Newer, more expensive transducers may incorporate annular array and dynamic focusing technology. These transducers form the ultrasound beam by adding together many small beams from an array of small crystals. Dynamic focusing will allow the operator to place any portion within the beam into maximum resolution without having to change transducers.

Deciding what frequency of transducer to use is easy. Use as high a frequency transducer as possible to maximize resolution while still allowing penetration to the needed depth. Remember, the higher the frequency of the transducer, the shorter

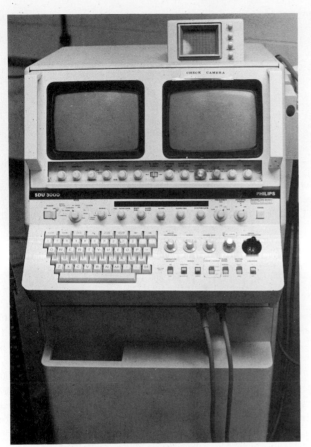

FIGURE 7–37. Mobile real-time ultrasound unit.

The ultrasound equipment controls will vary from machine to machine, but the concept of *time-gain compensation* is fairly universal. The echoes coming from acoustic interfaces close to the transducer are stronger than the echoes returning from farther away from the transducer. Time-gain amplification compensates for the progressive attenuation with depth in the ultrasound beam. Time-gain compensation (TGC) is operator dependent and is set for the best-looking uniform image.

The Ultrasound Image

As one begins using ultrasound, the need increases to re-study anatomy. The ultrasound image is a thin cross-sectional slice through the body in a new or different orientation. It will help to use a standard image orientation, which places the head or front of the animal on the left in the sagittal or longitudinal view and the animal's right on the screen's left on the transverse or axial view.

Ultrasound terminology is easy. *Echogenicity* refers to the strength or amplitude of the returning echoes. A structure that is *sonodense* or *echogenic* (bright) produces echoes. A structure that is *anechoic* or *sonolucent* (dark) produces few or no echoes. A structure is *hyperechoic* (brighter than) if it produces more echoes than adjacent structures. A structure is *hypoechoic* (darker than) if it produces fewer echoes than surrounding structures. An *isoechoic* (same as) structure has a level of echogenicity similar to that of adjacent structures. A structure that is complexly echogenic contains multiple different echogenicities and echo textures. Mixed echogenicity refers to an organ or structure with two echogenicities. Remember that echogenicity is a relative term. We can make any structure bright by adjusting machine control settings. Compare organs at the same depth and control settings to avoid misinterpretation of relative echogenicities.

the sound wavelength and the better the resolution. However, as the frequency increases, the depth of sound beam penetration decreases. For abdominal ultrasound in small dogs (15 kg or less) and cats a 7.5-MHz transducer is ideal. For middle-sized to large-breed dogs, a 5-MHz transducer works well. A guide for selecting a transducer is as follows:

High Frequency: Increase resolution
Increase attenuation
Decrease penetration
Low Frequency: Decrease resolution
Decrease attenuation
Increase penetration

Ultrasound Artifacts

Most people fail to take the time to fully understand ultrasound artifacts. They ignore artifacts because by definition an artifact does not contribute useful image information. This is not true of ultrasound artifacts. Ultrasound artifacts provide accurate clues to what makes up the ultrasound image.

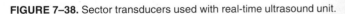

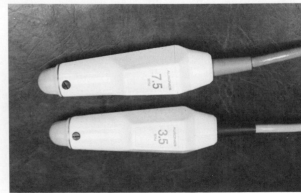

FIGURE 7–38. Sector transducers used with real-time ultrasound unit.

Reverberation Artifact

Reverberation is present when some of the returning sound is reflected from the transducer face or an internal interface and re-enters the patient. The second echo will have the same shape and be double the distance from the first echo. Reverberation echoes reflect from gas-filled structures and usually appear as high-amplitude parallel lines occurring at regular intervals. The distance between each line corresponds to the distance between the transducer and the gas interface. Each reverberation is weaker than the preceding one. Reverberation artifact can also be referred to as "dirty shadowing" and "comet tails" (Fig. 7–39).

Shadowing

Shadowing artifact occurs owing to inadequate sound beam penetration through a highly reflective or sound absorptive substance. Acoustic shadowing is an area of darkness or hypoechogenicity that occurs deep to gas or very dense material, such as bone, calcium or calculi. Very small objects cast an acoustic shadow only if they are within the focal zone or narrow portion of the ultrasound beam.

Acoustic Enhancement

If the ultrasound beam passes through an area with few tissue interfaces (low attenuation region), the emerging ultrasound beam will have more intensity than would be expected and will be brighter or more echogenic distal to the nonattenuating structure. The best example of this is the normal gallbladder surrounded by the hepatic parenchyma. The liver tissue distal or deep to the gallbladder appears brighter than adjacent hepatic tissue (Fig. 7–40). This artifact is seen deep to fluid-filled structures and is also referred to as "through transmission."

Refraction or "Edge Artifact"

This is a hypoechoic band or stripe at the margin of a curved structure due to the refraction or bending of the sound beam. The sound beam is deflected from its true path with an effect

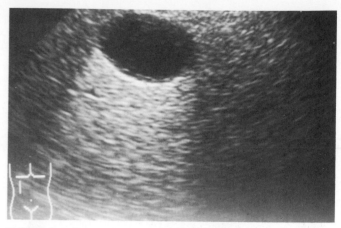

FIGURE 7–40. The bright echogenic band beneath the gallbladder represents acoustic enhancement. The ultrasound beam is not attenuated as much as it traverses the fluid-filled gallbladder as it is in the surrounding liver.

similar to shadowing. Edge artifact can create false hypoechoic masses in structures within its path.

Mirror-Image Artifact

The ultrasound machine places the returning echo on the viewing screen as a function of the time it took the echo to return. If the sound wave reverberates within a highly echogenic structure before returning to the transducer, the image will be duplicated on the screen distal to the original image. This is most commonly seen as a duplication of the gallbladder in mirror image.

Slice-Thickness Artifact

If the width of the ultrasound beam cuts through both the edge of a cystic structure and solid tissue, the solid tissue may look as if it is layered within the cyst. This artifact is responsible for the erroneous appearance of debris within the urinary bladder and gallbladder, although no debris is present. The erroneous appearance is the result of volume averaging of tissue by the ultrasound machine.

The Ultrasound Examination

A complete ultrasound examination requires at least 20 to 30 minutes to perform. When ultrasound is used for a quick answer to a question such as pregnancy versus pyometra, the examination will be shorter. When using ultrasound for abdominal disease diagnosis, a complete examination should be performed every time.

It is important to have a thorough understanding of the normal appearance of the various abdominal organs before trying to identify the abnormalities associated with disease. The ranking of small animal abdominal organs from least echogenic (darkest) to most echogenic (brightest) is as follows:

Least echogenic	Renal medulla
	Renal cortex
↓	Liver
	Spleen
	Prostate
Most echogenic	Renal sinus fat

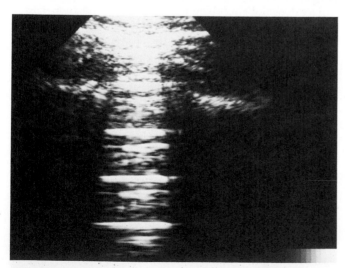

FIGURE 7–39. Reverberation artifact from the air-filled lung of a normal horse. The parallel evenly spaced echogenic bands represent reverberation between the transducer and the pleural surface.

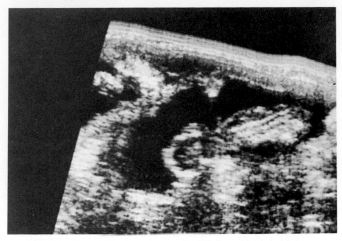

Remember that echogenicity is a relative term, and one must compare organs at similar control settings and similar depths to avoid misinterpretation.

Clinical Use

Large Animals. Ultrasound is most commonly used in horses for pregnancy diagnosis. It is used also for examination of the thorax and of tendons, and its use for abdominal diseases is increasing. The linear array scanner with a 3.0-MHz or 5.0-MHz scan head is most popular among veterinarians. Essentially, any superficial muscle or tendon can be examined. The use of ultrasound for examination of joints is currently being investigated.

Small Animals. Equipment designed for use in people is readily adaptable for use in small animals. The most common transducers used are 3.0, 5.0 or 7.5 MHz. Sector scanners are most popular because of their small contact area (Fig. 7–37).

Ultrasound has become a popular tool to diagnose cardiac diseases. M-mode and real-time studies are commonly used by veterinary radiologists and cardiologists in teaching institutions and in large or specialty practices. Valvular lesions, pericardial effusion and neoplasia are routinely diagnosed by cardiac ultrasound (often called echocardiography).

Great progress has been made in the past few years with abdominal ultrasound. The liver, spleen and the entire urinary system can be imaged and diagnoses are made routinely (Fig. 7–41). The non-invasive ultrasound technology often replaces the more dangerous invasive or surgical techniques used a few years ago. Several cardiac diagnoses can now be made using non-invasive ultrasound in an unanesthetized patient, rather than using an invasive angiocardiogram with injectable contrast medium in an anesthetized patient.

NUCLEAR MEDICINE

Many veterinary schools and several progressive specialized veterinary practices have nuclear medicine capabilities. Nu-

FIGURE 7–41 Ultrasonogram of a 52 day old canine fetus.

clear medicine can be divided into therapeutic and diagnostic procedures. Currently, veterinary therapeutic nuclear medicine involves the administration of radioactive iodine (^{131}I) for the treatment of hyperthyroidism and thyroid tumors. Diagnostic nuclear medicine involves the administration of radionuclides to the animal and detecting the electromagnetic radiation emitted from the animal with a gamma scintillation camera. Radionuclides are atoms with an unstable nucleus that undergoes radioactive decay. Radioactive decay is the transformation or disintegration of an unstable nuclide by spontaneous emission of electromagnetic radiation. Electromagnetic radiations that are of nuclear origin are termed gamma rays, in contrast to diagnostic radiations (x-rays), which originate from the electron cloud that surrounds the nucleus.

Diagnostic nuclear medicine does not generate visual images equivalent to those of diagnostic radiology but detects functional or physiological, pharmacological and kinetic data from the patient in image or numerical data form. Figure 7–42A and Figure 7–42B show a standard gamma scintillation camera,

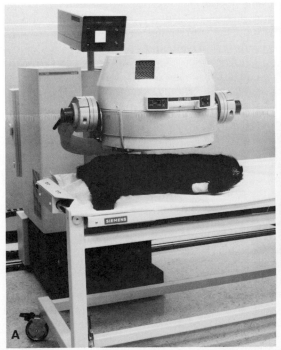

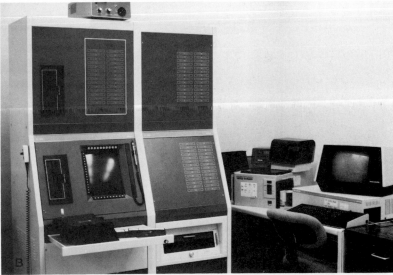

FIGURE 7–42. A, Gamma scintillation camera in position over a dog during a whole-body bone scan to check for metastatic neoplasia. B, Control panel monitor, nuclear medicine computer and matrix camera.

control panel and nuclear medicine computer. Common clinical uses of veterinary nuclear medicine include bone scanning to detect tumor metastasis to bone and radiographically undetectable bone injury or infection, lung scanning to detect pulmonary embolism and as a pulmonary function test, renal scans to assess kidney perfusion and function, and thyroid scans for the characterization of hyperthyroid patients and to detect metastasis. Other less common nuclear medicine studies include hepatobiliary scanning, brain scans, labeled white blood cell scans for the detection of occult infection, lymphoscintigraphy, nuclear angiography and scans to detect an unknown focus of blood loss.

The most commonly used radionuclide is technetium-99m (^{99m}Tc). This agent is commercially available from a disposable technetium generator. Technetium is administered in an ionic form as ^{99m}TcO$_4$ (pertechnetate) or bound to a specific organ-localizing pharmaceutical agent prior to administration. Technetium is the radiopharmaceutical of choice because it has a 6-hour physical half-life and emits a 140 keV gamma ray, which is appropriate for most imaging studies. The radioactive or physical half-life ($T_{1/2}$) of a radionuclide is the time required for the number of radioactive atoms to decrease by 50 percent.

Radiation safety practices are important with nuclear medicine. When working in a practice that uses nuclear medicine one should insist on receiving comprehensive instruction in radiation principles and safety. This chapter is meant only as an introduction.

The primary route of radionuclide administration to veterinary patients is intravenous. Latex examination gloves should be worn and careful injection techniques should be performed to be sure the entire dose is delivered intravenously and not perivascularly. This is especially important in equine bone scans for which a large dose of radionuclide is administered. The routes of excretion of the radioactive imaging agents vary with the agent used. Technetium is primarily excreted in urine, with a lesser amount in the feces. Animals should be housed in a separate restricted area of the hospital, and their stool and urine should be carefully collected and held for decay until the levels are below exempt quantities. Always wear latex examination gloves and limit contact with these patients

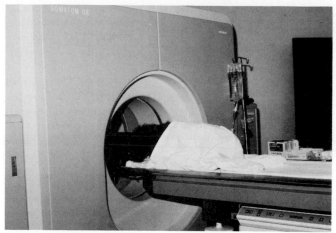

FIGURE 7–44. Dog in position for a head CT. The large circular gantry houses the x-ray tube and detectors.

to only that necessary for their care. Never eat or bring eating utensils (coffee cups, spoons and so forth) into a nuclear medicine area. The dose of radiation to the patient is small, but repeated physical contact or accidental ingestion of radionuclides may be harmful to the nuclear medicine technologist. Animals should be held until they pose no radiation threat to their owners or the population at large. This is generally 3 to 10 physical half-lives of the radiopharmaceutical, depending on specific state regulations.

COMPUTED TOMOGRAPHY (CT SCAN)

In the past several years there has been an expansion of the diagnostic imaging techniques available to veterinary patients. Most veterinary schools and several specialty practices have access to computed tomography or "CT scans." A CT scan is obtained by passing a very thin x-ray beam transaxially through the patient and measuring the x-ray attenuation at multiple sites in a thin slice of the patient's anatomy. The computer then reconstructs the transmitted x-ray data into a cross-sectional image on a video monitor. The image can then be captured on film or video tape or stored for later use on magnetic tape. The advantage of CT over standard radiography is the greatly improved radiographic contrast, spatial resolution, and cross-sectional anatomical presentation. The most common use of CT in veterinary medicine is head examinations for intracranial disease. CT allows the veterinarian a non-invasive look inside the skull of patients (Fig. 7–43).

When a CT scan is performed the patient is placed in VD or DV position on the long narrow movable CT table. The table then moves the patient through the circular gantry that houses the x-ray tube and detectors (Fig. 7–44). The table moves in a measured stepwise fashion. During each table step the CT scanner obtains a single cross-sectional slice of data. The patients need to be heavily sedated or under general anesthesia to prevent any motion and must be positioned perfectly straight. Most studies are performed twice on the same animal. The first study without contrast and the second following intravenous iodinated contrast administration. Urographic contrast agents are commonly used at a dose of 800 mg of iodine per

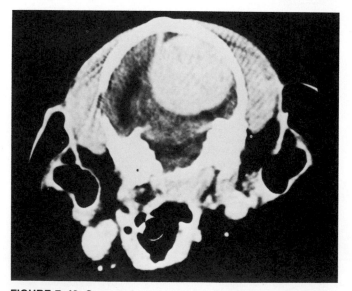

FIGURE 7–43. Computed tomogram of a dog brain showing a large contrast-enhancing brain tumor (meningioma) in the central cerebrum.

kg of body weight. Contrast will highlight vascular structures, and some neoplasms will have a characteristic contrast enhancement pattern. Besides brain studies, CT can be used to identify and characterize musculoskeletal, spinal, thoracic and abdominal disorders.

Recommended Reading

Barr F: Diagnostic Ultrasound in the Dog and Cat. Oxford, England, Blackwell Scientific Publications, 1990.

Bushong SC: Radiologic Science for Technologists. 4th ed. St. Louis, The CV Mosby Co., 1988.

Curry TS, Dowdey JE, Murry RC: Christensen's Introduction to the Physics of Diagnostic Radiology. 4th ed. Philadelphia, Lea & Febiger, 1990.

Douglas SW, Herrtage ME, Williamson HD: Principles of Veterinary Radiology. 4th ed. East Sussex, England, Bailliere Tindall, 1987.

Eastman-Kodak Company: The Fundamentals of Radiography. 12th ed. Rochester, NY, 1980.

Hall EJ: Radiobiology for the Radiologist. 3rd ed. Philadelphia, JB Lippincott Co., 1988, Chapters 1 and 24.

Herring DS: Symposium on Diagnostic Ultrasound. Vet Clin North Am (Small Anim Pract) 15:1105–1324, 1985.

Kleine LJ and Warren RG: Small Animal Radiography—Animal Health Technology. St. Louis, The CV Mosby Co., 1983.

Morgan JR and Silverman S: Techniques of Veterinary Radiography. 4th ed. Ames, IA, Iowa State University Press, 1987.

Rantanen NW: Diagnostic Ultrasound. Vet Clin North Am (Equine Pract) 2:1–258, 1986.

Stashak TS: Adams' Lameness in Horses. 4th ed. Chapter 4. Philadelphia, Lea & Febiger, 1987.

Steckel RR: Advanced Diagnostic Methods. Vet Clin North Am (Equine Pract) 2:207–480, 1991.

Ticer JW: Radiographic Technique in Veterinary Practice. 2nd ed. Philadelphia, WB Saunders Co., 1984.

8

Diagnostic Sampling and Treatment Techniques

MERLYN J. LUCAS and SUSAN E. LUCAS

INTRODUCTION

The trained veterinary technician has an important patient support role in many practices. Under the direction of the veterinarian, the skilled technician is able to obtain diagnostic samples and perform routine treatment procedures. This allows the veterinarian to concentrate more on medicosurgical decisions, making the practice more productive.

The blood sample is the basis for the routine clinical pathological evaluation of the health status of the animal. It is essential to collect blood samples with minimal damage to the vein. This is especially important when repeated sampling is needed.

In this chapter, blood sampling techniques using a needle and syringe will be described. Vacutainer tubes (Becton Dickinson Co., Rutherford, NJ) can also be used in all blood collection techniques described. This system makes collection and processing of blood much easier. When using the Vacutainer system, the tube is placed in the holder without piercing the rubber stopper. Once the needle is inserted under the skin, the tube is advanced into the holder so that the rubber stopper is pierced. When the vein is entered, blood is suctioned into the tube until the tube is approximately three quarters full. Proper-sized tubes must be used, since large tubes will collapse a small vein.

In all cases, blood samples must be handled carefully to prevent exposure to temperature extremes and rough handling. Blood samples taken with a syringe should not be forced through a small-gauge needle. This will often cause hemolysis of erythrocytes and give erroneous laboratory values.

SMALL ANIMAL SAMPLING AND TREATMENT TECHNIQUES

Sample Collection—Venipuncture

The site most commonly used for blood sample collection in the dog is the cephalic vein, which is located on the cranial surface of the foreleg. For esthetic reasons, it is usually best not to clip the hair over venipuncture sites; however, in long-haired animals, it may be necessary in order to identify the vein. After thorough wetting and cleansing with an antiseptic solution (70 percent alcohol), the hair can usually be parted so that the needle is introduced directly through the skin. If the right cephalic vein is to be used, the assistant should stand on the left side of the animal and place the left arm under the animal's chin to restrict movement of the head. Using the right hand, the assistant reaches across and grasps the animal's right foreleg distal to the elbow joint. The thumb is used to occlude the vein and to rotate it so that it lies on top of the outstretched leg. If an assistant is not available, a tourniquet placed just distal to the elbow joint may be used. The person collecting the sample grasps the foreleg of the animal and places the thumb alongside the vein. The syringe, which is held in the opposite hand, should be equipped with a small-gauge needle: a 12.7-mm, 25-gauge for small dogs, a 19.05-mm, 22-gauge for medium dogs, and a 2.5-cm, 20- or 21-gauge for large dogs. The needle should be thrust through the skin at a 20-degree angle and into the vein in one motion (Fig. 8–1). A gentle pull on the plunger allows blood to flow into the syringe

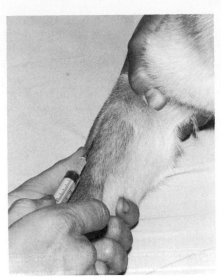

FIGURE 8–1. The cephalic vein is commonly used for canine venipuncture.

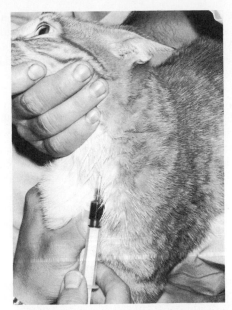

FIGURE 8–3. Jugular venipuncture in the cat.

(Fig. 8–2). When the necessary amount of blood has been collected, the digital pressure or tourniquet is released. The needle is quickly withdrawn, and digital pressure is immediately applied to the puncture site to prevent bleeding or hematoma formation.

The jugular vein is another site frequently used for collecting blood samples. The assistant restrains the animal in sternal recumbency and extends the head and neck. In cats, it may be helpful to grasp the front feet in one hand and extend them over the edge of the examination table while using the other hand to extend the head and neck. Unruly cats may be placed in a cat bag or wrapped in a large towel to restrain both front and hind legs (see Chapter 1). Rotating the head slightly often allows improved visualization of the vein. The person performing the venipuncture places the thumb in the jugular furrow at the thoracic inlet, which distends the vein. The jugular vein in shorthaired animals is generally easily visualized and is often located beneath the "cowlick" on the neck. Venipuncture is accomplished by inserting the needle in a cranial direction into the jugular vein (Fig. 8–3).

Other sites that may be used for blood sample collection in cats are the lateral saphenous, femoral and medial saphenous veins. The femoral vein is an effective puncture site for obtaining blood from cats. However, it is very mobile because of its loose subcutaneous support, and a hematoma may develop as a result of venipuncture.

Sample Collection—Urine

Catheterization

Male Canine. Passing a urethral catheter to obtain a urine sample is usually not difficult in a male dog. Proper catheterization requires an assistant to aid in restraining the animal. The dog is placed in lateral recumbency, and the rear leg on top is pulled forward and flexed by the assistant. The sheath of the penis is retracted enough to allow the end of the penis to protrude, and the glans penis is cleansed with an antiseptic soap and rinsed with saline. The distal 2 to 3 cm of the appropriately sized catheter (size 4 to 10 French, 45 cm long with the opposite end adapted to fit a syringe) is lubricated with sterile lubricating jelly. The catheter should not be removed entirely from its container while it is being passed, because the container allows the operator to handle the catheter without contaminating it. The catheter may also be passed with sterile gloved hands or by using a sterile hemostat. When the catheter reaches the caudal end of the os penis, resistance may be met because of the flexure of the urethral canal. Steady but gentle pressure should overcome this resistance. If the catheter cannot be passed on the first try, the catheter size should be re-evaluated. When the size of the catheter has been determined to be satisfactory, it should be gently rotated while being passed a second time. As it passes the sphincter of the bladder, there should be a flow of urine at the end of the catheter. A sterile syringe is used to aspirate urine from the bladder, and 2 to 5 ml of 50 percent nitrofurazone solution may be flushed into the bladder and along the urethral canal as the catheter is withdrawn.

Female Canine. Urinary catheterization of the female dog is

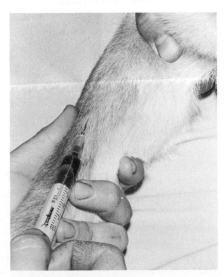

FIGURE 8–2. Successful canine venipuncture.

more difficult because of the positioning of the urethral orifice. The animal is restrained in a standing position by an assistant. Metal catheters are available in assorted sizes. The curved insertion end of the catheter is lubricated and is passed along the vestibular floor until it passes through the urethral opening and into the bladder. A female speculum and penlight or an otoscope fitted with a large speculum may be used to visualize the urethral opening (Fig. 8–4). After collection of the urine sample, 2 to 5 ml of 50 percent nitrofurazone solution may be flushed through the catheter into the bladder.

Male Feline. Catheterization of the male cat may require the use of a short-acting anesthetic, such as thiamylal sodium, or a rapidly cleared gas anesthetic, such as halothane, or both. However, extra care should be taken when severely ill or uremic cats are anesthetized. In many cases, sedating the uremic cat may be all that is required to accomplish catheterization. The anesthetized or sedated animal is placed on his back, with the hind legs pulled forward. The penis is drawn from the sheath and gently drawn backward. A sterile, flexible, plastic or polyethylene catheter (tomcat catheter) is passed through the urethral opening and into the bladder. The catheter should be kept parallel to the vertebral column. If resistance is met, the catheter should not be forced through the urethra, since a urethral calculus may be causing an obstruction. It may be necessary to inject 3 to 5 ml of sterile water or saline in order to flush out the concretions and pass the catheter.

Female Feline. Female cats may be catheterized by use of a plastic, blunt-ended tomcat catheter. It is necessary to first anesthetize the vestibular-vaginal vault by instilling 0.5 percent xylocaine. The lips of the vulva are cleansed, grasped and pulled caudally. A lubricated catheter is then inserted along the floor of the vestibule into the urethral orifice.

Bladder Expression

A second method of urine collection is by expression of the bladder. This procedure must be done with great care, especially if there is an obstruction in the urethra. Excessive pressure on the bladder may cause it to rupture. The bladder is located by palpation of the abdomen and gentle, steady pressure is applied. One hand may be used to express the bladder of cats and small dogs. In larger animals, it is often easier to use both hands by exerting gentle pressure on either side of the bladder. If pressure is applied to the bladder and no resulting flow of urine occurs, there is a possibility that urethral blockage exists, and another method of urine collection should be considered.

Cystocentesis

Urine specimens that are being collected for bacterial culture may be obtained by *cystocentesis*. This procedure is done only when the bladder is sufficiently full to be easily palpable. The skin is aseptically prepared, and the bladder is manually immobilized by abdominal palpation. A syringe (5 to 20 ml) with a needle attached (20- to 24-gauge, 3.75 to 5 cm long) is inserted through the abdominal wall and into the bladder. As much urine as possible is removed by gentle suction. A three-way valve may be attached to the syringe and needle to aid in the removal of urine. Care should be taken not to leave a large amount of urine in the bladder, since the pressure may cause urine to leak through the puncture site and into the abdominal cavity.

Free-Flow Collection

Collection of urine may also be achieved during normal voiding. Dogs frequently urinate when taken outside for a walk. A straightened wire coat hanger or a small-diameter aluminum rod may be bent into a circle at one end and a urine cup may be placed within the opening. As the animal begins to void, the cup is slipped into place to obtain the urine sample. Use of a metabolic cage (if available) may also prove beneficial. The animal is placed in a cage on a wire platform that is over a solid floor that slopes to a central funnel. A clean container is placed under the funnel to collect any urine that is voided. A solid plastic sheet placed in a litter box may be useful in obtaining urine samples from cats.

Fecal Collection

Fecal samples are most commonly obtained by picking them up with a wooden tongue depressor after the animal has defecated. A sample may also be collected by inserting a gloved, lubricated finger into the rectum and withdrawing any fecal material within reach. An enema may be used to obtain a sample, but soapy or oily enemas should be avoided because they will interfere with good examination of the feces. If the sample is to be kept for a few hours before examination, it should always be refrigerated.

Abdominocentesis

Abdominocentesis is a useful technique for removing excessive fluid from the abdominal cavity and for obtaining fluid for analysis of cellular appearance and chemical characteristics. An aspirating needle of sufficient length to enter the abdominal cavity without penetrating or damaging the abdominal organs is needed. A 16-gauge needle is generally adequate,

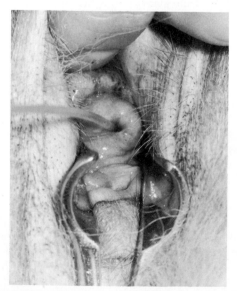

FIGURE 8–4. Close-up view of urine-filled catheter inserted into urethral opening of a bitch.

though this may vary slightly depending on the presence of fluid transudates or exudates. An alternative to the hypodermic needle is the use of a plastic "over-the-needle" intravenous catheter. The catheter and needle are inserted into the abdominal cavity. The needle is then removed, leaving the flexible catheter to remove abdominal fluid.

The animal is placed in left lateral recumbency. The puncture site should be chosen to avoid damaging major organs (spleen, liver, urinary bladder). A midline site 2.5 to 5 cm caudal to the xiphoid process is generally acceptable but not critical. The bladder is manually expressed, and the puncture site is aseptically prepared. Local anesthesia and sometimes sedation are required. The taut, drawn skin is displaced slightly, and the needle (with syringe attached) is inserted through the abdominal wall. By gently drawing back on the plunger, one creates a vacuum in the syringe, and as the abdominal cavity is entered, fluid will be drawn into the syringe. A test tube containing an anticoagulant, such as ethylene-diaminetetraacetic acid (EDTA), should be used to store the sample, since abdominal fluids often clot. If a large quantity of fluid is to be drawn off, the animal should be made to stand to aid in removal of the fluid.

Impression Smears

Tissue specimens obtained by biopsy are often prepared for cytological examination by means of an impression smear. The surface of the tissue collected is gently blotted with a paper towel to remove any blood or fluid. The cut surface of the lesion is gently touched to the surface of a clean, dry slide. Excessive pressure is avoided so that the number of cells left on the slide are not too numerous for examination. After several imprints have been made on the slide, the smears are either air-dried or fixed, and the slide is stained with a permanent stain (see Chapter 4). If an impression smear is needed from an open lesion, the lesion is carefully cleansed and a clean glass slide is pressed gently to the surface. The slide is then prepared in the previously described fashion.

ADMINISTRATION OF MEDICATION IN THE SMALL ANIMAL

Intravenous Administration

Administration of medication by intravenous injection ensures the most rapid method of drug absorption into the circulation and tissues. It may also be the method of choice for drugs that irritate the tissues. The most common sites for intravenous injections are the cephalic vein and the lateral saphenous vein. The techniques for venipuncture should be followed as was previously discussed under the section on Sample Collection—Venipuncture. Proper positioning of the needle in the vein is ascertained by aspirating a small amount of blood into the syringe. The digital pressure or tourniquet is released, and the medication is injected, usually slowly. If there are any small air bubbles in the syringe, it should be held so that the air bubbles float to the plunger end. The air bubbles and a small amount of liquid are then left in the syringe. The needle is quickly withdrawn, and the digital pressure is promptly applied to the injection site to prevent bleeding.

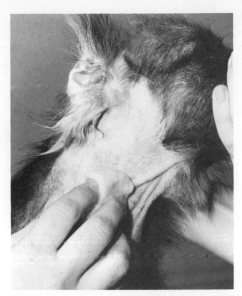

FIGURE 8–5. The site of jugular catheterization is aseptically prepared.

If an irritating drug is accidentally injected into the tissues surrounding the vein, physiologic saline solution can be instilled at the site to dilute the medication.

Occasionally, an animal will need repeated intravenous treatments for long-term fluid therapy. Placing a catheter in the vein ensures that the vein is readily accessible for each treatment. The preferred site of catheter placement is usually the jugular vein because the large size of this vein facilitates easy insertion of the catheter. The catheter is also more easily secured in place here than at other sites of the body. There are numerous catheters on the market, and insertion technique will vary according to type. Directions for use are generally included with the catheter and should be strictly followed. Prior to insertion, the skin site is clipped and aseptically prepared (Fig. 8–5). When the catheter has been successfully placed in the vein, it is secured by placing adhesive tape around the base in a butterfly manner (Figs. 8–6 and 8–7). The puncture site should be covered with a square of sterile gauze on which an antiseptic ointment has been liberally spread (Fig. 8–8). The catheter is then taped in place on the neck. Additional tape may be added to completely cover the

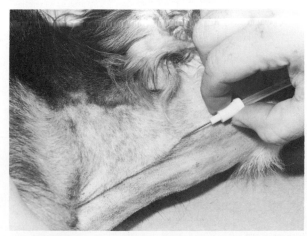

FIGURE 8–6. Insertion of catheter into jugular vein.

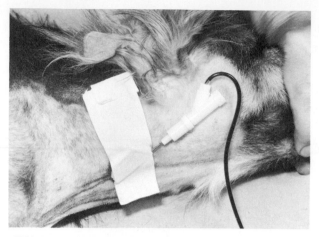

FIGURE 8–7. Adhesive tape is used to secure catheter in vein.

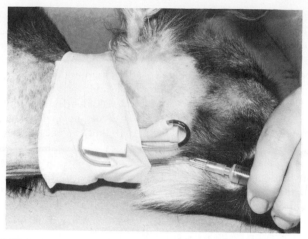

FIGURE 8–9. Completed canine jugular catheterization. Small amounts of heparinized saline should be injected periodically to prevent clotting in the catheter.

catheter, which makes it difficult for the animal to pull it loose (Fig. 8–9).

Subcutaneous Injections

Subcutaneous injections allow quick systemic action, since the drug is readily absorbed into the lymph and blood systems. It is also a commonly used route when vaccinating dogs and cats. Subcutaneous injection should be used for nonirritating drugs only. An ideal site for subcutaneous injection is the dorsal back area from the shoulder to the rump. The injection site may be prepared by parting the hair and cleansing the skin with 70 percent rubbing alcohol. A fold of skin is picked up, pinched and pinched again as the injection is made (Fig. 8–10). Gentle massage of the area aids in the absorption of the medication.

Intramuscular Injections

Slightly more irritating medications may be injected intramuscularly. Drugs given by this route should generally be smaller in volume, since muscular tissue cannot readily expand. One injection site is the semimembranosus and semitendinosus muscle mass (hamstring muscles) in the rear leg. The

site should be approached laterally with the needle angled in a slightly caudal direction to avoid damaging the sciatic nerve. The lumbar region is also commonly used for intramuscular injection. One method of choosing a site in the lumbar region is to place the thumb and second finger on the wings of the ileum and allow the first finger to fall naturally. The injection is given at the area of the point of the finger. It would be best to avoid the lumbar area if the patient is extremely thin or small.

After the injection site has been chosen, the skin is cleansed with 70 percent alcohol, and the muscles are grasped between the thumb and fingers. The needle is inserted perpendicularly, and the plunger of the syringe is retracted slightly to ensure that a vein has not been entered (Fig. 8–11). The medication is then injected, and the needle is withdrawn.

Topical Medications

Eye

When administering drops to a patient's eye, the hand holding the dropper rests on the animal's head. The other hand is used to evert the lower lid, and the drops are placed on the inner canthus without the dropper touching the eye. Ointment

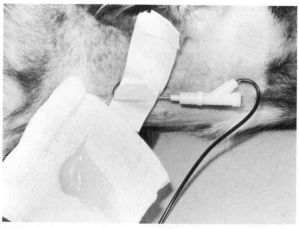

FIGURE 8–8. Sterile gauze with antiseptic ointment is used to cover the puncture site.

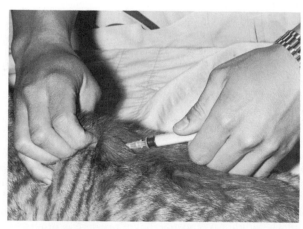

FIGURE 8–10. Subcutaneous injection of a cat.

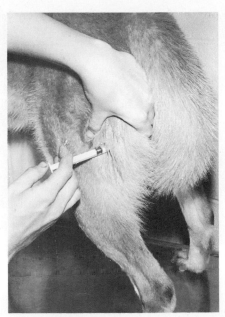

FIGURE 8–11. Intramuscular injection in the semitendinosus and semimembranosus muscles of the dog.

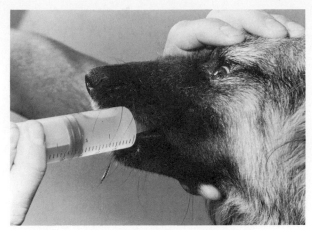

FIGURE 8–13. A syringe may be used to administer liquid medication perorally.

applied to the eye should be placed in a 3-mm-wide strip on the lower palpebral border (Fig. 8–12).

Ear

To administer medication to the ear, the canal is first straightened by pulling the earflap upward and backward. The nozzle or tube is inserted slightly downward and medially a short distance into the ear canal. After the medication has been administered, the base of the ear should be gently massaged to spread the medication over the lining of the horizontal and vertical ear canal.

Oral Medication

The most frequently used route for medicating the dog or cat is by mouth. Not only is this procedure less painful for the

animal, but it is also safe and convenient. Clients can easily be trained to use the techniques of peroral medication so that the animal will continue to receive necessary treatments at home.

There are three forms of peroral medications: liquids, tablets and capsules. Of the three, liquids are usually the easiest to administer. A syringe or small prescription bottle may be used to accurately measure the prescribed amount of medication. A pocket is formed by gently pulling out the animal's lower lip at the corner. Small amounts of liquid are then poured into the pouch (Fig. 8–13). The head should be tilted so that the nose is in a horizontal line with the eyes. Any greater angle of the head may result in difficulty in swallowing.

Stomach Tube

Liquids may also be administered by the veterinarian or technician by use of a stomach tube. Plastic tubing for this purpose is available in many sizes. A soft rubber catheter (22 French, 75 cm long for dogs; 12 French to 16 French, 40 cm long for cats) will also work well. Before the tube is passed, the distance from the animal's incisor teeth to the level of the eighth or ninth rib should be measured and marked on the tubing with tape or a ballpoint pen (Fig. 8–14). A partially used roll of adhesive tape or a wooden spacer-block should be inserted behind the canine teeth to hold the animal's mouth

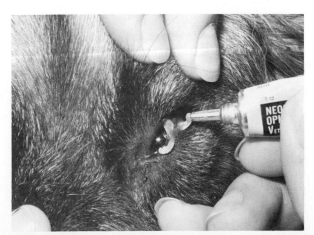

FIGURE 8–12. Ointment is applied to the dog's eye on the lower palpebral border.

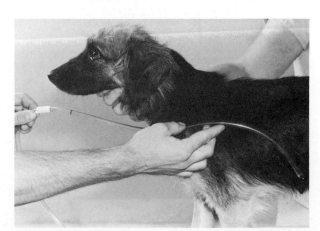

FIGURE 8–14. The stomach tube is measured to the level of the eighth or ninth rib before being passed.

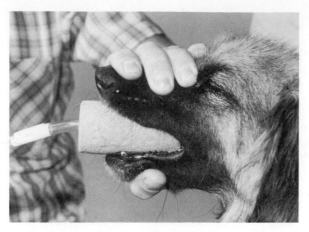

FIGURE 8–15. A roll of adhesive tape is used to hold the mouth open and prevent the animal from biting the tube.

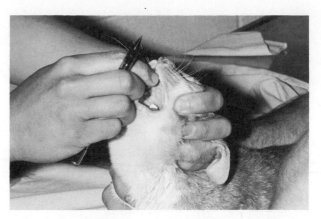

FIGURE 8–17. Placement of a tablet or capsule at the base of the tongue in a cat.

open (Fig. 8–15). The end of the stomach tube should be lubricated with water or a sterile lubricating gel inserted through the central hole in the tape roll or block, and pushed gently into the pharynx. As the animal swallows, the tube is advanced to the level previously marked. The neck should be palpated to be certain the tubing can be felt in the esophagus. A syringe or funnel may be attached to the end of the stomach tube and the medication administered slowly. When withdrawing the tube, it should be kinked in order to prevent stomach contents from being withdrawn and possibly inhaled.

Hand Pilling

The most frequently used forms of oral medication are tablets and capsules. The medication is held between the second and third fingers of the right hand while the left hand is used to open the patient's mouth. This is accomplished by grasping the upper jaw with the thumb on one side and fingers on the other and pressing the lips over the upper teeth. The thumb of the right hand may be used to press downward on the lower jaw in the space behind the incisors. A second option is to hold the medication between the thumb and second finger and use the third finger to open the animal's mouth. The pill is placed in the center on the base of the tongue (Figs. 8–16 and 8–17), and the animal's mouth is closed. A gentle tap on the nose or under the chin generally startles the animal into swallowing.

Fractious dogs and cats may be medicated by use of a curved hemostat or special pill forceps to place the pill over the base of the tongue. In the cat, a third option is to drop the pill deep into the mouth and then, by using a finger or the eraser end of a pencil, tapping the pill deeper, thereby stimulating the cat to swallow (Fig. 8–18). If the animal licks its nose, it is a good indication that the medication has been swallowed. Nasogastric intubation (passing a tube to the stomach via the nostrils) may be performed in the dog and cat. However, the small lumen of the nostrils restricts the types of solutions that can be administered by this route, which makes stomach tubing through the mouth more practical.

Pharyngostomy Tube

In animals whose condition requires repeated medications or feedings by stomach tube, the veterinarian may decide a pharyngostomy should be performed. A standard surgical pack, suture material and feeding tube (plastic or rubber) are needed for this procedure. A short-acting anesthetic or local anesthesia alone may be used, depending upon the condition of the patient and its ability to tolerate surgery. The area posterior to the angle of the mandible is aseptically prepared, and the mouth is held open with the aid of a speculum. A gloved index finger is inserted into the pharynx and placed in the location of the piriform fossa of the pharynx just posterior to the base of the tongue and lateral to the hyoid apparatus (Fig.

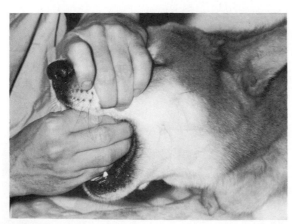

FIGURE 8–16. Tablets or capsules are placed in the center of the base of the tongue in a dog.

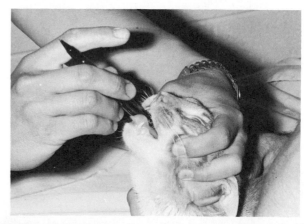

FIGURE 8–18. Tapping the pill over the base of the tongue stimulates swallowing.

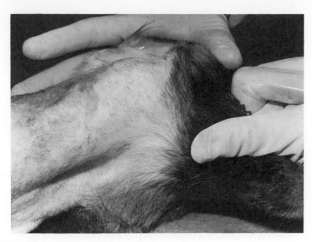

FIGURE 8 19. A gloved index finger is used to locate the incision site for a pharyngostomy

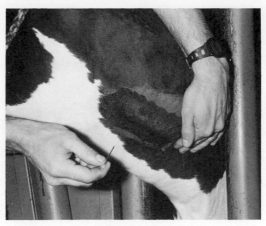

FIGURE 8–21. Digital pressure applied in the jugular furrow allows good visualization of the vein.

8–19). A curved hemostat is inserted through the mouth and is used to exert outward pressure on the skin at this location. A No. 11 or a No. 15 scalpel blade is used to incise the skin over the bulge and, using the hemostat, the tube is drawn through the incision site and placed in the esophagus (Fig. 8–20). After proper positioning of the stomach tube, the proximal end is sutured into place. This is accomplished by using a piece of adhesive tape as a cuff, which is sutured to the skin of the neck. The incision site should be cleansed daily, and the tube should remain capped when not in use. The incision site is generally allowed to heal by second intention after the tube is removed.

LARGE ANIMAL SAMPLING AND TREATMENT TECHNIQUES

Bovine Venipuncture

The choice of a venipuncture site in the bovine depends a great deal on the type of restraint available and the amount of blood needed. When collecting a blood sample via the jugular vein, the animal must be restrained by use of a halter or a halter and nose lead. If at all possible, the patient is placed in

a chute or stanchion with the head drawn upward and to the opposite side from which the blood will be drawn by use of the halter or halter and nose lead. The head is secured in this position by tying the restraint rope or ropes to a solid area such as the top bar of the stanchion. After cleansing the venipuncture site with 70 percent alcohol, the vein is occluded by applying digital pressure in the jugular furrow, which allows good visualization of the vein (Fig. 8–21). Using the opposite hand, a 14- or 16-gauge, 5- to 7.5-cm needle is pushed with one sharp motion through the skin at a 45- to 90-degree angle. When a flow of blood from the needle signals that the vein has been entered, the needle is threaded either upward or downward to the hub (Fig. 8–22). Keeping the vein occluded, a syringe is attached to the needle, and the necessary amount of blood is aspirated (Fig. 8–23). After releasing the pressure on the vein, the needle, still attached to the syringe, is withdrawn.

A second common site for bovine venipuncture is the ventral coccygeal vein, commonly referred to as the "tail vein." Once again, the animal must be confined to an area, such as a chute, in which it will be unable to move sideways. Tail restraint is applied with one hand by bending the tail directly forward at the base, and the venipuncture site is cleansed with 70 percent alcohol (Fig. 8–24). An 18- to 20-gauge, 2.5- to 3.75-cm needle attached to a syringe is held by the opposite hand and is inserted at a 90-degree angle to the skin on the midline be-

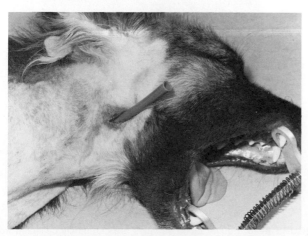

FIGURE 8–20. Completed pharyngostomy in the dog.

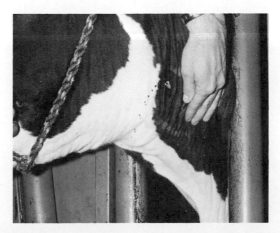

FIGURE 8–22. A flow of blood from the needle ensures proper placement of the needle in the vein.

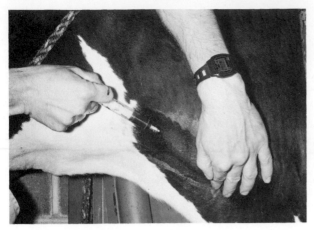

FIGURE 8–23. Successful bovine blood sample collection.

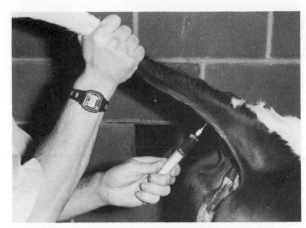

FIGURE 8–25. Adequate tail restraint is essential when obtaining a blood sample from this site.

tween the hemal arches of coccygeal vertebrae 4 through 7 (Fig. 8–25).

Equine Venipuncture

Routine equine blood samples are collected from the jugular vein as outlined for the bovine. The type of restraint needed will vary, depending upon the temperament of the animal. The vein is occluded and an 18-gauge, 3.75-cm needle attached to a syringe is used to collect the sample (Fig. 8–26). The right jugular vein is used whenever possible in order to avoid hitting the esophagus, which runs near the jugular groove on the left side. The head is turned away from the side of the venipuncture so that the vein is stretched and more easily identified.

Swine Venipuncture

Anterior Vena Cava

Blood samples from swine have traditionally been most often obtained from the anterior vena cava. The needle size required to obtain blood from this site depends upon the size of the animal—a 2.5-cm, 20-gauge needle may be used for pigs up to 11.25 kg in weight; a 3.75-cm, 18-gauge needle may be used for animals 11.25 to 22.5 kg; a 5-cm, 17- to 18-gauge needle may be used for pigs 22.5 to 56.25 kg; and a 6.25-cm, 17- to 18-

gauge needle may be used for weights up to 117 kg. In animals weighing more than 117 kg, it is necessary to use a 7.5- to 12.5-cm needle.

Use of the right anterior vena cava is preferred because both the phrenic nerve and thoracic duct lie near the exterior jugular vein on the left. Small hogs may be restrained in dorsal recumbency with head fully extended and front legs pulled caudally. Mature animals are restrained by a hog snare with head held in a straight line with the body and slightly elevated. The puncture site is made in the right jugular fossa in a depression just lateral to the anterior projection of the sternum. The appropriately sized needle, attached to a syringe, is inserted perpendicular to the plane of the neck and toward the left shoulder (Fig. 8–27). By remaining craniad to the first pair of ribs, puncture of the pleural cavity will be avoided. The needle should be inserted to its full length, which will usually cause it to pass through the vein. It is then gradually withdrawn while a slight negative pressure on the syringe is maintained. Withdrawal must be slow to allow time for the blood to travel through the long needle into the syringe. As blood enters the

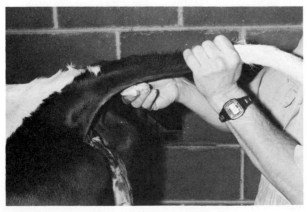

FIGURE 8–24. Preparation of the ventral coccygeal venipuncture site.

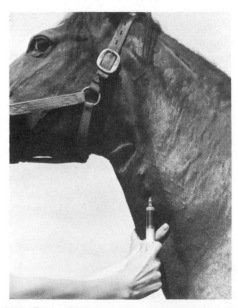

FIGURE 8–26. Equine blood samples are commonly collected from the jugular vein. The right jugular vein is preferred when possible.

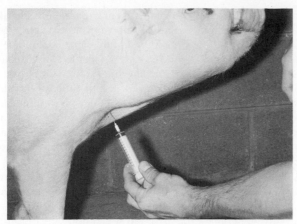

FIGURE 8–27. Proper positioning of the head aids in venipuncture of the anterior vena cava. The needle is inserted perpendicular to the plane of the neck and toward the left shoulder.

syringe, withdrawal is halted until the desired sample quantity has been collected (Fig. 8–28). If no blood appears in the syringe, the needle should be withdrawn slightly (not out of the skin) and redirected.

Brachiocephalic or External Jugular Veins

Collecting blood from the brachiocephalic or external jugular vein has become common. For simplicity, the following description will refer only to the brachiocephalic vein, even though the actual venipuncture may be made into one of the jugular veins, since the venipuncture point is near the location where the internal and external jugular veins join and become the brachiocephalic vein. The landmarks for collection from the brachiocephalic vein are established by first finding the deepest part of the right jugular fossa and then visualizing a transverse line through the manubrium sterni and shoulders, parallel to the ground. A second line is then visualized from the manubrium sterni toward the right scapula at a 45-degree angle to the transverse line that was previously described. The location where the second line crosses the deepest part of the right jugular fossa is where the needle is inserted through the skin. The needle should enter at a perpendicular angle, which

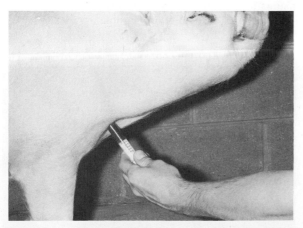

FIGURE 8–28. Slight negative pressure is maintained until the proper amount of blood is obtained.

is formed between the needle and the ventral surface of the extended neck. In the extended neck, the needle is directed caudodorsally and should not deviate toward either scapula. Since the brachiocephalic vein is superficial, negative pressure is applied to the syringe as soon as the skin is penetrated. The needle should continue to be advanced until blood starts to enter the syringe. As with collection from the anterior vena cava, the right side is preferred in order to avoid hitting the phrenic nerve or the thoracic duct, which lie near the external jugular vein. A 16- or 18-gauge, 3.75-cm needle is commonly used in pigs that weigh up to 90 kg. For larger swine, a 16- or 18-gauge, 5.0-cm needle is often used.

Ear Vein

A third site of venipuncture in swine is the ear vein. This vein is generally used for collecting small samples only, since sustained negative pressure on the syringe will collapse the vein wall. While the animal is being restrained by a hog snare, the vein is occluded by placing a strong rubber band or long-jawed forceps encased in rubber tubing around the base of the ear. The tip of the ear is grasped in one hand while a syringe attached to an 18- to 20-gauge, 2.5- to 3.75-cm needle is held in the other. The needle is inserted into the vein while slight negative pressure is maintained on the syringe, and the appropriate quantity of blood is drawn. The ear vein is commonly used for intravenous administration of medication. A 19- or 21-gauge butterfly catheter may be used for collection of blood or administration of medication.

Ovine and Caprine Venipuncture

Collection of blood from sheep can be frustrating, especially when considerable wool is covering the neck. Since it is often not possible to visualize the jugular vein in sheep, it is important to stretch the neck to one side in order to make venipuncture easier. One method that can be used requires the sheep to be placed in a sitting position on its rump. The person performing the venipuncture places one knee on the ground and stretches the neck of the sheep over the thigh of the other leg. The head of the sheep is held by the arm that is used to perform the venipuncture. The opposite hand is used to occlude the jugular vein. An 18- or 20-gauge, 2.5-cm needle is directed into the jugular furrow at a 20-degree angle to the skin (Fig. 8–29). If repeated attempts are unsuccessful, small pieces of wool can be plucked from the skin over the jugular furrow so that the vein can be visualized. This method is satisfactory for sheep that can be successfully placed on their rump.

Blood can also be collected from sheep in the standing position by backing the sheep into a corner and keeping it forced against one side of the pen. The operator stretches the neck by holding the head of the sheep to the side with the arm that is to perform the venipuncture. The other hand is again used to occlude the vein (Fig. 8–30). The method of venipuncture is the same as already described.

The procedure described previously for venipuncture of the jugular vein in the bovine can be applied to the goat. An alternative location for collection of blood in the goat is the cephalic vein. The previously described procedure for cephalic venipuncture in the dog may be adjusted to the goat.

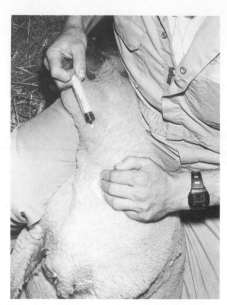

FIGURE 8–29. Stretching the neck to one side aids in venipuncture of the jugular vein.

Bovine, Equine and Ovine Urine Collection

Various stimuli may be used when one is attempting to collect urine samples from cows and heifers. Individual animals seem to respond to different types of stimulation. An often successful method of stimulating a cow to urinate is to stroke repeatedly beneath the area of the vulva. It is important not to hold the tail with the other hand as it may distract the animal. Several pieces of hay or straw can be used to stroke the vulva, which is sometimes effective to stimulate urination in some animals. If these methods fail, the lips of the vulva can be repeatedly flapped together to stimulate urination. It is best to collect a midstream sample in order to avoid contamination from the vestibule and vulva.

Catheterization can be easily performed by using a bent metal catheter or an artificial insemination pipette that has

been slightly bent approximately 2.5 cm from the tip. The skin around the vulva and the lips of the vulva are scrubbed with an antiseptic scrub and are rinsed with water containing an antiseptic solution at least three times. A sterile gloved hand is introduced into the vulva, and the fingers are slid along the ventral shelf of the vestibule in order to find the urethral orifice. The catheter is then introduced into the vestibule and directed into the urethral orifice by guiding it with one of the fingers of the hand that is in the vestibule. After introduction into the urethra, the catheter is gently advanced until it enters the bladder, which will be evident by a flow of urine.

Urine can be collected in the mare in a similar manner. Care should be taken to wrap the tail prior to the procedure to prevent the tail hairs from entering the vulva. The hair will not only contaminate the area, but it can also be irritating to the sensitive mucous membranes.

Urine can often be collected in the ewe by holding both nostrils and the mouth closed. After a short period of time, the ewe will struggle to get air and will eventually urinate at the same time. An assistant is needed to collect the sample.

Equine and Bovine Abdominocentesis

Samples of abdominal fluid that are needed for clinical pathological evaluation may be obtained by abdominocentesis. To perform this technique in the horse, a site behind the xiphoid on the midline is clipped and aseptically prepared. The area is then desensitized with 2 to 3 ml of a local anesthetic. Wearing sterile surgical gloves, the operator punctures the skin with a No. 15 blade while making certain to avoid incising any veins (Fig. 8–31). The blade is then rotated to form an entrance large enough for a sterile teat cannula to pass through. The cannula should be pushed through a square of sterile gauze before being inserted into the incision (Fig. 8–32). This will prevent any blood from dripping down the outside of the cannula and contaminating the sample. The cannula is then passed through the incision and into the abdomen. It is wise to allow a small amount of fluid to drip from the cannula before collecting the sample, because early fluid may contain blood or other contaminants. The sample is then collected by allowing fluid to drip into a sterile tube (Fig. 8–33). If there is not a large amount of fluid present, it may be necessary to attach a syringe to the cannula and withdraw fluid by maintaining gentle negative pressure on the syringe. It may also be necessary to redirect the cannula in order to get a flow of fluid.

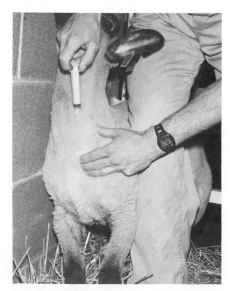

FIGURE 8–30. An alternate method of restraining the sheep for venipuncture.

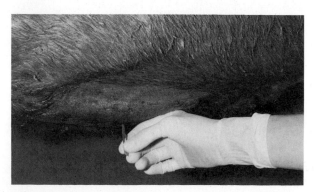

FIGURE 8–31. A No. 15 blade is used to create an entrance for a sterile teat cannula to pass through.

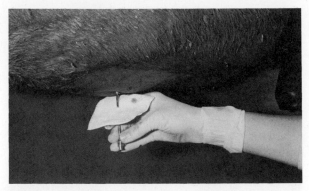

FIGURE 8–32. Sterile gauze prevents contamination of the sample.

Abdominocentesis can also be performed in a similar manner in the bovine. It is usually performed only on the right side of a standing animal, since most attempts on the left side end up in the rumen. Care should be taken to avoid the large "milk" veins along the ventral abdomen of many cows.

ADMINISTRATION OF MEDICATION IN LARGE ANIMALS

Bovine Intravenous Medication

Jugular Vein

Intravenous medication of cattle is most commonly administered in the jugular vein. The animal is restrained in a head catch with head drawn upward and to the opposite side from which the injection will be made. The injection site is cleansed with 70 percent alcohol, and the vein is occluded by applying digital pressure in the lower jugular groove. The opposite hand is used to sharply push a 14- or 16-gauge, 5- to 7.5-cm needle into the vein at a 45- to 90-degree angle to the skin. While keeping the vein occluded, the needle is threaded either upward or downward into the vein to the hub. The syringe is then attached, and the positioning of the needle in the vein is verified by aspirating a small amount of blood into the syringe. If medication is being administered by a simplex, the bottle of fluids can be lowered below the injection site in order to

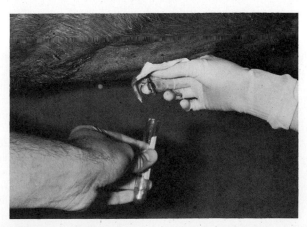

FIGURE 8–33. Abdominal fluid drips through the cannula into a sterile test tube.

observe blood flowing back into the simplex. Digital pressure on the jugular groove is released, and the medication is administered.

Occasionally, an animal will require repeated injections of large amounts of fluids. In such cases, it is wise to cannulate the jugular vein, which ensures easy access to the vein for each treatment. After clipping and scrubbing the skin, one performs the cannulation by placing a 10-gauge, 3.75-cm needle into the vein and threading an appropriately sized sterile polyethylene tube through the needle until approximately 50 cm of tubing is in the vein. The 10-gauge needle is removed, and a 15-gauge *blunted needle* is inserted into the tubing. Fluids should be started immediately to prevent blood from clotting in the tubing. The tubing should not be pulled from the vein while the 10-gauge sharp needle is still in place because the tubing could be severed by the bevel of the needle.

The tubing should be flushed occasionally with a solution of 0.5 ml heparin in 5 ml sterile saline between infusions of medication in order to prevent clotting. The tubing should be secured by placing a piece of white adhesive tape in a butterfly fashion around the blunted needle. The white adhesive tape is then sutured to the skin above and below the jugular groove with a nonabsorbable suture material. A square of sterile gauze covered on one side with a liberal amount of antiseptic ointment should be placed over the site at which the tubing enters the skin. The gauze square is secured by several wraps of white adhesive tape around the neck.

Subcutaneous Abdominal Vein

The subcutaneous abdominal vein (milk vein) can be used for administering small quantities of medication while the bovine is confined in the milking parlor. Tail restraint is essential. Care should be taken when using this vein, since large hematomas may result because of its ventral location and loose skin covering. Pinching the skin for several minutes after withdrawing the needle from the vein helps to prevent hematoma formation.

Coccygeal Vein

The ventral coccygeal vein ("tail vein") can be used for the administration of small quantities of nonirritating medications (see discussion of bovine venipuncture procedures). Caustic compounds injected into this region can cause vascular compromise and subsequent sloughing of the tail.

Equine Intravenous Medication

Jugular Vein

Medication given intravenously in the equine is administered in the jugular vein. Because the esophagus runs near the jugular groove on the left side, the right jugular is the preferred vein to use whenever possible. An 18-gauge, 3.75-cm needle is adequate for most injections, though a 14- or 16-gauge, 5- to 7.5-cm needle may be used when large quantities of medication are being given. If repeated infusions of large quantities are necessary, the jugular vein should be cannulated in the same manner as discussed for cattle, or it can be catheterized with a commercially available catheter. As in the cow, the skin over the jugular vein should be clipped and aseptically prepared prior to insertion of the catheter under sterile conditions. The catheter should be secured by placing a piece of white adhesive tape around the base of the catheter in a butterfly fashion. A sterile gauze covered on one side with an antiseptic ointment should be placed over the site at which the catheter enters the skin. White adhesive tape or elastic adhesive tape can then be used to secure the butterfly with several wraps around the neck of the horse.

When a single intravenous injection is to be made, the skin should be cleansed with alcohol prior to insertion of the needle. The needle should be inserted into the distended vein at a 90-degree angle to the skin. When blood flows from the needle, it should be directed in either a cranial or a caudal direction. The caudal direction will prevent caustic materials from seeping around the injection site, whereas the cranial direction will disperse the material and prevent local irritation of the inner surface of the vein. Care should be taken to ensure that the needle is in the jugular vein. Drugs injected into the carotid artery can cause severe reactions when they reach the brain in high concentrations. The resistance of needles smaller than 18-gauge will slow the flow of blood so that an arterial blood flow may be mistaken for venous flow.

Bovine Intramuscular Injection

The gluteal muscles are commonly used for intramuscular injections in cattle. Restraining the animal in a stanchion or while crowded in an alley is usually adequate for this procedure. The injection site may be cleansed with 70 percent rubbing alcohol. A 16- or 18-gauge, 3.75- to 5-cm needle is grasped, and a fist is formed with the same hand. The injection site is struck with the flat of the fist (Fig. 8–34); then, turning the hand slightly, the animal is struck again as the needle is popped through the skin perpendicular to the surface of the skin. Striking the animal in this manner lessens the animal's awareness of the needle being inserted. The needle should not be attached to a syringe as this procedure is taking place, since a sudden movement of the animal could cause the needle or syringe tip to break. After the needle has been firmly seated in muscle, the syringe is attached (Fig. 8–35). Slight negative pressure is applied to the syringe to be sure blood vessels have not been entered. The medication is then injected, and the

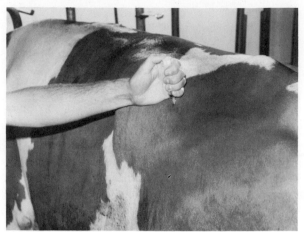

FIGURE 8–35. The syringe is attached after the needle has been securely placed in the muscle mass.

needle and syringe are withdrawn. This injection site works well with large groups of cattle when the animals can be crowded into a confined area and one can make the injection by reaching over a fence. Administration of large quantities of medication into the gluteal muscles is often avoided in dairy cows in which these muscles are thin, because of the possible complication of abscesses or cellulitis.

Other options are also available for intramuscular injections in cattle. The semitendinosus muscle may be used, though the operator may wish to apply tail restraint as the injection is given. The triceps also work well for small quantities of medication when the animal can be restrained from making lateral movements, as when in a stanchion. Injections in very young animals may be given in the lateral femoral muscle, though care must be taken to avoid damage to the sciatic nerve. The neck muscle in the area just anterior to the scapula can be used in heavily muscled animals such as bulls.

Equine Intramuscular Injection

Intramuscular injection technique in the horse is very similar to that used in cattle. The gluteal muscles halfway between the greater trochanter and the tuber coxae can be used. When using this area for injection, it is wise for the operator to stand on the side of the animal that is opposite the injection site and reach across the back. If the animal kicks, it will generally kick toward the side on which the needle is being inserted. A 16- or 18-gauge, 3.75- to 5-cm needle is generally used for injection. This site is not always preferred, since an injection complication would be esthetically unappealing.

The brachiocephalicus muscle in the neck is easily accessible and requires a minimum of restraint. However, this site is not commonly used for large quantities of medication as most horses are not heavily muscled in this area.

Medication that is not easily absorbed may be administered in the triceps muscle because the movement of the animal aids in the distribution of the drug. However, this site should not be used in horses that are to be harnessed or saddled within several weeks. Highly irritating drugs (injectable iron, vitamins A, D, and E, and so forth), which may cause abscesses, may occasionally be injected into the pectoral muscles, since this area will drain readily.

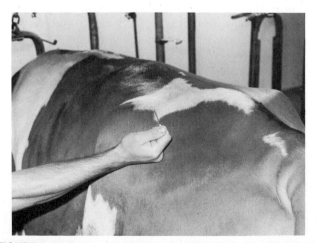

FIGURE 8–34. Striking the injection site with the flat of the fist distracts the animal from the insertion of the needle.

The semitendinosus muscle is often used when repeated intramuscular injections are required. The person making an injection in this region is vulnerable to being kicked and should take appropriate care.

Intramuscular injections in the rear quarters of racing horses should be avoided, as myositis may affect their performance. No more than 20 ml should be injected at any one site.

Bovine and Equine Subcutaneous Injections

Subcutaneous injections may be used for drugs that are not irritating to the tissues. The most desirable site for subcutaneous injection of small quantities in the bovine and equine is the middle area of the neck between the scapula and the ramus of the mandible. This area is easily accessible, and minimal restraint is required. The injection site is prepared by cleansing the skin with 70 percent rubbing alcohol. A fold of skin is picked up and pinched as the injection is given. An 18- or 20-gauge, 2.5- to 3.75-cm needle is adequate for subcutaneous injections. Gentle massage of the injection site will facilitate distribution and absorption of the medication. When administering a drug preparation that is not easily absorbed, the injection may be made just over or behind the spine of the scapula. The movement of the animal aids in the distribution of the medication, which will help to prevent abscesses from forming. This is a common site used for administration of large quantities of fluid. It is commonly used when administering the second 500-ml bottle of a calcium solution to a cow with milk fever.

Sheep and Goat Injection Sites

The jugular vein is the preferred site for intravenous therapy in the sheep and goat. When collecting blood or making intravenous injections, the goat is best restrained by an assistant who turns the head laterally. This allows good visualization and access to the jugular vein. The procedure described previously for intravenous injections and catheterization in the horse applies to the goat. Most intramuscular injections in the goat are administered in the semitendinosus and semimembranosus muscles. Few goats have enough muscle mass in other parts of their bodies for safe intramuscular injections. Intramuscular injections in the sheep are usually given in the semitendinosus or semimembranosus muscles and sometimes in the gluteal muscles.

Subcutaneous injections in both the goat and sheep are routinely administered in the neck or shoulder region. In show animals in whom appearance is important, the axillary or flank fold areas should be used for medications that may cause an irritation or blemish.

Swine Injection Sites

The dorsal neck muscle is a common intramuscular injection site in swine. It is usually one of the cleanest areas for injection and is easily accessible in animals confined in a farrowing crate or those crowded with a panel. Swine also seem to be less sensitive to pain in this area. A 16- to 18-gauge, 2.5- to 3.75-cm needle should be used. The insertion of the needle

and the injection of the medication is accomplished in one motion. The procedure must be quick to avoid excessive movement by the pig.

The medial side of the ham is often used in giving medication to small pigs that can be restrained by holding the hind legs. This is a common site for iron injection in young pigs. An 18- to 19-gauge, 1.25- to 2.5-cm needle is often used in small pigs. The posterior ham can be used in the standing adult for intramuscular injections. It should be avoided whenever possible, however, since it is a choice meat cut and is often a dirty site. If used, a 16- to 18-gauge, 3.75- to 5-cm needle is preferred.

Subcutaneous injections in the area just posterior to the base of the ear are also easily administered in swine confined in a farrowing crate or crowded with a panel. A 16- to 18-gauge, 2.5- to 5-cm needle is directed ventrally. The insertion of the needle and the administration of medication should be accomplished as quickly as possible. In small pigs, the axillary space or flank fold can be used if the pigs are held by their legs. A 16- to 18-gauge, 1.9- to 2.5-cm needle may be used.

Fluids are usually administered by the intraperitoneal route in pigs, since long-term intravenous therapy is impractical. These fluids should be warm and isotonic (see Chapter 20). In baby pigs held by their hind legs, a 16-gauge, 1.25- to 2.5-cm needle is inserted halfway between the midline and the flank. In standing adults, the paralumbar fossa should be used. Often a 16- to 18-gauge, 7.5-cm needle is required to penetrate through the thick muscle and fat into the peritoneum. Whenever the intraperitoneal route is used, the skin should be properly cleansed and disinfected prior to insertion of the needle.

Oral Medication of the Ovine and Caprine

The administration of boluses to sheep and goats is accomplished by use of a balling gun. The end of the balling gun should be smooth and preferably made of soft plastic. The head and neck of the animal can be straddled by one person to stabilize it. Often, it is best to have the animal in a corner so that it is unable to back up. The side of the mouth is pried open, and the balling gun is carefully slid into the mouth and over the base of the tongue, at which point the lubricated bolus is released.

Oral liquid medication can be administered by the use of a dose syringe, dosing bottle or stomach tube. A dose syringe that has a large bulb on its tip is preferred, since it prevents injuries to mucous membranes. The head of the sheep or goat should again be stabilized and held horizontally. The bulb end is introduced into the interdigital space and again over the base of the tongue, at which point the medication is delivered. If the animal coughs, its head should be lowered to prevent aspiration into the trachea.

A stomach tube can be readily passed in a restrained sheep or goat by using a tape roll or appropriately sized syringe case whose end has been smoothed (Fig. 8–36). A lubricated 9.5-mm diameter foal tube is passed through the speculum device and over the base of the tongue into the esophagus (Fig. 8–37). Care must be taken to visualize or feel the passing of the tube through the esophagus to ensure placement of medication in the rumen. If any doubt exists regarding the location of the tube, either it should be passed again or air should be blown into the tube so that an assistant listening with a stetho-

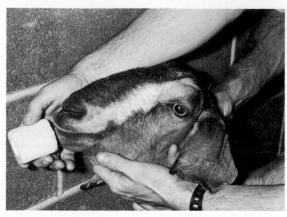

FIGURE 8–36. A tape roll is inserted into the animal's mouth to facilitate passing the stomach tube.

scope over the left paralumbar fossa can hear air bubbling through the rumen contents.

Oral Medication of the Bovine

Boluses are usually passed in the bovine with a balling gun (preferably with a soft plastic bolus chamber). The animal is restrained in a head catch. The operator reaches over the head and places the hand in the interdigital space to open the mouth and introduce the balling gun. The lubricated bolus is placed over the base of the tongue. An alternative method is to grasp the nose by its septum with the thumb and the first finger of one hand and then pull upward. This usually causes the animal to open its mouth so that the balling gun can be introduced.

Large numbers of boluses can be delivered by a multiple delivery balling gun or a Frick speculum placed over the base of the tongue. A stomach tube or any appropriate plunger-like device can be used to expel the boluses. A Frick speculum or wooden block can be used for passing a stomach tube in the bovine. It is often best to place the stomach tube end in the speculum before introducing it into the mouth. The tube can then be rapidly passed once the speculum is properly placed. As in the small ruminant, it is essential to be sure that the tube has been placed in the rumen before any medication is administered. When large quantities of fluids are given, a ruminant

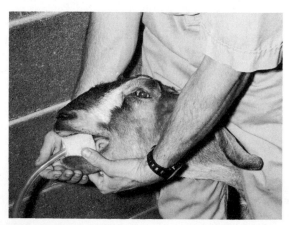

FIGURE 8–37. The stomach tube is passed through the center of the tape roll and into the esophagus.

may sometimes regurgitate stomach contents. When this occurs, the tube is removed and the head is lowered from the horizontal position so that fluid is not aspirated into the trachea. When withdrawing a stomach tube, it is important to kink the tube or to place a thumb over the end of the tube to prevent medication or rumen contents from entering the trachea.

COLLECTION PROCEDURES FOR MILK CULTURES AND SOMATIC CELL COUNTS

In order to reduce the number of contaminating organisms in milk samples used for culturing, proper milk collection techniques must be utilized. Sterile, disposable plastic or autoclaved glass tubes are used to collect samples. A waterproof system of labeling the tubes should be used to identify the cow and quarter. Increased numbers of somatic cells (mostly neutrophils and some sloughed epithelial cells) are a normal part of the inflammatory process. The increased numbers of somatic cells are useful in determining the inflammatory status of an individual quarter or herd. The best time to collect milk samples for culture or for determination of somatic cell count is either prior to milking or at least 6 hours after milking. Samples for somatic cell counts should be taken after milk letdown has occurred.

Table 8–1
INTERPRETATION AND GRADING OF THE CALIFORNIA MASTITIS TEST

Symbol	Suggested Meaning	Description of Visible Reaction
N	Negative	Mixture remains liquid with no evidence of formation of a precipitate.
T	Trace	A slight precipitate is formed, which is best seen by tipping the paddle back and forth and by observing the mixture as it flows over the bottom of the cup. Trace reactions tend to disappear with continued rotation of the paddle.
1	Weak positive	A distinct precipitate forms, but there is no tendency toward gel formation. With some milk, the reaction may disappear after prolonged rotation of the paddle.
2	Distinct positive	The mixture thickens immediately, and a gel formation is suggested. As the mixture is swirled, it tends to move toward the center, which exposes the outer edge of the cup. When the swirling is stopped, the mixture levels out and covers the bottom of the cup.
3	Strong positive	A gel is formed, which causes the surface of the mixture to become convex. Usually, there is a central peak that projects above the main mass, even after the rotation of the paddle is stopped.

Procedure

Brushing loose dirt off the udder is preferred to washing, since residual water can cause contamination of the sample. One or two streams of milk should be discarded from each teat. Each teat end should then be cleansed with a separate cotton or cloth gauze pledget or similar material soaked in 70 percent alcohol. Scrubbing should continue until no visible dirt is seen on the gauze. The end of the teat should be thoroughly dry prior to collection of the sample. Teats on the far side of the cow are cleansed first to prevent contamination of the near side. The milk tube is held so that the cap can be easily removed without contaminating the opening of the tube. The cap should be held with the inner surface downward and the tube held as horizontal as possible to minimize contamination. Care should be taken to avoid touching the tube with either the cow's teat or the hand of the sampler. Samples should be taken with minimal pressure starting with the quarters nearest the collector. The hands of the collector should be washed in disinfectant between sampling cows.

The sample should be cooled soon after collection and should be maintained in a cool state until delivered to the laboratory. The samples should be cultured immediately or held at 4 to 5°C until it is convenient to do so. However, for best results, samples should be cultured within 24 hours. If the samples cannot be cultured within 24 hours, they should be frozen as soon as possible after collection.

California Mastitis Test

A simple and very useful cowside field test for subclinical mastitis is the California Mastitis Test (CMT). Abnormally high numbers of somatic cells are detected by the CMT and by several laboratory tests. The CMT is more subjective in interpretation than other tests but is easy to perform and inexpensive and provides immediate results.

Procedure for the CMT

The CMT uses a white plastic paddle with four shallow cups for each of the four quarters of the cow. Approximately 2 ml of milk are tested. This is the amount that remains in each cup when the paddle is turned to a nearly vertical position. An equal amount of CMT reagent is added to each cup. The paddle is gently rotated in a circular motion to thoroughly mix the milk and reagent. An interpretation is made after about 10 seconds while continuing to rotate the mixture. Interpretations should be made quickly, since the precipitate tends to disappear after 20 seconds.

The interpretation of the CMT has five categories, which are based on the amount of precipitate formed (Table 8–1). The CMT reagent also contains a pH indicator (bromcresol purple). The mixture becomes a dark purple when the milk is alkaline. Alkaline milk is a reflection of decreased secretory activity, which occurs at drying off or as a result of inflammation.

Recommended Reading

Coles EH: Veterinary Clinical Pathology. 4th ed. Philadelphia, WB Saunders Co., 1986.

McCurnin DM and Poffenbarger EM (editors): Small Animal Physical Diagnosis and Clinical Procedures. Philadelphia, WB Saunders Co., 1991.

Kirk RW and Bistner SI: Handbook of Veterinary Procedures and Emergency Treatment. 4th ed. Philadelphia, WB Saunders Co., 1985.

9

Small Animal Emergency Care

STEVEN L. WHEELER

INTRODUCTION

The term emergency is defined by the Veterinary Emergency and Critical Care Society (VECCS) as a sudden generally unexpected occurrence, or set of circumstances, demanding urgent action. An emergency arises whenever the patient needs immediate attention. The underlying disease process may have been present for some time, with the animal only recently becoming symptomatic. This occurs frequently with chronic renal failure or congestive heart failure. Alternatively, some owners may be aware of a problem over a period of days, weeks, or even months, without seeking attention. At some point, the problem assumes a critical nature to the owner (and may, in fact, be so for the patient), and the animal is presented as an emergency.

The client's definition of an emergency may or may not coincide with the medical definition. However, there are several considerations that may alter the medical definition—if an owner is extremely upset about a situation (laceration, intractable diarrhea, coughing, and so forth) or the circumstance is an emergency to that person despite the fact that the patient may be stable and may not even require medical attention. It is also difficult to assess the true nature of an animal's condition over the telephone. Therefore, errors will invariably be made in deciding that an "emergency" can wait until morning, or occasionally a healthy animal will be seen because the

situation sounded critical. It is unquestionably better to err toward the latter situation.

If the veterinary technician is monitoring calls, all questionable emergencies should be referred to the veterinarian. Situations such as status epilepticus, an animal who has been hit by a car and is in shock or gastric dilatation are unequivocal emergencies, but there are many "gray" areas that should be left to the discretion of the clinician. Generally speaking, a veterinary emergency is any condition that the owner is convinced is an emergency. If there is the possibility that an emergency exists, it should be recommended to the client that the animal be seen immediately.

There is also a distinction between intensive care and acute emergency care. However, with the advent of emergency care clinics that may serve as intensive care centers in evenings and on weekends for local veterinary clinics, the differences may be less than the similarities. Certainly there are many areas of overlap. There may be a preponderance of monitoring and nursing in an intensive care unit, but one must always be prepared for an emergency, such as a cardiac arrest. The training and duties of personnel for both facilities should be similar, given the nature of the patients.

Emergency clinics are becoming rather commonplace, especially in urban areas. The types of cases vary, but fall into a fairly narrow range (Table 9–1). Given that an emergency is in part defined by an owner, an emergency clinic may still have its share of patients affected with routine medical problems, such as dermatological conditions, otitis externa or kennel cough. Although the definition of an emergency has obviously been expanded and somewhat distorted, taking care of these routine problems also provides a very real service.

The author gratefully acknowledges the original contribution by Johanna Kaufman, D.V.M., M.S., upon which portions of this chapter are based.

Table 9–1 CASES SEEN IN AN EMERGENCY CLINIC DURING A 6-MONTH PERIOD	
Condition	**Number of Cases**
Vomiting	53
Diarrhea	65
Hemorrhagic diarrhea	20
Hit by car	50
Laceration	43
Dog bite wounds	20
Cat abscess	25
Urethral obstruction	20
Ethylene glycol toxicity	6
Renal failure	3
Addison's disease	2
Diabetic ketoacidosis	2
Hemangiosarcoma	4
Feline cardiomyopathy (saddle thrombus)	3
Feline pyothorax	2
Feline mediastinal lymphosarcoma	4
Feline anemias	
Hemobartonella	5
Myeloproliferative disorders	3
Diaphragmatic hernia	2
Gastric dilatation or volvulus	8
Pyometra	2
Dystocia	6
Otitis externa	10
Seizures	15
Toxicities (miscellaneous)	3
DIC	2
Warfarin poisoning	1
Thromboembolic disease secondary to heartworm	2

EMERGENCY SERVICE

The purpose of an emergency service is actually twofold. The primary responsibility is to provide care and support. The secondary responsibility is to perform enough diagnostic procedures to treat the patient appropriately, as well as to furnish baseline data to the referring veterinarian who will see the animal the next morning.

One must be aware that an emergency situation represents only one point in time during the entire progression of a disease process. Therefore, to treat without obtaining preliminary baseline data may "cover the tracks" and impede the diagnostic work-up that will follow the initial care. Veterinarians will have individual preferences for what they consider a minimum data base, and the technician should become familiar with it. The minimum recommended data base for all emergency cases should include body weight, packed cell volume (PCV), total solids and urine specific gravity (USG). Some emergencies will call for a more extensive minimum data base. As an example, an animal might present with acute bloody diarrhea, which can result from a variety of causes, including parvovirus, coronavirus, hemorrhagic gastroenteritis or gastrointestinal parasites. Many clinicians will want to obtain a complete blood count (CBC) or a PCV, a total solid determination, white blood cell (WBC) count, and fecal flotation before treatment is instituted. There are also instances when a

diagnostic procedure is therapeutic. A dyspneic cat with pleural effusion falls into this category. Thoracocentesis (aspiration of the chest cavity for removal of fluid) is the treatment of choice and is essential for the patient's survival if the effusion is severe. Although removing the fluid so that the animal can breathe easier is the primary goal, the nature of the fluid will distinguish among various disease processes, such as pyothorax, feline infectious peritonitis, chylothorax or pleural effusion secondary to cardiac disease or neoplasia. The technician should save an aliquot of fluid in a sterile manner during the procedure so that it can be used for diagnostic purposes after the initial crisis is over.

In many cases, the diagnostic effort is dictated by the animal's clinical presentation. The minimum data base required by the veterinarian will be different for an animal that is hit by a car and is in shock than it will be for a patient that has been chronically ill and is presented in a moribund state. In any case, needless stress should be avoided, and the primary goal of emergency medicine is to stabilize the patient. Therefore, extraneous diagnostic procedures are to be avoided.

One need not have an entire laboratory in order to deal with emergencies successfully. However, there are certain items that are virtually essential for effectively dealing with all emergency situations. They include an x-ray machine, an electrocardiograph and a laboratory that is capable of performing some rudimentary procedures, which include a CBC, and blood glucose and blood urea nitrogen (BUN) determinations. In addition, there should be a centrifuge, a refractometer and a microscope. The refractometer will be used to determine USG and total serum solids. The microscope can be used for WBC differentials, effusions or cytological studies, urine sediment studies and fecal examinations. The veterinarian will decide what tests are necessary for short-term emergency treatments, but all clinics that deal with emergencies should be able to perform basic diagnostic procedures.

Many times the first contact that the technician has with the client is over the telephone. The call may involve merely asking for information or asking if a given situation warrants the animal's being seen by the veterinarian. It is impossible to list the many and varied situations that arise. The role of the technician will be defined by experience as well as by clinic policy.

First Aid

The technician may be called on to administer first aid. Many times, instructions on how to administer first aid will be given over the telephone to a client. Again, the awareness of certain clinical entities and their significance, as well as what the client can do before arriving at the clinic or must do in order to transport the animal to the hospital, are essential. An example is the animal that has been observed ingesting a toxic substance. One can advise the owner to give 3 percent hydrogen peroxide to induce vomiting. In many instances, this is more effective and works more rapidly than the administration of ipecac (5 to 20 ml), and it is readily available in the home. Another example is an animal that has been hit by a car, resulting in a fractured spine. The owner should be advised on the best way to transport the animal without producing further spinal injury (i.e., use a board to transport the animal).

When an animal arrives at the clinic, the technician should immediately assess the patient. There are situations in which there is not time to wait to be seen or even time to wait to speak with the veterinarian to see what protocol should be followed. A quick assessment of the patient's status will help to determine whether the animal is a true emergency or is relatively stable and does not require immediate attention. Less than a minute is required to observe an animal in this fashion. Color, pulse character, capillary refill time, respiratory rate and respiratory character can be assessed in a few seconds. If an animal is presented in a moribund state, the technician should insert a thermometer as the preceding baseline parameters are being assessed. Evaluating the patient in this way will permit the formation of rational treatment priorities. It will also help the veterinarian to know the seriousness of the situation, in the event that he or she is involved in something that must be interrupted.

There are certain priority treatments for seriously ill or injured patients. The first priority is to make sure that there is a patent airway and to make sure that the animal is breathing. Mucus, vomitus or blood may occlude the animal's airway. If the animal is awake, but is dyspneic because of debris in the oral cavity, the foreign material should be removed manually. Many times, suction will help if there is a copious discharge. If the animal is apneic (not breathing) or hypoventilating, it should be intubated to establish a patent airway (see Chapter 11). After establishing a patent airway, the next priority is breathing. Conditions that may interfere with breathing include pneumothorax, pleural effusion, pulmonary contusions, diaphragmatic hernia, fractured ribs and head trauma. For discussion of the treatment of these conditions, refer to the section on Common Emergencies in this chapter.

The cardiovascular system should next be assessed and supported. The patient should be evaluated for shock and, if necessary, treated. Hemostasis is also important. After these life-threatening areas have been addressed, the patient as a whole should be attended to.

Hemostasis can be achieved under most circumstances by the use of a pressure wrap or tourniquet. Pressure wraps work quite well for foot pad lacerations and other lacerations on the extremities that may bleed profusely. For bleeding that is more severe, it may be necessary to use a tourniquet in conjunction with a pressure wrap. The pressure wrap usually consists of gauze squares or cotton, or both of these materials, and gauze wrap and adhesive tape. It is virtually impossible to apply a pressure wrap too tightly on a *short-term* basis (less than 3 hours). This is not true of a tourniquet, which should not be left on longer than a few minutes without relieving the pressure occasionally. There are rare instances in which larger vessels or arteries are exposed. The veterinarian may wish to ligate them before the pressure wrap is applied and the animal is stabilized. One should then attend to fractures. This procedure will be detailed later.

The main goal in first aid is to establish priorities so that life-threatening matters are attended to quickly and vigorously. Assessment of the patient is critical in order for this to be correctly applied. One can only stress that there will be instances when the technician is alone, or there is no time to contact the veterinarian to institute life-saving procedures.

Cardiopulmonary Resuscitation

Cardiopulmonary arrest (CPA) is a sudden cessation of effective cardiac output with accompanying ventilatory failure. Either cardiac or respiratory arrest may occur initially; however, ventilatory or circulatory failure will soon follow.

Although the prognosis for recovery is poor in most cases of CPA, with early recognition and appropriate therapy, a successful outcome can be attained. The greater the time interval between recognition of CPA and institution of cardiopulmonary resuscitation (CPR), the poorer the chances for successful outcome. Signs of CPA include apnea (lack of breathing), cyanosis (blue mucous membranes), absent pulses or apex beat, dilated pupils and unconsciousness. Agonal respirations (forceful but ineffective breathing) also indicate that CPA is present. Once CPA is diagnosed or even suspected, CPR should be immediately initiated.

The technician should become familiar with the principles of CPR. The "ABCs" of CPR, or Basic Life Support, consist of assessing Airway patency, Breathing for the animal, and maintaining Circulation through external thoracic compressions. The primary emphasis in CPR should be on performing optimal Basic Life Support, since this aspect of CPR is most important in obtaining a successful outcome. Advanced Life Support consists of the "D, E" portion of CPR and includes Diagnosis of electrocardiographic abnormalities and therapy with Emergency drugs. Intensive care monitoring, or Prolonged Life Support, is implemented after successful CPR.

Basic Life Support

Airway

The first priority in CPR is to establish an airway. Any vomitus or other foreign matter should be removed from the oral cavity. Traction should be applied on the tongue and an endotracheal tube should be placed to establish a patent airway. In rare cases with hemorrhage, fractures, or edema secondary to oral trauma, a tracheostomy may be necessary. If a tube is not immediately available, it is possible to hold the animal's mouth shut and forcefully breathe into the nostrils (Fig. 9–1). This obviously is not ideal but may help to deliver some oxygen until an endotracheal tube is procured.

Breathing

After an airway is established, assisted ventilation is begun. Ideally, the animal should be ventilated with 100 percent oxygen supplied from an anesthetic machine. The anesthetic system should be free of any anesthetic gases. If oxygen is not available, ventilation with room air (21 percent oxygen) may

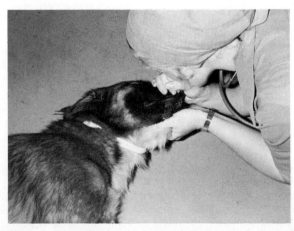

FIGURE 9–1. The lungs can be expanded by blowing in the nostrils. This may be performed on an animal in respiratory arrest before the arrival of an endotracheal tube.

be accomplished with an *Ambu bag* (Fig. 9–2). If this equipment is not available, by blowing into the endotracheal tube, one can ventilate the animal with expired air (about 16 percent oxygen). Since less oxygen will be delivered to the lungs with room or expired air, ventilation with 100 percent oxygen is preferred. Hypoxia (low blood oxygen) may blunt the beneficial effects of chemical and electrical therapy. The chest should be observed for expansion during artificial ventilation. Peak inspiratory pressure should be about 20 cm of water. Higher airway pressures can result in lung trauma and should therefore be avoided.

Circulation

After two quick breaths are delivered, the carotid or femoral arteries should be palpated for a pulse. If a pulse is present but the animal is not breathing, ventilation should be continued at a rate of 12 to 20 times per minute. If no pulse is palpated, the diagnosis of cardiac arrest is confirmed and thoracic compression should be started immediately. In people, forward blood flow during CPR was considered to be the result of compression of the heart between the sternum and the spine. However, echocardiographic and cineangiographic studies have indicated that cardiac size changes little during external compression and that forward blood flow results from an increase in intrathoracic pressure. In animals weighing more than 7 kg, chest compression is performed with the animal in dorsal recumbency (Fig. 9–3). Because of the larger ventrodorsal dimension of the thorax, this body position will maximize the increase in intrathoracic pressure. Compression is applied over the distal one third of the sternebrae with the heel of the hand and with enough force to compress the thorax 30 to 40 percent of its diameter.

In cats and dogs weighing less than 7 kg, direct cardiac compression is possible. Experimental studies have demonstrated that increased oxygenation occurs when the animal is placed in lateral recumbency and compression is applied by squeezing the thorax in the area of the fourth to fifth intercostal spaces between the thumb and fingers (Fig. 9–4).

Larger increases in intrathoracic pressure occur with simultaneous ventilation and chest compression than with compressions interrupted by ventilation. Simultaneous compression and ventilation are performed by ventilating the animal at the same time that the chest is compressed. Expiration coincides with the noncompressive phase of chest compression.

Since cardiac output is enhanced, simultaneous ventilation

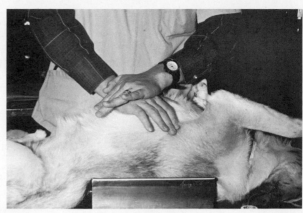

FIGURE 9–3. Dogs weighing more than 7 kg should be placed in dorsal recumbency to perform external cardiac compression. Enough pressure should be applied with the heel of the hand over the distal one third of the sternum to compress the chest by 30 to 40 percent of its diameter.

and compression are recommended rather than interrupting chest compressions to deliver ventilation. Another advantage of simultaneous ventilation and compression is that higher inspiratory pressures can be delivered without causing trauma to the lungs. With simultaneous compression and ventilation, a peak inspiratory pressure of 40 cm of water may be used. The rate of chest compressions should be 80 to 120 per minute, using the lower end of the range for larger dogs and the higher end of the range for smaller dogs and cats. Compression should be interrupted following every 10 compression and ventilation cycles and a ventilation given without simultaneous compression. This interposed ventilation leads to improved blood oxygenation.

Abdominal compressions interposed between chest compressions will improve cardiac output in CPR. Interposed compressions are performed by compressing the abdominal area during the noncompressive (relaxation) phase of the chest compression cycle. While the chest is being compressed, abdominal compression should be in the noncompressive phase. Interposed abdominal compressions act to improve venous return to the heart to improve cardiac output in CPR.

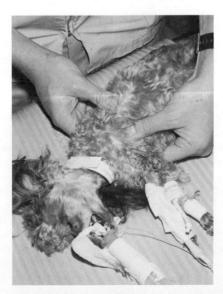

FIGURE 9–4. Cats and dogs weighing 7 kg or less should be placed in lateral recumbency to perform external cardiac compression. The thorax should be compressed between the thumb and fingers.

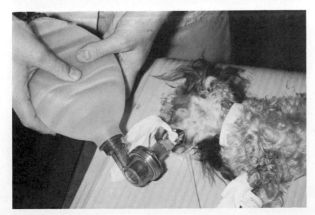

FIGURE 9–2. Animals can be ventilated with room air (21 percent oxygen) with an Ambu bag.

Table 9–2

THERAPEUTIC RECOMMENDATIONS FOR ADVANCED LIFE SUPPORT BASED ON ELECTROCARDIOGRAPHIC RHYTHM DURING CPR

EMD	Ventricular Asystole	Ventricular Fibrillation
1. Naloxone 1 ml/animal IV or IT 2. Epinephrine (1:1000) 0.2 mg/kg IV 0.4 mg/kg IT	1. Atropine 0.02–0.04 mg/kg IV or IT 2. Epinephrine (1:1000) 0.2 mg/kg IV 0.4 mg/kg IT	1. Defibrillate 0.5–1.0 watt sec/kg external 0.2–0.4 watt sec/kg internal 2. Repeat initial defibrillation dosage 3. Defibrillate at two times initial dosage 4. Epinephrine (1:1000) 0.2 mg/kg IV 0.4 mg/kg IT 5. Defibrillate at 100 watt sec 6. Lidocaine 0.25 mg/kg IV or IT 7. Defibrillate 100 watt sec

Advanced Life Support

The three principal electrocardiographic (ECG) rhythms in CPA are ventricular asystole, electromechanical dissociation (EMD), and ventricular fibrillation. In ventricular asystole, there is no mechanical or electrical cardiac activity, signified on the ECG by a flat line. In EMD, there is electrical activity but no corresponding mechanical contraction of the heart. Electrocardiographically, EMD appears as slow rhythm with wide bizarre complexes. In ventricular fibrillation, there is an uncoordinated ventricular contraction that results in ineffective cardiac output. The recommendations for drug therapy based on the type of rhythm present are summarized in Table 9–2. These guidelines are modified from recommendations for human CPR made by the American Heart Association.

CPR drugs may be delivered by the intravenous (IV), intracardiac (IC), or intratracheal (IT) routes. The IC route is not recommended for drug administration because it requires that thoracic compression be interrupted, is difficult to perform, and can cause lacerations of coronary vessels and the lungs, leading to hemothorax, pneumothorax, and hemopericardium. Because of decreased cardiac output, it is very difficult to establish an IV line during CPR. If drugs are administered intravenously, delivery of drugs into a central IV line (i.e., jugular catheter) is preferred over peripheral IV infusions because of decreased flow to the periphery during CPR.

The IT route is recommended for all emergency drugs except for sodium bicarbonate in CPR. Sodium bicarbonate should not be given IT because it will inactivate lung surfactant, leading to decreased lung function. To administer IT drugs, the anesthetic machine or Ambu bag is disconnected from the endotracheal tube, and a male urinary catheter or an intravenous extension tube is passed down the endotracheal tube (Fig. 9–5). Drugs should be diluted with saline to a final volume of 5 to 10 ml prior to IT administration.

It is no longer recommended that large doses of fluids be administered to routine arrest patients. Large volumes of fluids have been shown to decrease coronary perfusion during CPR. Only if the patient has preexisting acute blood loss or severe dehydration is fluid therapy indicated. Guidelines for bicarbonate therapy during CPR have also changed. With good Basic Life Support, metabolic acidosis does not become a problem until 15 minutes into CPR. Sodium bicarbonate therapy can cause complications, such as increased binding of oxygen to hemoglobin leading to decreased delivery of oxygen to tissues, constriction of coronary arteries, cardiac arrhythmias, and paradoxical central nervous system acidosis.

Bicarbonate therapy is rarely necessary if good basic life support is performed, and it should be used only after adequate ventilation and compression have been instituted unless a specific preexisting indication (e.g., hyperkalemia) is present. Bicarbonate should not be administered concurrently with catecholamines or calcium, since it inactivates the former and precipitates the latter. Bicarbonate therapy should be considered after 10 to 15 minutes into CPR. Initially, bicarbonate should be given at a dose of 1 mEq/kg, followed by a dose of 0.5 mEq/kg every 10 minutes thereafter.

Ventricular fibrillation is best treated with prompt electrical defibrillation to convert the cardiac rhythm to ventricular asystole. Unfortunately, most veterinary hospitals do not possess electrical defibrillators. Chemical defibrillators include lidocaine, bretylium, and acetylcholine–potassium chloride. Although acetylcholine-potassium has been shown to be beneficial in dogs, it is not commercially available. Lidocaine, at a dose of 1.0 mg/kg in dogs and 0.25 mg/kg in cats, and bretylium, at a dose of 5 mg/kg in both dogs and cats, can be used.

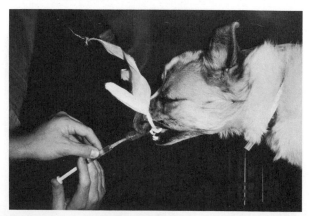

FIGURE 9–5. All emergency drugs except sodium bicarbonate may be administered by the intratracheal (IT) route during CPR. A male urinary catheter or intravenous extension tube is passed down the endotracheal tube to administer drugs.

Unfortunately, with chemical defibrillation alone, the chances for successful defibrillation are remote.

Prolonged Life Support

Unfortunately, even if the animal is successfully resuscitated, frequently subsequent cardiac arrests occur in the immediate post-resuscitation period. Accordingly, the patient should be closely monitored following an arrest. If possible, ECG, ventilatory pattern, neurological function, serum electrolytes, acid/base status, central venous pressure, body temperature and urine output should be monitored in the post-resuscitation period. Cerebral edema is commonly encountered in patients following a successful resuscitation and should be treated with corticosteroids and mannitol. If possible, oxygen administered by either an oxygen cage or nasal catheter should be given in the period following cardiac arrest.

Shock

A discussion of the pathophysiology of shock is beyond the scope of this chapter. However, it is important for the technician to understand the basic underlying causes, signs and treatment. Shock has been described as "the rude unhinging of the machinery of life." It has a variety of causes—trauma, hypovolemia, severe hemorrhage or sepsis—but the ultimate outcome is always the same—cardiovascular collapse. A vicious cycle is created by lack of tissue perfusion, including myocardial perfusion, which enhances the detrimental metabolic effects of shock. Tissue acidosis and venous pooling result both from the insufficient supply of cellular nutrients and from waste removal. This further impairs the cardiac output, and without treatment, the effects of shock can become irreversible and fatal (Fig. 9–6).

Clinical Signs

Since prompt therapy is vital to a successful outcome, the technician who is able to recognize shock may be instrumental in saving a patient's life. The parameters of mucous membrane color, heart rate, pulse character, capillary refill time and tem-

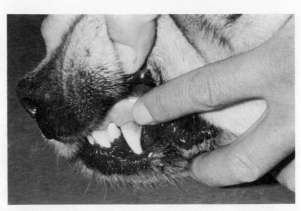

FIGURE 9–7. Capillary refill time can be used to assess peripheral tissue perfusion. One presses on the gums to blanch the membranes. The normal amount of time for the color to return is less than 2 seconds.

perature are critical in assessing this state. This is true not only for determining whether a patient is in shock on entry but also for using the changes in these values to monitor the animal's response to treatment.

Mucous membrane color is generally pink in a normal animal, and the capillary refill time is less than 2 seconds. Capillary refill time may be evaluated by applying digital pressure to the gum or inner surface of the lip and observing how rapidly the pink color returns to the tissue (Fig. 9–7). An animal in shock will have pale mucous membranes in most instances. They may take on a bluish tinge (cyanosis), especially if the animal is dyspneic or has not been respiring effectively. The capillary refill time may be slower than normal. This reflects compromised tissue perfusion. The color and refill time in traumatic, hypovolemic or hemorrhagic shock should be contrasted with those of an animal in septic shock. Here, the inciting cause is endotoxins that are released by the cell walls of gram-negative bacteria. In the initial stages, the color may be injected, and capillary refill time can be faster than normal. During this time, the animal is usually febrile. As shock progresses, the color becomes pale or muddy, and the refill time is prolonged.

The heart rate is elevated in shock as the heart tries to increase cardiac output. Heart rates of large dogs in shock may be as high as 200 beats per minute. In conjunction with this, the pulse character is thready (weak), reflecting the ineffectiveness of the heartbeat. Both heart rate and pulse character are easily obtained and are accurate reflections of a shock state. With effective shock therapy, heart rate will decrease and pulse quality will improve.

The temperature is usually subnormal, though one should remember that it may not have had time to fall if the animal is seen immediately after a traumatic event. However, temperatures may be as low as 35°C. Because of peripheral vasoconstriction, extremities may be cold and thus may be used as a method of assessing and monitoring shock. The difference between the rectal temperature and the toe-web temperature is easy to obtain. In the normal animal, it is not greater than 3.1°C (±1.9 degrees). As the animal responds to treatment, the temperature of the extremities will warm (Fig. 9–8). The patient's attitude is a good indicator as well, and animals will become much more alert and responsive as they return to a normal state.

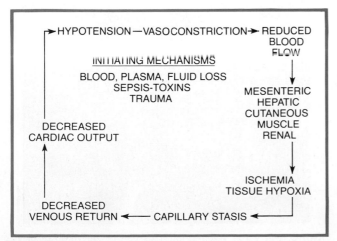

FIGURE 9–6. Flow chart depicting the "vicious cycle" created and the conditions that predispose to or result from shock.

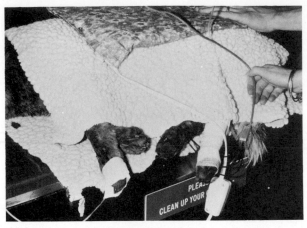

FIGURE 9–8. The patient under the fleece pads is hypothermic and is in shock. A temperature probe is placed between the digits on the front foot. Comparing the toe-web temperature with the rectal (core) temperature reflects the patient's peripheral perfusion and can be used to assess the response to treatment for shock.

Treatment

The treatment for shock varies to a certain extent based upon the type of shock and the veterinarian's preference. However, the mainstay and absolutely essential treatment involves the use of fluids. Crystalloid fluids are used; the type is not critically important in the initial treatment, though balanced electrolyte solutions, such as lactated Ringer's solution or 0.9 percent sodium chloride, are generally used (see Chapter 10). Vigorous administration is required to re-establish the blood volume necessary for an effective cardiac output. Dogs can require as much as 90 ml/kg to be delivered rapidly. Cats have been given less, and fluid treatment for cats has been closer to 40 ml/kg in the past. However, recent studies have shown that cats can tolerate as large an amount as dogs can without suffering fluid overload. Pressure bags are valuable for delivering large volumes of fluids (Fig. 9–9). This amount of fluid should be used only as a guideline and should be modified according to each patient. Not all shock patients require the large doses of fluids listed above. Additionally, in patients with concurrent pulmonary contusions, head trauma, or congestive heart failure, excessive volumes of fluids are contraindicated. Fortunately, close patient monitoring will help determine the amount of fluids to administer to a shock patient. Pulse quality, heart rate, mucous membrane color, attitude and rectal to toe-web temperature difference should be monitored frequently. Fluid administration can be slowed or even stopped when the above parameters indicate patient improvement.

The use of corticosteroids in all types of shock is controversial. They are known to stabilize cellular membranes as well as to enhance cardiovascular performance. Dexamethasone sodium phosphate and prednisolone sodium succinate are the two forms of rapidly acting corticosteroids that are recommended for shock.

The addition of glucose to the fluids is indicated in septic shock, because the patient is usually hypoglycemic. Blood glucose levels may be lower than 45 mg/dl. If there is any question about an animal's status, a blood glucose determination with glucose test strips (Chemstrip BG, Boehringer Mannheim Di-

agnostics, Indianapolis, IN) should be made so that proper fluids can be administered. Dogs with parvovirus are predisposed to sepsis and should be monitored for hypoglycemia and treated if necessary.

The use of sodium bicarbonate is another controversial subject. Many veterinarians use it routinely in shock. Others feel that, as the basic underlying pathological condition is corrected by vigorous fluid therapy, the tissue acidosis will correct itself. Bicarbonate therapy, however, is not without detrimental side effects. Experimental studies of hypovolemic shock in dogs have demonstrated a poorer outcome when sodium bicarbonate has been administered.

Crystalloid fluids (e.g., lactated Ringer's solution) are indicated in hemorrhagic shock unless too much blood has been lost. A general rule of thumb is that if an animal's PCV is less than 20, it should be transfused with whole blood. This generalization must also be modified by clinical judgment, because the hematocrit does not change initially during blood loss, since both red cells and plasma are lost at the same rate. Therefore, an animal could lose as much as one half of its blood volume quickly and require whole blood, even though the blood loss would not yet be reflected by a change in the PCV. The technician should always make an initial determination of PCV and total protein on any severely traumatized or bleeding animals. If total protein declines below 3 g/dl, plasma or colloidal fluids (Dextran 70 or Hetastarch) should be given unless the animal is also anemic. In the latter case, whole blood should be given.

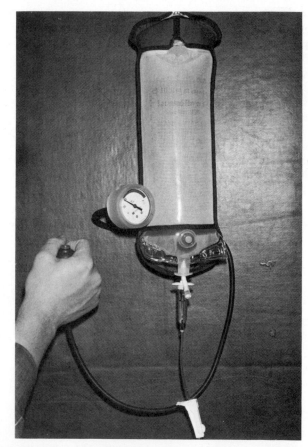

FIGURE 9–9. Large volumes of fluids can be delivered quickly to effectively treat shock by using a pressure bag.

COMMON EMERGENCIES

Trauma—Hit by Car

No matter how stringent leash laws are in any community, there will always be animals hit by cars. There is a great deal of variability in the amount of trauma sustained; some animals will be completely unscathed, whereas others will not even survive long enough to be transported to the hospital.

In traumatized patients, injuries to the respiratory, cardiovascular, and central nervous systems are frequently life-threatening if not treated immediately, while injuries to intra-abdominal organs and the musculoskeletal system, although serious, are not likely to cause death acutely. Accordingly, diagnosis and treatment should be prioritized, with attention first given to organ systems with injuries that are more likely to be life-threatening and later to other injuries.

Respiratory System

Respiratory complications are fairly common in trauma. They include pneumothorax, hemothorax (blood in the thoracic cavity), pulmonary contusions, diaphragmatic hernia and flail chest. Pneumothorax can be life-threatening. This is another example in which a diagnostic procedure is therapeutic. If the veterinarian has a high index of suspicion that there is a pneumothorax, thoracocentesis is indicated. Air can be withdrawn from the chest with a 20-gauge needle, extension tube, three-way stopcock and syringe (Fig. 9–10). This allows a substantial amount of air to be withdrawn with minimal manipulation or stress to the patient. It is recommended that this apparatus be set up at all times so that it is immediately available for emergencies. If the thorax continues to fill with air (Fig. 9–11), the veterinarian may want to place a chest tube so that the animal can be attached to a continuous suction device (e.g., Pleur-evac [Deknatel, Inc.] or a Heimlich valve [Becton-Dickinson, Inc.]) (Fig. 9–12).

A hemothorax can be similarly relieved. Thoracic radiographs may be indicated, but many times the animal is not stable enough to withstand the stress of x-rays. In these cases, a chest tap will be therapeutic as well as diagnostic.

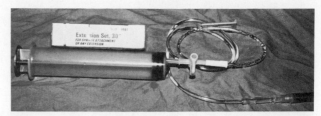

FIGURE 9–10. The equipment used to tap a chest for either air (pneumothorax) or fluid (hydrothorax) consists of a large syringe, a three-way stopcock, extension tubing and a needle. The stopcock allows large volumes of air or fluid to be drained without repositioning the needle.

Pulmonary contusions occur when there is bleeding into the lung. Pulmonary contusions are frequently seen in animals with pneumothorax and hemothorax. Treatment of pulmonary contusions includes supportive therapy with oxygen and avoidance of excessive intravenous fluid volumes that increase bleeding into the lung.

Diaphragmatic hernia occurs when there is a tear in the diaphragm that allows the abdominal organs to enter the thoracic cavity. In many instances, diaphragmatic hernias occur together with other chest injuries, such as pneumothorax and pulmonary contusions. Although diaphragmatic hernias ultimately require surgical repair, the animal should be stabilized first. Pneumothorax and pulmonary contusions should be treated as outlined above. If respiratory distress is still present, suspending the animal momentarily in a head-up vertical position may move the abdominal organs back into the abdominal cavity and provide some respiratory relief.

A particularly dangerous form of diaphragmatic hernia (and luckily a less common one) occurs when the left side of the diaphragm is ruptured, and the stomach is herniated into the thoracic cavity. The stomach may fill with air rapidly and, if not reduced, this condition will be fatal. The bloat can be relieved either by stomach tube or by trocharization. A patient with this type of condition should have surgery as soon as possible.

Flail chest occurs when there are both proximal and distal rib fractures on at least two consecutive ribs, allowing a seg-

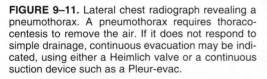

FIGURE 9–11. Lateral chest radiograph revealing a pneumothorax. A pneumothorax requires thoracocentesis to remove the air. If it does not respond to simple drainage, continuous evacuation may be indicated, using either a Heimlich valve or a continuous suction device such as a Pleur-evac.

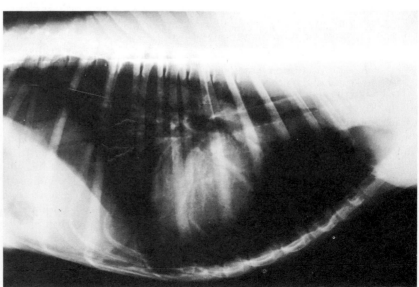

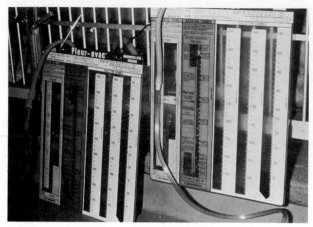

FIGURE 9–12. A Pleur-evac is used for continuous suction drainage of either air or fluid. Fluid is retained in the collection chamber.

ment of the chest wall to move paradoxically and thereby interfere with ventilation. Like diaphragmatic hernias, flail chest may occur together with other chest injuries that will need to be treated. Initial therapy with narcotic analgesics will improve ventilation in dogs with flail chest or fractured ribs. Specific treatment for flail chest is directed at stabilizing the flail segment. Initially, this is performed by applying a snug, but not constrictive, chest wrap. Better stabilization can be attained by applying an external aluminum frame and securing the flail segment to the frame by placing nylon sutures around the ribs of the flail segment.

Central Nervous System

Brain trauma may have occurred. If the owner reports that the animal was unconscious following a traumatic incident, brain trauma is likely to be present. Signs of brain trauma include depression, coma and seizures. Pupils may be constricted, dilated or unequal in size. Treatment for brain trauma is focused on decreasing the swelling of the brain. The use of corticosteroids is indicated, and oxygen is also helpful in reducing cerebral edema. The use of mannitol is controversial: If there has been hemorrhage, mannitol is likely to exacerbate the cerebral hemorrhage. However, mannitol is beneficial in reducing simple edema. Since intracranial hemorrhage is uncommon in dogs and cats with head trauma, mannitol given at a dose of 1 gm per kg intravenously is indicated.

Abdominal Cavity

Trauma to the abdominal organs is also possible. There can be rupture of the bladder, ureters or urethra, especially when a fractured pelvis has been sustained. Fractures (i.e., torn or ruptured capsules) of the spleen or liver will cause abdominal hemorrhage, and significant blood loss can occur. Perforation of the intestines is rare unless there has been a penetrating wound (i.e., gunshot or knife wound).

The clinical signs vary with abdominal trauma. The animal may appear normal initially or on palpation may have an extremely tender abdomen. If a significant amount of blood is being lost into the peritoneal cavity, the animal may be in severe shock. Patients with urinary tract damage may or may not have a painful abdomen. Many times, the pain is referable to bony fractures. There can be bloody urine, blood dripping from the urethra or anuria. One should keep in mind that

there can be severe damage to the urinary tract (e.g., ruptured ureter), and the animal may be observed to urinate normally. In contrast, there can be gross hematuria without any significant damage when there may have been bladder bruising or ruptured vessels, and the problem will resolve without surgical intervention. Any animal that has been hit by a car should be observed carefully for the ability to urinate. When the animal does urinate, it should be noted in the record. This prevents slip-ups in communication from developing into panic situations.

If the veterinarian suspects abdominal hemorrhage, abdominocentesis can be performed. The abdomen should be tapped in four quadrants before concluding that there is no hemorrhage (see Chapter 8). In contrast to blood in the thorax, this blood need not be removed. In fact, the animal will be able to autotransfuse itself. However, if there is significant bleeding, the animal should be treated for hemorrhagic shock, and may even require a transfusion.

If leakage of urine into the abdomen is suspected, abdominocentesis should be performed. Urine leakage is confirmed if the creatinine of the abdominal fluid is significantly elevated when compared with the serum creatinine.

Musculoskeletal System

After the animal has been stabilized, lacerations and fractures should be attended to. Lacerations or abrasions should be clipped and cleansed. A sterile lubricant jelly may be applied to the wound before clipping. This will prevent hair from sticking to tissues and will make it easier to irrigate and cleanse the wound. Fractures of distal extremities (i.e., distal to elbow or stifle joint) need to be stabilized. Otherwise, a simple fracture could become an open one if the animal struggles or tries to bear weight. The type of stabilization will depend on the type of fracture as well as on the veterinarian's preference. Open fractures should be vigorously cleansed as already outlined before stabilization is attempted. The technician should become familiar with the various temporary stabilization devices such as Robert Jones bandages, casts and different splints (see Chapter 13).

Poisoning

A poison is any substance that is noxious to the body. An animal need not be poisoned maliciously; it may eat something in the owner's home or find something while roaming. A history of having observed the animal ingest a suspect substance is extremely helpful. There are poison control centers located in many large cities that are staffed 24 hours a day. The poison control number should be posted in the clinic to be readily available.

If the substance has been ingested recently, an emetic may be indicated. Vomiting should not be induced if the substance ingested is caustic or the animal is not fully conscious. Apomorphine works well to induce vomiting in a clinical setting. Hydrogen peroxide (15 ml per 5 kg body weight) or a tablespoon of salt also causes vomiting. These substances can be used in the clinic, or the client can be advised over the telephone to administer them before bringing in the animal. If the time elapsed has exceeded that for gastric emptying (less than ½ hour for liquids and 1 to 4 hours for solids), induction of vomiting will be of no benefit. However, the administration of charcoal may help in absorbing toxic substances. This should be done with a mouth speculum and a stomach tube. Fractious animals may have to be sedated for this procedure. If the type of poison is known, there may be a specific antagonist that can be used. Examples are atropine for organophosphates, vitamin K for warfarin, and ethanol for ethylene glycol (antifreeze) toxicities.

Acute Abdomen

There are many different disease entities that will result in an acute abdomen, that is, one demanding immediate medical attention. Although the clinical signs are referable to the abdomen, they may vary. An animal may or may not be vomiting, the abdomen may be splinted and painful or it may be distended with either gas or fluid. A diagnostic work-up will be necessary in order to treat the patient properly (to rule out acute pancreatitis, peritonitis and so on).

Gastrointestinal Obstruction

A gastrointestinal obstruction will usually cause vomiting, so this will be the primary complaint. Many foreign bodies or intussusceptions (in which the bowel telescopes on itself) can be detected on abdominal palpation. However, this is not always the case, and x-rays may be necessary to establish the diagnosis. The animal's state of hydration should be noted; if it is vomiting excessively, there may be severe dehydration. Hydration status can be clinically evaluated in several ways (see Chapter 10). The moistness of the mucous membranes gives an indication. However, if an animal has just vomited, the gums may be wet despite dehydration. Another indicator is skin turgor (Fig. 9–13). When the skin of a normal animal is lifted up, it returns to its normal position in less than a second. As an animal becomes dehydrated, fluid leaves the interstitial tissues, and the skin loses some of its elasticity. This causes it to return more slowly. There are several pitfalls to be aware of in using this method. The most important one is that it is impossible to detect dehydration by this method unless the animal is already 5 percent dehydrated (see Chapter 10). It is also difficult to use in an obese animal (who will always seem well hydrated) and in emaciated, very young or very old animals (who will always seem somewhat dehydrated). The PCV and total protein determination will help to augment the clinical determination, as will USG. All three values will be elevated in a dehydrated animal.

In any case, the animal with an obstruction should be given nothing by mouth. Diagnosis and stabilization are necessary before surgery is performed.

Peritonitis

Peritonitis (inflammation of the lining of the abdominal cavity) can be caused by a variety of insults—rupture of any abdominal organ, which can contaminate the peritoneal cavity, severe pancreatitis or penetrating wounds. There can be a chemical peritonitis in which there is no bacterial contamination, but the visceral surfaces are severely inflamed; this is the case with a ruptured gallbladder or with a ruptured urinary bladder. The patient's clinical status will depend on the sever-

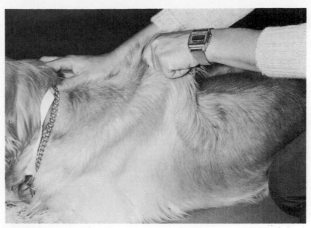

FIGURE 9–13. Skin turgor is used to obtain an estimate of the patient's hydration status. The skin is picked up and released. It should return within 1 second. The minimum amount of dehydration that can be appreciated by this method is 5 percent.

ity and duration of the disease. The first clinical sign is an extremely painful abdomen. Animals may hold themselves in a splinted position ("tucked-up" position) and may be extremely resentful of palpation. The mucous membranes may be normal or pale, but as the disease continues, they may become hyperemic and injected. This is especially true in septic peritonitis. If the animal is septic, it may also be in shock.

The patient should be evaluated, and any shock should be treated vigorously. If sepsis is suspected, blood glucose levels should be measured since the animal may be hypoglycemic. The veterinarian may wish to perform abdominocentesis in order to examine any fluid that is in the abdomen, which may aid in a diagnosis. For this procedure, the hair is clipped and the area is aseptically prepared. Fluid is obtained with a needle and syringe (see Chapter 8).

Penetrating Abdominal Wound

If there is a penetrating abdominal wound (e.g., gunshot or knife), one is always safer in expecting that contamination has taken place and treating aggressively rather than taking a "wait and see" attitude. Many veterinarians feel that an animal with a penetrating abdominal wound should undergo exploratory surgery even if it appears stable on entry. The philosophy that peritonitis is a serious and often fatal disease, which is more easily treated in the initial stages than after there have been gross contamination and tissue responses, results in fewer fatalities. This especially holds true with gunshot injuries.

Pancreatitis

Most dogs with pancreatitis will vomit profusely. The abdomen is usually tender. These animals are best treated aggressively with intravenous fluids and given nothing by mouth.

Gastric Dilatation or Volvulus

The syndrome of gastric dilatation or volvulus is common in the large and giant breeds of dogs, especially those with deep chests. It is seen in Great Danes, Irish wolfhounds, German shepherd dogs, Irish setters, St. Bernards, and Doberman pin-

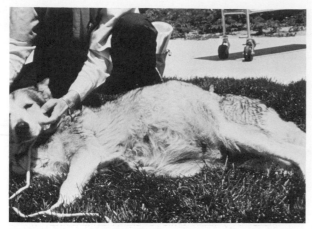

FIGURE 9–14. A dog with a gastric dilatation has a distended abdomen and may be extremely depressed or in shock.

schers. However, it may occur in smaller breeds. Many times, an owner will phone to say that the dog is depressed and has been wretching frequently but not producing vomitus. The owner may also report that the abdomen is distended (Fig. 9–14).

Gastric dilatation or volvulus, or both, are life-threatening. If signs such as those described are related over the telephone, the owner should be advised to come in immediately, and the veterinarian should be notified at once.

In these conditions, the stomach becomes distended with food, liquid and air, and the cardiac sphincter of the stomach acts as a one-way valve so that the animal cannot vomit. Sometimes the stomach rotates so that both esophagus and pylorus are occluded (volvulus). It is impossible to distinguish between these two entities clinically or even by passing a stomach tube.

Shock is an important aspect of gastric dilatation, because the stomach becomes so distended that it can occlude return of blood to the heart by the caudal vena cava and azygous vein. Therefore, one of the first procedures to be performed in these patients is insertion of an intravenous catheter and administration of shock doses of fluids. The use of bicarbonate is again controversial. It has been shown that animals with gastric dilatation or volvulus can be acidotic or alkalotic or can have normal blood gases. Therefore, unless blood gases can be measured, the use of bicarbonate is not justified and may even be contraindicated. The use of corticosteroids may be helpful, especially in shocky animals.

Decompression of the stomach is essential. Every veterinary clinic should have a stomach tube available (Fig. 9–15A). A mouth speculum can be made from a 5-cm roll of adhesive tape so that the animal cannot bite the tube. This may be taped in place (Fig. 9–15B). The tube is then passed with a small amount of lubricant on the tip. Positioning the dog with the front portion of the body elevated will facilitate passage of the tube. Many times, the tube will not pass at the cardia. This does not necessarily indicate that there is volvulus. Forcefully blowing into the tube may allow passage.

If initial attempts at passing the tube are unsuccessful, relieving some of the excess gas by trocharization will usually allow passage of the tube. The right lateral abdomen is clipped and aseptically prepared over the area of greatest resonance. Insertion of 18-gauge needles allows the gas to escape. Few complications are seen with this method, and it may make passage of

the stomach tube feasible. Once the tube has been passed, food, fluid and gas will escape. The stomach should then be lavaged with copious amounts of warm fluids until the returning fluid is relatively clear.

If it is impossible to pass a stomach tube, decompression will have to be achieved by gastrotomy (opening into stomach) as an emergency surgical procedure. If this is necessary, the animal can remain with the open stoma until it is stable for surgery.

Many animals respond dramatically to decompression in conjunction with treatment for shock. If the stomach has twisted on its axis, surgery is absolutely indicated. However, even if there has been only a simple dilatation, the animal is predisposed to a repeat episode, and prophylactic gastropexy surgery is strongly recommended. Animals should be monitored carefully for signs of re-bloating. A tape measure can be used periodically to evaluate the girth diameter. The veterinarian may wish to place a pharyngostomy tube extending into the stomach to prevent recurrence of dilatation (see Chapter 8).

Renal Failure

Animals in renal failure may be presented as emergencies with the complaint of vomiting. The veterinarian will recommend the rudimentary diagnostic procedures to determine the cause of vomiting to be uremia. One will be aided by history, BUN and USG as an emergency minimum data base. It is further necessary to distinguish between acute and chronic or end-stage renal failure, since the prognosis and response to treatment vary greatly.

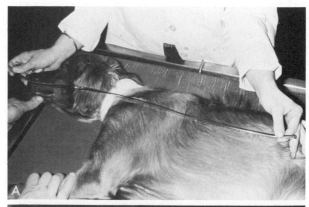

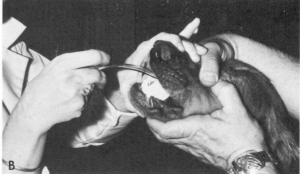

FIGURE 9–15. Gastric intubation. A, The tube should be premeasured to the end of the last rib before it is passed. B, A roll of tape can serve as a speculum in order to prevent the dog from biting the tube.

Obstetrical Problems

Dystocia (difficult birth) is virtually always an emergency. It is much more common in dogs than in cats. The first contact is usually made over the telephone with a worried owner and a variety of situations. The dog may have been in labor for an extended period, a prolonged period may have elapsed between the birth of the young or the young may be lodged in the birth canal. The animal may also be overdue on the calculated date of parturition.

Normal *parturition* (delivery) is divided into three stages. *Stage 1* involves the nesting behavior that is seen 12 to 24 hours prior to whelping. The animal may be restless, panting or shivering. The rectal temperature will usually drop to about 36°C to 37°C. The length of time from stage 1 is usually 6 to 12 hours but can go to 36 hours in animals who are whelping for the first time. *Stage 2* involves straining, abdominal contractions and delivery. In most cases, the maximum time between pups is less than 4 hours, and the maximum total time for delivery of the litter is 12 hours. There should be no more than 2 hours between the rupture of the allantoic membrane (first water bag) and delivery of the first pup. *Stage 3* involves the expulsion of the placenta. This should take place within 12 hours of the end of parturition. These guidelines may assist telephone communications with worried clients.

Reasons for dystocia include uterine inertia, birth canal narrowing, such as pelvic fractures, or fetal dystocia in which the fetus is too large to pass through the canal. One should suspect dystocia if there is prolonged labor without delivery, prolonged gestation (greater than days 66 to 68), abnormal vaginal discharge or a history of previous dystocia or trauma.

If medical therapy (consisting of oxytocin and calcium or glucose) is not effective, surgery must be performed. The role of the technician is extremely important, since the pups must be managed as soon as the surgeon delivers them. The amnion (second water bag) should be removed from the pups' faces and the noses and mouths wiped and cleared of secretions. The pups should be warmed with a towel and stimulated by rubbing. If they do not start breathing, a few drops of doxapram hydrochloride on the tongue will act as a respiratory stimulant. If anesthesia has been used, it will affect the pups. Many veterinarians induce bitches with oxymorphone (a narcotic), which can be reversed easily. If this drug has been used, a reversal agent such as naloxone can be placed on the tongue or injected intraperitoneally. The pups should be kept warm under a heating lamp until the bitch is awake enough to take care of them.

Feline Urethral Obstruction

Feline urethral obstruction is a potentially life-threatening condition that occurs fairly frequently in male cats. The inability to urinate causes an accumulation of electrolytes and waste products that may rapidly become toxic. Potassium is the primary electrolyte that can cause severe problems, especially with the cardiovascular system (i.e., cardiac arrhythmias).

The first contact may be made over the telephone. The owner's complaint is often that the cat is spending a lot of time straining in the catbox. The distinction between a simple cystitis and actually being blocked can be made only by palpation of the bladder. Therefore, it is better to err on the side of being too cautious and to advise all owners with this history to bring the cat into the clinic. Alternatively, the problem may have been going on for a longer time, with the owner describing signs of anorexia, depression and vomiting in the cat.

The manner in which the case is handled will depend on the clinical status of the patient. Cats that have been blocked only for a short time and are stable may only need to have the obstruction relieved. However, those animals that have been unable to urinate for longer (greater than 24 hours) may require intensive treatment. Hyperkalemia (increased serum potassium) can cause severe cardiac arrhythmias and should be treated. These cats may also be acidotic, which can cause the potassium to be even higher, since it is driven out of the cells in exchange for hydrogen ions. Therefore, one of the treatments involves the use of bicarbonate (1.0 mEq/kg intravenously). If arrhythmias are severe, intravenous regular insulin (0.5 units/kg) will also drive potassium back into the cells. It should be used in conjunction with glucose (1.0 g per unit of insulin intravenously initially, followed by another 1.0 g per unit of insulin to be given in the intravenous fluids over the next 6 hours) in order to avoid the possibility of hypoglycemia (low blood glucose levels).

Cats that are extremely ill require no sedation in order to relieve the blockage. Others may be healthy enough that it is easier and less stressful to both patient and veterinarian to use chemical restraint. Massaging the tip of the penis may loosen the plug that is usually composed of mucus and struvite crystals. If this is not effective, a sterile lubricated catheter is passed while sterile saline is simultaneously flushed retrograde. There are several ways to restrain the cat manually and to extrude the penis so that the veterinarian or technician can pass the urinary catheter (Fig. 9–16). After the obstruction is relieved, the bladder may be irrigated with a sterile saline solution in order to clear it of as many crystals and debris as possible (Fig. 9–17). The catheter may or may not be sutured in place, depending on the clinical status of the patient. Patient status will also determine the use of intravenous fluids. Animals that have become azotemic (uremic) should unquestionably be given fluids. This is especially important for cats that may undergo a post-obstruction diuresis and may be unable to take in as many fluids as they are losing in the very dilute, copious urine produced after the obstruction is relieved. An Elizabethan collar is necessary to prevent the cat from pulling out the urethral catheter during the recovery period.

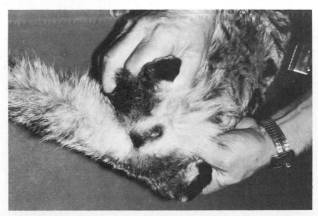

FIGURE 9–16. Method of restraint for a cat with a urethral obstruction. The cat is on its back, and the hindlimbs are held.

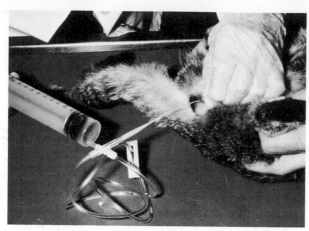

FIGURE 9–17. A catheter is inserted in the penis, and sterile saline is used to flush the obstruction retrograde. Following removal of the obstruction, the bladder can be lavaged.

Electrical Shock

Electrical shock is usually seen in young animals that bite or chew on electrical cords. They may or may not have burns on the tongue and gums and may look entirely normal on presentation. However, pulmonary edema is a severe and fairly common complication that ensues. If the animal is normal, it should still be monitored carefully for 12 to 24 hours for the development of pulmonary edema. If edema is already present, the use of oxygen, diuretics and corticosteroids is indicated.

Metabolic Crisis

Diseases that are a result of deranged metabolism may have an insidious onset. However, the animal may be presented as an emergency if it decompensates. Examples of these diseases are diabetes mellitus, renal failure and Addison's disease. Much of the treatment (even supportive) depends on rudimentary diagnostic procedures before therapy can begin (see Introduction).

Heat Stroke

Heat stroke is a fairly common occurrence in the summer. An animal that has been left in an unventilated car or one that has been exercising vigorously may be a victim of heat stroke. Rectal temperatures can exceed 41°C. The most important therapy involves cooling the animal. This can be attained by using cold water baths, intravenous fluids and cold water enemas. One should constantly monitor the temperature. Once it has come down to 40°C, cooling measures should be stopped. If they continue, many times the temperature will continue to plummet, and the problem becomes hypothermia with temperatures as low as 35°C. These animals should be monitored once they are stabilized. One of the complications of heat stroke is disseminated intravascular coagulation (DIC). In the early stages of this blood coagulation disorder, there is coagulation of the blood within small vessels. Later in the disease, the blood does not clot because clotting factors have been consumed. During this phase, the animal may bleed excessively

and become anemic. Therefore, the animal should be checked for petechiae or for a sudden drop in the PCV.

Status Epilepticus

Status epilepticus (continuous seizures) must be treated as an emergency. If an animal is constantly having seizures or is having more than six seizures an hour, it should be attended to by a veterinarian. One can use diazepam intravenously in 5-mg increments up to a total dose of 1.0 mg per kg to control these seizures. If this is not effective, intravenous pentobarbital is titrated to effect.

MONITORING THE CRITICAL PATIENT

Several parameters may be used to monitor the critical care patient. They include temperature, pulse, respiration and urinary output. These have been discussed in the previous sections of this chapter. To reiterate, monitoring temperature during shock is extremely important, and rectal versus toe-web temperatures may be used. Assessment of respiration should include its rate and character. The color of the mucous membranes should be checked frequently. Monitoring cardiovascular performance includes measuring heart rate and rhythm as well as character of the pulse. Electrocardiograph monitoring should be used if available. Urinary output is also a good way of monitoring an animal's response to treatment for shock. Normal urinary output is between .25 to .50 ml per kg per hour. When an animal being treated for shock does not urinate within a few hours, the bladder should be palpated. If it is not palpable, one may suspect urinary tract trauma.

Supportive treatment may include the use of thoracic tubes, indwelling catheters (intravenous as well as urinary), tracheostomy tubes or gastrostomy tubes. Thoracic tubes should be used if a pneumothorax or hemothorax is not amenable to one-time treatment. These can be attached to 60-ml syringes with a stopcock, Heimlich valves (Becton-Dickinson, Inc.) or Thor-Klex (Davol, Inc.). Management of chest tubes is critical for two reasons. First, if there is not a tight seal or a tube becomes disconnected from the valve or the stopcock, air is allowed into the chest and re-establishes the pneumothorax. For this reason, it is always best to wire stopcocks onto the chest tube. Second, any foreign body allows the possibility of bacterial contamination. Extreme caution and aseptic technique should be practiced with any chest tube.

Tracheostomy tubes should be used if there is upper airway obstruction. Indications include laryngeal edema, severe laryngoplegia or tumors or abscesses that occlude the upper airway. Once inserted, management is extremely important. Many times secretions can act as a plug so that the initial problem of respiratory obstruction is compounded. Many animals die with a tracheostomy tube in place because the tube has not been properly managed (Fig. 9–18). They should be suctioned frequently (once every 4 hours for the first 24 hours after initial placement and once every 6 to 8 hours thereafter). The equipment used for this (extension tubing, syringes) may be reused if it is left soaking in a solution such as Nolvasan (Fort Dodge) between uses. Prior to suctioning the artificial airway, this equipment should be rinsed with sterile saline.

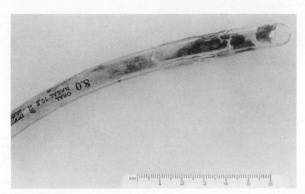

FIGURE 9–18. This endotracheal tube was used as an emergency tracheostomy tube. A plug of mucus became lodged, and the animal died of respiratory failure. Cleaning and suctioning a tube will prevent such an occurrence.

Sterile surgical gloves should be worn by the person performing tracheostomy care. Animals with tracheostomies should also be monitored carefully for development of respiratory infections, since the tracheal defenses are compromised by the use of the tracheostomy tube.

CONCLUSION

The technician's role in handling emergencies is critical. Communication on the telephone is important, and one must have the knowledge to answer questions correctly and have the judgment to know when an animal must be seen immediately. A well-trained technician aiding a veterinarian with critical patients is invaluable in terms of placing catheters, stabilizing patients, performing diagnostic procedures, assessing treatment response and monitoring.

Recommended Reading

Kirk RW and Bonagura JD (editors): Current Veterinary Therapy XI. Philadelphia, WB Saunders Co., 1992, pp 68–158.

Kirk R and Bistner S: Handbook of Veterinary Procedures and Emergency Treatment. 4th ed, Philadelphia, WB Saunders Co., 1985.

Murtaugh RJ and Kaplan PM: Veterinary Emergency and Critical Care Medicine. St. Louis, Mosby-Year Book, 1992.

Stamp GL (editor): Emergency Medicine and Critical Care. 1. Semin Vet Med Surg (Small Anim) 3(3):183–254, 1988.

Stamp GL (editor): Emergency Medicine and Critical Care. 2. Semin Vet Med Surg (Small Anim) 3(4):255–312, 1988.

10

Small Animal Medical Nursing

T. MARK NEER

INTRODUCTION

Small animal medical nursing consists of attending to the total needs of a medical illness. The nursing process can be viewed as a traditional exercise in problem solving. Problem solving can be divided into several components: data collection, data interpretation, implementation of a plan and evaluation of the response to the plan. The veterinary technician should apply each of these steps to small animal medical nursing.

The cornerstone of data collection for the technician is *observation*. Effective observation requires an understanding that many clinical problems are dynamic processes that are capable of rapid change. If change is to be recognized, careful, detailed and systematic observation is required. The precise system and nature of patient monitoring will vary, depending on the specific clinical situation; however, the evaluation of all patients should take place according to a regular and reliable schedule. An important part of any system of observation is to establish an accurate baseline for whatever parameters are being serially monitored.

Observations by the veterinary technician are invaluable in providing optimal medical care for the ill animal. In many instances the technician has observed the patient for longer periods of time than has the veterinarian. Thus, the technician may be able to recognize changes that are not readily apparent to the veterinarian during routine daily physical examination. Also, the manifestations of certain significant medical problems, such as pain, can be subtle. Dogs may manifest pain by being restless or uneasy without displaying any other sign of discomfort.

Data interpretation by the veterinary technician consists of recognizing and correctly interpreting the observations that have been made. Stated differently, the technician must recognize and define clinical problems. A clinical problem is anything that interferes with the well-being of the animal patient or anything that requires treatment or further diagnostic evaluation. Examples of clinical problems that might be recognized by the technician include diarrhea, vomiting, anorexia and respiratory distress.

It is important to document that a problem exists before implementing a diagnostic or therapeutic plan. For example, the technician may suspect increased water consumption, but before an extensive evaluation is initiated it may be wise to accurately measure the water consumed over a 24-hour period. In certain instances, documentation of a problem may simply consist of repeating a clinical determination or measurement.

Formulation, organization and implementation of a diagnostic or therapeutic plan is the next step in the total nursing process. Usually, this occurs following consultation with the attending veterinarian. For nursing to be optimally effective, a mechanism should exist for the ready exchange of information between technician and veterinarian. A team approach to animal health care is the ultimate goal, with veterinarian and technician each contributing their unique skills and abilities to the task of returning the patient to health.

The need for thorough observation does not end once the diagnostic or therapeutic plan has been initiated. Frequently, the plan is modified because of a changing clinical situation or because of the response to the specific plan.

When implementing any diagnostic or therapeutic plan, it is important to remember that the quantity and nature of nursing care should always be individualized. One patient may readily accept a specific procedure, whereas another will resist to the point that the intended benefit is lost. Although excessive intervention may be detrimental to certain animals, this should not be construed as an excuse for medical neglect. The fundamental principle is that if a patient is not meeting a requirement for survival, the technician must intervene promptly. Certain animals require tremendous amounts of attention and affection from the technician simply to maintain their will to live during periods of separation from the owner.

Each technician and each animal hospital should establish and maintain consistent standards of nursing care. Veterinary technicians have a professional and moral obligation to every animal patient to provide the following basic necessities:

1. A clean, comfortable environment, as free of stress as possible.
2. Food and water at all times unless restricted for medical reasons.
3. Adequate exercise and grooming care unless restricted for medical reasons.
4. Suffering should be relieved promptly and humanely.
5. Every patient should be treated humanely and with dignity at all times.

GENERAL CARE

Grooming and bathing are aspects of the general care of the animal patient that are important for several reasons. First, a clean and well-groomed animal has an enhanced sense of well-being and potentially will recover from an illness more rapidly. Second, a clean animal is much less likely to develop severe contact dermatitis from urine scalding and fecal soiling of the skin, which, if it does occur, becomes another clinical problem to manage. Third, grooming and medicated baths are recommended for the prevention or treatment of many dermatological problems. Bathing with shampoo that contains an insecticide is a useful adjunct in the control of ectoparasites. Finally, the cleanliness of the patient at the time of discharge is an indication to the owner of the overall quality of the health care provided.

Every animal hospital should have an adequate collection of grooming and bathing equipment and supplies, that is, combs, brushes, scissors, towels for drying, electrical dryers and a selection of shampoos appropriate for different situations. Care must be taken to prevent the spread of infectious problems, such as dermatomycosis, from one animal to another via grooming instruments. These instruments should be thoroughly cleansed in an appropriate disinfectant solution after each use.

When clipping or removing hair from an animal for medical reasons, it is important to obtain the owner's permission, whenever possible. This is particularly important in animals used for show purposes. In certain breeds, such as the Afghan hound, regrowth of hair is extremely slow.

Bathing

The basic technique for bathing dogs and cats is self-evident; however, the following points warrant emphasis. The eyes should be protected from chemical injury by instilling a drop of mineral oil or a small amount of boric acid ophthalmic ointment prior to bathing. Care should be exercised to prevent water from entering the external ear canal. This can be accomplished by placing a small piece of cotton in each ear. Remember to remove the cotton when the bath has been completed. Thermal injury from excessively hot water can be prevented by constantly monitoring the water temperature. Thorough rinsing with clean water prevents irritation of the skin from residual shampoo. The axillary and scrotal regions of longhaired dogs are particularly vulnerable to residual shampoo irritation. If a cage dryer is used, caution must be exercised in order to prevent overheating (hyperthermia). Shampoos containing insecticides should be used only with the approval of the attending veterinarian because of the possibility of cumulative toxicity or drug interactions. If insecticidal dips are used, correct dilutions are necessary to avoid toxic reactions. If a complete immersion bath is contraindicated, localized soiling of the animal may be handled with a sponge bath.

Exercise

Moderate exercise is beneficial for the general care of the animal patient. Exercise should take place in a secure, controlled and safe environment so that injury or loss of the animal does not occur. Contraindications to exercise include many, but not all, respiratory, cardiovascular and musculoskeletal problems. The decision whether to restrict exercise or not should be made following consultation with the attending veterinarian. Moderate exercise can be considered the simplest and most basic form of physical therapy and can be a useful means of reducing peripheral edema and improving muscle tone and strength.

Feeding

The animal health technician plays a particularly pivotal role in ensuring that each patient remains in a positive energy balance, in which caloric intake exceeds metabolic requirements. As stated earlier, the technician is in an excellent position to observe complete or partial anorexia (loss of appetite) and to take appropriate action to rectify the situation. In certain instances, merely substituting a more palatable food will solve the problem. Familiarity with the home feeding regimen will aid in the selection of palatable alternative diets. In certain instances, it may even be advisable for the owner to prepare food at home and bring it to the hospital. It is helpful to stock a variety of types of food, such as canned, semimoist and dry, in a variety of flavors to satisfy even the most discriminating patient. Although not suitable for long-term nutritional maintenance, meat-flavored baby food may be used to stimulate an animal's appetite. In other instances, personalized attention at the time of feeding will increase food intake. Hand feeding will usually be sufficient, but forced feeding may be required in selected cases. Forced feeding consists of manually placing boluses of food in the caudal pharynx in order to stimulate the swallowing reflex. High-calorie density supplements, such as Nutrical (Evsco), may facilitate meeting the caloric requirements of the patient but by no means will they meet the animal's daily requirements by themselves. In many animals requiring forced feeding for an extended period, gastric gavage is preferred, because it is less stressful (both to the patient and to the veterinary technician). The technique for gastric gavage (stomach tubing) is discussed in Chapter 8. Other methods of enteral nutrition are being used with increased frequency. These include feeding by way of nasogastric, pharyngostomy, gastrostomy and jejunostomy tubes. Specially tailored complete diets may be administered through these routes to ensure adequate nutrition in a variety of disease states, such as hepatic lipidosis in cats and renal failure. One such complete diet, which can be forced through a 60-cc syringe, is Prescription Diet A/D (Hills).

Nail Trimming

Nail trimming (pedicure) is an important general care technique. Excessive nail length results in altered gait and the potential accentuation of lameness problems. Excessively long nails are more likely to be traumatically avulsed. Finally, untrimmed nails can become ingrown (usually into the footpads) resulting in cellulitis or abscess formation.

A sturdy, durable nail trimmer is required for this procedure. Two common types are available (Resco and Whites nail trim). In order to avoid cutting pigmented (black) nails too short in the dog, the cutting surface of the nail trimmer should be held parallel to the palmar (plantar) surface of the digital foot pads, and the nail is cut in this plane. In cats, the nails can be exposed by grasping the paw between the thumb and index finger and sliding the skin on the dorsum of the paw away from the nails (Fig. 10–1). Once exposed, the nails can be trimmed as described for the dog. Since certain animals vehemently resent handling of their feet for nail trimming, it is a good practice to routinely give a pedicure to any animal anesthetized or tranquilized for any procedure. If the blood vessel in the nail is inadvertently severed ("the quick is cut"), silver nitrate sticks can be used to stop the hemorrhage by means of chemical cautery. If the owner is receptive, it is desirable to provide instructions in the proper technique of nail trimming so that this routine task can be accomplished at home.

Ear Cleaning

The external ear canal may accumulate cerumen, exudate or cellular debris as a sequela to otitis externa or a foreign body (e.g., grass awn), which then requires cleaning. Certain breeds, notably poodles, Bedlington terriers and Kerry blue terriers, also may accumulate excessive hair in the external ear canal. The initial and essential step in the treatment of any external ear problem is complete and thorough cleaning of the entire ear canal. Frequently, satisfactory cleaning requires the administration of a short-acting general anesthetic or heavy tranquilization. The first step is to remove any hair that is present, and if excessive wax is present, a cerumenolytic agent (i.e., dioctyl sodium succinate [Cerusol, Burns-Biotech Labs]) can be instilled to soften the wax. Excessive wax and debris can then be removed by using a soft rubber bulb syringe and a

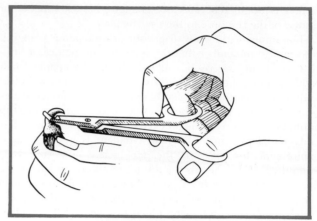

FIGURE 10–1. Schematic diagram depicting pedicure technique in the cat.

dilute disinfectant solution to lavage the external ear canal. Balls of cotton and cotton applicator sticks can be used to gently wipe the wax from the external ear canal. Some of this debris should be suspended in mineral oil and smeared on a microscope slide to be examined under low power for the presence of *Otodectes* (ear mites). Cleaning the horizontal ear canal should be done gently and with extreme caution in order to prevent damage to the tympanic membrane or the packing of debris deep into the horizontal canal (Fig. 10–2). If the ear canal contains purulent debris, a sample should be obtained for cytological evaluation (smear) and bacterial culture prior to instrumentation and cleaning. If bacterial growth is observed, antibiotic sensitivity should be evaluated *in vitro* (see Chapter 6). If the cytological preparation reveals the presence of yeast *(Malassezia)*, appropriate therapy should be initiated. Some practitioners advocate the use of pulsating streams of water from a dental hygiene apparatus (Water Pik, Teledyne Inc.) to clean the external ear canal. Approximately 5 ml of povidone-iodine (Betadine, Purdue-Frederick) or Nolvasan solution (Fort Dodge Laboratories) is added to approximately 236 to 384 ml of warm water. The stream of water should be applied in a rotating motion and directed parallel to the external ear canal. The excess water and debris can be caught in an ear irrigation basin or similar vessel. An inexpensive alternative is the use of a rubber bulb syringe to manually loosen debris and aid in flushing the ear canal. This technique is not recommended if the tympanic membrane is not intact.

Regardless of the technique employed to clean the external ear canal, a second otoscopic examination should be performed to evaluate the completeness of the ear cleaning. Once the ear canal is sufficiently clean, the canal should be carefully dried with clean cotton swabs, and the initial dose of prescribed otic preparation instilled.

Anal Sacs

The anal sacs are reservoirs for the secretions produced by the anal glands. The anal glands line the walls of the anal sacs and produce a foul-smelling fluid that varies from serous to pasty in consistency and brown to off-white in color. The anal sacs are paired structures, approximately 1 cm in diameter, that lie between the internal and external anal sphincter muscles on either side of the anal canal. Each sac opens into the

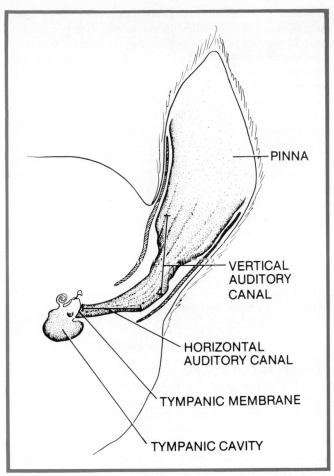

PINNA

VERTICAL AUDITORY CANAL

HORIZONTAL AUDITORY CANAL

TYMPANIC MEMBRANE

TYMPANIC CAVITY

FIGURE 10–2. Schematic diagram of the anatomy of the canine ear.

lateral margin of the anus by a single duct, at approximately the four and eight o'clock positions of the anus.

Clinical signs associated with impacted anal sacs include excessive licking of the perineum, "scooting" or dragging the perineum on the floor, abnormal carriage of the tail or vague indications of pain or discomfort in the perineal region.

The anal sacs are best expressed by inserting a lubricated, gloved forefinger into the rectum. The distended sacs are immobilized between the forefinger and the thumb, which remains external to the anus. The sacs are generally found in a ventrolateral location. Gentle pressure is applied until the secretions are forced through the ducts. Since the ducts as well as the one are occasionally compressed with this technique, if the sac cannot be expressed with gentle pressure, the finger and thumb are repositioned and pressure is reapplied. Paper toweling or cotton placed over the anus can be used to prevent the extremely unpleasant liquid from soiling the patient, the environment or the technician!

Bedding

The optimal means of keeping an ambulatory dog clean is by the appropriate use of bedding and exercise runs. Several types of bedding are routinely used in small-animal practice. They include newspaper, other types of paper products, blankets and towels. It is important that the bedding material se-

lected be either disposable or readily and effectively cleaned between uses. Since occasionally dogs will ingest their bedding, it is also important that the material be safe and nontoxic. Most dogs are extremely reluctant to urinate or defecate in their cage; therefore, keeping the cage and patient clean is facilitated by regular use of exercise runs. Specifically, dogs should be placed in the runs several times a day for an adequate period of time. Dogs should be run individually to prevent fight injuries, and the run should be inspected periodically to be certain that it is secure and free of sharp edges.

Generally, cats are easier to keep clean than dogs during periods of hospitalization. Cats will use litter pans and groom and clean themselves unless they are seriously ill. Litter should be changed daily, and pans or trays should be either disposable or constructed of materials that will allow thorough cleaning and disinfection between uses. It is unnecessary to place cats in exercise runs unless the hospital stay is unusually long.

Decubital Sores

Keeping the nonambulatory patient clean and free of associated problems is far more challenging. Prevention and management of *decubital sores* (bedsores) and urine scald are extremely important aspects of the care of recumbent patients. Animals suffering from various neurological or orthopedic problems can be recumbent for prolonged periods and require special care. Urine and fecal soiling can cause serious problems that can complicate recovery from the underlying condition. Scalding due to urine or diarrhea can be prevented by a light topical application of a protective compound, such as Aquaphor (Beiersdorf, Inc., Norwalk, CT) or petrolatum (e.g., Vaseline) to susceptible perineal or inguinal areas.

Decubital sores not only complicate recovery but also can be a source of sepsis, which can lead to the demise of the patient. The best treatment for decubital sores is *prevention*. Decubital sores develop over bony prominences as the result of continuous pressure and damage to the overlying skin. Various types of bedding have been advocated to reduce the frequency and severity of decubital sores. They include the use of air or water mattresses, foam padding, synthetic fleeces, grids or grates and straw. The material should either be disposable or have an impermeable surface that does not retain moisture or microorganisms and can be thoroughly cleaned. A potential problem with impermeable surfaces is that urine and moisture tend to remain in contact with the skin and can exacerbate the problem. Therefore, care should be taken to keep the skin surface as dry as possible. This is why, for long-term management, straw is beneficial since adequate cushioning is available for the animal and also urine drains through the straw away from the patient.

Other routine measures that help to prevent decubital sores include frequent turning of the patient from side to side, intermittent use of slings or carts to prevent continuous pressure over the bony prominences and frequent baths to keep the skin clean.

Once decubital sores have developed, they should be thoroughly cleaned with a surgical scrub. Surgical debridement of necrotic tissue may be necessary. Following cleaning, the area should be completely dried. Soaking the affected area two to four times daily with a mild astringent will aid in keeping the decubital sore dry. A 1:40 astringent solution of aluminum acetate (Burow's solution) may be made by dissolving one packet (Domeboro solution, Dome Laboratories) per pint of warm water. Ideally, the area of the decubital sore should be padded to prevent further pressure injury; however, the sore itself should remain exposed to the air to prevent retention of moisture. One way of accomplishing this is to fashion a "donut" from foam rubber and to fix this to the skin by means of adhesive tape. Unfortunately, it is difficult to maintain these pads in the proper location for long periods of time.

Topical antimicrobial agents should be applied judiciously, since many contain ointment or cream bases that form an occlusive dressing that will retain moisture. Furthermore, it is questionable how beneficial they are in controlling an infected decubital sore.

Routine Immunization Program for Dogs and Cats

One of the greatest areas of advancement in veterinary medicine in the last 50 years is in the prevention of infectious diseases. The purpose of any vaccination program is to prevent clinical disease by preventing or limiting infection (Schultz, 1982). The vaccination program can also be the foundation of a complete well-animal health maintenance program. At the time of vaccination, owners should be counseled regarding nutrition, parasite control and matters regarding reproduction. Chapter 31 provides a complete overview of canine and feline preventive health programs and vaccination recommendations.

A physical examination by the veterinarian at the time of vaccination is extremely important, since a number of conditions will potentially influence the immunization procedure, such as pregnancy, debilitation and fever.

Numerous factors influence the patient's ability to respond to vaccination. Factors that are of practical significance include colostral antibodies, vaccine type, route of administration, age of the patient, nutritional status of the patient and concurrent infection or drug therapy.

Colostral Antibodies

In pups and kittens, approximately 95 percent of their circulating immunoglobulins come from absorption of colostrum (first milk) shortly after birth. These circulating immunoglobulins provide essential temporary protection, but they also have the ability to interfere with more permanent protection. Interference occurs because the vaccine does not reach the appropriate cells to stimulate the active immunity process. Consequently, it is necessary for the level of circulating immunoglobulins derived from the colostrum to be reduced before successful vaccination is possible. In puppies born to bitches that have received vaccinations against canine distemper and infectious canine hepatitis, this period of uncertain response to vaccination may extend to 14 weeks of age. Thus, the last dose of vaccine should be administered at 14 to 16 weeks of age in order to optimize the success of the vaccination program. Colostral immunoglobulins to canine parvovirus may last for at least 16 weeks in puppies; therefore, the last dose of vaccine for parvovirus should be given no earlier than 16 weeks of age. In the Rottweiler and Doberman breeds, it is suggested that the last dose of parvovirus vaccine be given at 18 weeks of age.

An alternative technique to prevent or reduce the blocking effect of colostral antibodies upon canine distemper vaccination is to use measles virus vaccine. Approximately 50 percent of puppies at 6 weeks of age will not respond to canine distemper virus vaccination, whereas the vast majority will respond to measles virus vaccine. Measles virus vaccine prevents clinical disease but does not prevent infection. Measles virus vaccine should be considered a temporary method of preventing canine distemper until the dog can respond to the canine distemper vaccine. There is no reason to use vaccines containing measles virus in dogs older than 16 weeks of age. There are no known public health dangers associated with the use of measles virus–containing vaccines. Measles virus vaccine does not provide protection against infectious canine hepatitis.

Methods of overcoming the effects of colostral (maternal) antibodies are not absolute. Therefore, research is continuing in this area. Although colostral antibodies interfere with the immunization process, colostrum is extremely important for the protection of the neonate against a number of potentially harmful microorganisms. Therefore, pups and kittens should never be deliberately deprived of colostrum.

Type of Vaccine

The type of vaccine is very important in formulating a successful vaccination program. Viral vaccines can be either *inactivated* or *modified live* virus vaccines. Since live virus vaccines depend on viral replication in the recipient animal to provide protection, the vaccine must be handled strictly according to the instructions supplied by the manufacturer. Inactivated vaccines are less labile; however, in general they must be administered several times to get an adequate protective response. It is impossible to state that one type of vaccine is categorically better than another; therefore, in the future, both inactivated and modified live virus types of vaccine will continue to be used.

In order to achieve the optimal response, the entire dose of vaccine should be given as recommended; thus the dose should not be split and given to more than one animal. Different vaccine products should not be mixed in the same syringe prior to administration. Frequently, vaccines contain preservatives that will interfere with another vaccine.

Route of Administration

The route of administration specified in the manufacturer's instructions should be followed. With certain viruses, significant differences in response occur, depending on the route of administration. For example, with measles virus and some rabies virus vaccines, the intramuscular route is much more effective than the subcutaneous route. Therefore, the manufacturer's recommendations must be understood and followed for all vaccines.

With certain viruses—for example, feline viral rhinotracheitis, calicivirus, and feline infectious peritonitis—vaccines that produce local immunity have been developed. These vaccines are given by the intranasal and intraocular routes. An example of a bacterial disease for which an intranasal vaccine has been developed is *Bordetella bronchiseptica.* The basis for this approach is the concept that if the vaccine is administered by the same route that natural infection takes, greater protection will be achieved. Unfortunately, these vaccines can produce mild clinical disease.

Age of Patient

Age of the animal is important, not only because of the persistence of colostral antibodies, but also because of the relative immaturity of the immune response in the puppy and kitten during the first 2 weeks of life. This phenomenon is at least partially due to the hypothermia that exists during this period. Optimal functioning of the cells of the immune system depends on a normal body temperature.

Orphaned pups should not be vaccinated during the first 2 weeks of life. Instead of being vaccinated, pups and kittens should be given *immune serum,* either by parenteral injection or by mouth. The immune serum can be mixed with artificial milk replacer.

Age of vaccination is also important in older patients. It has been shown that certain older dogs (greater than 7 years of age) do not respond as well to vaccination as do younger animals. Consequently, annual revaccination is particularly important in these patients to ensure adequate protection.

Nutritional Status

An animal in poor nutritional condition may not respond adequately to vaccination. Generally, caution should be exercised in giving modified live virus vaccines to debilitated animals. However, a debilitated animal should be vaccinated if it is to be hospitalized. Although there is a chance the animal may not respond to the vaccination, it is also possible that the animal will be protected from infection with a virulent organism. If a debilitated dog or cat is vaccinated, vaccination should be repeated when the patient's nutritional status has improved so that immunity is more certain. Every veterinary hospital should establish a specific vaccination policy and protocol and adhere to it at all times. This will prevent errors of omission that could result if the vaccination policy is not clearly defined.

Concurrent Disease or Therapy

Occasionally, dogs and cats presented for vaccination are incubating an infectious disease. A detailed history of possible exposure to infected animals as well as a complete physical examination may suggest this situation. However, it is impossible to definitively diagnose most infections in the incubation stage. Therefore, if there is a history of exposure to an infected animal, the owner should be informed that there is a risk of their animal's developing disease despite vaccination.

Certain infections and diseases may be associated with alteration of the immune system and may interfere with successful response to vaccination. Examples include dogs infected with demodectic mange and cats infected with feline leukemia virus or feline immunodeficiency virus.

Furthermore, it has been suggested that certain virus vaccines may increase the susceptibility of the recipient animal to other agents or may alter the natural history of infection with other agents. These interactions have been proposed for canine distemper virus vaccine and canine parvovirus as well as canine adenovirus type 1 (CAV-1) vaccine and the canine distemper virus.

Modified live virus vaccines are not recommended in dogs and cats receiving immunosuppressive agents. Drugs that suppress the immune system are frequently given to animals with cancer or autoimmune diseases, such as immune-mediated hemolytic anemia. Commonly used immunosuppressive agents include cyclophosphamide, azathioprine, methotrexate and corticosteroids. When corticosteroids are used at anti-inflammatory dose levels (less than 2 mg per kg body weight), the response to virus vaccines is not altered. Other drugs that are not used exclusively as immunosuppressive agents (i.e., levamisole) may also alter the response to vaccination.

Program Guidelines

When all of the clinical factors discussed are considered, along with economic factors, it is safe to conclude that there is no single perfect vaccination program. Nonetheless, certain general guidelines are possible. Usually, the first vaccination should be administered when the animal is between 6 and 8 weeks of age. Animals should be revaccinated at 10, 12, and 16 to 18 weeks of age. Revaccination should occur annually for the entire life of the animal. Although annual revaccination is probably unnecessary for certain viral diseases, for others it is of critical importance.

Geriatric Nursing

With improved veterinary care, pets are enjoying an increased life span; consequently, the number of geriatric patients seen in small-animal practices is increasing. The geriatric patient can be presented with a number of problems that directly influence the nursing process. These problems are generally related to or are secondary to degenerative diseases and other geriatric changes, such as arthritis, deafness and blindness.

Dogs with arthritis or other degenerative diseases of the musculoskeletal system may be suffering from chronic pain. Therefore, these animals are likely to react aggressively when an affected body part is touched or manipulated. Dogs suffering from central nervous system disorders (such as a brain tumor or cerebral infarction) may also display aggressive behavior.

Deafness is another disorder that frequently accompanies old age. It is easy to surprise or startle a deaf, older dog, and certain dogs will instinctively respond by biting. Therefore, when approaching a deaf dog, it is important that the patient be able to see you before you attempt to handle it or perform a procedure.

Blindness can occur in older dogs from cataracts, retinal degeneration, glaucoma and other diseases. As is the case with deaf dogs, blind dogs should be approached cautiously. It is best to move slowly and speak as you approach the dog. Generally, elderly dogs and cats show less response to external stimuli. They appear to be less interested in their surroundings and frequently remain inactive for prolonged periods. In fact, they tend to resent any interference and react aggressively when disturbed. Some dogs forget previous training and may fail to respond to basic commands. Finally, the geriatric dog or cat is resistant to changes in daily routine. The stress of hospitalization alone can sometimes cause rapid deterioration. Obviously, it is impossible to correct or reverse many of the changes associated with aging; however, a willingness to provide gentle, compassionate nursing care is of paramount importance.

Pediatric Nursing

The clinical situation that best illustrates the skills required in pediatric nursing is the hand-rearing of orphaned puppies or kittens. The first step is to determine the caloric requirements of the puppy or kitten. During the first week of life, these requirements are approximately 27 calories per kg per day; 32 to 36 calories per kg per day during the second week; 36 to 41 calories per kg per day during the third week; and 41 to 45 calories per kg per day during the fourth week. A number of artificial milk replacers (Esbilac, Borden; Unilac, Upjohn) are available for use in puppies. These products provide approximately 30 to 40 calories per approximately 29.5 ml. KMR (Borden) is an artificial replacement for queen's milk (see Table 10–1 for formula dosage). The following formula can be used as a short-term emergency supplement in puppies: 8 ounces of cow's milk mixed with 2 egg yolks and 1 teaspoon of corn oil. For an emergency formula in kittens, 4 ounces of cow's milk can be mixed with 2 egg yolks and 1 drop of multivitamins. Once the total daily requirement has been calculated, this amount can be divided into four equal feedings. Frequent feedings are necessary to prevent over-distention of the stomach and subsequent emesis and aspiration pneumonia. Generally, it is faster and easier to use gavage via an orogastric tube than to bottlefeed.

The technique for gavage is to use a soft rubber feeding tube (French sizes Nos. 8–16). The tube is marked with a marking pen or tape at a point equal to the distance between the tip of the nose and the eighth rib. The tube is advanced into the pharynx and down the esophagus to the level of the midthorax. A syringe can be used to inject the artificial milk replacer slowly. The stomach capacity of puppies and kittens can be calculated at 9 ml per kg of body weight, and this amount should not be exceeded in a single feeding.

If the puppies or kittens are vigorous nursers, an alternative technique would be to use Pet Nursettes (Borden) or human premature baby bottle nipples. This technique is slower but may satisfy the pups and kittens more, so that the incidence of littermate nursing on each other will be reduced.

The neonatal puppy is essentially poikilothermic (body temperature varies with ambient temperature). Therefore, it is imperative that the ambient temperature of the whelping box be maintained between 30°C and 33°C. If hypothermia occurs, it will reduce feeding by the neonate and may enhance the pathogenicity of certain viruses, such as canine herpes. In order to detect hypothermia in neonates, it is desirable to use a low-reading clinical rectal thermometer.

Table 10–1
ORPHAN FORMULA DOSAGE FOR PUPPIES AND KITTENS

Age (weeks)	Dosage* (ml/100 g body weight/day)
1	13
2	17
3†	20
4	22

*Divide and feed four times daily.
†Begin to feed solid food.

Ideally, puppies and kittens should nurse during the first 24 hours of life to ensure maximal transfer of protective immunoglobulins. If the neonate has not nursed, it is recommended that between 1 and 5 ml of serum be obtained from the dam and either injected subcutaneously or mixed with milk replacer and administered orally.

A highly effective monitoring technique during the neonatal period is to weigh the neonates frequently. Puppies should gain approximately 10 to 20 percent of their birth weight daily for the first week of life. Postage or food scales should be used to weigh each animal two or three times daily, especially during the first 2 weeks of life. Weight loss or failure to gain weight each day may be the first sign of illness.

PRACTICAL NURSING PROCEDURES

In many veterinary practices, it is the responsibility of the veterinary technician to monitor the patient's vital signs (i.e., temperature, pulse and respirations).

Temperature

One routine method for determining the body temperature of a small animal is to use a standard mercury-in-glass clinical rectal thermometer. Veterinary thermometers differ from those used in humans in that the storage reservoir for the mercury is short and spherical rather than elongated. Human thermometers can be used in dogs and cats without difficulty. Thermometers can be calibrated in Fahrenheit or Celsius degrees. A Fahrenheit reading can be converted to Celsius by using the formula degrees C = degrees F − 32 × ⁵⁄₉.

When taking the patient's temperature, one should first shake the thermometer so that the mercury is below the constriction in the glass tube. The thermometer is well lubricated with petrolatum, mineral oil or a mild soap and is inserted into the rectum with a gentle twisting motion. The thermometer is advanced into the rectum beyond the bulb and is held in place for the minimum period of time stated on the thermometer. The patient is restrained in order to prevent the thermometer from being broken. The thermometer is withdrawn, and the bulb and stem are wiped clean with an alcohol-soaked cotton swab. The thermometer is held horizontally and rotated until the magnified scale is clearly visible. Because of the constriction in the glass tube, the level of the mercury does not fall until it is shaken down. Finally, the thermometer should be stored in an antiseptic solution (e.g., benzalkonium chloride). Hot water should not be used for cleaning thermometers.

Certain diseases that produce fever display a diurnal pattern (i.e., the temperature fluctuates) during the day. If the patient's temperature is taken just once per day, the periods of fever may not be recognized. If this situation is suspected, a temperature chart may be kept by taking and recording the temperature at regular intervals, for example, every 4 hours.

The normal rectal temperature in the dog is 38.9°C. The normal rectal temperature in the cat is 38.6°C. Excitement or activity can elevate the temperature above these limits. In rare clinical situations (i.e., rectal laceration or rectal prolapse), it may not be possible to measure the rectal temperature. In these situations, the temperature may be taken in either the

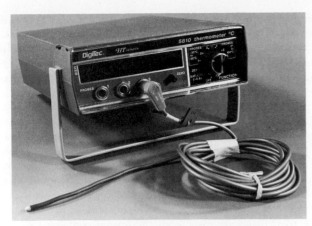

FIGURE 10–3. Digital electronic thermometer.

axilla or the external ear canal. The temperature recorded in these sites will be significantly lower than the simultaneous rectal temperature. In general, 2°C can be added to an axillary or ear canal temperature to approximate rectal temperature. These alternative techniques for determining the body temperature are useful when the same site is used serially in an individual patient, and the results are compared. The temperature is taken by placing the bulb of the thermometer deep in the axilla or ear canal for several minutes.

Recently, electronic thermometers and thermocouples have come into widespread clinical use (Fig. 10–3). These devices allow continual monitoring of the body temperature in critically ill animals. An infrared thermometer has been developed that records accurate body core temperatures by focusing the infrared beam upon the tympanic membrane. This thermometer is helpful in those patients with very low rectal temperatures or in those for which taking a rectal temperature is contraindicated (Exergen Veterinary Infrared Tympanic Temperature Scanner, Newton, MA).

Pulse

The rate and character of the pulse are valuable means of assessing the cardiovascular status of the patient. The pulse can be palpated in any artery located close to the body surface. The pulse is most commonly felt in the femoral artery. The femoral artery is usually palpated on the medial aspect of the thigh, proximal to the stifle. Palpation of the femoral pulse requires practice and can be difficult in a trembling patient or in a patient with short, heavily muscled legs. Alternate sites for taking the pulse are the palmar aspect of the carpus and the ventral aspect of the base of the tail. The *normal pulse rate* in adult dogs is 60 to 160 beats per minute, up to 180 beats per minute in toy breeds and 220 beats per minute for puppies. The maximum rate in cats is 240 beats per minute.

The heart rate can be counted by palpation or auscultation at the point of maximal intensity of the heart beat. The point of maximal intensity is located at the sternal border between the left fourth and sixth intercostal spaces. If the pulse rate is taken at the same time as the heart rate and the pulse rate is less, it is called a *pulse deficit*. A pulse deficit generally indicates a cardiac dysrhythmia.

The dog can have heart and pulse rates that are "regularly irregular." Characteristically, the heart and pulse rates in-

crease with inspiration and decrease with expiration. This normal variation is called *sinus arrhythmia*.

In addition to taking the pulse rate, it is also beneficial to evaluate the pulse pressure and character of the pulse. Decreased pulse pressure may indicate systemic hypotension (drop in blood pressure) secondary to a process such as hypovolemic shock. Instrumentation for the non-invasive measurement of blood pressure in the dog and cat that is very accurate has been developed (Dinamap 8300, Critikon, Tampa, FL) (Fig. 10–4).

Respiration

The respiratory rate should be counted when the animal is at rest but not sleeping. Respiration involves both an inspiratory and expiratory phase. When counting the respiratory rate, it is necessary to count either inspirations or expirations, but not both. The normal rate in the dog is between 15 and 30 breaths per minute. Smaller breeds tend to have a more rapid rate of respiration than larger breeds. The rate in cats is between 20 and 30 breaths per minute. In addition to determining the rate, it is important to characterize the respiratory status of the patient by inspection.

Several terms are used to describe respiratory function. *Tachypnea* refers to very rapid breathing. *Hyperpnea* indicates a condition in which the respiration is deeper and more rapid than normal. *Depth of respiration* indicates the volume of air inspired with each breath. Increased depth of respiration indicates a greater demand for oxygen. Shallow respiration can be due to either metabolic derangement (e.g., acidosis) or mechanical injuries (e.g., fractured ribs). *Dyspnea* is a term used to indicate the subjective impression of increased difficulty or distress in breathing.

All hospitalized patients should have their vital signs monitored at least once per day. Depending on the underlying problem and the status of the patient, it may be necessary to monitor the patient more frequently. The temperature, pulse

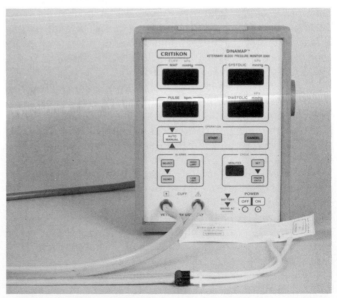

FIGURE 10–4. Dinamap 8300 (Critikon, Tampa, FL), instrument for noninvasive measurement of blood pressure.

and respiration rate should be recorded in the medical record every time they are taken. This will facilitate recognition of abnormalities as early as possible. Furthermore, serial observations will permit recognition of clinical trends.

Administration of Medications

It is important for the animal health technician to be familiar with several basic principles of clinical pharmacology. These principles are important when considering the route of administration of various drugs. Drugs can be administered parenterally (e.g., by injection), orally or topically. The parenteral techniques routinely used in veterinary medicine include the intravenous, intramuscular and subcutaneous routes. The specific techniques used to administer drugs by these various routes are discussed in Chapter 8. This discussion will be concerned with the selection of an appropriate route in various clinical situations.

In choosing the route of administration, a variety of factors must be considered. First, the pharmacological properties of the drug should be considered. Certain drugs are not adequately absorbed when given by a certain route (e.g., gentamicin is poorly absorbed from the gastrointestinal tract). Similarly, insulin must be given by injection because it is destroyed in the gastrointestinal tract. Other drugs cannot be given by a certain route because they produce severe tissue reactions (e.g., thiamylal sodium causes sloughing of the skin if it is given subcutaneously). Another pharmacological factor to consider is the rate of absorption. If an animal is critically ill, the route of administration that will provide the earliest onset of action is preferred. For example, an animal with a severe, overwhelming infection should receive an antibiotic intravenously rather than orally.

It is also important to consider the patient when considering the route of administration. For example, it is generally unadvisable to administer oral medications to a vomiting patient or to an animal with severe respiratory embarrassment. The temperament of the patient should also be considered. In a fractious animal, it may be impossible to administer drugs topically, orally or intravenously. Subcutaneous or intramuscular injections may be the only feasible routes of administration. Finally, convenience and compliance of the client will influence therapeutic decision. Obviously, the topical and oral routes are preferred for treatment at home.

The principal advantages of the oral route are convenience and reduced risk of infection or abscess caused by faulty injection technique. Disadvantages of the oral route include the potential for inhalation of liquid medications and the potential for animals to spit out the medication so that the prescribed dose is not absorbed.

Advantages of parenteral injections include, in general, more rapid absorption and greater assurance that the prescribed dose is accurately delivered.

The major advantage to topical medication is that systemic effects are reduced and safety is thus increased. The major disadvantage is that most systemic illnesses do not respond to topical medication alone.

Whenever any drug is administered, it is essential to record the treatment (drug, dose, time) and route of administration completely and accurately in the medical record. The notation should be made immediately after administering the medication. If this procedure is consistently followed, patient care will improve, because it is less likely that treatments will be omitted or inadvertently repeated. In addition to improving the level of patient care, it should also be remembered that this policy is important because the medical record is a legal document, and every treatment should be recorded in case of subsequent litigation.

It is also of utmost importance that all medications, either those used in the hospital or those dispensed for use at home, be labeled correctly. The dispensing label information should include the complete name of the drug, the size or concentration of the drug, the number of tablets or capsules or milliliters of drug dispensed, the dose and frequency of administration, the name of the client and the name of the hospital. If potentially toxic drugs are dispensed, child-proof containers should be used, as determined by state and federal regulations.

Fluid Therapy

The veterinary technician generally will not be called upon to formulate a fluid order in a hospitalized patient without supervision of the attending veterinarian. However, familiarity with certain fundamental points will allow the technician to participate actively in this essential process.

The total volume of fluid required to treat an animal can be approximated by considering the volume of fluid needed to rehydrate the patient, the volume of fluid needed for maintenance requirements and the volume of fluid needed to correct ongoing losses:

1. Dehydration deficit—estimate as percentage from chart found in Table 10–2
2. Maintenance requirement—60 ml per kg body weight per day
3. Contemporary (ongoing losses)—estimated volume lost in diarrhea or vomitus in milliliters

Sensible losses are roughly equivalent to urine output. *Insensible losses* represent the fluid lost in the feces and during respiration. *Contemporary losses* are due to ongoing problems (i.e., vomiting and diarrhea).

The hydration status, and thus the rehydration requirement, can be assessed by the following physical examination criteria: skin turgor, dryness of the mucous membranes, capillary refill time and the degree of sinkage of the eyes into the bony orbit. Several laboratory criteria are beneficial, particularly if they are followed serially. These criteria include the hematocrit, the

Table 10–2 DIAGNOSIS OF DEHYDRATION—PHYSICAL EXAMINATION FINDINGS	
Percent Dehydration	**Clinical Signs**
<5%	Undetectable
5%–6%	Skin slightly doughy, inelastic consistency
6%–8%	Skin definitely inelastic, eyes very slightly sunken in orbits
10%–12%	Increased skin turgor, eyes sunken in orbits, prolonged refill time, dry mucous membranes
12%–15%	Shock and imminent death

total protein determination and urine specific gravity (SG). Finally, serial body weights can be valuable in determining changes in hydration status. One pound of body weight is equivalent to one pint or 480 ml of fluid.

By using the physical examination findings mentioned, the degree of dehydration is estimated as a percentage of body weight (Table 10–2). Thus, an animal that shows only a slight alteration in skin turgor is approximately 5 to 6 percent dehydrated. Skin turgor is evaluated by pinching a fold of the skin and subjectively assessing the rate at which it returns to its normal position. An animal that is 10 to 12 percent dehydrated will display pronounced changes in skin turgor; dry, tacky mucous membranes; prolonged capillary refill time and eyes that are sunken into the orbits. The physical alterations associated with dehydration are a continuum so that an animal that is 8 percent dehydrated should have abnormalities midway between the end points described. It should be stressed that physical examination findings are at best very crude indicators of the degree of dehydration. The quantitative value of these parameters is improved if they are carefully and critically assessed over time.

The laboratory criteria used to assess the degree of dehydration evaluate the extent of hemoconcentration. Thus, the higher the hematocrit and the total protein determination, the more hemoconcentrated and thus dehydrated the patient. These laboratory tests are useful in detecting relative changes and do not necessarily measure the absolute hydration status of the patient. If the concentrating ability of the kidneys is normal, a urine SG greater than 1.035 in the dog and 1.040 in the cat provides further evidence that the patient may be dehydrated.

Since changes in body weight over short periods are caused by changes in fluid balance rather than by the loss or gain of body mass, an accurate daily weight can also be helpful in assessing changes in the hydration status of the patient.

The most reliable means of establishing the degree of dehydration is to make a collective judgment based on as many of the criteria mentioned as possible.

Once the degree of dehydration has been estimated, it can be used in calculating the volume of fluids needed to rehydrate the patient. The percent dehydration is multiplied by the body weight in kilograms and then by 1000. This is the number of milliliters needed to rehydrate the patient.

Generally, the volume required to rehydrate the animal is not replaced immediately. One procedure is to administer approximately 80 percent of this volume over the first 24 hours and the remaining 20 percent over the next 24 hours. In addition to the volume required for rehydration, the maintenance requirement must also be incorporated in the calculation of the daily fluid order. The maintenance requirement consists of estimates of both sensible and insensible losses.

As already mentioned, sensible losses refer to the urine output. Insensible losses represent the fluid lost from the body via the gastrointestinal and respiratory tracts. Although sensible and insensible losses will vary somewhat depending on the clinical setting, a useful clinical approximation is 60 ml per kg per day. If the animal is not taking any liquids by mouth, a volume equivalent to the sensible and insensible losses (e.g., the maintenance requirement) should be included in the daily fluid order.

Most animals with problems requiring fluid therapy do not resolve these problems immediately upon initiation of fluid therapy. Therefore, contemporary or ongoing losses must also be considered in determining the daily fluid order. For example, if a patient has gastroenteritis, the volume of fluid lost with each episode of vomiting and diarrhea should be estimated and added to the rehydration and maintenance volumes. The volume of diarrhea and vomitus is frequently underestimated; therefore, it has been recommended that the visual estimate be *doubled* to more accurately reflect the actual volume lost.

Routes of Fluid Administration

Oral fluid administration is the preferred method because of reduced expense, ease of administration and safety. Contraindications to oral fluid administration include vomiting and severe, life-threatening fluid imbalances that require immediate correction.

Many conditions respond well to subcutaneous administration of fluids. Fluids given subcutaneously should be warmed to body temperature and must be isotonic with extracellular fluid. Isotonic fluids have an osmotic pressure approximately equal to that of extracellular fluid. Never give dextrose solutions with a concentration greater than 2.5 percent subcutaneously; sloughing of skin and abscess formation are common sequelae. The volume and rate of subcutaneous fluids that can be given will vary from patient to patient. A rough guideline for total daily volume is approximately 60 ml per kg. Absorption of subcutaneous fluids will occur over 6 to 8 hours; therefore, this total daily dose can be divided and given every 6 to 8 hours. It is necessary and desirable to administer this divided dose in as many sites as possible. Subcutaneous fluid administration is safe and easy; however, it is not the recommended route of administration when prompt correction of severe deficits is required.

The intraperitoneal route of fluid administration is not recommended. Peritonitis and intra-abdominal abscess formation may result from this form of fluid therapy. The rate of absorption of intraperitoneal fluids is roughly equivalent to the rate of absorption of subcutaneous fluids.

Signs of volume overload include restlessness, hyperpnea (increased respiratory rate), serous (watery) nasal discharge, chemosis (edema of the ocular conjunctiva) and pitting edema. Volume overload can be due to either an excessive total volume or an excessive rate of fluid administration. Decreased cardiac function or decreased plasma protein can predispose to a volume overload state. If volume overload is suspected, the lungs should be auscultated for evidence of pulmonary edema, and the central venous pressure should be determined. Prior to the development of pulmonary edema or elevated central venous pressure, weight gain may be seen. Therefore, it is advisable to weigh the animal three times daily while intravenous fluid therapy is being used, especially in those patients who are less able to handle a fluid load (such as patients with cardiac or renal disease).

Fluid therapy is a dynamic process that must be reassessed at frequent intervals and adjusted in order to obtain the maximum results. The technician's role in clinically assessing the patient is important in making appropriate adjustments.

Central Venous Pressure

The measurement of central venous pressure is a useful aid in evaluating the fluid status of a patient. When used and interpreted properly, it can substantially reduce the likelihood of excessive fluid administration. Measurement of the central venous pressure is a simple technique that can be performed in all veterinary practices.

In order to measure the central venous pressure, an indwelling intravenous catheter is placed in the cranial vena cava via the external jugular vein. It is very important that the catheter tip be located in the cranial vena cava at the level of the right atrium. If the intravenous catheter is properly placed, a 2- to 5-mm fluctuation in central venous pressure will be noted with each respiration.

Next, a sterile three-way stopcock is attached to the intravenous catheter. The open line of the three-way stopcock is connected to the intravenous fluid source. The intravenous fluids are used to prime the manometer, that is, the manometer is filled to overflowing with the intravenous fluids. With the patient in lateral recumbency, the zero point of the manometer is positioned at the level of the sternum (Fig. 10–5). The central venous pressure is equal to the level of intravenous fluid in the manometer once equilibrium has been established. In order to improve accuracy, this determination should be repeated a total of three times. If the pressure is high, prevent blood from entering the manometer, since a blood clot may alter the measurements.

The following points are important considerations when measuring and interpreting central venous pressure measurements: Serial measurements should be performed with the same zero point and the patient in the same position. If the catheter is obstructed because of blood clots or kinking, the central venous pressure will be falsely elevated. Obstruction

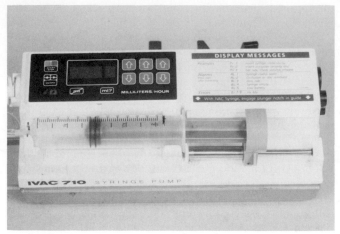

FIGURE 10–6. IVAC 710 Syringe Pump (IVAC, San Diego, CA), fluid pump used for the administration of small volumes and slow rates of fluid to the cat and small dog.

should be suspected if the level of the manometer does not fluctuate with respiration. Since continuous recording is not possible, pressure measurements are made intermittently. If intravenous fluids are not being administered between central venous pressure measurements, the catheter should be flushed with heparinized saline. Heparinized saline is prepared by adding 5 U of heparin per ml of saline. When evaluating the central venous pressure, it is better to evaluate trends rather than single measurements. Usually, changes of less than 3 cm of water are not significant. Using the sternum as the zero point, normal central venous pressure in the dog and cat varies between 0 and 5 cm of intravenous fluid. If the central venous pressure is consistently greater than 8 to 10 cm of intravenous fluid, volume overload is suspected and fluid administration should be slowed or stopped.

The chance of inadvertent fluid overload can be reduced by using indwelling intravenous catheters and administering fluids over prolonged periods of time rather than using rapid bolus techniques. In addition, Minidrip (Travenol Laboratories, Inc.) and Buretrol (Travenol Laboratories, Inc.) administration sets can be used in cats and small dogs. Also, syringe pumps are useful in administering fluids to cats and very small dogs (IVAC 710 Syringe Pump, San Diego, CA) (Fig. 10–6).

Several basic types of fluid are routinely used in small animal practice. They include physiologic (0.9 percent) saline, 5 percent dextrose in water and extracellular fluid replacement solutions such as lactated Ringer's solution or Ringer's solution. Combinations of these basic fluid types are also used. These basic parenteral fluid types can be supplemented with concentrated solutions of electrolytes and dextrose to produce the desired fluid composition appropriate for the specific clinical situation (Table 10–3).

Frequently, antimicrobials are added to intravenous fluids for administration. A number of the commonly used antimicrobials are incompatible with certain fluids (Table 10–4). The physical incompatibilities include things such as precipitation of the drug out of solution and chemical inactivation. In addition to these incompatibilities, it has been noted that when certain drugs are mixed in infusion solutions, inactivation occurs. For example, when carbenicillin is added to a solution containing gentamicin, the gentamicin is inactivated. As a gen-

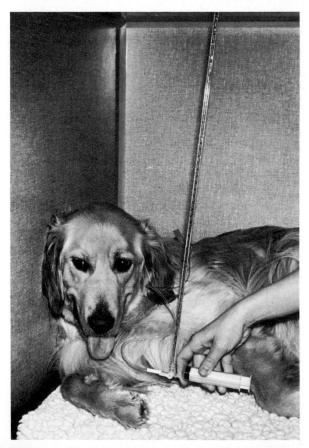

FIGURE 10–5. Use of a manometer to measure central venous pressure in a dog.

Table 10–3
BASIC FLUIDS

Fluid Type	Fluid Composition per Liter					
	NA^+	CL^-	K^+	CA^{++}	LACTATE	KCAL
Lactated Ringer's solution	130	109	4	3	28	9
Ringer's solution	147	156	4	5	0	0
0.9% saline	154	154	0	0	0	0
2.5% dextrose in ½ normal saline	77	77	0	0	0	85
5% dextrose in lactated Ringer's solution	130	109	4	3	28	179
5% dextrose in water	0	0	0	0	0	179

eral rule, it is undesirable to mix multiple drugs either in a syringe or in intravenous fluids. Frequently, the interaction is visible upon mixing, but other times it will not be observed prior to administration.

Blood Transfusion

Blood transfusion is an effective fluid replacement but a potentially hazardous form of treatment. Therefore, clear indications for its use must be present. The effectiveness of transfusion is temporary. Consequently, every effort must be made to identify and correct underlying problems.

Severe blood loss is an indication for transfusion therapy. Massive hemorrhage can occur following trauma or surgery. Measurement of the packed cell volume (PCV) can be misleading immediately following acute blood loss, because of compensatory vasoconstriction and splenic contraction. The PCV may remain normal for as long as 6 hours after an acute bleeding episode, but the total protein will decrease soon after the bleeding episode and therefore it can be used as an early indicator of blood loss. As the intravascular volume is restored by the redistribution of body fluids, the PCV will drop. Collectively, the following clinical parameters are better indicators of acute hemorrhage than the PCV: total protein, pulse pressure, depth and rate of respiration, mucous membrane color, capillary refill time, urine production, central venous pressure and arterial blood gases.

In the treatment of chronic anemia, blood is used primarily for its oxygen-carrying capabilities and should not be considered definitive therapy. The decision to transfuse should be based on clinical signs (e.g., respiratory distress and weakness) rather than an arbitrarily determined PCV or hemoglobin concentration. Some animals with chronic anemia have been shown to be able to increase oxygen delivery at the tissue level by means of biochemical changes within the red cells. Thus, one dog with a PCV of 12 may be well compensated, whereas another with the same PCV will be severely compromised and will require a transfusion.

Transfusions are indicated to stop or prevent bleeding resulting from decreased number of platelets or abnormal platelet function. Large quantities of blood are needed to significantly raise the platelet count; therefore platelet-rich plasma is the preferred method to replace platelets. Since platelets survive for less than 12 hours in stored blood, freshly drawn blood should be used. Transfusion therapy is also useful in the treatment of hereditary or acquired bleeding disorders, for example, hemophilia or disseminated intravascular coagulation (DIC). As with platelets, some coagulation factors are labile, so transfused blood should be less than 12 hours old. The basis for this use is to provide adequate concentrations of the deficient coagulation factor at the bleeding site.

Transfusion of blood is indicated in autoimmune hemolytic anemia only in life-threatening situations. Transfusion of a patient with autoimmune hemolytic anemia can initiate or accelerate a hemolytic crisis and increase production of antibodies directed against red blood cells (RBCs). Therefore, if transfusion is necessary as a lifesaving measure, only the absolute minimum number of RBCs should be administered. An initial replacement volume of not more than 12 ml/kg body weight would be acceptable in this situation.

Transfusions to correct leukopenia (low white blood cell [WBC] count) or hypoproteinemia (low serum protein) are of equivocal long-term benefit.

There are eight canine blood groups. Blood groups are designated by the presence of specific *canine erythrocyte antigens* (e.g., CEA-1, CEA-2, CEA-3, and so forth). Any of these erythrocyte antigens can stimulate antibody production if it is transfused into a recipient that is negative for that particular antigen. CEA-1 is the most powerful stimulus for such antibody production. Reactions to CEA-2 are less pronounced; however, they can still be of clinical significance. Reactions to the other canine erythrocyte antigens are generally clinically insignificant. Antibodies directed against CEA-1 and CEA-2 do not occur naturally; consequently, clinically significant adverse reactions do not occur on initial transfusion.

Since 60 percent of dogs have either CEA-1 or CEA-2 antigens, transfusion with blood from a random donor (i.e., untyped donor) has a 24 percent chance of stimulating CEA-1 or CEA-2 antibody production. On subsequent repeated random transfusions, the incidence of transfusion reactions is about 15 percent. Besides the possibility of transfusion reactions, other problems associated with the transfusion of untyped blood include decreased survival of transfused cells in the recipient and hemolytic disease of newborn pups born to dams sensitized by transfusion.

Unfortunately, blood typing sera are not readily available. Therefore, in many veterinary practices it is necessary to use

Table 10–4
PHYSICAL INCOMPATIBILITIES OF ANTIMICROBIALS IN INTRAVENOUS SOLUTIONS

Antimicrobial	Incompatible With
Amphotericin B	Normal saline
Cephalothin sodium	Lactated Ringer's solution, calcium gluconate, calcium chloride
Chloramphenicol sodium succinate	Vitamin B complex with vitamin C
Chlortetracycline hydrochloride, oxytetracycline hydrochloride, tetracycline hydrochloride	Lactated Ringer's solution, sodium bicarbonate, and calcium chloride
Penicillins	Dextrose-containing solutions with pH greater than 8 (i.e., added sodium bicarbonate)
Penicillin G potassium	Vitamin B complex with vitamin C

and apply to the affected part. As the temperature of the towel decreases, the towel can be rinsed with hot water and reapplied. Twenty minutes is an adequate period of time for this form of heat treatment.

In most traumatic injuries, *early* application of cold will reduce swelling and muscle spasm. Towels or cloths soaked in either cold water or ice water and wrung lightly are a means of applying cold to an animal patient. Alternatively, commercial cold packs or ice packs can be used; however, they should be used with caution in order to prevent cold-induced injury. Fifteen to 20 minutes are usually required for treatment.

If peripheral edema is present, massage may be beneficial. The technique for therapeutic massage consists of gentle stroking and light kneading of the involved area. An attempt should be made to direct the peripheral edema from the involved area toward the heart. This will enhance venous return of the edematous fluid.

Active movement should be encouraged as soon as it can be accomplished safely and without pain. Active movement can be accomplished by swimming the patient in a whirlpool or bathtub. Most animals will swim with encouragement and then actively exercise a body part that otherwise would not be exercised. A towel or sling can be used for support and to keep the animal upright. When appropriate, therapeutic exercise can occur on any nonslippery surface. If the patient is not able to ambulate without assistance, a towel or sling can provide the necessary support. Active therapeutic exercise is of greater benefit than passive exercise.

Although not widely used in veterinary practice, electrical stimulation is beneficial in the treatment of some neuromuscular diseases and neurogenic atrophy.

Owners of animals that would benefit from physical therapy are usually willing to perform physical therapy at home. However, the owner must be carefully instructed on how to perform the treatments and why it will be beneficial to the patient. The technician is usually the best person in the practice to demonstrate the proper technique.

Oxygen Therapy

The primary indication for oxygen therapy is *hypoxia,* which refers to a deficiency of oxygen at the tissue level. Tissue hypoxia may be due to a reduction in perfusion (reduced blood flow) or a reduction in oxygen content of the blood. Hypoxia is probably more common than is recognized in veterinary medicine, since a caged animal at rest will not show signs until the oxygen content of the blood is severely reduced.

Hypoxia can be manifested in a variety of ways, and the veterinary technician must be alert to identify these changes. Abnormalities that may be noted in the cardiovascular system include tachycardia or dysrhythmias. An increased respiratory rate, open-mouthed breathing and dyspnea may also be noted. *Dyspnea* is the term used to indicate subjective difficulty or distress in breathing. With severe hypoxia, central nervous system changes may be noted and include drowsiness, altered motor abilities or increased excitability. Finally, cold extremities may indicate an inadequate supply of oxygen at the tissue level. *Cyanosis* is not a reliable indicator of hypoxia, especially if the animal is anemic. Cyanosis refers to dark bluish or purplish discoloration of the skin and mucous membranes.

Although the basic defect in hypoxia is decreased oxygen availability at the tissue level, it can occur by a variety of mechanisms. For example, it can result from lung disease, decreased cardiac output or severe anemia.

In small-animal practice, oxygen therapy is used primarily in the following clinical situations: pulmonary edema, severe bronchopneumonia, upper airway disease in brachycephalic breeds such as English Bulldog and Boston terrier, pulmonary trauma, atelectasis of lung lobes and shock.

Methods of oxygen therapy include oxygen cages, human pediatric incubators, masks, nasal catheters, endotracheal tubes and intratracheal catheters.

Oxygen Cage

Oxygen cages for veterinary use are sold commercially. These cages permit control of not only the oxygen concentration but also temperature and humidity (Fig. 10–8). These cages are useful in animals able to ventilate without assistance. However, they are expensive and consume large amounts of oxygen. Surplus human pediatric incubators are a less expensive means of providing similar therapy to small dogs, cats or exotic animal patients. Oxygen cages and incubators should be flushed (filled) with oxygen after they have been opened.

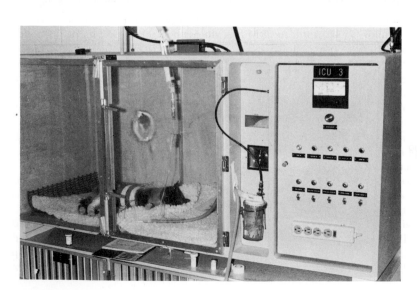

FIGURE 10–8. Small animal oxygen cage.

Some units are equipped with entry ports that allow access to the patient without excessive loss of oxygen.

Mask Induction

In certain circumstances, masks can be used to administer oxygen. Masks are available in a variety of sizes and shapes suitable for use in dogs and cats. If an oxygen mask is used, it is important to provide a high oxygen flow rate in order to prevent excessive accumulation of carbon dioxide. Administration of oxygen via a mask is suitable for short periods of time only and only in selected patients. Some patients will resist the use of an oxygen mask, and the resultant stress will negate any beneficial effect of the oxygen.

Intratracheal Catheter Induction

An alternative means of oxygen administration that is both inexpensive and effective is the intratracheal catheter. This technique is reserved for critically ill patients. The skin is aseptically prepared, and a local anesthetic is administered over the trachea in the midcervical area. An intravenous catheter (14-, 16-, or 18-gauge) is introduced into the trachea and is advanced to a point craniad to the bifurcation of the trachea. The delivered oxygen should be humidified and administered at a flow rate of between 0.5 liter and 4 liters per minute. The flow rate should be adjusted, depending on the size of the animal.

Nasal Catheter Induction

Nasal catheters can also be used to administer oxygen for brief periods to severely depressed animals. In this technique, a small (5 to 8 French) soft rubber feeding tube or urinary catheter is inserted through the external nares to the level of the caudal nasopharynx. The catheter can be coated with a topical anesthetic cream, or topical anesthetic drops can be instilled in the nostril to facilitate passage. Adhesive tape is attached to the catheter, and the tape is sutured to the forehead. An Elizabethan collar should be used to prevent the patient from dislodging the catheter.

An inspired oxygen concentration of 30 to 40 percent is adequate for animals requiring oxygen therapy. Excessively high oxygen concentrations can result in oxygen toxicity. Neonatal kittens appear to be particularly susceptible to retinal changes induced by oxygen toxicity.

Respiratory Physical Therapy

Physical therapy of the respiratory system is a valuable adjunct to other forms of therapy for diseases of the lungs and airways. Appropriate physical therapy is also useful as a preventative measure in patients at high risk for the development of pulmonary disease. Secondary bronchopneumonia is a common complication in patients with atelectasis. Stimulation of the cough reflex by compressing the trachea will expand the lungs maximally and prevent atelectasis. Regular turning of recumbent patients will enhance drainage and circulation and thus prevent hypostatic congestion.

Percussion (coupage), also known as tapping or clapping, is a technique of striking the animal's chest in order to loosen bronchial secretion and thus facilitate drainage. The chest is struck with the hand held slightly cupped with fingers and thumb closed so that a cushion of air is trapped between the technician's hand and the chest wall. Best results come from using both hands alternately in rapid sequence for several seconds, moving from ventral to dorsal on the lung fields. When done properly, this is a noisy procedure; however, it is not painful to the patient. An electric hand vibrator can be used to set up fine vibration that will also aid the drainage of secretions. If the animal is ambulatory, a brief walk after coupage will aid in mobilization of respiratory secretions.

Whenever possible, animals with pulmonary problems should be maintained in an upright position (i.e., sternal recumbency). If necessary, slings or supports should be used to maintain this posture. This position will decrease the amount of hypostatic congestion that develops.

Topical Therapy

Topical therapy plays an important role in the treatment of dermatological disease. It can be used to treat a specific disease—for example, sarcoptic mange. More frequently, however, topical therapy is used either in conjunction with systemic medications or as a form of symptomatic therapy when the diagnosis is unknown.

Plain tap water is one of the most effective topical agents. Depending on how water is used, it can either hydrate or dehydrate the skin. Frequent wetting of the skin will stimulate evaporation from the skin and thus cause dehydration. This approach can be useful in managing any acute moist dermatitis ("hot spot"). In contrast, if a film of oil (e.g., Alpha Keri, Westwood Pharmaceuticals, Inc.) is applied immediately after soaking with water, evaporation is slowed or stopped, and the skin remains moist.

Soaks

Soaks are an effective means of handling localized acute eruptions. Soaks can be applied with moist towels or by placing the animal in a water-filled basin or tub. Soaks for local acute dermatosis should be applied for 10 to 15 minutes three or more times daily. The involved area should be kept constantly moist, and the warm temperature of the soak should be maintained by adding hot water as needed. Some of the solutions commonly used for soaks in veterinary medicine include water, aluminum acetate (Burow's solution, Domeboro solution, Dome Laboratories) and magnesium sulfate (1:65 solution in water, 1 tablespoonful per 1000 ml of water).

Astringents

Astringents precipitate proteins on the surface of an area of acute damage and form a beneficial covering. These agents do not penetrate deeply. Aluminum acetate is an excellent mild astringent. Another effective astringent is tannic acid. Tannic acid is combined with salicylic acid and alcohol in several products to form a potent astringent. These combination products are especially useful as part of the management of localized acute moist dermatitis; however, this agent should be applied only once to an involved area.

Baths

Cleansing baths are an important part of topical dermatological therapy. Baths aid in the removal of dirt, debris and scale. A variety of effective mild cleansing soaps or detergents are available. Mild dishwashing detergents or soaps (e.g., Joy and Palmolive liquid) are effective and inexpensive. If a milder, less irritating product is desired, a balanced pH soap, such as Johnson's Baby Shampoo (Johnson & Johnson), can be used. If an even milder product is needed, vegetable oil soaps (coconut oil) are the most bland. Regardless of how mild the soap or detergent, it should always be thoroughly rinsed out of the coat with copious volumes of clean water.

A medicated bath can be applied as a shampoo or as a rinse applied to the animal following a routine cleansing bath. Medicated baths contain ingredients that enhance the actions of routine cleansing shampoos. Medicated shampoos should be lathered into the coat for 10 to 15 minutes. This allows the medicated component of the shampoo time for effect or limited absorption. Types of medicated baths used in small animal practice include colloidal oatmeal, tar-sulfur, sulfur-salicylic and benzoyl peroxide products. Colloidal oatmeal (Aveeno, Cooper Care, Inc., and Epi-Soothe cream rinse, Allerderm, Inc.) baths are used for their soothing and antipruritic properties. Tar-sulfur shampoos (Lytar, Dermatologics for Veterinary Medicine, Inc., and Allerseb-T, Allerderm, Inc.) are used in the management of oily, flaky seborrheic conditions. While sulfur and salicylic shampoos (Sebalyte, Dermatologics for Veterinary Medicine Inc., and Sebolux, Allerderm, Inc.) are used in the management of dry, flaky seborrheic conditions, benzoyl peroxide shampoos (Oxydex, Dermatologics for Veterinary Medicine, Inc., and Pyoben, Allerderm, Inc.) are useful in the treatment of superficial pyoderma (bacterial skin infection), excessive crusting and debris problems and oily seborrheic conditions. The underlying condition and the individual response to the medicated bath determine the required frequency of application.

Dips and Rinses

Dips or rinses use water as a means of delivering various antifungal or antiparasitic agents to the skin. Although applied to the skin, some of these agents have the potential to cause systemic toxicities. Clipping the hair and using cleansing baths helps to obtain greater penetration in animals with excessive scale or crust. Dips that are useful in the treatment of dermatophytosis (ringworm) include dilute sodium hypochlorite solution, dilute Nolvasan solution (Fort Dodge Laboratories), dilute iodine solutions or lime sulfur solutions. Antiparasitic products used as dips or rinses include chlorpyrifos (Dursban), pyrethrins, pyrethroids, organophosphates (malathion) and carbamates. Amitraz (Mitaban, Upjohn Co.) is useful in the treatment of generalized demodectic mange.

Powders

Powders are occasionally used in veterinary medicine as drying agents and vehicles for parasiticides and to reduce friction and irritation. When used as a drying agent, powders may be in the form of true powders, shake lotions or pastes. Components that improve the drying action of various powdered products include talc, zinc oxide, cornstarch and tannic acid.

Carbaryl powders are a valuable part of flea control programs in the dog and cat. Labels should be checked carefully to be certain that the specific product is safe for dogs and cats. The powder must be worked down into the hair coat to increase the parasiticidal effect. This can be accomplished by rubbing the hair coat against the grain as the powder is applied. The powder should be applied to the entire body, excluding the face. Fractious or frightened cats can be treated by wrapping them in a thick bath towel and medicating small sections until the entire animal has been covered. Flea sprays can be used similarly.

Creams and Ointments

Creams and ointments are also used in the topical treatment of dermatological problems. The area of treatment should be clipped, if not hairless, and protected from immediate removal by licking. For practical and economic reasons, the area to be treated should be relatively small. Ointments are thicker than creams and leave a greasy feeling when applied to the skin. Ointments and creams soften, lubricate and protect the skin and aid in the removal of scale and crusts. Ointments and creams form an occlusive covering and, therefore, are not indicated for moist or oozing skin lesions.

Topical creams and ointments can be used to treat localized dermatophytosis (ringworm). They can be used as the sole type of therapy or as an adjunct to oral therapy or topical rinses. Creams and ointments must be restricted to small lesions because of expense and convenience. Effective topical fungicidal products used in veterinary medicine contain miconazole and thiabendazole. Since the use of ointments and creams alone is often insufficient to clear the infection or prevent reinfection, rinses or dips are important.

Otic Preparations

Most topical otic preparations contain various combinations of antibiotic, anti-inflammatory, fungicidal and parasiticidal agents. Topical antimicrobial agents are indicated whenever infection is present. Chloramphenicol, neomycin, polymyxin and gentamicin are the commonly used antibiotics in these combination otic preparations. Neomycin and gentamicin have been reported to cause ototoxicity when used for prolonged periods in dogs with ruptured eardrums. (Gentamicin is inactivated by pus; therefore, the ears must be thoroughly cleaned before use.)

Corticosteroids are used in these combination products because they decrease inflammation and the build-up of discharge and, consequently, decrease self-trauma by the animal. The antifungals are useful in treating dermatophytes and yeast organisms such as *Malassezia pachydermitis (Pityrosporon)*. Thiabendazole and miconazole are effective topical antifungal agents.

Certain drugs owe their efficacy to their ability to alter the pH in the ear canal. Acetic acid (dilute vinegar solution) and Domeboro Otic (Dome Laboratories) are specific examples. Remember not to use products that lower the pH with gentamicin because the effectiveness of gentamicin is significantly reduced in an acid environment.

Products that contain rotenone in oil or thiabendazole are used to treat ear mites. It is essential that treatment for ear mites be continued for at least 3 weeks and that all animals in the household be treated. Otic instillation of ivermectin, as a one-time application (on occasion, two to four treatments may be needed), has also been shown to be effective in the treatment of ear mites.

INFECTIOUS DISEASES

This section will discuss a number of common medical problems of dogs and cats. It is not intended to be a comprehensive review of internal medicine. Rather, a number of specific problems have been selected that illustrate or emphasize important aspects of medical nursing.

Canine Respiratory Disease Complex

Synonyms for canine upper respiratory disease complex include kennel cough and infectious tracheobronchitis. This complex is composed of a number of different disease processes. Causative factors include viral and bacterial agents as well as predisposing environmental factors. These factors may occur singly or in combination. The diagnosis of this complex is usually based on historical and physical examination findings rather than on laboratory tests. This problem is most often self-limiting, and the duration of signs generally is no more than 2 weeks.

Treatment involves nursing care and the correction of any environmental factors that may have predisposed to the illness. The dog should be kept in a warm space that is well ventilated and free of drafts and should be fed a highly palatable diet. Appetite will be enhanced if eyes and nose are kept free of accumulated discharge. If anorectic, the patient should be hand-fed or force-fed. Intravenous or subcutaneous fluid therapy is occasionally necessary. Steam or vaporizer therapy may provide symptomatic relief. Steam therapy can be performed by placing the dog in a steam-filled bathroom several times a day. Alternatively, cold mist vaporizers can be used several times a day.

The decision to use antitussive (cough suppressant) therapy should be based upon the frequency of coughing and how prolonged the episodes are. If codeine-derivative cough suppressants are used to excess, depression and anorexia will result.

Treatment with antibiotics usually is not indicated unless there is evidence of lower respiratory or systemic involvement—for example, fever. If antibiotic therapy is instituted, a complete regimen of 10 to 14 days at full therapeutic doses should be completed. The selection of an antibiotic would ideally be based on the results of culture and sensitivity testing. If these are not available, chloramphenicol trimethoprim-sulfonamide combination or tetracyclines are usually effective. The use of systemic products containing both antibiotics and corticosteroids is not indicated. Likewise, the intratracheal injection of any product is inappropriate therapy.

Owing to the highly contagious nature of the causative organisms, an infected dog should be isolated from other hospitalized patients. If possible, hospitalization should be avoided. Once an outbreak occurs in a kennel or veterinary hospital, control is difficult. Ideally, the area should be kept vacant for approximately 2 weeks, and appropriate preventative measures should be instituted, consisting of the implementation of an effective vaccination protocol for every hospitalized patient. All dogs should preferably be vaccinated at least 10 days prior to exposure. Yearly revaccination of all patients should be a consistent hospital policy. Although parenteral immunization is widely used, studies suggest that intranasal vaccines are more efficacious in preventing infection. Vaccination is recommended more often than yearly for animals at high risk of exposure to the causative agents (such as frequent boarding or dog shows). The commonly used disinfectants, such as chlorhexidine (Novalsan) and benzalkonium (Roccal), effectively kill the causative bacteria and viruses.

Feline Respiratory Disease Complex

The principal components of the feline respiratory disease complex are feline viral rhinotracheitis and feline calicivirus. Less frequently incriminated agents include feline reovirus, feline pneumonitis (Chlamydia psittaci), Mycoplasma and various bacteria.

Clinical signs of this complex include fever, cough, paroxysms of sneezing and hypersalivation. As the infection progresses, mucopurulent ocular and nasal discharge, lacrimation and open-mouthed breathing can be seen. Ulceration of the tongue, hard palate and nasal pad have been reported with feline calicivirus. The severity of signs and the mortality rate are greatest in young (less than 1 year of age), nonvaccinated cats and kittens. The severity of the clinical signs will vary widely from patient to patient. The variability results from a number of interacting factors, which include the virulence of the virus, the infecting dose of virus and the general health and immune status of the infected cat.

Diagnosis is based primarily on history and clinical signs rather than on laboratory findings. Occasionally, laboratory confirmation of the diagnosis by means of virus isolation or the demonstration of serum antibodies is indicated. The additional expense of laboratory confirmation is only justified when dealing with groups of cats having a chronic history of feline respiratory disease complex.

Treatment will vary, depending on the severity of signs. Some cats will show only mild, transient signs, and they require no treatment. Secondary bacterial infection will occasionally be a sequela to the feline respiratory disease complex, and therefore a broad-spectrum antibiotic may be indicated in the very young kitten (<12 wk of age).

General nursing care is of much greater importance than antibiotics in typical cases. Whenever possible, infected cats should be treated at home rather than in the hospital.

A vital part of nursing care is to gently clean away accumulated ocular or nasal discharge. If the nostrils are kept patent, the cat is more likely to continue eating. In order to ensure that this happens, the owner should indulge his pet and provide highly palatable foods. Strongly flavored or odorous foods are more likely to stimulate the appetite of an anorectic cat. Steam therapy is frequently useful and can be achieved by placing the cat in a steam-filled bathroom or by using a vaporizer.

In cats that become completely anorectic, subcutaneous or intravenous fluids may be required until the appetite returns to normal. Force feeding or repeated syringe feedings may be attempted; however, in certain cats, the associated stress may negate any beneficial effect. Alternatives that appear to be better tolerated include nasogastric or pharyngostomy tubes. These procedures should be reserved for severely cachectic cats.

Proper care of the eyes is required to prevent serious injury and subsequent blindness. In most instances, a broad-spectrum antibiotic ophthalmic ointment is preferred. If pneumonitis is suspected, tetracycline ophthalmic ointment is the treatment of choice. Corticosteroids should not be used under any circumstance if feline respiratory disease complex is suspected. Specific antiviral and mucolytic ophthalmic preparations may be indicated in cases with corneal ulceration.

The virus is usually transmitted following direct contact with an infected cat. Sneezing with subsequent aerosolization of the virus will spread the virus a distance of approximately 15 to 20 cm. Fomite transmission via hands, clothing, litter boxes and food and water dishes is a more significant means of transmission than aerosolization in veterinary hospitals. The agents responsible for the feline respiratory disease complex are sensitive to hypochlorite disinfection.

The best way to prevent outbreaks of feline respiratory disease complex in hospitalized cats is to have an effective immunization protocol. Adequate ventilation will reduce the likelihood that infection will spread within the hospital. The humidity should be maintained between 30 and 50 percent. Disposable food trays and litter pans and autoclavable water dishes should be used. Cats should not be moved from one cage to another unless absolutely necessary during an outbreak. Cages should be thoroughly cleansed with a dilute hypochlorite solution. Finally, since the infection can be spread via hands and clothing, meticulous hygiene on the part of all hospital personnel is essential. It is important to understand that up to 80 percent of the cats that go through this respiratory complex remain lifelong carriers of the organism(s). They can pose a risk to other cats or can experience a recrudescence of the complex in stressful situations.

Canine Distemper

Canine distemper is an important viral disease of dogs because of the ubiquitous nature of the virus and the mortality associated with infection. The severity of signs will vary from a transient, subclinical infection to a severe fatal disease that involves several different organ systems. This variability is due to the differing virulence of various virus strains and differences in host immunity.

The initial phase of the infection is associated with fever, transient anorexia, lethargy and a mild serous ocular discharge after an approximate 9- to 14-day incubation period. Obviously, these signs are not specific for canine distemper. Later, as the virus spreads to the respiratory and gastrointestinal systems, mucopurulent ocular and nasal discharge, coughing, diarrhea and occasionally vomiting are noted. Many dogs are anorectic at this point and become severely dehydrated. Involvement of the central nervous system may occur and can be the only signs manifested by some dogs. These dogs may develop seizures or other evidence of neurological disease. Some dogs will seemingly recover from the severe respiratory and gastrointestinal signs, but weeks or months later they develop neurological signs that either are fatal or require euthanasia because of their severity.

Although the virus may survive in the environment for weeks at near-freezing temperatures (0 to 4°C), it is susceptible to heat, drying and ultraviolet light. Routine disinfection is usually effective in destroying the virus in a hospital or kennel.

Feline Panleukopenia

Feline panleukopenia is a potentially severe, highly contagious parvoviral disease of cats. Synonyms are feline distemper and infectious enteritis.

The typical clinical signs associated with feline panleukopenia include lethargy, anorexia, vomiting and diarrhea after a 7-day incubation period. Characteristically, the feces are yellowish, semiformed to fluid in consistency and may be blood-tinged. Severe dehydration may be present. Cats will occasionally hang their heads over water bowls but will not drink. The temperature may be elevated or subnormal. Feline panleukopenia can be an acute disease. Rarely, development of signs is so rapid that the owner may suspect malicious poisoning. Kittens and young cats appear to be more severely affected.

Diagnosis of feline panleukopenia is based on the presence of the clinical signs described above in the presence of a low total leukocyte count (less than 2000 WBC per mm³). The low total white blood cell count is primarily due to low numbers of neutrophils. The diagnosis of feline panleukopenia can be confirmed by virus isolation and serological and histopathological characteristics.

Treatment is primarily supportive, since specific antiviral drugs are not available. The cornerstone of successful therapy is the correction of fluid and electrolyte imbalances and prevention of sepsis by the use of broad-spectrum antibiotics. Symptomatic control of vomiting and diarrhea is usually indicated. Another complication the technician should be alert to is the development of hypoglycemia (low blood glucose). This may be manifested by the development of extreme weakness and/or seizure activity.

The prognosis for recovery is good if the cat survives the initial 3 to 6 days of severe clinical signs. The prognosis for kittens and young cats is guarded. A rising WBC count indicates a more favorable prognosis. It can exceed 50,000 per mm³ with a significant left shift during the recovery phase.

If the queen is infected during pregnancy, fetal death or congenital defects in the kitten may result. The fetus is susceptible to the virus because most tissues have high cell-proliferation rates. If the fetus is infected just prior to or immediately after birth, the development of the cerebellum may be affected. These kittens show balance and coordination problems beginning at about 3 to 4 weeks of age.

Fortunately, because of the availability of excellent vaccines, feline panleukopenia is currently an infrequent clinical problem.

Feline Leukemia Virus and Feline Immunodeficiency Virus Infection

These two distinct retroviral infections in cats may cause similar clinical signs. Feline leukemia virus (FeLV) has been recognized for many years and may cause immunosuppression and/or neoplasia. Lymphosarcoma and bone marrow disorders are the more common disorders associated with FeLV.

The virus is transmitted between cats by direct contact through grooming, sharing food dishes and fighting. The virus is easily killed in the environment, and isolation of an infected cat is adequate to prevent transmission to susceptible cats. Although most cats that are exposed to the virus successfully eliminate the infection, 1 to 3 percent of cats in single-cat households and up to 30 percent of cats in multiple-cat households will become persistently infected with the virus. These infected cats are then at risk for the development of the plethora of FeLV-related diseases. Feline leukemia virus infection can be identified by an in-hospital test. There are many such in-hospital tests now on the market and available to the practicing veterinarian. There are several vaccines available for the prevention of FeLV, and as many as 70 percent of cats will be protected with a successful immunization program.

Feline immunodeficiency virus (FIV), also called T-lymphotrophic T cell lentivirus (FTLV), is a recently identified virus of cats that causes primarily immunosuppression. Common clinical signs of infection with this virus include gingivitis, chronic diarrhea, generalized lymphadenopathy, fever, conjunctivitis, rhinitis and dermatitis. It is notable that all of these signs may be seen in cats infected with FeLV. Feline immunodeficiency virus is found nationwide and, indeed, worldwide. Most cats infected with this virus will not become immune, which differs from FeLV infection. The disease is spread by inoculation of the virus through cat bites. Transmission of the virus by direct contact through grooming, sharing of food dishes and close contact is less than what is seen with FeLV. No treatment or vaccine is available for this disease. Commercial kits detecting antibodies to this virus are available for in-hospital testing.

Pet-Associated Zoonoses

A zoonosis is a disease of animals that is transmissible to humans under natural conditions. The technician is frequently questioned by clients about the public health significance of animal diseases. Hospitalized animals may represent potential sources of zoonotic infection. Thus, these infections may be considered occupational diseases.

It is beyond the scope of this section to discuss all the pet-associated zoonoses; however, several of the more important infections will be described. It is important to stress that when questions about human medical care arise, a physician should be consulted.

Canine brucellosis occurs rarely in humans. Transmission from an infected dog to a human can occur by contact with blood, urine, semen, milk and infected tissues. Vaginal discharges, aborted fetuses and placental material following abortion contain large numbers of bacteria. Infection in humans can be an insidious, chronic disease that resembles infection with other strains of *Brucella* or it can result in relatively mild flu-like symptoms.

Toxoplasmosis can be acquired by human exposure to cat feces containing infective oocysts. Cats are an obligate host in the life cycle of *Toxoplasma*. *Toxoplasma* oocysts can remain viable in the environment for as long as 6 months under ideal conditions. The following recommendations to reduce the exposure hazard from toxoplasmosis-infected cats should be followed: Plastic gloves should be worn when cleaning litter pans or handling potentially contaminated soil. Children's sand-boxes should be covered and basic principles of sanitation should be followed. Immunodeficient people and women of childbearing age should exercise extreme caution to reduce the risk of exposure. Women contemplating pregnancy should have their antibody status determined by a physician. Those with a significant titer against toxoplasmosis are probably protected from reinfection. Antibody titers in cats are of little value, since they do not indicate which cats are actively shedding infective oocysts. A recently developed ELISA test, currently available through the University of Georgia and Colorado State University Veterinary Schools, identifies IgM and IgG antibodies in a cat's serum and can provide evidence for an acute or recent infection in a cat. It should be stressed to the concerned client that eating raw or improperly cooked meat is probably the most common source of human toxoplasmosis.

Campylobacter and *Salmonella* are bacteria that can produce pet-associated zoonosis. Pets appear to be relatively infrequent sources of *Campylobacter*. When pets are incriminated, it is usually a stray or recently adopted puppy or kitten that has had recent diarrhea. The incidence of *Salmonella* infection acquired from pets is unknown. Animals can be asymptomatic shedders of this organism for an average of 6 weeks. Since the route of transmission is the fecal-oral route, good sanitation is important.

Reports of human leptospirosis attributed to vaccinated pets have appeared in medical literature. The *Leptospira* bacteria that are used for routine immunization may not protect against subclinical infection and shedding of the organisms in the urine. Since transmission is via infected urine, good sanitation is essential.

Visceral and cutaneous larval migrans are due to the migration of animal parasite larvae in human hosts. The technician plays an important role in prevention by educating clients about the risks posed by pets infected with intestinal parasites. Treatment of infected animals and reducing environmental contamination will reduce the incidence of these problems.

Plague is an infectious disease of animals that is transmitted to humans by the bite of an infected ectoparasite, usually the flea. Although the majority of cases in humans result from exposure to infected wild rodents, domestic cats have been associated with a number of infections in humans. Infections have been reported in persons employed in veterinary hospitals. Cats with suppurative lymphadenitis (infected draining lymph nodes) should be considered plague suspects, and caution should be exercised by the veterinary technician when handling exudates or treating draining wounds.

Cat-scratch disease is a disease of humans that usually is associated with cat scratches or close contact with cats. Rarely, exposure to cats has not occurred and other injuries are incriminated, for example, splinters, thorns, dog scratches and so on. The causative agent is a small gram-negative bacterium. It is presumed that cats simply act as vectors for the disease, since they are not ill. Multiple cases in the same household have occurred over a period of months or even years.

Rabies is an acute, fatal viral disease of the central nervous system that affects all mammals. Rabies is transmitted by infected secretions, usually saliva. In the United States, the skunk and bat are the most important sources of human exposure. However, raccoons, foxes and unimmunized dogs and cats may also represent a hazard. In most areas of the world, the dog is the most important vector of rabies.

CARDIOLOGY

Congestive Heart Failure

Congestive heart failure is a clinical term used to describe the state when the heart is unable to maintain adequate cardiac output. Because of decreased cardiac output, the body's tissues do not receive sufficient blood supply for normal function. The decreased cardiac output and the resultant increase in pressures within the vessels entering the heart stimulate complex compensatory mechanisms that contribute to the clinical signs of congestive heart failure. The term *congestive heart failure* does not indicate a specific etiology.

Tachycardia and cardiomegaly (heart enlargement) are general signs associated with congestive heart failure. However, depending on the principal site of involvement, signs of left-sided or right-sided heart failure will predominate.

Left-sided heart failure results from dysfunction of the left atrioventricular valve (mitral valve) or ventricle or both. Clinical signs associated with left-sided heart failure include cough, exertional dyspnea, orthopnea, and at times syncope. Characteristically, early in left-sided heart failure the cough occurs in paroxysms and at night or in the early morning. The cough in left-sided heart failure is usually secondary to the development of pulmonary edema or occurs because the left atrium has enlarged and compressed the left mainstem bronchus. Exertional dyspnea refers to labored breathing associated with increased activity. This may be manifested as decreased exercise tolerance or reluctance to exercise. *Orthopnea* means difficult or labored breathing in the recumbent position. Pulmonary edema refers to the accumulation of abnormal fluid in the interstitial spaces and alveoli of the lungs. It can be detected by auscultating rales (crackles) in the lungs or by observing the characteristic pattern on chest radiographs. Syncope, or fainting, results from decreased cardiac output to the brain.

Right-sided heart failure results from a pathological condition of the right atrioventricular valve (tricuspid valve), the right ventricle or both. Clinical signs associated with right-sided heart failure include hepatic enlargement, ascites, pleural effusion and subcutaneous edema. Increased pressure in the abdominal veins results in congestion and enlargement of the liver. Increased hydrostatic pressure in capillaries results in leakage of fluid and the subsequent development of ascites, pleural effusion and subcutaneous edema. Subcutaneous edema is a relatively rare sign in the dog and is seen late in the course of the condition. (See Table 10–6 for list of signs seen with left and right heart failure.)

Certain cardiovascular problems result in both left-sided and right-sided heart failure. Obviously, the signs described are not specific for heart disease. Consequently, when evaluating a patient for cough or ascites, the conditions to rule out should include noncardiac problems.

Mitral Insufficiency

Mitral insufficiency resulting from chronic mitral (left atrioventricular) valvular fibrosis is the most frequently diagnosed form of heart disease in the dog. It is followed in prevalence by chronic tricuspid (right atrioventricular) valvular fibrosis, which causes tricuspid insufficiency. Valvular insufficiency is a term used to indicate functional incompetence (leakage) of

Table 10–6
CLINICAL SIGNS OF LEFT- AND RIGHT-SIDED HEART FAILURE

Congestive Signs—left
1. Pulmonary congestion and edema resulting in: cough, tachypnea, dyspnea, orthopnea, pulmonary crackles, tiring, hemoptysis, cyanosis
2. Secondary right heart failure
3. Cardiac arrhythmias

Congestive Signs—right
1. Systemic venous congestion:
   High CVP (central venous pressure)
   Jugular vein distention
2. Liver and spleen enlargement
3. Fluid in chest cavity (pleural effusion) causing: dyspnea, orthopnea and cyanosis
4. Fluid in abdominal cavity (ascites)
5. Subcutaneous edema
6. Fluid in pericardial sac (pericardial effusion)

the valve with subsequent regurgitation (backward flow) of blood from the ventricle into the atrium during ventricular systole.

The signs associated with chronic mitral insufficiency are those of left-sided heart failure, for example, cough, exertional dyspnea and pulmonary edema. The specific cause of mitral valvular fibrosis is unknown; however, it appears to be associated with aging. Certain breeds appear to be predisposed, the majority of these being small breeds of dogs (e.g., miniature poodles). Mitral insufficiency as a cause of left-sided heart failure is much less common in the cat. The diagnosis of chronic mitral insufficiency is based on the clinical history, auscultation of the heart and lungs, thoracic radiography and electrocardiography. Although the traditional treatment for this condition has included the use of cardiac glycosides (e.g., digoxin), recent evidence indicates that cardiac contractility is normal to increased in the majority of these dogs, and therefore digoxin is not indicated until late in the course of the failure state.

Initially, the use of diuretics such as furosemide (Lasix), a sodium-restricted diet and exercise restriction are the primary mode of therapy. Later in the disease progression, treatment with vasodilators such as hydralazine (Apresoline), captopril (Capoten) and enalapril (Vasotec) is advocated. These drugs work by decreasing the resistance against which the heart has to pump. As more long-term data are accumulated, we may find in dogs, as in people, that vasodilators may help to prolong survival of dogs with heart failure if they are begun earlier in the disease state.

Heartworm Disease

Heartworm disease, caused by *Dirofilaria immitis*, is characterized principally by the presence of right-sided heart failure. The adult parasites lodge in the right atrium, right ventricle, right ventricular outflow tract, pulmonary arteries and venae cavae. The major effect of heartworm disease is to produce pulmonary hypertension (increased blood pressure in pulmonary arteries), which results in right-sided heart failure.

Heartworm disease has a geographical distribution. The

highest incidences of infection occur along the southeastern Atlantic and Gulf coasts. Gradually, heartworm disease has spread to most of the eastern and midwestern United States. Small endemic areas have also been reported in the western United States. With the increased travel of dogs from one region to another, heartworm disease is possible anywhere.

Mosquitoes are an intermediate host for the parasite. The disease is spread by mosquitoes ingesting microfilariae (immature parasites, the L_1 larvae) from the blood of an infected dog. The microfilariae undergo maturation within the mosquito to become an infective larva. Infective larvae (L_3 stage) enter the dog through the skin puncture wound produced by the mosquito and migrate to subcutaneous tissue, muscle or fat. Two more molts occur within the dog's body, and the young adult heartworm arrives in the heart approximately 110 days after infection. The adult female heartworms begin producing circulating microfilariae 6 to 7 months after infection.

The most practical method to detect heartworm disease is to observe the presence of circulating microfilariae in the peripheral blood. The microfilariae of a nonpathogenic filarial worm, *Dipetalonema reconditum,* must be differentiated from those of *Dirofilaria immitis.* The most useful diagnostic characteristics of the microfilariae of *Dipetalonema reconditum* are the blunt shape of the head and the serpentine progressive movement demonstrated in direct blood smears. There are three basic tests used to detect microfilariae. They include the direct smear, modified Knott test and filter tests. Each test has its advantages and disadvantages; however, if cost, sensitivity and ease of species identification are considered, the modified Knott test is preferred.

It has been estimated that as many as 25 to 65 percent of dogs with heartworm disease have no circulating microfilariae. This is referred to as occult heartworm disease. If heartworm disease is suspected based upon history, physical examination, radiography and electrocardiography, yet circulating microfilariae are not present, a serological test for detection of adult heartworm antigens should be performed.

The treatment of heartworm disease can be divided into three phases. The first phase is to kill the adult heartworms (adulticidal therapy) that are present in the heart and blood vessels. The next phase is to eradicate the circulating microfilariae (microfilaricidal therapy). Finally, preventative medication (prophylactic therapy) is administered to those dogs at risk of developing heartworm disease. This would include any dog residing in or traveling to an endemic area.

Adulticide therapy consists of administering thiacetarsamide sodium (Caparsolate, Abbott Laboratories) intravenously. The recommended regimen is to administer the drug twice per day for 2 days. If the injection takes a perivascular route, swelling, inflammation and tissue necrosis will occur. If it is suspected that extravasation has occurred, the area should be infiltrated with sterile saline and dexamethasone immediately. Thiacetarsamide may produce renal and hepatic toxicity. The adult heartworms will die slowly over a 2- to 3-week period. Fever, coughing and, in more severe cases, dyspnea and hemoptysis (coughing up blood) are the signs observed as the worms die and pass to the lungs (pulmonary thromboembolism). Prednisone therapy (1 mg/kg) is the accepted therapy for pulmonary thromboembolism. Aspirin therapy (5 mg/kg once daily) is recommended in dogs with moderate to severe heartworm disease to reduce thromboembolism. It may be started 1 week before treatment and continued 4 to 6 weeks after treatment.

In order to minimize the development of clinical pulmonary thromboembolism, it is important to restrict exercise for 3 to 4 weeks following adulticide therapy. If the signs associated with pulmonary thromboembolism are severe, hospitalization and administration of bronchodilators, anti-inflammatory drugs and antibiotics are recommended. Disseminated intravascular coagulation (DIC) may occur in dogs with severe clinical signs. Treatment of advanced DIC is usually unsuccessful.

Microfilaricide therapy is begun 3 weeks following adulticide therapy. Ivermectin (Ivomec), 50 µg/kg orally once, is the current accepted method of treatment for microfilaria, even though it is not FDA-approved for this function.

Heartworm disease may be prevented with the use of one of several products. Some of these also have protective activity against some endoparasites. Table 10-7 lists the products currently available for heartworm prevention in the dog.

Cardiomyopathy

Cardiomyopathy is a general term that merely indicates that the basic pathological lesion involves the heart muscle. Cardiomyopathies can be primary or secondary. Primary cardiomyopathies indicate that the myocardial disease is not due to any recurrent or preexisting cardiovascular or systemic disease. Primary cardiomyopathies in cats are further subdivided into hypertrophic, dilated and restrictive forms. Secondary cardiomyopathies in dogs and cats are less frequent and are due to diseases such as infection, metabolic disorders (e.g., uremia), endocrine problems (e.g., hyperthyroidism) and infiltrative processes (e.g., neoplasia).

Hypertrophic cardiomyopathy is characterized by increased thickness of the myocardium and a small left ventricular lumen. Clinical signs are seen in middle-aged cats of all breeds. The most prominent sign is the sudden development of respiratory distress secondary to pulmonary edema. Hindlimb paresis (weakness) and severe pain may also be present. These hindlimb signs are due to aortic thromboembolism (blood clots) disrupting the blood supply to the hindlimbs. This prob-

Table 10–7 CURRENTLY AVAILABLE HEARTWORM PREVENTATIVES			
Trade Name	**Ingredient(s)**	**Company**	**Anti-parasitic Activity**
Multiples	Diethylcarbamazine	Multiple	Roundworms Heartworm prevention
Filaribits	Diethylcarbamazine	SmithKline Beecham	Roundworms Heartworm prevention
Filaribits-Plus	Diethylcarbamazine Oxibendazole	SmithKline Beecham	Hookworms Roundworms Whipworms Heartworm prevention
Heartgard-30	Ivermectin	MSD-Agvet	Heartworm prevention
Interceptor	Milbemycin oxime	Ciba-Geigy	Heartworm prevention Hookworms

lem can usually be diagnosed easily if femoral pulses are found to be poor or absent. Diagnosis of cardiomyopathy is based on history, physical examination, radiography, electrocardiography and echocardiography. If echocardiography is not available, nonselective angiocardiography may be necessary for diagnosis. The basic initial therapeutic approach is to use diuretics (e.g., Lasix, Hoeschst-Roussel Pharmaceuticals), cage rest, oxygen therapy and beta-adrenergic blockers, such as propranolol (Inderal, Ayerst Laboratories). Long-term management consists of diuretics, beta blockers, a sodium-restricted diet (feline H/D, Hills), aspirin and restricted activity. Aspirin is used to reduce the likelihood of aortic thromboembolism.

Dilated cardiomyopathy is characterized by extreme ventricular dilation and moderate atrial enlargement. This results in impaired pump function of the ventricle. This type of cardiomyopathy is also known as *congestive cardiomyopathy*. Signs of right-sided heart failure usually predominate. In addition, cats may show a gradual onset of lethargy and anorexia and at times may be presented dehydrated, hypothermic and in cardiovascular shock. Respiratory distress secondary to pleural effusion and aortic thromboembolism resulting in hindlimb paresis are also occasionally seen. The basic therapeutic approach is to mechanically remove as much fluid as possible from the pleural cavity (thoracocentesis), digitalize the cat (digoxin therapy) and administer diuretics. Aspirin is used as a preventative measure against aortic thromboembolism. Vasodilators, such as nitroglycerin ointment (Nitrol ointment, Kremers-Urban Co.), may have a role in the management of dilated cardiomyopathy.

Some cats with dilated cardiomyopathy have low plasma taurine levels, and cardiac function will increase with oral taurine supplementation of 250 to 500 mg daily. Cardiac function usually improves over a period of months, and if cats are placed on a diet containing ample taurine, cardiac drugs and taurine supplementation may eventually be discontinued. It should be stated that since this association of low taurine levels and cardiomyopathy in the cat has been made, almost all commercial and prescription diets have adequate levels of taurine now, so that low-taurine dilated cardiomyopathy is much less common than it used to be.

Restrictive cardiomyopathy is the least common form of primary feline cardiomyopathy. A synonym is endomyocardial fibrosis. Respiratory distress is the most common clinical sign. Diagnosis is similar to the other forms of primary cardiomyopathy. Response to therapy is generally poor.

Primary cardiomyopathies in the dog are categorized as dilated (congestive), boxer cardiomyopathy, Doberman pinscher cardiomyopathy and hypertrophic cardiomyopathy.

Dilated cardiomyopathy is most common in large and giant breed male dogs aged 4 to 6 years; however, English cocker spaniels and schnauzers are also affected. Presenting signs often include weakness, lethargy, respiratory distress, cough, anorexia, weight loss, and possible ascites and syncope. The left ventricle and atrium are dilated with decreased contractility. Diagnosis is confirmed by physical examination, radiography, electrocardiography and echocardiography. Treatment consists of diuretics, a low sodium diet, arteriolar dilators and positive inotropes, such as cardiac glycosides. The long-term prognosis is guarded in that most dogs with the dilated form of cardiomyopathy have an average life span of 6 to 8 months after the diagnosis has been made.

A specific cardiomyopathy occurs in boxers. These dogs may be asymptomatic or present with syncope and episodic weakness. Arrhythmias are common and may cause sudden death. Diagnosis is confirmed by the same methods as those used in dogs with dilated cardiomyopathy. Treatment with diuretics and antiarrhythmics, such as propranolol, may be useful; however, prognosis is still poor.

Doberman pinschers may present with a primary cardiomyopathy that is similar to congestive or dilated cardiomyopathy. Ventricular contractility is often severely compromised, and atrial arrhythmias are common. These dogs are often in fulminant congestive heart failure and require supportive care with oxygen, diuretics, positive inotropes, and vasodilators. Prognosis is poor.

Hypertrophic cardiomyopathy is the most uncommon primary cardiomyopathy. It is most often seen in German shepherd dogs and other large breeds. Presenting signs are referable to cardiac disease, and sudden death may occur. Treatment with diuretics and propranolol may improve cardiac output and clinical signs.

ENDOCRINOLOGY

Canine hyperadrenocorticism (Cushing's syndrome) is a disorder that results from the excessive production of cortisol by the adrenal cortex. The clinical signs of canine hyperadrenocorticism include polyuria, polydipsia, abdominal distention, polyphagia, muscular weakness, dermatological changes and reproductive problems (anestrus and testicular atrophy). Cushing's syndrome can result from excessive production of adrenocorticotropic hormone (ACTH) by the pituitary gland (pituitary-dependent hyperadrenocorticism) or from a functional tumor of the adrenal cortex. Pituitary-dependent hyperadrenocorticism is by far the most common, comprising approximately 80 percent of the cases. Diagnosis is based on measurements of the plasma cortisol levels following stimulation with ACTH or suppression with dexamethasone. Treatment is different for these two conditions. If a functional tumor is present, the recommended treatment is surgical removal. The drug used to treat Cushing's syndrome caused by excessive ACTH production is mitotane (Lysodren, Bristol Laboratories). Side effects associated with the use of mitotane include anorexia, lethargy, vomiting and depression.

Hypoglycemia

Canine hypoglycemia is a clinical problem associated with a variety of diseases rather than a specific diagnosis itself. The signs associated with hypoglycemia include weakness of the rear legs, generalized weakness, focal or diffuse muscle twitching, incoordination, blindness, generalized seizures and behavioral changes. These behavioral changes include aggressive behavior and anxiety as evidenced by incessant running, barking and loss of bowel and bladder control. These signs tend to be episodic, regardless of the cause of hypoglycemia. Hypoglycemia should be considered a differential diagnosis in any dog that is having seizures or is presented in a coma.

The first step in evaluating a patient with suspected hypoglycemia is to verify or document that hypoglycemia exists. Improper handling of blood samples may result in falsely low blood glucose levels. The blood glucose level can be lowered if the serum is not removed from the clot or if the specimen is stored at room temperature for a prolonged period. It is preferable to remove serum from the clot within 10 to 15 minutes of drawing the blood sample. If this cannot be done, use of sodium fluoride tubes may be helpful.

Once hypoglycemia has been verified, the signalment, history, clinical findings and further laboratory tests may be needed to reduce the long and rather diverse list of conditions that may cause hypoglycemia. Functional beta-cell tumors (insulinomas of the pancreas), nonpancreatic tumors, hypoglycemia-ketonemia in pregnant bitches, glycogen storage diseases, septic shock, juvenile and neonatal hypoglycemia, canine parvoviral diarrhea and excessive insulin administration in diabetic patients are all examples of diseases that may cause hypoglycemia.

Hypothyroidism and Hyperthyroidism

Hypothyroidism is one of the most common endocrine disorders in the dog, but it is rare in the cat. Some of the common clinical signs include oily seborrhea, alopecia, thickened skin, weight gain, lethargy, and cold intolerance. There are some breeds with an apparent increased incidence of hypothyroidism, and these are listed in Table 10–8. The thyroid-stimulating hormone (TSH) stimulation test is the most accurate diagnostic test available for assessment of thyroid gland function. This test involves drawing blood before and 6 hours after TSH administration, and then measuring the serum T_4 levels on each sample. Most normal animals should increase their baseline T_4 level by $2\times$ and exceed $3\mu g/dl$ at the 6-hour sampling. Treatment of hypothyroidism consists of supplementation with thyroxine (T_4).

Hyperthyroidism is the most common endocrinopathy affecting cats older than 8 years of age, but it is rare in the dog. The most common clinical signs of hyperthyroidism are weight loss despite a good appetite, restlessness, hyperactivity, and diarrhea. In many cases a thyroid nodule can be palpated in the ventrocervical region of the neck. The diagnosis can usually be confirmed by documenting an elevated serum T_4 level. Treatment may consist of medical therapy with methimazole (Tapazole, Eli Lilly and Co.), surgical removal of the thyroid nodule and/or radioactive iodine (^{131}I).

Diabetes Mellitus

This endocrinopathy is seen in the older dog and cat, and it is more common in the female dog and the male cat. Common clinical signs include excessive water intake (polydipsia), urination of large volumes of urine (polyuria), weight loss in spite of a good appetite, and rapidly developing lens opacities (cataracts) in the dog. If the dog or cat is ketoacidotic, then weakness, vomiting, depression and possibly coma may develop. The diagnosis of diabetes mellitus is made by documenting hyperglycemia, glucosuria and $\pm$ ketonuria or ketonemia (if animal is ketoacidotic).

The technician's role in the treatment of patients with this endocrinopathy is twofold: (1) management of the ill ketoacidotic diabetic in the hospital and (2) education of clients concerning home management and treatment of their pets.

The ketoacidotic diabetic represents a true challenge for the veterinarian and technician alike, and it is important that they

Table 10–8
BREEDS OF DOGS WITH AN APPARENT INCREASED INCIDENCE OF HYPOTHYROIDISM
Afghan hound
Airedale
Beagle
Boxer
Brittany spaniel
Chow chow
Cocker spaniel
Dachshund
Doberman pinscher
English bulldog
Golden retriever
Great Dane
Irish setter
Irish wolfhound
Malamute
Miniature schnauzer
Newfoundland
Pomeranian
Poodle
Shetland sheepdog

work in unison so that optimal patient care is achieved. The technician's role involves closely monitoring vital signs, making sure fluids are given at the proper rate, frequent blood glucose determinations and administration of short-acting (regular/crystalline) insulin. Because the ketoacidotic patient requires such close monitoring, the technician plays a major role in the minute-to-minute and hour-to-hour evaluation of the patient, so that minor changes in the patient's condition can be recognized early and the veterinarian be informed. Because of the complexity of the ketoacidotic diabetic, all of these functions should be done under the direct supervision of a veterinarian.

The second aspect of diabetic management involves the instruction of the client concerning home management of the pet. This can be a time-consuming function, and the technician who has a good understanding of diabetes management can be a tremendous asset to the veterinarian. Examples of areas in which the client should be instructed and/or shown include how to (1) mix the insulin, (2) read the syringes, (3) draw up the insulin into the syringe, (4) give the subcutaneous injection and (5) read urine test strips for urine glucose measurement. In addition, the client needs to be instructed (1) about the type of diet to be fed and how much and when to feed, (2) *not* to give the insulin if the pet does not eat in the morning and (3) if the pet has a seizure, to give the animal Karo syrup orally and call the hospital immediately. All of these items can be compiled into a handout that the technician can develop with the aid of the veterinarian. This handout can then be given to the client, who can refer to it as needed at home.

THERIOGENOLOGY
Postpartum Disorders in the Bitch

The postpartum bitch may be presented to an animal hospital for a variety of serious problems following whelping. These problems include mastitis, metritis and eclampsia.

Mastitis refers to inflammation of one or more mammary glands. In severe cases, affected glands are hot and painful, and the patient is systemically ill. Bitches with septic mastitis are depressed, anorectic and reluctant to care for the puppies. In less severe cases, the bitch may not be symptomatic; however, the puppies may fail to gain weight or may show signs of septicemia. Systemic antibiotics are used to treat mastitis. Since the affected glands produce abnormal milk, and the antibiotics excreted in the milk may be harmful to the puppies, it is recommended that the puppies be hand-reared.

Severe mastitis may progress to abscess formation or gangrenous mastitis. Surgical drainage and treatment may be required in these cases.

Stasis of milk in the mammary glands can occasionally result in enlarged, painful mammary glands. Galactostasis may be observed during pseudopregnancy or at the time of weaning when the body is attempting to resorb milk. Unlike mastitis, dogs with galactostasis are not systemically ill. Treatment consists of application of cool towels and compresses to decrease inflammation. Care should be taken not to massage the glands, since this can stimulate additional milk letdown.

Metritis is a uterine disease of the immediate postpartum period. Signs usually develop within the first week of whelping. Metritis is associated with retained placentas, retained fetuses and dystocia. Clinical signs suggestive of metritis include fever, depression and reduced interest in the puppies. A foul-smelling, brown or reddish-brown vaginal discharge may be present. The normal discharge following whelping is nonodorous and greenish. The diagnosis is based on history, clinical findings and laboratory results. Laboratory tests that are useful include vaginal cytological studies, CBCs and bacterial cultures.

Initial therapy consists of replacing fluid deficits, treating shock, if present, and initiating antibiotic therapy after cultures have been obtained. Medical drainage of the uterus can be attempted in valuable breeding bitches. In severe cases, ovariohysterectomy may be indicated to save the bitch's life.

Hypocalcemia (eclampsia) usually occurs 2 to 3 weeks postpartum in small bitches with large litters but occasionally can occur before birth. Presenting signs include weakness and trembling and may proceed to tonic convulsions. The temperature is usually elevated during convulsions.

Diagnosis is based on clinical signs in a lactating female. Treatment includes removing the young for 12 to 24 hours, treating the dam with intravenous 10 percent calcium gluconate and seeing that the dam receives oral calcium lactate or calcium gluconate and vitamin D at home. If the condition recurs, the young should be weaned.

Canine Brucellosis

Canine brucellosis is primarily an infection of the reproductive tract, though other organ systems may be involved. *Brucella canis* has been isolated from dogs with discospondylitis and chronic recurrent fever. Brucellosis is a frequent cause of infertility and other reproductive problems in both males and females.

Definitive diagnosis requires demonstration of the organism by a culture of blood or body fluids. Serological tests can be diagnostic as well. The rapid slide agglutination test is an easy, readily available test; however, false-positive results occur. The rapid slide agglutination can be used as a screen, with positive tests being confirmed using an alternative technique (e.g., agar gel immunodiffusion).

The mode of transmission is venereal. However, infection can also result from the ingestion of infected material, for example, aborted fetuses, placentas and vaginal discharge. Because of these means of spread, brucellosis can quickly become a kennel-wide problem.

Although a variety of antibiotic combinations have been recommended, therapeutic success cannot be guaranteed. Following antibiotic therapy some dogs will continue to harbor the organism and represent a risk to other dogs. Canine brucellosis is considered a possible zoonotic disease. For these reasons, some experts advocate removal of all infected dogs from the premises. Other experts feel that this position is extreme and instead recommend castration or ovariohysterectomy and antibiotic therapy for infected pet dogs.

Since treatment is not always successful, prevention is emphasized. All dogs should be tested prior to breeding or prior to introduction into a kennel.

Pyometritis

Pyometritis is a uterine disease that occurs during the luteal phase of the reproductive cycle. It occurs in both bitches and queens. Pyometritis may be part of a complex that initially starts with cystic changes in the endometrium and endometrial hyperplasia. Prior estrogen therapy may predispose to pyometritis.

Clinical signs are variable. A vaginal discharge may or may not be present, but, if present, the color of the discharge can be green, yellow or reddish brown. Bitches with pyometritis will frequently be polydipsic and polyuric. Affected animals can be severely depressed and septic or can be clinically normal.

An enlarged uterus on radiographs and leukocytosis with a left shift are considered diagnostic. Fluid therapy to correct fluid and electrolyte deficits followed by ovariohysterectomy is the treatment of choice in nonbreeding animals. In valuable breeding bitches, medical treatment with prostaglandin $F_{2-alpha}$ has been advocated in order to preserve the breeding life of the patient. Treatment with prostaglandin $F_{2-alpha}$ is expensive and potentially dangerous; therefore, it should be strictly reserved for dogs of significant breeding value.

Canine Prostatic Disease

Prostatic disease is occasionally seen in older intact male dogs. Clinical signs include straining to urinate (stranguria), painful urination (dysuria), blood in the urine (hematuria) and/or difficulty in defecation. The conditions that affect the prostate include benign prostatic hypertrophy, bacterial prostatitis, prostatic abscess, prostatic cyst and prostatic neoplasia.

The following noninvasive techniques are used to evaluate the prostate: rectal palpation, routine radiology, sonography (ultrasound), urethrography, cytological studies and bacterial cultures of prostatic washes or the prostatic fraction of the ejaculate. Frequently, it is difficult to differentiate neoplasia, infection and hypertrophy, using these noninvasive techniques. Consequently, surgical exploration and biopsy may be required to establish a definitive diagnosis.

Treatment varies, depending on the specific process. Dogs with benign prostatic hypertrophy respond to castration. Although estrogen therapy reduces the size of the prostate in benign prostatic hypertrophy, it is not recommended because of possible adverse reactions. Prostatic abscesses and cysts require surgical drainage. Bacterial prostatitis and prostatic abscesses are treated with antibiotics. Prostatic neoplasia is generally highly malignant, and treatment is directed toward palliation rather than cure. Some dogs with prostatic cancer may benefit from castration because the tumors possess testosterone receptors.

GASTROENTEROLOGY

Acute Gastroenteritis

Acute gastroenteritis is one of the more common problems seen in canine practice. Some examples of conditions that may cause this problem include dietary indiscretion, viral gastroenteritis, bacterial gastroenteritis, gastrointestinal foreign bodies, gastrointestinal parasites, intussusception, ingestion of toxins, acute pancreatitis and hypoadrenocorticism. The clinical history, signalment and physical examination may suggest the diagnosis. Frequently, response to symptomatic therapy is used to assess whether further diagnostic study is warranted. The intensity and degree of symptomatic and supportive care is determined by the severity of clinical signs.

The fundamental decision whether to hospitalize the patient is based on a number of factors. They include the hydration status of the dog, the severity and frequency of vomiting and diarrhea, the presence or absence of blood in the vomitus or stool and the presence of fever or profound lethargy. Non–patient-related factors to be considered include the client's ability to provide adequate care for the patient at home and the ability of the client to pay for hospitalized care.

Clinical management of outpatients consists primarily of dietary restriction, the administration of locally acting gastrointestinal medications and the use of fluid therapy when indicated. Dietary restriction is the most important aspect of the symptomatic care of acute gastroenteritis. The objective is to rest the gastrointestinal tract. This is accomplished by withholding all food for 12 to 24 hours, depending on the details of the case. If vomiting is severe, water is also withheld. If diarrhea is present and vomiting has not occurred, warm electrolyte-containing solutions can be given by mouth. During this period of symptomatic therapy, it is imperative that the patient be observed closely to prevent ingestion of foreign material and to detect any worsening of clinical signs.

After food has been withheld for the prescribed period, small, frequent, bland meals should be offered. These meals should be low in fat, low in fiber and easily digested and absorbed. These criteria are met by prescription diets, such as Prescription Diet I-D (Hills), and by homemade diets, such as cottage cheese and boiled rice. These diets should be warmed before feeding. These frequent, small, bland meals should be continued for 2 to 3 days. If the patient is doing well, the regular diet and feeding schedule can be gradually reintroduced over the next 3 to 5 days. If clinical signs recur during this process, the dog should be re-evaluated. Further diagnosis, evaluation and more intensive supportive therapy may be warranted.

Although a vast number of locally acting preparations are available for the treatment of acute gastroenteritis, most have not been proved effective in controlled clinical trials. An over-the-counter preparation containing bismuth subsalicylate (Pepto-Bismol) has been shown to shorten the duration of symptoms in humans with experimental viral enteritis. It is theorized that the beneficial response is not due to the coating action of the product but rather to the salicylate-inhibiting prostaglandin synthesis. Prostaglandins play a role in diarrhea by affecting both motility and secretory activity of the gastrointestinal tract. The recommended dose of Pepto-Bismol in the dog is 2.2 ml per kg of body weight three or four times daily. The technician should be aware that Pepto-Bismol may cause the stool to be dark to black in color, giving the false impression that melena is present when it truly is not.

In animals who are slightly to mildly dehydrated, some form of fluid therapy is appropriate. Fluids can be administered by mouth if the patient is not vomiting. Commercial water and electrolyte solutions, such as Gatorade, can be used to restore hydration and correct electrolyte imbalances. Alternatively, a homemade solution can be prepared inexpensively. One formula that has been recommended consists of 3.5 g of sodium chloride, 2.5 g of sodium bicarbonate, 1.5 g of potassium chloride and 20 g of glucose added to 1 liter of water. Approximately 13.6 ml per kg per day of this solution will meet the maintenance requirements of the patient.

If the dog is mildly to moderately dehydrated or is vomiting, subcutaneous fluids are indicated. Lactated Ringer's solution is the fluid of choice. If signs have been prolonged, the lactated Ringer's solution can be supplemented with potassium chloride. Generally, the dose of subcutaneous fluids is 4.5 to 9.0 ml per kg of body weight administered at multiple sites. This can be repeated if necessary.

Client education is an essential part of the symptomatic care for acute gastroenteritis. The client should be informed that a definitive diagnosis has not been established and that merely the symptoms are being treated. If the animal is getting worse or if the signs persist longer than 36 to 48 hours, the animal should be re-evaluated. The technician should have a concerned, caring attitude during the outpatient visit so that if signs persist, the client will not hesitate to return or call for additional help. In many practices, it is standard procedure to telephone the client in order to receive follow-up progress reports. This ensures close client contact and thus improves the chances of successful management of the problem.

If initial clinical signs are severe or if there is no response to symptomatic therapy, hospitalization is necessary. A major indication for hospitalization is the need for intravenous fluid therapy. Details about intravenous fluid therapy have been discussed earlier.

Dogs with severe acute gastroenteritis may also benefit from the parenteral administration of an antibiotic. Damage to the mucosal barrier of the intestines and altered intestinal motility may result in bacteremia. The parenteral route is preferred in order to provide effective tissue antibiotic levels. This is necessary because of potential decreased intestinal absorption. Oral administration of antibiotics is not recommended in the vomiting patient. Antibiotics of choice in an adult animal would be a combination of ampicillin and gentamicin. Spectinomycin is a safe alternative for puppies since nephrotoxicity is less than with gentamicin. Specific therapy is indicated if an etiologic agent is identified by fecal culture, such as erythromycin for the treatment of *Campylobacter* and chloramphenicol for the treatment of *Salmonella* or *Yersinia*.

The oral administration of aminoglycoside antibiotics (neomycin, gentamicin, kanamycin) is controversial. The proposed justification is that since the aminoglycosides are poorly absorbed from the gut, they will sterilize the gut and prevent absorption of harmful bacteria through the damaged intestinal wall. The counterargument is that this practice may actually do harm. In certain species the aminoglycosides have been shown to damage the intestinal mucosa. It has been demonstrated that complete sterilization of the gut with any antibiotic or combination of antibiotics is impossible. Instead, oral antibiotics may alter the normal population of bacteria in the intestinal tract so that disease-producing organisms may predominate. In certain bacterial gastroenteridities, antibiotics may prolong the shedding of the infective organism in the feces.

Medications that alter the motility of the gastrointestinal tract may be indicated in cases of severe gastroenteritis. Improved understanding of the pathophysiology of intestinal motility has resulted in the more rational use of medications that are used to symptomatically treat vomiting and diarrhea. Anticholinergics decrease the resistance to intestinal flow and thus are of questionable efficacy in treating diarrhea. Antispasmodics are of minimal benefit as well.

Narcotics and narcotic-like drugs increase the rhythmical segmental contractions of the bowel, slow the passage of ingesta and thus help to control diarrhea. These drugs should be used cautiously because of potential problems. Generally, they are reserved for more chronic or severe cases that are unresponsive to conservative therapy. A major disadvantage of the narcotic derivatives is that they can cause central nervous system depression. The decreased ingesta flow rate may result in increased absorption of toxins and altered bacterial flora in the gut. These compounds are contraindicated in the presence of intestinal obstruction.

Drugs used for the treatment of acute vomiting can be divided into several categories (Table 10–9).

Drugs that have been used to decrease gastric acidity include anticholinergics. Anticholinergics probably have no effect on acid secretion. Antacids do not decrease the secretion of acid; however, they neutralize the acid that is produced. Antacids must be given frequently, since their duration of action is brief. Paradoxically, if antacids are not given frequently, total daily acid secretion increases. Antacids administered according to a two or three times per day schedule are probably of no value and may, in fact, be harmful. In most practices, more frequent administration is not practical. Drugs that block H_2 (histamine) receptors inhibit secretion of gastric acid. Cimetidine (Tagamet, SK&F Lab Co.) works by this mechanism. Phenothiazine-derivative tranquilizers—for example, chlorpromazine—work on the vomiting center of the central nervous system. These drugs are effective at controlling vomiting at much lower doses than the usual tranquilizer doses. These agents should be used with caution in dehydrated patients because of their blood pressure–lowering effects. Other antihistamines act by inhibiting a neural center involved in vomiting called the chemoreceptor trigger zone. Vomiting induced by certain drugs, for example, digoxin, is mediated by this center. Vomiting caused by motion sickness or vertigo may also respond to drugs in this group.

When the patient has improved, oral fluids and frequent, small, bland meals can be instituted. After discharge from the hospital, the dog can be treated as already described under outpatient management.

Table 10–9
ROSTER OF COMMONLY USED DRUGS FOR THE TREATMENT OF ACUTE GASTROENTERITIS

Narcotics
  Lomotil (diphenoxalate, atropine)
  Donnagel-PG (opium, atropine, hyoscyamine, kaolin, pectin)
  Imodium (loperamide)
  Diban (opium, atropine)
  Parapectolin (paregoric, pectin, kaolin)
Tranquilizers
  Thorazine (chlorpromazine)
  Darbazine (prochlorperazine, isopropamide)
  Tigan (trimethobenzamide)
Anticholinergics
  Atropine
  Secopolamine
  Methscopolamine
  Robinol-V (glycopyrrolate)
  Centrine (aminopentamide hydrogen sulfate)
  Diathal (diphemanil methylsulfate, penicillin, dihydrostreptomycin, chlorpheniramine maleate)
  Darbazine (prochlorperazine, isopropamide)
  Biosol-M (methscopolamine, neomycin)
  Amoforal (kanamycin, aminopeptamide hydrogen sulfate, pectin)
  Sulkamycin tablets (phthalylsulfacetamide, neomycin, belladonna alkaloids, pectin)
Locally Active Agents
  Kaopectate (kaolin, pectin)
  Kao-forte (kaolin, pectin)
  Pepto-Bismol (bismuth subsalicylate)
Smooth Muscle Relaxants ("Antispasmodics")
  Oct-Vet (isometheptene)
  Novin (dipyrone)
  Jenotone (aminopropazine)
  Myoquin-65V, Neopavin (ethaverine)
Antihistamines
  Dramamine (dimenhydrinate)
  Bonine (meclizine)
H_2 Blockers
  Tagamet (cimetidine)

Canine Viral Enteritis

The two most important causes of viral enteritis in the dog are canine coronavirus and canine parvovirus. Other viral agents can occasionally produce gastroenteritis. They include canine distemper and canine rotavirus.

Clinical signs vary from subtle lethargy and anorexia to severe, rapidly fatal hemorrhagic gastroenteritis. Dogs of any age can be affected; however, the more severe cases typically occur between 6 and 20 weeks of age. On physical examination, the pups are usually febrile, depressed and dehydrated. Vomiting or diarrhea may be observed. The stool may be watery, watery with flecks of blood or severely hemorrhagic. Occasionally, infected dogs will display abdominal tenderness or pain. The presence of fever is more commonly associated with parvovirus than with coronavirus. A history of vaccination does not rule out viral enteritis, since maternal antibodies may have prevented a protective immune response to the vaccination. It should be noted that the gastroenteritis and clinical disease secondary to coronavirus infection is much less severe than that seen with parvovirus infection.

Hemograms are usually normal with coronavirus enteritis but may be abnormal with parvovirus enteritis. Transient leukopenia is present in roughly one third to one half of dogs with parvovirus infections. Severely leukopenic patients may develop secondary infections because of a compromised immune system.

Plain abdominal radiographs do not reveal specific changes. Gastrointestinal contrast study changes may mimic small bowel obstruction. Abnormalities include dilated loops of bowel, tremendously prolonged passage time and gas-capped fluid lines.

Definitive diagnosis is possible by several techniques. The viruses may be detected in the stool by electron microscopy. An ELISA performed on the feces can detect parvoviral antigen and can be used to demonstrate the virus in the feces during the period of active viral shedding. This period corresponds to the clinical illness.

It should be stressed that the treatment of canine viral gastroenteritis is supportive, since there are no effective antiviral agents. This treatment includes aggressive intravenous fluid therapy, antibiotics, injectable anti-emetics and keeping the animal clean and comfortable. One other complication seen with parvovirus infection, to which the technician should be alert, is the development of hypoglycemia. If profound weakness and/or seizures develop, a blood glucose level should be determined.

A myocardial form of canine parvovirus has been described in young pups. This form of the disease is characterized by sudden death in otherwise healthy pups; however, it appears to be becoming less common. This may be due to the fact that most pups have maternal antibodies at the critical period when they are susceptible to the myocardial form.

Both canine parvovirus and coronavirus are highly contagious. The major route of the infection is fecal-oral. Dogs showing clinical signs will shed large numbers of viral particles for 1 week to 2 weeks. The canine parvovirus is hardy; therefore, once the environment is contaminated, infective virus will survive for prolonged periods. The virus has been shown to remain infectious in dog feces held at room temperature for longer than 6 months.

Good sanitation will reduce the numbers of infective virus in the hospital environment. Dilute hypochlorite (chlorine bleach and water, diluted to a ratio of 1:32) solutions have significant viricidal properties. Since the virus is ubiquitous, however, the best means of prevention is an appropriate immunization program.

NEPHROLOGY-UROLOGY

Canine Uroliths

A *urolith* is a pathological stone formed from mineral salts found in the urinary tract. Clinical signs depend on location, number, size, shape and whether there is concurrent urinary tract infection. Urolith classification is generally based upon the predominant mineral component, for example, phosphate or urate. In the dog, greater than 90 percent of the uroliths are located in the bladder and urethra, and less than 10 percent are located in the kidneys. Although uroliths can occur in any breed, some breeds suspected to be at greater risk include the miniature schnauzer, dalmatian, dachshund, pug, English bulldog, Welsh corgi, basset hound, Pekingese and Scottish terrier.

If the urolith is located in the bladder, there may be no clinical signs, but more commonly stranguria, increased frequency of urination (pollakiuria) and hematuria will be seen. If the urolith is in the urethra, there may be frequent attempts to urinate and dribbling of urine. If the urethra is completely obstructed by the stone or stones, abdominal distention, pain, anorexia, depression and vomiting will be observed.

Laboratory findings generally are not specific for uroliths. Radiology, including contrast studies such as cystograms and pneumocystograms, may be necessary to establish the diagnosis. Generally speaking, uroliths are managed surgically. A prescription diet (S/D, Hills) has been advocated as a means of medically treating phosphate uroliths. The diet is high in sodium and low in protein and phosphorus and has an acidifying effect on urine. Dissolution of the uroliths occurs over a period of weeks. Unfortunately, this medical approach has several important limitations. A prescription S/D diet is effective in the dissolution of only phosphate calculi and is not recommended as a long-term maintenance diet.

The overall recurrence rate for bladder stones is high, approximately 25 percent. Therefore, efforts to reduce the chance of recurrence are very important. The first step is to analyze the mineral composition of the stone, since different stone types are managed differently. It is also important to determine whether infection is present and, if so, which antibiotics are most likely to be effective.

Several preventative measures are appropriate regardless of the stone type. These include elimination of any infection and stimulation of increased urine output. The urine output can be increased by salting the diet and thereby increasing water intake.

Depending on the specific stone type, it may also be desirable to initiate dietary therapy and modify the urine pH. Ammonium chloride is commonly used to acidify the urine, and sodium bicarbonate is used to alkalinize it.

Since the recurrence rate for uroliths is high, client education is extremely important. First, long-term therapeutic compliance will be achieved only if the importance of these measures is stressed to the client. Second, the owner should be aware of signs that indicate recurrence of the problem.

Feline Urological Syndrome

Feline urological syndrome is the term used to describe a condition of unknown etiology in cats characterized by dysuria, hematuria, pollakiuria, urinating in uncommon places and occasionally urethral obstruction. Urethral obstruction, if it occurs, is potentially fatal because of the associated severe metabolic derangements. The emergency treatment of feline urethral obstruction is covered in Chapter 9.

Since recurrence of the urethral obstruction is frequent, some clinicians prefer to routinely use indwelling urethral catheters for a brief period of time following relief of the obstruction. The justification for the use of indwelling catheters is to maintain urine flow without the trauma associated with recatheterization and manual compression of the bladder. Indwelling urethral catheters should be used judiciously because of the risk of ascending urinary tract infection and catheter-induced injury to the bladder or urethra. Complications associated with the use of indwelling catheters can be minimized if an appropriate catheter is selected. Commercially manufactured polypropylene catheters (Sovereign tomcat catheters and open-end tomcat catheters, Sherwood Medical Industries) can be either too short or too long. Therefore, care should be taken to select a catheter with an appropriate length. Soft, flexible polyvinyl catheters, such as Sovereign sterile disposable feeding tube and urethral catheter, are preferred because of decreased damage to the urethral and bladder mucosa. In order to pass these catheters, they are kept frozen until immediately before use. This will make the catheter sufficiently rigid to allow passage in a male cat. The catheter should be well lubricated prior to passage.

Indwelling urethral catheters are generally secured by suturing the catheter to the prepuce. Adhesive tape is attached longitudinally and transversely to the end of the catheter. If the catheter is wet when the tape is applied, it may not stick. Two simple interrupted sutures on either side of the prepuce penetrate the tape and thus prevent movement of the catheter. If analgesia is required to place the sutures, the prepuce can be numbed by applying an ice cube for 1 minute or 2 minutes. When the catheter is sutured in place it should be done in such a way that there is no chance of kinking. An Elizabethan collar can be used to prevent the cat from removing the indwelling catheter.

In order to prevent ascending urinary tract infection, sterile technique is required when placing and maintaining the indwelling catheter. The collection apparatus should be a closed, sterile system. The entire system—catheter, plastic tubing and collection bottle—must be sterile initially and must be kept sealed to prevent bacterial contamination. Povidone-iodine ointment should be applied several times a day at the point at which the catheter exits the urethra.

Indwelling urethral catheters should be used for as brief a time as possible. The prophylactic use of antimicrobials does not reduce infection. If infection does develop, it is frequently caused by an organism resistant to the prophylactic antimicrobial.

Since the recurrence rate for feline urological syndrome is high, preventative measures are an important aspect of its medical management. Unfortunately, since the etiology of feline urological syndrome is unknown, preventative measures are largely empirical. The most frequently recommended preventative measures include providing an ample supply of fresh, potable water, cleaning the litter pan frequently and lightly salting the food in order to increase water intake and thus urine volume. Exclusive feeding of diets that contain 20 mg of magnesium per 100 kcal or less and that maintain a urine pH of 6.4 or less is the most important preventive measure. Certain diets, such as C/D or Feline Maintenance (Hills), meet this requirement. Although urinary acidification with ammonium chloride has been recommended, it should be emphasized that some diets, such as the ones mentioned above, cause urinary acidification, and additional acidifiers are contraindicated. The basis of acidifying the urine is to increase the solubility of this crystalline material, which is incriminated as the cause of feline urological syndrome.

If ammonium chloride is used with a nonacidifying diet, it should be thoroughly mixed with the food in order to improve palatability. It should also be administered with every meal. Any change in diet or introduction of a food additive—for example, ammonium chloride or salt—should be done gradually over several days. This will reduce the chances of the cat's rejecting the new or altered food. Enteric-coated ammonium chloride tablets are not effective in the cat.

Chronic Renal Failure

Animals in renal failure should be fed diets containing reduced quantities of high-quality protein and adequate nonprotein calories. This can be accomplished by using prescription diets such as K/D (Hills). K/D is a moderate protein-restricted diet available for dogs in canned, semimoist and dry forms. Feline K/D is a canned product suitable for use in uremic cats.

If desired, homemade diets can be used (Lewis et al., 1987). The following is a recipe for a moderately low-protein diet for dogs:

> ¼ lb. regular ground beef
> 1 hard-boiled egg, finely chopped
> 2 cups cooked rice without salt
> 3 slices white bread, crumbled
> 1 tsp. calcium carbonate
> Balanced vitamin and mineral supplement

The meat should be braised, retaining the fat, and thoroughly mixed with the other ingredients. This recipe will meet the daily requirements of a 13.5-kg dog.

The following is an example of a homemade protein-restricted diet for cats:

> ¼ lb. liver
> 2 large eggs, hard boiled
> 2 cups cooked rice without salt
> 1 T vegetable oil
> 1 tsp. calcium carbonate
> Balanced vitamin and mineral supplement

Dice and braise the liver, retaining fat. This recipe provides a total of 635 kcal per pound.

Many animals with renal failure are anorectic because of nausea and vomiting. Small, frequent meals are recommended to reduce the nausea. If the animal can tolerate food orally but is not eating, feeding by means of an orogastric tube is recommended. The diets described can be administered through a stomach tube if the ingredients are thoroughly mixed with water in a kitchen blender.

Supportive therapy for chronic renal failure includes the use of phosphorous binders, anabolic steroids, sodium bicarbonate, sodium chloride, calcium and vitamin D metabolites. The use of these treatments should be based on documented abnormalities, since the inappropriate or incorrect use of these agents can do more harm than good.

ORTHOPEDICS

Canine Hip Dysplasia

Hip dysplasia refers to a developmental problem of the canine coxofemoral joint. Subluxation of the femoral head leads to abnormal wear and eventual degenerative joint disease. The acetabulum is more shallow than normal, and the femoral head is flattened.

The etiology of hip dysplasia is multifactorial. Genetics and environmental factors such as nutrition appear to be important. Hip dysplasia is seen in most large breeds and is inherited by a polygenic mode of inheritance. This means that many genes are responsible for its development. It is also quantitative in its expression. In other words, affected dogs can show slight or severe changes. As is characteristic for traits with a polygenic mode of inheritance, hip dysplasia is modified by environmental factors. For example, it has been suggested that dogs fed a high-calorie diet during growth have an increased incidence, whereas dogs fed a low-calorie diet have a decreased incidence.

The Orthopedic Foundation of America in Columbia, MO, is an organization established to evaluate the hip radiographs of potential breeding dogs. Radiologists identify those dogs with radiographically normal hip joints. Unfortunately, because of the factors mentioned, breeding two radiographically normal dogs does not ensure normal progeny. It is better to evaluate entire families (siblings and progeny) when selecting dogs to be included in a breeding program to decrease the incidence of hip dysplasia. It is also important to recognize that good hip joints should not be the sole criterion for selection. Other traits, such as disposition, working ability and conformation, should also be considered.

The clinical signs of hip dysplasia vary tremendously from occasional slight discomfort to a severe disabling disease. It should be remembered that the clinical signs of hip dysplasia do not always correlate with the severity of hip dysplasia detected radiographically.

Dogs with hip dysplasia will respond differently to varying levels of exercise. Some dogs are most comfortable with minimal activity, yet others do best with a regular regimen of moderate exercise. Swimming is an excellent form of exercise, since muscle tone is increased with the hip joints in a non–weight-bearing position. Any exercise program should be instituted gradually. Forced sudden activity such as ball playing or rough play should be discouraged. Severely affected dogs should be treated symptomatically with analgesics and anti-inflammatory drugs.

Several surgical procedures have been advocated for the treatment of hip dysplasia. They include procedures such as pectineus myotomy, pelvic osteotomy, excision arthroplasty and total hip prosthesis. A discussion of these surgical procedures is beyond the scope of this chapter.

Intervertebral Disk Disease

Intervertebral disk disease is a relatively common problem affecting the spinal cord of chondrodystrophoid and other breeds. Breeds commonly affected include dachshunds, Pekingese, cocker spaniels, poodles, pugs and beagles. The chondrodystrophoid breeds tend to develop signs at an earlier age than the non-chondrodystrophoid breeds.

The intervertebral disks are structures located between the vertebrae and function as a shock-absorbing system. The disk itself is composed of two parts—the firm fibrous outer anulus and the softer inner nucleus. In intervertebral disk disease, the anulus undergoes degeneration and the nuclear material protrudes or is completely extruded. The result is compression of the spinal cord with the subsequent development of neurological signs. These signs vary from simple pain to complete paralysis.

Intervertebral disk disease can be managed either conservatively with cage confinement and anti-inflammatory drugs or more aggressively with neurosurgery. Management decisions are based on the history, the neurological signs and the wishes of the owner.

If conservative therapy is elected, the technician plays a vital role. Extreme care should be taken in handling the patient because movement may result in the extrusion of additional disk material and worsening of signs. In order to reduce handling, these patients should be placed in lower cages whenever possible. Since these patients are frequently in severe pain, gentle, compassionate care is essential. Many cases will benefit from some of the physical therapy techniques described earlier.

Dogs with intervertebral disk disease receiving anti-inflammatory drugs, such as dexamethasone, may develop secondary problems, such as gastrointestinal hemorrhage or acute pancreatitis. Consequently, these patients should be observed closely for fever, anorexia, abdominal pain and hemorrhagic vomiting and diarrhea.

Recommended Reading

Feldman EC and Nelson RW: Canine and Feline Endocrinology and Reproduction. Philadelphia, WB Saunders Co., 1987.

Lewis LD, Morris ML and Hand MS: Small Animal Clinical Nutrition III. Topeka, KS, Mark Morris Associates, 1987.

Schultz RD: Theoretical and practical aspects of an immunization program for dogs and cats. JAVMA 181:1142–1149, 1982.

11

Veterinary Anesthesia

JANYCE L. CORNICK

INTRODUCTION

Anesthesia is a necessary part of veterinary medicine for restraint, elimination of pain sensation during surgical and medical procedures, control of seizure activity and humane euthanasia. Anesthesia is an area in which veterinary technicians can contribute significantly to their employers and their patients.

Anesthesia is defined as total loss of sensation in a body part (local anesthesia) or in the entire body (general anesthesia), which results from administration of a drug (or drugs) that depresses the activity of part or all of the nervous system. The safe and effective use of anesthetic agents requires a general understanding of their pharmacological actions and the refinement of several technical and interpretive skills for a variety of animal species. Anesthesia requires a thorough preanesthetic evaluation of every patient, formulation of an anesthetic plan based on the patient, the surgical or medical procedure to be performed, drug availability, and the experience of the anesthetist. Careful patient monitoring will be required throughout the anesthetic period.

Five topics will be discussed in this chapter, including (1) anesthetic pharmacology, (2) anesthetic equipment, (3) anesthetic monitoring and ventilatory support, (4) anesthetic management of selected domestic species and (5) anesthetic emergencies.

PHARMACOLOGY OF ANESTHETIC AGENTS

Preanesthetic agents are an important part of safe patient management. Drugs most commonly used as preanesthetic agents

in veterinary medicine include anticholinergic agents, tranquilizers, sedatives, opioids, and combinations of an opioid with a tranquilizer or sedative (neuroleptanalgesic combinations). These agents are used in the practice of anesthesia to (1) aid in animal restraint; (2) allay apprehension and/or minimize pain; (3) decrease the quantity of potentially more severe cardiopulmonary depressant drugs used to produce sedation, analgesia or general anesthesia; (4) produce a safe, smooth and uncomplicated induction, maintenance and recovery from general anesthesia; (5) minimize the adverse and potentially toxic effects of concurrently administered drugs used for general anesthesia; and (6) minimize autonomic reflex activity.

Anticholinergic Agents

These agents are used to prevent bradycardia associated with increased vagal tone and to prevent excessive upper airway and salivary secretions. Atropine and glycopyrrolate are the two most commonly used drugs. Although atropine is more economical to use, glycopyrrolate offers some advantages, including a longer duration of action, less tendency to promote cardiac arrhythmias and perhaps less suppression of intestinal motility (Short, 1987). Glycopyrrolate appears to increase heart rate less than does atropine; this may be beneficial in animals with heart disease in which the increase in myocardial oxygen consumption associated with a profound increase in heart rate could be detrimental. Glycopyrrolate, unlike atropine, does not cross the placental barrier, thus having no effect on the fetus during cesarean section.

Although many veterinarians use anticholinergic agents as a routine part of a preanesthetic regimen, their use has become more selective and is based on the needs of the individual patient, the anticipated response to the anesthetic agents, and the tendency to develop bradycardia or excessive salivation. Procedures that may increase vagal tone include traction on abdominal organs and procedures involving the neck, throat and eye. Anesthetic agents that promote bradycardia include opioids, xylazine, barbiturates and gas anesthetics. Dissociative agents, such as ketamine, may cause excessive salivation, which may be minimized by using an anticholinergic agent.

The use of anticholinergic agents is controversial in large animal species. They are never used routinely in horses because of the resulting ileus and subsequent colic. Nor are they recommended for use in ruminants because the secretions become more viscid and difficult to clear from the respiratory tract. Anticholinergic agents may be used in swine in conjunction with drugs known to promote bradycardia or excessive salivation. Anticholinergic agents should be used in horses and ruminants only when life threatening bradycardia develops. (See Table 11–5 for normal ranges for heart rate.)

Tranquilizers and Sedatives

These agents are used to depress the central nervous system to aid in restraint and to reduce anxiety and struggling. This action helps to minimize stress during both induction and recovery and to reduce the requirements for the more potent agents used for induction and maintenance of anesthesia.

Tranquilizers used in veterinary medicine include phenothiazines such as acepromazine (PromAce, Fort Dodge), butyrophenones such as droperidol (Innovar-Vet, Pitman-Moore) and benzodiazepines such as diazepam (Valium, Hoffmann-LaRoche) and zolazepam (Telazol, AH Robbins). Acepromazine calms animals and decreases motor activity; however, animals may be readily aroused by external stimuli, especially animals that are highly excitable or apprehensive. Acepromazine itself does not provide analgesia but may enhance the analgesic effects of concurrently used drugs. Acepromazine has a long duration of action and is dependent on metabolism by the liver; thus acepromazine should be avoided in patients with liver disease and in geriatric and pediatric patients. Other side effects and contraindications are listed in Table 11–1.

Butyrophenones have a mechanism of action and side effects similar to those of the phenothiazines but do not promote seizure activity. They should not be used in horses because of the high incidence of an excitatory response.

Benzodiazepine tranquilizers produce minimal tranquilization and may even increase excitability in dogs, cats and horses. Diazepam is rarely used alone but is useful for potentiating the effect of concurrently used premedication (such as opioids), for providing muscle relaxation in association with the dissociative drugs (such as ketamine) and for reducing the requirements for induction agents (such as barbiturates). Because of minimal cardiopulmonary effects, diazepam is useful in geriatric and pediatric animals and animals with heart disease. Benzodiazepines have anticonvulsant activity and are useful in patients with a history of seizures or any neurological disorder. Diazepam is usually used intravenously because its carrier, propylene glycol, causes pain when given intramuscularly.

Xylazine (Rompun, Haver) and detomidine (Dormosedan, SmithKline Beecham) are classified as sedatives and produce excellent calming, muscle relaxation and analgesia. Because of the profound cardiovascular effects (Table 11–1), xylazine should be used only in healthy dogs and cats and should always be used with an anticholinergic agent in these species. Thermoregulation is impaired in cats for several hours following xylazine administration, so extremes in environmental temperature should be avoided. Xylazine and detomidine are used most frequently in horses. Xylazine is also used in ruminants; large and small ruminants are sensitive to xylazine, and low doses must be used (Table 11–2). A reversal agent, yohimbine, is available for use in veterinary medicine (Table 11–2).

Opioids

Opioids are commonly used in veterinary medicine to produce analgesia and sedation. In horses and cats, they should be used in conjunction with a tranquilizer or sedative because excitement is likely when pure opioids, such as morphine or oxymorphone, are used. Opioids promote bradycardia which is responsive to anticholinergic agents, but depression of cardiac contractility is minimal. Opioids produce respiratory depression; thus, apnea and hypoventilation during general anesthesia are more likely to occur when opioids are used. Ventilatory support may be required to alleviate this effect, especially in animals with underlying respiratory abnormalities (such as pneumonia or diaphragmatic hernia).

Thermoregulation is impaired by opioids, which may delay the return of normothermia following anesthesia. External stimuli should be minimized prior to general anesthesia in animals that have received opioids because they are hyper-responsive, especially to noise. An advantage of opioids is the availability of opioid antagonists (such as naloxone) to reverse their effects (Table 11–2).

Neuroleptanalgesia is defined as a state of profound central nervous system depression and analgesia produced by the combination of a tranquilizer or sedative with an opioid agent (see Tables 11–2 and 11–9). Animals may become unconscious but remain responsive to external stimuli. These drug combinations provide more profound analgesia and calming than is the case when either agent is used alone and may provide adequate analgesia and restraint for procedures such as radiography, wound debridement, suturing of skin lacerations and ear treatment. When a neuroleptanalgesic combination is used for premedication, dosage requirements of the agents used for induction and maintenance are greatly reduced.

Dissociative Agents

Dissociative agents are usually used as part of an induction or maintenance protocol, but they may be used alone in cats as a premedication to produce immobilization for intravenous catheter placement and short non-invasive procedures and to facilitate induction of general anesthesia. They will be discussed in more detail in the following paragraphs.

Induction agents are incorporated into an anesthetic plan to facilitate smooth and rapid transition from consciousness to unconsciousness for maintenance of general anesthesia. Agents most commonly used include the ultrashort-acting barbiturates, guaifenesin, dissociative agent combinations, and gas anesthetics via mask delivery. *Agents for maintenance* of anesthesia are most commonly the gas anesthetic agents. Effective

Table 11-1
EFFECTS OF ANESTHETIC DRUGS USED FOR PREMEDICATION AND INDUCTION

Drug	Cardiovascular	Pulmonary	Adverse Effects	Contraindications
Premedications				
Acepromazine	Hypotension Antiarrhythmic effect	Minimal	Penile paralysis (stallions) Lowers seizure threshold Promotes hypothermia	Liver disease History of seizures Dehydration Hypovolemia Shock Heart disease Geriatric patients Pediatric patients

Diazepam	Minimal	Minimal	Hypotension if injected
			  too rapidly
			Burns when given IM
				Should not use alone
				  because excitement is
				  possible

Xylazine/detomidine	Bradycardia
	Conduction disturbances
	Hypotension
	Arrhythmias with
	  halothane anesthesia
	  in dogs and cats
		Respiratory depression	Impaired
			  thermoregulation
			Hyperglycemia
			Profound muscle
			  relaxation may
			  exacerbate upper
			  respiratory
			  abnormalities
				Heart disease
				Geriatric patients
				Pediatric patients
				Ruminants require *low*
				  doses

Opioids	Minimal
	Bradycardia that is
	  responsive to
	  anticholinergic
	  administration
		Respiratory depression	Impaired
			  thermoregulation
			  (panting in dogs)
			Hyperresponsive to
			  external stimuli
			Excitement in cats and
			  horses (pure agonists)
				Use with tranquilizer or
				  sedative in horses and
				  cats

Induction Agents				

Barbiturates	Myocardial depression
	Arrhythmias
	Hypotension
		Respiratory depression
		  (apnea)
			Excessive salivation
			Laryngospasm
			Tissue necrosis with
			  perivascular injection
				Heart disease
				Liver disease
				Geriatric patients (low
				  doses)
				Pediatric patients (low
				  doses)
				"Sight" hounds
				  (methohexital only)
				Obese animals (dose on
				  lean weight)

Ketamine/tiletamine	Increase in heart rate
	  and blood pressure
	Some direct myocardial
	  depression
		Minimal
		Apneustic breathing
		May cause apnea when
		  given IV
			Profuse salivation
			Muscle rigidity when
			  used alone
			Convulsions with high
			  doses
			Poor visceral analgesia
				Never use alone except
				  in cats
				Must have good sedation
				  prior to administration
				  in horses (IV only)
				Animals with seizure
				  history

Guaifenesin	Minimal	Minimal	Tissue necrosis with perivascular injection	

Table 11–2
DOSAGES* (mg/kg) OF COMMONLY USED ANESTHETIC AGENTS FOR PREMEDICATION AND CHEMICAL RESTRAINT

Agent	Dog	Cat	Horse	Cow	Goat/Sheep	Pig
Anticholinergics						
Atropine	0.02–0.04	0.02–0.04	—	0.04 (max. 20 mg)	0.04	0.04
Glycopyrrolate	0.011	0.011	—	—	—	0.003
Tranquilizers						
Acepromazine	0.055–0.22	0.11–0.22	0.022–0.088	0.044–0.088	0.044–0.088	0.22
Diazepam	0.22	0.22	0.022–0.088	0.022–0.088	0.022–0.088	0.22–0.44
Sedatives						
Xylazine	0.44–1.1	0.44–1.1	0.44–1.1	0.022–0.11	0.022–0.066	1.1–2.2
Detomidine	—	—	0.01–0.02	—	—	—
Opioids						
Oxymorphone	0.11–0.22	0.055–0.011†	0.011–0.044†	—	—	—
Butorphanol	0.11–0.44	0.22–0.44	0.011–0.044	0.011–0.022	0.022–0.044	0.22–0.33
Morphine	0.44–1.1	0.11–0.22†	0.044–0.11†	—	—	0.44–0.88
Meperidine	0.44–1.1	0.22–0.44†	0.22–0.66†	—	—	0.44–1.1
Pentazocine	0.22–0.44	0.11	0.44–0.88	—	—	—
Buprenorphine	0.01–0.015	0.01–0.015	0.01–0.02	—	—	—
Neuroleptanalgesic Combinations						
Droperidol/fentanyl (Innovar)	1 ml/15–30 kg	—	—	—	—	1 ml/23 kg
Acepromazine	0.22	0.22	—	—	—	—
Oxymorphone	0.11–0.22	0.055–0.11	—	—	—	—
Acepromazine	0.22	0.22	0.044	—	—	—
Butorphanol	0.22	0.22–0.44	0.022	—	—	—
Xylazine	0.22	0.22	0.66	0.022	0.022	—
Butorphanol	0.11–0.22	0.22–0.44	0.022–0.044	0.022–0.055	0.022	—
Reversal Agents						
Yohimbine‡ (alpha₂ antagonist)	0.11	0.11	0.11	0.11	0.11	0.11
Naloxone (opioid antagonist)	0.0066	0.0066	0.005–0.022	—	—	0.0066

*Most agents may be used IV or IM. As a general rule, use higher dose range IM and lower dose range IV.
†Use these opioids in these species *only* in conjunction with a tranquilizer or sedative.
‡Administer yohimbine "to effect" in large animal species. Calculate recommended dose and give in ¼ increments until reversal of sedation is observed.
Adapted from Muir WW: Handbook of Veterinary Anesthesia. St. Louis, The CV Mosby Co, 1989, pp. 20–21.

anesthetic maintenance for short periods of anesthesia may be achieved using various combinations of those drugs used for induction.

Ultrashort-Acting Barbiturates

This group of drugs includes thiamylal and thiopental (thiobarbiturates) and methohexital (oxybarbiturate). They may be used without preanesthetic medication to produce rapid loss of consciousness; however, because of some undesirable cardiopulmonary effects (see Table 11–1), it is safer to use premedications to facilitate intravenous injection and to decrease the dosage required to achieve unconsciousness. The degree of respiratory depression associated with barbiturate administration is related to dosage and rate of administration. One should be prepared to intubate and provide ventilatory support if apnea occurs.

Detrimental cardiopulmonary effects are more likely to occur when large doses are administered rapidly and when higher concentrations are used. Although solutions up to 10 percent in strength are used in large animals, it is preferable to use a solution no stronger than 5 percent in small animals and safest to use a 2 percent solution. More dilute solutions

will decrease the likelihood of adverse effects and cause less tissue necrosis with accidental perivascular injection. Should perivascular administration occur, 2 percent lidocaine diluted 1:9 with sterile saline should be infiltrated into the injection site. Barbiturates are metabolized by the liver and should be avoided in animals with liver disease. Sighthounds (greyhounds, Irish wolfhounds, whippets) are unable to metabolize thiobarbiturates effectively, resulting in a prolonged recovery. An alternative induction method for sighthounds is with methohexital (6 to 11 mg/kg), which acts in much the same way as the thiobarbiturates but is effectively metabolized. Excitement during recovery may be more pronounced with methohexital administration, especially following short procedures, so preanesthetic tranquilization is indicated.

Dissociative Agent Combinations

Dissociative agents produce immobilization and superficial analgesia. Swallowing and ocular reflexes remain intact, and muscle tone is increased. These agents may be administered intramuscularly or intravenously; however, intramuscular administration requires higher doses and results in a prolonged recovery. The intramuscular route is most commonly used in cats, dogs, small ruminants and swine and is *never* used in horses.

Concurrent administration of an anticholinergic agent may be needed in some species (cats, dogs, swine) owing to excessive salivation. Although some direct depression of heart function occurs, an increase in sympathetic tone compensates for this effect by increasing heart rate and arterial blood pressure. This effect on heart rate and blood pressure offers an advantage over the thiobarbiturates for use in debilitated and septic patients or patients with heart disease. Since elimination of ketamine depends on both liver metabolism and renal excretion, high dosages should be avoided in animals with liver or kidney disease.

Ketamine offers an alternative method of induction for sighthounds and is most commonly used in combination with diazepam for this purpose. *Telazol* (AH Robbins) is a commercial drug combination containing equal parts of zolazepam (benzodiazepine) and tiletamine (dissociative), which may be used for both induction and maintenance of anesthesia. Although approved only for intramuscular use, intravenous administration of very low doses provides an effective method for induction and for short-term anesthesia (Table 11–3).

Guaifenesin is an intravenously administered central-acting muscle relaxant that potentiates the effects of concurrently used preanesthetic and anesthetic agents, allowing for lower dosages of these agents to be used. Guaifenesin is used in large animals as part of an induction protocol and may also be incorporated into the anesthetic plan for maintenance of anesthesia with injectable agents. Cardiopulmonary effects are minimal, and there is a wide margin of safety. Excessive dosages may result in paradoxical muscle rigidity of the forelimbs and neck and an apneustic breathing pattern, which is more likely to occur in young animals. Administration is best performed through an indwelling venous catheter because large volumes must be administered and perivascular injection is caustic to tissues.

Inhalation Anesthetics

Agents used in veterinary medicine include isoflurane, halothane and methoxyflurane. These agents produce general anesthesia, which includes unconsciousness, muscle relaxation and analgesia, and are suitable for use in all species. Advantages include more rapid control of changes in depth of anesthesia and a more rapid recovery. However, these agents produce profound effects on cardiopulmonary function and patients must be closely monitored throughout the anesthetic period. The use of gas anesthetics requires more complex and expensive equipment than that used with injectable techniques, and an understanding of this equipment is necessary to use the agents safely and effectively.

Some properties of the gases (Table 11–4) must be reviewed to appreciate the anesthetic vaporizers used to deliver the gases and the speed at which they exert their anesthetic effect. *Vapor pressure* of a gas determines the maximum concentration that may be achieved in the carrier gas (such as oxygen) at any given temperature. For example, methoxyflurane, with a low vapor pressure (23 mm Hg), may only reach a maximum concentration of 3.5 percent at room temperature, while halothane and isoflurane, both with vapor pressures of approximately 240 mm Hg, may reach a maximum concentration of 32 percent at room temperature. This means that a precision vaporizer (see discussion of equipment), which delivers a precise concentration of anesthetic gas according to settings on the vaporizer, is required to avoid potentially lethal concentrations of isoflurane and halothane. On the other hand, methoxyflurane may be used with a nonprecision vaporizer for which exact concentration settings are absent, since it is impossible to achieve the same excessive concentrations possible with the other two agents.

Solubility determines the speed of induction and recovery of the anesthetic gas and is most frequently defined as its distribution between blood and gas phases. Methoxyflurane with a

---

Table 11–3

DRUGS (mg/kg)* COMMONLY USED FOR INDUCTION OR FOR SHORT-DURATION ANESTHESIA

Agent	Dog	Cat	Horse	Cow	Sheep/Goat	Pig
1. Thiamylal	8.8–13	8.8–13	6.6–11	4.4–11	4.4–11	8.8–11
2. Thiopental	8.8–13	8.8–13	6.6–11	4.4–11	4.4–11	8.8–13
3. Guaifenesin	44–88	—	66–132	66–132	66–132	44–88
4. Ketamine	—	2.2–18	—	—	2.2–6.6	2.2–6.6
5. Telazol	2.2–11†	2.2–11†	—	4.4–11	2.2–11	4.4–11†
6. Guaifenesin/thiamylal	33–88	—	44–88	44–88	—	33–88
	2.2–6.6	—	2.2–6.6	2.2–6.6	—	2.2–6.6
7. Guaifenesin/ketamine	33–88	—	44–88	44–88	44–88	—
	1.1	—	1.1–1.5	0.6–1.1	0.6–1.1	—
8. Acepromazine/ketamine	0.11	0.22†	—	—	—	0.44†
	11.0	4.4–11†	—	—	—	2.2–6.6†
9. Xylazine/ketamine	0.66–1.1†	0.66–1.1†	1.1	0.044–0.088†	0.044†	2.2–4.4†
	2.2–11†	4.4–22†	2.2	2.2–6.6†	2.2–6.6	2.2–11†
10. Diazepam/ketamine	0.25	0.25	—	—	0.25–0.55	0.22–0.44
	5.0	5.0	—	—	4.4	4.4
11. Xylazine/telazol	0.44†	0.66†	1.1	0.022–0.11†	0.044–0.088†	0.66–1.1†
	6.6†	2.2–6.6†	1.1–2.2	2.2–6.6†	2.2–6.6†	4.4–6.6†
12. Xylazine/guaifenesin/ketamine	(See Tables giving specific species protocol.)					

*Dosage is for intravenous use unless otherwise designated.
†Indicates protocols that may be used intramuscularly in some species.
Adapted from Muir WW: Handbook of Veterinary Anesthesia. St. Louis, The CV Mosby Co, 1989, p. 76.

Table 11–4
CHARACTERISTICS OF COMMONLY USED INHALATION AGENTS IN VETERINARY MEDICINE

Agent	Vapor Pressure (mm Hg)	Solubility Coefficient	MAC Values				Induction		Maintenance	
			DOG	CAT	HORSE	PIG	SA	LA	SA	LA
Isoflurane	240	1.4	1.5%	1.6%	1.3%	1.47%	2–4%	4–5%	1–3%	2–3%
Halothane	244	2.4	0.87%	1.19%	0.9%	1.25%	2–4%	3–5%	0.5–1.5%	1–2%
Methoxyflurane	23	13.0	0.23%	0.16%	0.3%	*	2–3%	†	0.2–1%	†

*Value not available.
†Methoxyflurane is not used routinely in large animals.
SA = small animal, LA = large animal.

very high solubility is dissolved to a high degree in the blood. This delays the development of a tension (partial pressure) of anesthetic gas in the blood, which is essential for the gas to pass into the brain and render the patient unconscious. This high solubility of methoxyflurane is manifested clinically as a very slow induction of and recovery from general anesthesia, making it undesirable for use as an induction agent. Halothane is much less soluble than methoxyflurane, and isoflurane is the least soluble of the three. Both halothane and isoflurane may be used effectively to achieve induction of anesthesia via mask delivery, and the recoveries are much more rapid.

Minimum alveolar concentration (MAC) is a measure of anesthetic potency by which the gas anesthetic agents may be compared and is used as a guide to deliver adequate but not excessive concentrations for surgical procedures. MAC is defined as the minimum concentration of anesthetic in the alveoli at 1 atmosphere that prevents a response in 50 percent of patients exposed to a painful stimulus. The MAC values have been determined for the commonly used gas anesthetics for many animal species (see Table 11–4). For most surgical procedures in most species, 1.5 to 2.0 times MAC is adequate to maintain a surgical plane of anesthesia. Factors that may decrease the MAC requirement include age (older patients require less), hypothermia, administration of other depressant drugs (such as opioids, tranquilizers), anemia, and diseases such as septicemia.

The anesthetic gases cause a dose-dependent depression of heart function, with isoflurane causing the least effect on the heart at clinically used concentrations. All three gases cause respiratory depression, and ventilation should be assisted (see Ventilatory Support) to minimize the development of hypercapnia and atelectasis. Halothane has the additional undesirable characteristic of sensitizing the heart to catecholamines, which can result in the development of arrhythmias. Methoxyflurane is less likely to induce arrhythmias, and isoflurane does not have this effect. Isoflurane, although more expensive than halothane, is the safest and most versatile anesthetic gas because it may be used in young, old, debilitated and diseased patients with the least detrimental effects.

ANESTHETIC EQUIPMENT

Anesthetic equipment should be organized in a specific location in the hospital, usually the surgery preparation area. This area should be quiet and away from the mainstream hospital traffic. Once the technician knows what anesthetic drugs and equipment the veterinarian wishes to have available, adequate supplies should be stocked and maintained.

Basic equipment and supplies that should be available to provide anesthesia include needles and syringes, intravenous catheters, tape for securing catheters, heparinized saline (2 units of heparin per milliliter of 0.9 percent saline), endotracheal tubes in a variety of sizes, laryngoscope, lubricant for the endotracheal tubes, ophthalmic lubricant, an oxygen source and method of delivery, an apparatus for manual ventilation (i.e., Ambu bag [see Fig. 11–19] or anesthesia machine) and a selection of anesthetic agents. If gas anesthesia is used in the practice, an anesthesia machine, breathing systems and a selection of rebreathing bags and face masks should be available. An emergency drug box (discussed under Anesthetic Emergencies) should also be accessible in this area.

Catheters

Intravenous administration equipment and catheters are covered in Chapter 8. As a general rule of anesthesia, dependable venous access, as with an intravenous catheter taped or glued securely in place, should be available in all anesthetized patients. An intravenous catheter provides a route of administration for polyionic fluids to maintain homeostasis, for additional drugs to maintain anesthesia, which is especially important when injectable techniques are used, and for emergency drug administration if cardiopulmonary arrest occurs.

Endotracheal Tubes

The endotracheal tube provides the connecting link between the patient's airway and the anesthetic equipment. Although it is not essential to place an endotracheal tube when injectable anesthesia is utilized, tubes must be available in rare instances when respiratory arrest dictates the need for artificial ventilation and delivery of oxygen or when the risk of regurgitation and aspiration is increased (as in patients who have not adequately fasted, who have a history of vomiting or who are pregnant). Some veterinarians prefer to place an endotracheal tube routinely during injectable anesthesia as a precautionary measure. Cuffed tubes (Fig. 11–1) are most commonly used and provide for an effective seal within the airway to prevent aspiration and to facilitate effective ventilatory support. Cuffed tubes are available in a wide variety of sizes according to internal diameter (ID) in millimeters, with sizes 2.5 to 14 mm ID

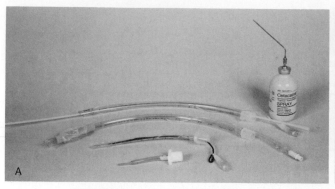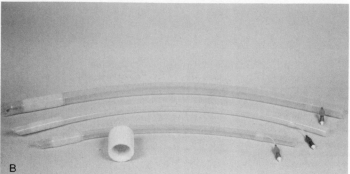

FIGURE 11–1. A, Representative sizes of cuffed endotracheal tubes appropriate for use in small animals, small ruminants and swine. Notice that the top tube and the third tube from the top contain two types of stylets in place as they might be used clinically to facilitate intubation. A noncuffed Cole tube is included at the bottom of the picture. Also pictured at the right is topical anesthetic spray (Cetacaine, Cetylite Industries Inc, Pennsauken, NJ) for desensitizing the larynx prior to intubation. B, Cuffed tubes (Bivona, Gary, IN) used for horses and cattle. An oral speculum, which is placed between the equine incisors to facilitate intubation, is also pictured.

appropriate for dogs, cats, swine and small ruminants and sizes 16 to 30 mm ID for large ruminants and horses. Noncuffed (Cole) tubes (Fig. 11–1) are used in very small patients (such as newborn kittens and puppies, ferrets, birds) because they preserve a larger airway diameter.

Laryngoscopes

Laryngoscopes facilitate intubation in many species and are especially beneficial in small ruminants, swine and cats. These instruments consist of a battery-containing handle with a detachable blade. Blades come in a variety of shapes and sizes. Two styles commonly used in veterinary anesthesia are shown in Figure 11–2.

Anesthetic Machines

The primary purposes of an inhalation anesthetic machine and breathing system are to deliver oxygen, to deliver a controlled amount of an inhalation anesthetic agent and to provide a method for assisting ventilation. The variability of anesthetic machines, which are offered in a wide variety of types and sizes by numerous manufacturers, presents a challenge to the veterinary anesthetist; however, all machines have the same basic components (Fig. 11–3) (Dorsch and Dorsch, 1984A; Hartsfield, 1987).

The four basic components of an anesthetic machine are a *compressed gas source* (oxygen and sometimes nitrous oxide); the *pressure regulator,* which reduces and controls the pressure of gas leaving the compressed gas source to a lower pressure that will not damage the flowmeter; the *flowmeter,* which precisely controls the flow of gas entering the patient's breathing system; and the *vaporizer,* which facilitates delivery of a controlled concentration of an inhalation anesthetic agent into the patient's breathing system.

Another feature on some machines is the pressure gauge, which reflects the amount of gas remaining in the compressed gas tank (Fig. 11–3). Specifically, a full oxygen tank maintains a pressure of approximately 2200 pounds per square inch (psi), and that pressure decreases proportionately as the tank empties. An oxygen flush valve, which is included on most anesthetic machines, delivers oxygen directly and rapidly (35 to 75 liters/minute) to the common gas outlet of the machine, thus bypassing the vaporizer and quickly filling the breathing system with pure oxygen (see Figs. 11–3 and 11–6).

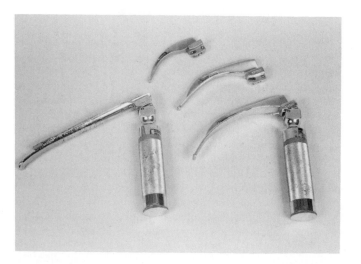

FIGURE 11–2. Laryngoscopes used in veterinary medicine. The three blades to the right are different-sized McIntosh blades. The blade to the left is a Miller blade, which is long enough to facilitate intubation of small ruminants and swine.

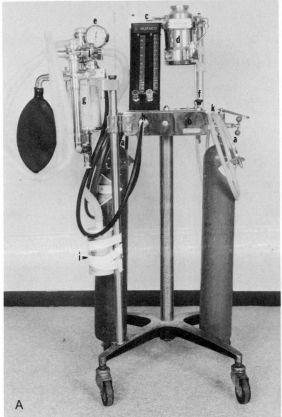
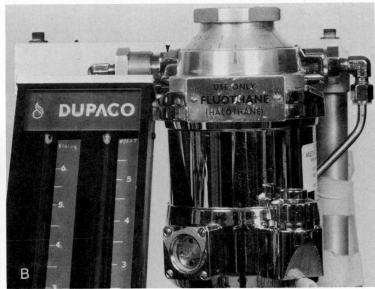

FIGURE 11–3. A, A basic veterinary anesthetic machine with a circle breathing system for use in animals between 7 and 135 kg. The basic machine components include compressed gas sources for both oxygen and nitrous oxide (a), built-in pressure regulator (b), flowmeters (c), and a precision vaporizer (d) located out of the system. Also note the pressure manometer (e), oxygen flush valve (f), soda lime canister (g), and the common gas outlet (h), which delivers oxygen and anesthetic gas to the breathing system. Also notice that a waste gas–capturing device (i), located below the breathing system, is connected by corrugated tubing to the "pop-off" valve (j). The hoses that attach at the back of the machine (k) allow connection to a central hospital gas pipeline system. B, A "Fluothane" Tec (Fluotec 3, Matrx Medical Inc, Orchard Park, NY) vaporizer showing calibration of output in volumes percent. The vaporizer is set at 0.5 percent. Note the button at the left of the vaporizer (arrow), which is a locking mechanism that must be depressed to activate the control dial.

Older machines may flush through the vaporizer (Fig. 11–4), which presents an inherent danger if the flush valve is engaged while the vaporizer is turned on. The flush valve may be used to quickly decrease the inhalation anesthetic concentration present in the breathed gases for a rapid decrease in anesthetic depth and/or rapid recovery from anesthesia. Use of the flush valve should be avoided as a method of filling the rebreathing bag unless a change in depth of anesthesia is desired.

Vaporizers convert a volatile liquid inhalation anesthetic into a vapor for delivery into the patient's breathing system. Classification of vaporizers is a complex task, and more detailed descriptions are available (Hartsfield, 1987; Dorsch and Dorsch, 1984B; Bednarski, 1991). Most newer vaporizers (precision) provide precisely determined vapor concentrations according to the settings on the vaporizer, regardless of temperature and incoming gas flow rate (see Fig. 11–3). Nonprecision vaporizers are low-efficiency vaporizers that volatilize the anesthetic without producing a precisely known vapor concentration, and their output varies with temperature and gas flow rate through the vaporizer (Fig. 11–4). A more specific set of

criteria exists for classification of vaporizers, and this includes method for regulating output concentration, method of vaporization, location of vaporizer in relation to the breathing system, method of temperature compensation and agent specificity (Hartsfield, 1987; Dorsch and Dorsch, 1984B, Bednarski, 1991).

Location of the vaporizer may be out of the breathing system (out-of-the-system) or in the breathing system (in-the-system) as illustrated in Figure 11–5. There is an inherent danger in the use of an in-the-system vaporizer. While an out-of-system vaporizer can never deliver a concentration higher than what is set on the vaporizer dial (because fresh gas flow passes through the vaporizer one time only), an in-the-system vaporizer receives, in addition to fresh gas flow, a gas mixture containing anesthetic gas not taken up by the patient; therefore, vapor concentration in the breathed gas may increase over time. This increase is exacerbated by low fresh gas flows, which allow exhaled gases already containing anesthetic vapor to recirculate more times, and by ventilation, with greater ventilation resulting in increased vaporization. The latter effect theoretically provides a built-in safety factor *if* the animal is

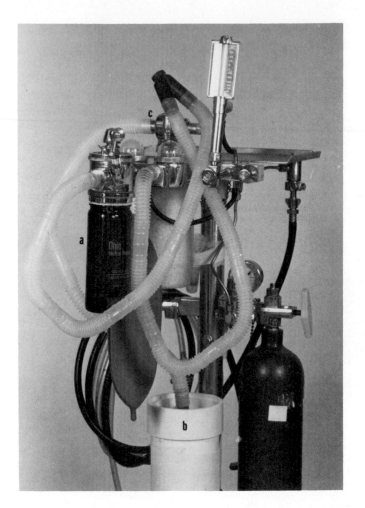

FIGURE 11–4. A basic veterinary anesthetic machine with a circle breathing system. The nonprecision vaporizer (a) is located within the breathing system for delivery of methoxyflurane. Note the mounted scavenger system (b), which is connected to the pop-off valve (c).

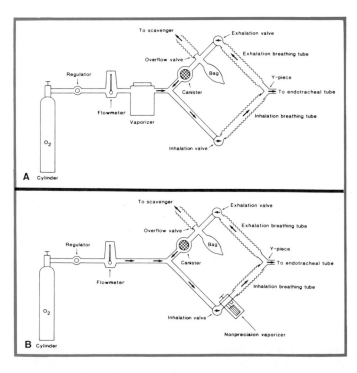

FIGURE 11–5. A, Diagram of the relationship of an out-of-the-system precision vaporizer to the various components of an anesthetic machine and a circle breathing system. (Reprinted with permission from Hartsfield SM: Machines and breathing systems for administration of inhalation anesthetics. *In* Short CE [ed]: Principles and Practice of Veterinary Anesthesia. Baltimore, The Williams & Wilkins Co., 1987, p. 403. © 1987, The Williams & Wilkins Company, Baltimore.) B, Diagram of the relationship of an in-the-system nonprecision vaporizer to the various components of an anesthetic machine and a circle breathing system. (Reprinted with permission from Hartsfield SM: Machines and breathing systems for administration of inhalation anesthetics. *In* Short CE (ed): Principles and Practice of Veterinary Anesthesia. Baltimore, The Williams & Wilkins Co., 1987, p. 403. © 1987, The Williams & Wilkins Company, Baltimore.)

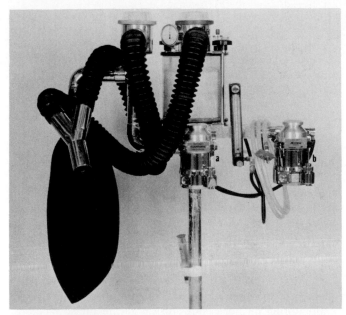

FIGURE 11–6. Large animal anesthetic machine with circle breathing system. This machine is equipped with both a halothane (a) and an isoflurane (b) precision vaporizer, which may be used interchangeably.

breathing spontaneously, because as anesthetic depth increases, ventilation becomes depressed, allowing anesthetic concentration in the breathed gases to decrease.

Breathing Systems

The most commonly used breathing system is the circle rebreathing system, meaning that the patient rebreathes the gas mixture within the circle (Figs. 11–3 through 11–6). Three sizes are available, including pediatric (<7 kg), standard adult circle (7 to 135 kg) (see Fig. 11–3) and large animal (>135 kg) (Fig. 11–6). These systems vary in internal volume owing to differences in diameter of the connecting Y-piece, breathing tubes, breathing tube connectors, one-way valves and the size of rebreathing bags used (Hartsfield, 1987).

Gases move in one direction owing to the presence of one-way valves, and carbon dioxide produced by the animal is neutralized by soda lime or barium hydroxide lime contained in the absorbent canister (see Figs. 11–3 and 11–6). Most absorbent granules contain an indicator dye, which becomes visible owing to a color change as the granules become exhausted. Although no set guidelines exist for when to change the absorbent granules, a general rule is that a strong color indicates the point of clinical exhaustion and should be changed when the color shift is present in two thirds of the absorbent (Dorsch and Dorsch, 1984C).

Rebreathing bag selection may be made by multiplying the patient's tidal volume (10 ml/kg) times six. Rebreathing bags available for animals <135 kg include 1-, 2-, 3-, 5- and 6-liter sizes, and for animals >135 kg, they include 15-, 20- and 30-liter sizes.

Fresh gas flow rates vary with personal preference. A setting that just meets the patient's metabolic oxygen needs (small animal = 8 to 10 ml/kg/minute; large animal = 2 to 3 ml/kg/minute) is termed a "closed" circle system, in which the overflow or "pop-off" valve is closed and flow rates are adjusted to maintain a constant volume in the rebreathing bag. Although this system is more economical, retains more heat and humidity and causes less environmental pollution, hypoxia may develop if the patient is not closely monitored. The system must be flushed two to four times during the first 15 minutes of anesthesia, and every 30 minutes thereafter, to prevent nitrogen (which is exhaled by the patient) from building up within the system. In a "semiclosed" circle system, defined by fresh gas flows of three times the patient's metabolic oxygen needs (small animal = 30 ml/kg/minute; large animal = 6 ml/kg/minute), the "pop-off" valve is open. Although these flow rates are less economical and result in more pollution, they ensure greater patient safety. Regardless of the flow rate used for maintenance, flow rates for mask induction and for a short period following intubation and connection to the breathing system (2 to 5 minutes) should be increased (except for in-the-system vaporizers) to facilitate delivery of anesthetic gas to the patient and to aid in denitrogenation of the patient. A rate of two to three times the calculated maintenance flow rate will be adequate.

Non-rebreathing systems are also used in veterinary medicine for patients weighing less than 7 kg. Non-rebreathing (NRB) systems are simple to use and inexpensive, do not require carbon dioxide absorbent, and impart minimal resistance to breathing. Disadvantages include decreased economy and increased pollution due to the high flow rates required to remove carbon dioxide and a greater loss of heat and humidity. Flow rates vary according to the particular system used but are approximately 100 to 300 ml/kg/minute with a minimum flow of 500 ml/minute. A commonly used NRB system in veterinary medicine is the Bain coaxial system (Fig. 11–7).

In veterinary hospitals in which inhalation anesthetics are used, it is important to minimize environmental exposure of attending personnel to waste gases. Reduction of environmental pollution is facilitated by scavenging the waste gas exiting through the pop-off valve, checking equipment frequently for

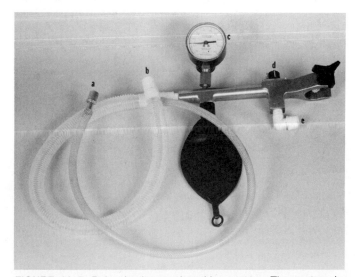

FIGURE 11–7. Bain circuit nonrebreathing system. The system is attached (a) to the common gas outlet of the anesthetic machine, and the patient connection end is shown (b). This system is also equipped with a pressure manometer (c), a "pop-off" valve (d), which remains open except during assisted ventilation, and an interface for connection to a waste gas scavenging system (e).

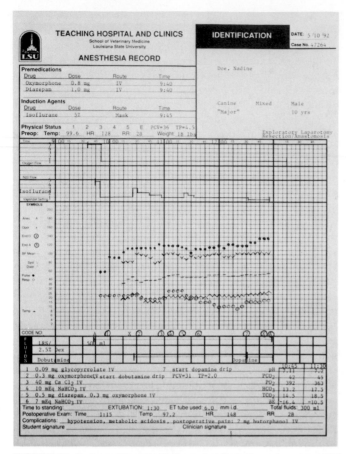

FIGURE 11–8. A sample anesthetic record that allows for sequential recording of heart rate, respiratory rate, and arterial blood pressures. Also included is a summary of the preanesthetic findings and the dose, route and time of administration of drugs used.

leaks (see under Preparation of Equipment and Supplies) and practicing techniques that minimize environmental pollution (Dorsch and Dorsch, 1984D; Paddleford, 1987; Muir et al., 1989). Although a cause-and-effect relationship has not been clearly demonstrated, studies of operating room personnel suggest that exposure to trace anesthetic gases may be a contributing factor in spontaneous abortion, congenital abnormalities, cancer, hepatic disease, renal disease and neurological disease (Dorsch and Dorsch, 1984D; Paddleford, 1987). Scavenging systems must include the gas-capturing device, the interface and the disposal system, and detailed descriptions are available (Dorsch and Dorsch, 1984A, 1984D; Paddleford, 1987). Considerations that help to minimize waste gas exposure include the following:

1. Fill vaporizers at the end of the work day when fewer people are present, taking care to avoid spillage.

2. Use low-flow techniques when possible.

3. Have patients recover in well-ventilated areas and leave the patient attached to the breathing system as long as possible so that expired gases can be scavenged.

4. Do not turn on vaporizer until patient is connected to the machine.

5. When disconnecting patient from machine, turn off vaporizer and occlude Y-piece until patient is reconnected.

6. Use mask or chamber inductions only when considered necessary for the safety of the patient or for unrestrainable patients.

MONITORING

Intraoperative monitoring is essential to successful anesthesia because chemical restraint and general anesthesia impose a great stress on homeostasis in both normal and debilitated patients. Since irreversible brain and cellular changes occur in 3 to 5 minutes following the cessation of blood flow that occurs with cardiac arrest, vital signs should be assessed and recorded every 5 minutes. Life-threatening changes must be detected early so that action can be taken to avoid permanent damage to the patient.

The anesthetic record is a concise method for recording time of administration and doses (in milligrams) of anesthetic agents used and physiological data measured throughout the anesthetic period. The record serves as a legal document, prompts the anesthetist to evaluate and record the patient's vital signs at regular intervals, permits recognition of trends in one or more of the recorded parameters that might signal an impending problem and provides information for any subsequent anesthetic procedures in the same patient (Fig. 11–8).

Monitoring includes both physical and technical methods. Physical methods parallel those skills involved in performing a physical examination plus assessment of muscle tone and eye reflexes. Technological methods use sophisticated equipment to quantify various aspects of homeostasis. Monitoring should focus on the cardiovascular and pulmonary systems, the central nervous system and body temperature because these systems are most affected by anesthetic drugs and surgical procedures. The preanesthetic physical status of the patient (see Preanesthetic Evaluation, below), the anesthetic protocol used, the procedure to be performed and the anticipated duration of anesthesia help to determine the sophistication of monitoring techniques used.

Cardiovascular system monitoring involves integrated assessment of heart rate and rhythm, pulse quality, capillary refill time (CRT) and mucous membrane color. Heart rate and

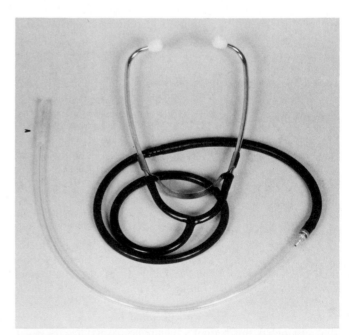

FIGURE 11–9. Esophageal stethoscope (arrow), which allows auscultation of heart sounds during the anesthetic monitoring period. The device may be coupled to a stethoscope or to an amplifier for transmission of audible heart sounds.

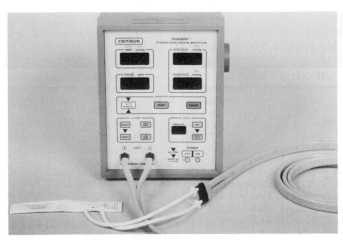

FIGURE 11-10. Oscillometric peripheral pulse monitor for indirect monitoring of systolic, diastolic and mean arterial blood pressures. This monitor also records pulse rate (Dinamap, Critikon, Tampa, FL).

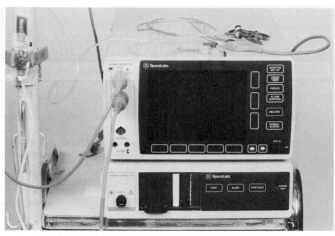

FIGURE 11-12. A computerized electrocardiograph monitor for recording a continuous electrocardiogram. The monitor is also equipped with a pressure transducer (a), which may be connected (b) to a catheter placed in a peripheral artery for direct measurement of systolic, diastolic and mean arterial blood pressures. This monitor will also continuously record body temperature (c: probe not shown) (Spacelabs Inc, Redmond, WA).

rhythm may be assessed by external auscultation or with an esophageal stethoscope in small animals (Fig. 11-9). During the surgical procedure, direct auscultation may be difficult, especially in large animals, and palpation of a peripheral pulse is more reliable. Peripheral pulses used to assess rate and quality include the femoral, dorsal metatarsal, digital and lingual arteries in dogs; femoral artery in cats and swine; facial, transverse facial, and dorsal metatarsal arteries in horses; and auricular, digital, coccygeal, and dorsal metatarsal arteries in ruminants. A continuous electrocardiogram (ECG) determines whether cardiac rate and rhythm are normal and aids in early detection of arrhythmias. Lead II is used in small animals, and a base-apex lead placement, recorded in lead II, is useful in large animals. Lead placement for a base-apex ECG (right arm over heart; left arm over jugular furrow; left leg over point of shoulder) will yield a large positive R wave. It is important to remember that a normal ECG only indicates normal electrical activity and yields no information regarding heart contractility or tissue perfusion.

Adequate perfusion is assessed by subjective evaluation of mucous membrane color, CRT (normal <2 seconds) and

pulse quality. Arterial blood pressure may be measured by either direct or indirect methods. Indirect methods, which include the oscillometric pulse monitor (Fig. 11-10) and the ultrasonic Doppler apparatus (Fig. 11-11), require placement of an inflatable cuff on a peripheral artery. These methods are easy to use but are less accurate than direct methods and are not applicable to all species or breeds because of variations in limb shape and/or size.

For direct pressure monitoring, a catheter is placed in a peripheral artery and connected via heparinized saline-filled tubing to a pressure transducer (Fig. 11-12) or aneroid manometer (Fig. 11-13). Direct methods require more technical skill and knowledge of the equipment. The aneroid manometer is relatively inexpensive and gives a continuous value for mean arterial pressure, whereas a pressure transducer records mean, systolic and diastolic arterial pressures but requires expensive equipment. Blood pressure monitoring aids in the assessment of depth of anesthesia and adequacy of tissue perfusion; a minimum of 60 mm Hg mean arterial pressure should be maintained in all patients to ensure adequate perfusion to vital organs (brain, heart, lungs, kidneys) (Haskins, 1987). Normal values for arterial blood pressure are listed in Table 11-5.

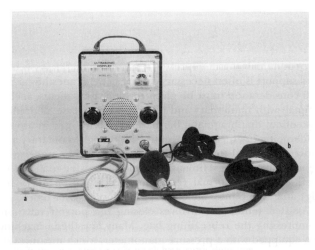

FIGURE 11-11. Ultrasonic Doppler apparatus for indirect monitoring of systolic arterial blood pressure. An electronic activated crystal (a), positioned distal to an occlusive cuff (b), senses blood flow in a peripheral artery, which is audibly broadcast.

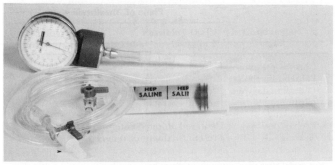

FIGURE 11-13. An aneroid manometer for the direct measurement of mean arterial blood pressure. The device is attached (arrow) to a catheter placed in a peripheral artery, and the air-water interface with the connecting tubing should be placed at the level of the patient's heart.

Table 11–8
PHYSICAL STATUS CLASSIFICATIONS AS DEFINED BY THE AMERICAN SOCIETY OF ANESTHESIOLOGISTS

Classification	Definition	Example
I	Normal animal admitted for elective surgery	Elective castration
II	Animal with slight to moderate systemic disturbance	Obesity, dehydration
III	Animal with major systemic disturbance which limits activity but is not incapacitating	Heart disease, anemia, severe fracture
IV	Animal with very severe systemic disturbance that could lead to death if surgical and/or medical intervention is not applied	Frequent arrhythmias, ruptured bladder, internal hemorrhage, severe pneumothorax
V	Animal in a moribund state which will probably die despite surgical and/or medical intervention	Prolonged gastric dilatation, volvulus, severe trauma with shock

an anesthetic protocol. The animal should be *fasted* prior to anesthesia; the duration varies between species (Table 11–7). Neonates, birds and patients under 2 kg should not be fasted because of limited glycogen stores and high metabolic rates.

Preparation of Equipment and Supplies

Selection of an anesthetic protocol is based on several factors, including the animal's temperament and physical status, the procedure to be performed, the available anesthetics, the familiarity of personnel with the drugs available and the amount of assistance. Suggested protocols utilizing both inhalation and injectable techniques for the common domestic species are listed in Tables 11–9 to 11–13.

An anesthetic preparation check list should be devised to optimize organization so that anesthetic induction and maintenance will be smooth and uncomplicated. Preparations may be completed after the animal has been premedicated and should include the following:

1. Organize necessary supplies for intravenous catheterization, including appropriate catheters, tape, heparinized saline and antiseptics for sterile preparation of the skin site.
2. Organize equipment for endotracheal intubation, including appropriately sized tubes that have been checked for cuff leaks, laryngoscope, stylet and topical anesthetic spray if needed for the particular species, oral speculum for large animal species, gauze or tape to secure tube in place, sterile lubricant to facilitate passage of the tube into the trachea and a syringe to inflate the endotracheal tube cuff.

3. Prepare the anesthesia machine and select a breathing system according to the animal's size (see selection criteria in the section on Anesthesia Equipment):
   a. Fill vaporizer and check the oxygen supply.
   b. Evaluate soda lime absorbent and refill if material is exhausted.
   c. Turn on flowmeter to check for free movement of indicator.
   d. Close pop-off valve and pressurize the breathing system to 40 cm H_2O (on pressure manometer) using the

Table 11–9
SUGGESTED PROTOCOLS FOR CHEMICAL RESTRAINT AND GENERAL ANESTHESIA IN DOGS

NEUROLEPTANALGESIC COMBINATIONS FOR CHEMICAL RESTRAINT

1. Acepromazine:	0.22 mg/kg IV (maximum: 4 mg)
Oxymorphone:	0.22 mg/kg IV (maximum: 4 mg)
2. Acepromazine:	0.22 mg/kg IV (maximum: 4 mg)
Butorphanol:	0.22 mg/kg IV
3. Atropine:	0.044 mg/kg SC
Xylazine:	0.22 mg/kg IV followed by:
Butorphanol:	0.11–0.22 mg/kg IV

For animals in which acepromazine and xylazine should be avoided:

4. Diazepam:	0.22 mg/kg IV
Oxymorphone:	0.22 mg/kg IV (maximum: 4 mg)
5. Diazepam:	0.22 mg/kg IV
Butorphanol:	0.22 mg/kg IV

PROTOCOL FOR PHYSICAL STATUS 1 AND 2 ANIMALS

Premedication:	Acepromazine: 0.11 mg/kg IM (maximum: 2 mg)
	OR
	Acepromazine: 0.11 mg/kg IM (maximum: 2 mg) plus
	Butorphanol: 0.22 mg/kg IM
Induction:	Thiamylal: 11.0 mg/kg IV "to effect"
Maintenance:	Halothane, isoflurane, or methoxyflurane

PROTOCOL FOR PHYSICAL STATUS ≥3 ANIMALS

Premedication:	Neuroleptanalgesic combinations number 4 or 5 listed above. Alternate administration of ¼ calculated dose of each drug beginning with opioid until total dose has been administered or until desired degree of sedation is achieved.
Induction:	Mask with isoflurane
	OR
	Ketamine: 2.2–4.4 mg/kg IV "to effect"
Maintenance:	Isoflurane (if available). Halothane may be used but delivered concentrations should be minimized.

INJECTABLE PROTOCOLS FOR SHORT-DURATION ANESTHESIA*

1. Atropine:	0.044 mg/kg SC	
Xylazine:	0.66–1.1 mg/kg IV or IM	
Ketamine:	6.0–12.0 mg/kg IV or IM	
2. Diazepam:	0.25 mg/kg	Mix and inject IV.
Ketamine:	5.0 mg/kg	Provides 10–15 minutes of anesthesia.
3. Atropine:	0.044 mg/kg SC	
Xylazine:	0.44–0.88 mg/kg IV or IM	
Telazol:	4.4–11.0 mg/kg IV or IM	

*Protocols 1 and 3 may be used IV or IM. Use higher dose range when administering IM. The IM route will be slower in onset of effect and will give a longer duration of anesthesia and a longer recovery.

Table 11–10
SUGGESTED PROTOCOLS FOR CHEMICAL RESTRAINT AND GENERAL ANESTHESIA IN CATS

PROTOCOL FOR PHYSICAL STATUS 1 AND 2 ANIMALS

Premedication:	Acepromazine: 0.066 mg/kg	
	Ketamine: 15 mg/kg	Mix and give IM.
Induction:	Mask with halothane or isoflurane	
	OR	
	Ketamine: 2.2–4.4 mg/kg IV "to effect"	
Maintenance:	Halothane or isoflurane	

PROTOCOL FOR PHYSICAL STATUS ≥ 3 ANIMALS

Premedication: (*if* needed)	Butorphanol: 0.44 mg/kg SC	
Induction:	Mask with isoflurane	
	OR	
	Diazepam: 0.25 mg/kg	Mix and give IV "to
	Ketamine: 5.0 mg/kg	effect."
Maintenance:	Isoflurane (if available). Halothane may be used, but delivered concentrations should be minimized.	

INJECTABLE PROTOCOLS

1. Butorphanol: 0.44 mg/kg
   Telazol: 6–11 mg/kg   Mix and give IM.
2. Atropine: 0.044 mg/kg
   Xylazine: 1.1 mg/kg
   Ketamine: 22 mg/kg   Mix and give IM.
3. Diazepam and ketamine may be used as above to provide 10–15 minutes of anesthesia.

oxygen flush valve. This may be accomplished by placing thumb over the patient connection. The system should maintain pressure if no leaks are present.

    e. Connect machine to waste gas scavenging system.

4. Calculate oxygen flow rate according to patient size and breathing system used.
5. Organize fluids for administration and calculate appropriate administration rate (see below).
6. Calculate dosage for induction drugs. Withdraw drugs from bottles into labeled syringes.

Endotracheal Intubation

Endotracheal intubation techniques in a variety of species are described in Table 11–7. Several principles should be remembered when performing intubation in any species:

    1. Inject air into cuff before use to check the cuff's ability to hold volume.

    2. Always have two or three tube sizes readily available for each patient in case the first selection is too small or too large.

    3. For cats, dogs, small ruminants, and swine, positioning the animal in sternal recumbency so that the head and neck are in a straight line offers the best visualization of the larynx for successful intubation. Some anesthetists prefer dorsal recumbency to perform intubation in swine. Horses and adult cattle are usually intubated while positioned in lateral recumbency with the head, neck and back placed in a straight line to facilitate introduction of the tube into the larynx (Figs. 11–15 and 11–16). Horses may also be intubated via the ventral mea-

tus of the nasal cavity (a smaller tube must be used) with the head positioned as described above, and this position may be indicated for procedures involving the oral cavity. This method is especially applicable in foals and may be performed in the awake foal with minimal sedation to facilitate a rapid method of induction with inhalation anesthetics (Fig. 11–17).

    4. A stylet with an atraumatic tip may be necessary in some situations. A rigid stylet will provide support for very flimsy tubes and will facilitate proper placement. In species such as small ruminants, swine and sometimes cats, an atraumatic stylet such as a dog urinary catheter will facilitate introduction of the tube into the larynx. These species have a sensitive larynx, which is prone to laryngospasm. Visualization is poor in small ruminants and swine owing to their narrow oral cavity, and use of both a laryngoscope and a stylet is especially beneficial. In adult cattle, one can introduce a nasogastric tube into the trachea by digitally palpating the laryngeal opening. The endotracheal tube is then guided over the smaller and longer

Table 11–11
SUGGESTED PROTOCOLS FOR CHEMICAL RESTRAINT AND GENERAL ANESTHESIA IN HORSES

STANDING CHEMICAL RESTRAINT

1. Xylazine:	0.44–0.66 mg/kg IV	(Give xylazine first.)
Butorphanol:	0.022–0.044 mg/kg IV	
2. Detomidine:	0.022 mg/kg IV	
3. Acepromazine:	0.022–0.044 mg/kg IV	(Give acepromazine 20 minutes prior to
Xylazine:	0.44 mg/kg IV	administration of
Butorphanol:	0.022 mg/kg IV	other agents.)

PROTOCOLS FOR INDUCTION OF ANESTHESIA PRIOR TO MAINTENANCE WITH AN INHALATION AGENT

1. *Premedication:* *Induction:*	Xylazine: 1.1 mg/kg IV	(Give xylazine and wait 3–5 minutes
	Ketamine: 2.2 mg/kg IV	before administering ketamine.)
2. *Premedication:*	Xylazine: 0.44 mg/kg IV	
	OR	
	Acepromazine: 0.044 mg/kg IV	
Induction:	5% guaifenesin IV "to effect"	
	Thiamylal bolus: 4.4 mg/kg IV	
3. *Premedication:*	Xylazine: 0.22–0.44 mg/kg IV	(This protocol works well in old,
Induction:	5% guaifenesin "to effect"	debilitated, and colic patients.)
	Ketamine: 1.5–1.8 mg/kg IV	

INJECTABLE PROTOCOLS FOR INDUCTION AND MAINTENANCE OF GENERAL ANESTHESIA

Xylazine and Ketamine as listed above provides 8–12 minutes of anesthesia. Duration of anesthesia may be extended by:

1. Administering butorphanol (0.022 mg/kg IV) or diazepam (0.055 mg/kg IV) prior to ketamine administration.
   OR
2. Simultaneous administration of 50% of the original dose of xylazine and ketamine at 15–20 minute intervals. Do not repeat more than two times.
   OR
3. Administering a combination of 1 liter of 5% guaifenesin containing 1 mg/ml of ketamine and 0.5 mg/ml of xylazine. The combination is administered at a constant drip (approximately 2.2 ml/kg/hr) until the procedure ends.

Table 11-12
SUGGESTED PROTOCOLS FOR CHEMICAL RESTRAINT AND GENERAL ANESTHESIA IN RUMINANTS

CATTLE

Premedication: Xylazine: 0.022–0.066 mg/kg IM (may not be required depending on animal's temperament and available restraint)

Induction: 1 liter of 5% guaifenesin plus 2 mg/ml of thiamylal (give until animal assumes recumbency and can be intubated)

OR

1 liter of 5% guaifenesin given "to effect" followed by a bolus of ketamine (1.1–2.2 mg/kg IV) (indicated for debilitated cattle or cattle with gastrointestinal disorders)

Maintenance: Halothane

INJECTABLE PROTOCOLS FOR INDUCTION AND MAINTENANCE OF ANESTHESIA

1. 1 liter 5% guaifenesin plus 2 mg/ml thiamylal may be used for induction and maintenance: 1 liter will provide induction and 30–45 minutes of anesthesia for a 500-kg animal. If a second bottle is required, only 1 mg/ml of thiamylal should be added to the guaifenesin.
2. 1 liter 5% guaifenesin plus 1 mg/ml of ketamine plus 0–50 mg of xylazine (total). Omit xylazine if the animal was premedicated with xylazine. This combination may be used for induction (2.2–4.4 ml/kg) and maintenance (2.2 ml/kg/hour), and 1 bottle may last 30–90 minutes depending on the animal's size and type of procedure.

SHEEP AND GOATS

Premedication: Acepromazine: 0.055–0.11 mg/kg IV or IM
Diazepam: 0.22–0.55 mg/kg IV
(usually not required because animals are easy to restrain)

Induction: Thiamylal: 11 mg/kg IV (Give "to effect" to facilitate intubation.)

OR

Diazepam (0.25–0.5 mg/kg) plus ketamine (4.4 mg/kg): Mix and give IV "to effect" to facilitate intubation. (This combination is good for debilitated, old, or diseased animals.)

Maintenance: Halothane or isoflurane

INJECTABLE PROTOCOLS FOR INDUCTION AND MAINTENANCE OF ANESTHESIA

1. Xylazine: 0.11 mg/kg IM followed in 15 minutes by: Ketamine: 11.0 mg/kg IV
(This combination provides 30–45 minutes of anesthesia. The recovery is prolonged but may be shortened by reversing the xylazine.)
2. Diazepam and ketamine as described above under induction provides 5–10 minutes of anesthesia.
3. Telazol: 2.2–6.6 mg/kg IV or IM provides 20–30 minutes of anesthesia.

nasogastric tube and into the trachea. *The use of a wire or any sharp instrument as a stylet is not advised; severe and even fatal tracheal trauma could result!*

5. The conservative use of a topical anesthetic agent in the laryngeal area (see Fig. 11–1), specifically in cats, swine and small ruminants, will facilitate intubation with minimal trauma.

6. Adequate anesthesia and muscle relaxation are important for successful intubation. This will avoid unnecessary laryngeal trauma and excessive autonomic nervous system stimulation, which may give rise to cardiac arrhythmias.

7. The endotracheal tube should be long enough to reach midway between the larynx and carina so that accidental dislodgment does not occur. It should not be too long because this can increase the risk of endobronchial intubation, and an excessive tube length that extends beyond the oral cavity constitutes dead space, which can contribute to hypercapnia.

8. Proper tube placement may be assessed by (a) visualization of the tube passing between the arytenoid cartilages (not applicable in horses and cattle), (b) condensation of respiratory gases on the inside of the tube with expiration, (c) only one tubular structure (trachea) palpable in the neck region, (d) auscultation of lung sounds during assisted ventilation and (e) absence of vocalization.

9. The cuff should be inflated just enough to form an effective seal within the trachea. This can be assessed by closing the pop-off valve, assisting ventilation, and listening for air escaping around the cuff and/or checking for the smell of anesthetic gas.

10. Secure tube to patient by tying gauze tightly around the tube and then securing it around the head (cats, brachycephalic breeds) or to the upper or lower jaw. This is usually not necessary in horses and adult cattle.

Fluid Administration During Anesthesia

Fluid administration is important to the maintenance of homeostasis during anesthesia and provides venous access for the delivery of agents used intraoperatively for supportive therapy (such as antibiotics, inotropic agents), for maintenance of anesthesia (injectable anesthetic agents) and for cardiopulmonary resuscitation. Imbalances may occur owing to blood loss, drying of exposed tissues, removal of effusions and the hypo-

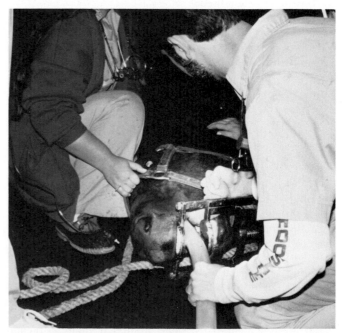

FIGURE 11–15. Positioning a horse to facilitate endotracheal intubation using the blind technique. An oral speculum is positioned between the incisor teeth to hold the mouth open, and the tongue is pulled out of the mouth.

Table 11–13		
SUGGESTED PROTOCOLS FOR CHEMICAL RESTRAINT AND GENERAL ANESTHESIA IN SWINE		
Premedication:	Atropine: .044 mg/kg IM	Can mix and give as one injection.
	Xylazine: 1.1–2.2 mg/kg IM	
	Ketamine: 2.2–4.4 mg/kg IM	
	OR	
	Atropine: .044 mg/kg IM	Can mix and give as one injection.
	Xylazine: 1.1 mg/kg IM	
	Telazol: 6.0 mg/kg IM	
Induction:	Mask with halothane or isoflurane to facilitate intubation.	
Maintenance:	Halothane or isoflurane	
Injectable Protocols for Maintenance of Anesthesia		
Premedication:	See above protocols. These combinations will facilitate catheter placement in an ear vein.	
Induction and	1 liter of 5% guaifenesin plus 1 mg/ml xylazine and 1 mg/ml ketamine	
Maintenance:	Drip at an approximate rate of 2.2 ml/kg/hour.	

tensive effects of anesthetic agents. The following guidelines will keep fluid therapy during anesthesia simple and effective:

1. Fluids most commonly used are polyionic isotonic crystalloid solutions, such as lactated Ringer's solution (LRS). For neonates (less than 1 month of age), very small patients and birds, use 5 percent dextrose or supplement LRS with 5 or 10 ml of 50 percent dextrose per 100 ml of LRS for a dextrose concentration of 2.5 percent or 5 percent, respectively.

2. For healthy animals during routine procedures the following fluid rates are suggested: *small animals, 10 to 20 ml/kg/hour; large animals, 5 to 10 ml/kg/hour. Exceptions to the foregoing fluid rates include:*

   a. Increase the administration rate in animals with pre-existing dehydration, excessive intraoperative blood loss, or hypotension, and during cardiopulmonary resuscitation.

   b. Decrease the administration rate in animals that have significant cardiac or renal disease or are hypoproteinemic. These situations make the animals more prone to the development of pulmonary edema because they are unable to handle the additional fluid load.

3. Blood lost during surgery should be replaced at a volume of three times the approximate loss in addition to the basic fluid rate during anesthesia. Ideally, when blood loss is significant, the PCV and total protein should be monitored to avoid excessive dilution. An acute decrease in PCV below 20 percent should be treated with packed red cells or whole blood. Total protein should not decrease below 3.5 g/dl because of the increased risk of developing pulmonary edema.

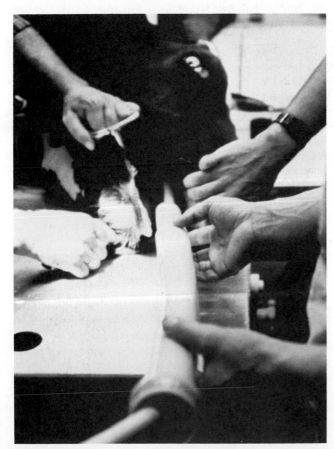

FIGURE 11–16. Endotracheal intubation of adult cattle requires placement of an oral speculum, digital palpation of the larynx and introduction of a nasogastric tube into the trachea to guide the endotracheal tube into the trachea.

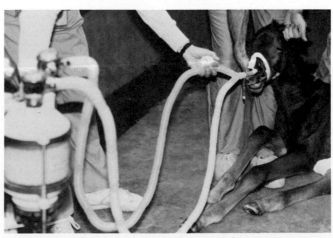

FIGURE 11–17. Newborn foal with an endotracheal tube introduced through the ventral meatus of the nasal cavity into the trachea for induction of anesthesia with isoflurane.

Induction and Maintenance

Guidelines for induction and maintenance are as follows:

1. Turn on oxygen flow a few minutes prior to connection of the patient to the breathing system to fill the system with oxygen.

2. Connect endotracheal tube to breathing system and turn on vaporizer to appropriate induction setting (see Table 11–4).

3. Assess pulse rate and quality.

4. Assess respiration. If animal is apneic or rate is slow, assist ventilation.

5. Apply ophthalmic ointment.

6. Reduce vaporizer settings to appropriate maintenance concentration as indicated by patient's anesthetic depth.

7. Begin intravenous fluid administration.

8. Begin monitoring and instrument with available technical monitoring equipment.

9. Record all pertinent information on anesthetic record and begin recording vital signs every 5 minutes (see Fig. 11–8).

10. When using injectable techniques in horses and adult cattle, procedures should be limited to 1 hour. For procedures lasting longer than 1 hour, an oxygen source should be available to insufflate oxygen (10 to 15 liters/minute) into the nares to prevent the development of hypoxia due to hypoventilation and atelectasis.

Padding and Positioning of the Patient

Proper padding and positioning depend on the procedure to be performed and the particular species.

1. Dogs, cats, neonates of all species and all small species should be placed on a covered heating pad or circulating water blanket when available to minimize hypothermia. *Never* place the animal directly on a heating pad or a water blanket.

2. When securing limbs to the surgery table, do not apply ties too tightly and do not apply excessive traction to the forelimbs. Both actions may result in neurological damage.

3. Ensure that the head and neck are positioned to avoid kinking of the endotracheal tube or disconnection from the breathing system.

4. Assure that appropriate expansion of the thorax is not compromised.

5. For horses and adult cattle, adequate padding, such as a thick foam pad, water-filled pad or air dunnage bag, is essential to prevent the development of postoperative myositis and neuropathy. For procedures in the field, a grassy area offers the best padding. The down eye should be protected and the head padded if possible.

6. For horses and cattle in lateral recumbency, the upper front and hind limbs should be supported so that they are parallel to the table surface. The down forelimb should be pulled forward to avoid entrapment of the brachial plexus between the rib cage and humerus.

7. Always remove the halter from horses during general anesthesia to avoid damage to cranial nerves by the metal connectors.

8. Ruminants should be placed in right lateral recumbency *when possible* so that the rumen is on the up side. During lateral

recumbency, the neck should be elevated with a soft pad so that the head angles downward to promote flow of saliva and regurgitation (if it occurs) out of the oral cavity.

9. Because of the high incidence of regurgitation in mature ruminants, an endotracheal tube should be placed and the cuff inflated (even if injectable anesthetics are used) prior to positioning the animal (especially in dorsal recumbency).

Recovery

Guidelines for recovery from anesthesia vary according to species.

Dogs and Cats

1. Flush breathing system with pure oxygen and continue oxygen delivery for 5 to 10 minutes.

2. Deflate cuff (*if* the animal is not at risk for regurgitation) and extubate only *after* swallowing is observed. Suction the oral cavity prior to extubation if excessive secretions have collected. Maintain the tube in place as long as possible in brachycephalic breeds, which are prone by conformation to upper airway obstruction following anesthesia.

3. Position animal in sternal recumbency with the head extended if possible. This is especially important in brachycephalic breeds.

4. Most animals are hypothermic following general anesthesia, and an external heat source will hasten recovery and the return to normothermia. Hot water bottles, heating pads or a circulating water blanket may be used, but *never* place them directly on the patient's skin.

5. Changing the animal's position and rubbing the body will hasten recovery.

6. Use analgesics (such as opioids) postoperatively if there is evidence of pain (vocalization, thrashing) or if the procedure was invasive (such as orthopedic surgery, thoracotomy).

7. Some patients may need continued intravenous fluid therapy (e.g., patients with renal disease, dehydration) and the suggested maintenance rate is 60 ml/kg/24 hours.

8. Check animal frequently until it can maintain sternal recumbency and stand unassisted.

Horses

1. When inhalation anesthesia is used, the horse should be placed in a padded dark room and allowed to recover unassisted. Extubate with the cuff deflated when swallowing is observed. A safer method to ensure a patent airway throughout recovery is to extubate when anesthesia is discontinued and place a smaller noncuffed tube into the trachea via the nasal passage and secure it to the muzzle with tape. This tube may be left in place until the horse is standing.

2. If available, insufflate oxygen (10 to 15 liters/minute) via the recovery tube for 15 to 30 minutes following the end of anesthesia.

3. For recoveries in the field, the halter should be replaced so that the animal can be assisted during recovery. The eye should be covered to minimize external stimulation.

4. Some horses have a rough recovery regardless of the technique used. Administration of a sedative such as xylazine or a

tranquilizer such as acepromazine or diazepam in low doses will quiet the animal until it is ready to rise unassisted.

Ruminants

1. If inhalation anesthesia is used, 100 percent oxygen should be administered for 5 to 10 minutes after anesthetic delivery is discontinued.

2. Ruminants should be positioned in sternal recumbency as soon as possible to promote eructation and minimize the chance of regurgitation.

3. Extubation should be performed with the cuff *inflated* only after swallowing is observed.

4. A stomach tube should be passed to decompress the rumen if bloat has developed intraoperatively.

5. Ruminants generally recover smoothly from general anesthesia and minimal assistance is required.

Swine

1. Continue oxygen for 5 to 10 minutes after anesthetic delivery has been discontinued when inhalation techniques have been used.

2. Extubate with the cuff deflated (unless there is evidence of regurgitation) when swallowing is observed.

3. Position animal in sternal recumbency as soon as possible and allow the animal to recover in a cool and quiet environment.

ANESTHETIC EMERGENCIES

Anesthesia causes a stress to homeostasis, including respiratory and cardiac depression, which may increase the risk of cardiopulmonary arrest, especially in high-risk patients. Cardiopulmonary arrest is the sudden cessation of ventilation and effective circulation that requires rapid emergency intervention (cardiopulmonary resuscitation) in order to prevent death. Physical status categorization alerts the anesthetist to the likelihood that complications that may lead to arrest could occur in a particular patient and stresses the importance of careful monitoring throughout the anesthetic period. Complications may occur at any time during the anesthetic period, including induction, maintenance and recovery.

Cardiopulmonary resuscitation (CPR) is subdivided into four phases, including readiness and prevention, recognition and basic cardiac life support, advanced cardiac life support and postresuscitative care.

Readiness and Prevention

Hospital personnel should be prepared to handle cardiopulmonary arrest by identifying an area in the hospital that is well lighted and stocked with emergency equipment and drugs (Table 11–14; Figs. 11–18 and 11–19). Staff members to be involved in resuscitation should have an assigned role, which should be practiced periodically in mock drills to improve response time and the quality of treatment.

Prevention, as it applies to anesthetic-related cardiopulmonary arrest, involves recognition of high-risk patients and the

Table 11-14
READINESS CHECKLIST FOR CARDIOPULMONARY RESUSCITATION

- Well-lighted area with adequate work space
- Clippers
- Emergency drugs (see Table 11–16)
- Endotracheal tubes
- Tracheostomy tubes
- Face masks
- Method for artificial ventilation (anesthesia machine or Ambu bag)
- Oxygen source
- Gauze for securing endotracheal tube
- Needles and syringes
- Laryngoscope
- Aspiration device
- Intravenous catheters
- Intravenous fluids
- Electrocardiograph machine
- Defibrillator

application of appropriate and effective monitoring of all anesthetized patients. Clinical signs that may indicate an impending arrest include cyanosis; changes in respiration, such as apnea, tachypnea, dyspnea or a marked abdominal effort associated with breathing; and changes associated with the cardiovascular system, such as bradycardia, tachycardia, weak, irregular or absent pulse, pale mucous membranes and increased CRT. Hypothermia may increase the risk of arrest by contributing to the development of bradycardia and excessive anesthetic depth. A body temperature less than 30°C (86°F) predisposes to life-threatening ventricular arrhythmias. Recognition and correction of some potentially life-threatening problems are listed in Table 11–15.

Recognition and Basic Life Support

Early recognition of cardiopulmonary arrest, if prevention was ineffective, is critical to successful resuscitation and is optimized by effective patient monitoring. The initial actions to be taken in the arrest of an anesthetized patient is to discontinue

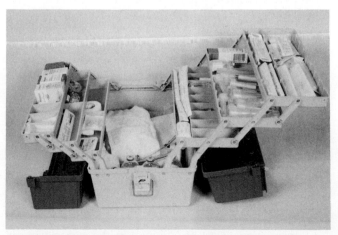

FIGURE 11–18. Example of a utility box used to organize emergency equipment and drugs for anesthetic emergencies.

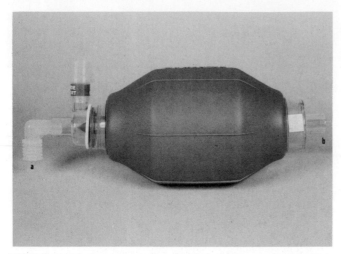

FIGURE 11-19. Ambu bag, which may be used to ventilate patients during cardiopulmonary arrest. The bag is attached to the endotracheal tube (a) and squeezed to deliver a breath. Some Ambu bags are equipped with tubing for connection to an oxygen source (b).

delivery of the anesthetic agent, flush the breathing system with pure oxygen and increase the fluid administration rate. Reversal of anesthetic agents, such as opioids or xylazine, may also be indicated in the anesthetized patient with cardiac arrest. The basic life support techniques should be initiated concurrently and include the following:

1. *Airway.* If the animal is not already intubated (as with injectable techniques), an endotracheal tube is placed. If the animal is already intubated, the tube should be checked for proper placement and patency. If an endotracheal tube cannot be placed or is not patent owing to an obstruction, a tracheostomy should be performed or the tube changed, respectively.

2. *Breathing.* Breathe for the patient using the anesthesia machine or an Ambu bag (see Fig. 11-19), preferably with 100 percent oxygen, at a rate of 20 breaths per minute performed simultaneously with every third to sixth chest compression, depending on the compression rate.

3. *Circulation.* If a pulse or heartbeat cannot be detected, external cardiac compressions should be initiated, the goal being to maintain adequate blood flow to the brain and heart until normal heart rhythm can be restored. In most animals, compressions are performed with the animal in lateral recumbency at the level of the costochondral junction between the fourth and eighth ribs at a rate of 80 to 120 per minute. In barrel-chested dogs, such as the brachycephalic breeds, compressions may be more effective placed in a ventrodorsal direction with the animal stabilized in dorsal recumbency. Abdominal wrapping or interposed rhythmic abdominal compressions may help to improve forward blood flow by increasing the intrathoracic pressure generated.

Advanced Life Support Techniques

These techniques include diagnosis of the type of arrest, the use of emergency drugs and/or defibrillation and internal cardiac massage.

1. *Drugs.* Venous access is critical in the successful treatment of cardiac arrest. Although a central venous catheter

(placed via the jugular vein) offers the most effective route for drug administration, such catheters are not placed routinely, and placement following arrest is difficult and time-consuming. Drugs may be given by a peripheral venous catheter, if effective blood flow has been established by compression techniques, and a fluid bolus should follow administration of every drug used. The tracheal route via the endotracheal tube is effective for epinephrine, atropine and lidocaine administration. Dosages should be twice those given intravenously, the dose should be diluted in 3 to 10 ml of saline and several rapidly applied ventilations should follow administration to ensure distribution to the pulmonary vasculature. The intraosseous route (via the tibial tuberosity, greater tubercle of humerus, trochanteric fossa of femur, wing of ilium) may also be used for fluid and drug administration if venous access cannot be achieved. Table 11-16 lists some of the commonly used emergency drugs, indications for their use and dosages.

2. *Electrocardiogram.* An electrocardiogram should be recorded as soon as possible during the course of resuscitation to identify the type of arrest so that specific therapy for conversion to normal rhythm can be applied. The three types of cardiac arrest include ventricular asystole, ventricular fibrillation and electromechanical dissociation. Figure 11-20 illustrates the three types of arrest, and Table 11-17 lists the specific treatment steps for each type of arrest.

3. *Fluid therapy.* Cardiac arrest is a rapidly vasodilating disease process, and fluid therapy, most often with an isotonic polyionic solution such as LRS, is essential. Never use dextrose-containing fluids during resuscitative efforts because dextrose may exacerbate brain damage. It is recommended that fluids be given rapidly as calculated boluses so that overhydration, which may predispose to pulmonary and cerebral edema, is avoided. For cats, boluses of 20 ml/kg are recommended, and for dogs and most other species, boluses of 40 ml/kg are recommended. These boluses may be repeated as needed throughout resuscitation to maintain an effective circulating volume. Three to 7 percent hypertonic saline (4 ml/kg) has been shown to be beneficial in resuscitation efforts, in conjunction with isotonic fluid administration, to rapidly restore vascular volume and decrease the risk for development of pulmonary and cerebral edema.

4. *Internal cardiac massage.* If external techniques and drug administration have not established effective circulation in 5 minutes or if the heart has not resumed normal rhythm in 10 minutes, a thoracotomy and internal massage should be performed at the left fourth or fifth intercostal space. This procedure should be performed immediately in very large or barrel-chested animals or in animals with fractured ribs or pneumothorax.

Postresuscitative Care

Patients may suffer arrest again following successful resuscitative efforts. Careful monitoring of the ECG, pulse quality, respiratory pattern, body temperature, and central nervous system (pupillary responses, mentation, seizure activity) is essential for several hours after the primary event. Neurological damage may become evident 24 to 48 hours after the arrest, so serial neurological examinations should be performed. Oxygen therapy should be administered for a period of time, depending on the condition of the patient.

Table 11–15
DIFFERENTIAL DIAGNOSIS AND TREATMENT OF COMPLICATIONS THAT MAY OCCUR DURING ANESTHESIA

Abnormality	Potential Causes	Treatment
Bradycardia	Excessive anesthetic depth Drugs: opioids, xylazine, gas anesthetics Hyperkalemia Vagal reflex (intubation, oculocardiac reflex) Visceral manipulation Hypothermia Terminal stages or hypoxia Exogenous and endogenous toxemias	Correct underlying cause if possible Administer anticholinergic agent Administer sympathomimetic agent Dopamine: 2–20 µg/kg/minute* Dobutamine: 2–20 µg/kg/minute* Ephedrine: 0.05–0.5 mg/kg bolus* Isoproterenol: 5–10 µg/kg/minute*
Tachycardia	Drugs: ketamine, thiobarbiturates, Anticholinergics, sympathomimetics Hypokalemia Hyperthermia Inadequate anesthetic depth Hypercapnia, hypoxemia Anemia, hypovolemia Hyperthyroidism, pheochromocytoma Anaphylaxis	Correct underlying cause if possible

Atrial and ventricular premature contractions	Light anesthesia
	Deep anesthesia
	Hypoxia, hypercapnia
	Hypovolemia
	Exogenous catecholamine therapy
	Digitalis toxicity
	Hypokalemia
	Hyperkalemia
	Hypercalcemia
	Certain anesthetics (xylazine, halothane, thiobarbiturates)
	Endocarditis or myocarditis
	Severe hypothermia
	End-stage visceral organ failure
	Intracranial disorders
		Correct underlying cause if possible
		Evaluate anesthetic depth
		Check anesthetic machine and oxygen flow
		Assist ventilation
		If arrhythmia persists and meets one or more of the following criteria:
		(1) >20 per minute
		(2) increasing in frequency
		(3) multifocal
		(4) occurring in runs
		(5) causing significant effect on pulse
		Treat arrhythmia as follows:
		(1) turn off anesthetic gas
		(2) increase fluid administration rate
		(3) administer lidocaine IV (maximum: 4 doses)
		    dog: 2.2 mg/kg
		    cat, horse: 0.5 mg/kg

Hypotension	Hypovolemia (i.e., blood loss)
	Sepsis
	Shock
	Drugs (thiobarbiturates, inhalants)
		Increase fluid administration rate
		Decrease anesthetic concentration
		Administer sympathomimetic agents
		    Dopamine: 2–20 µg/kg/minute*
		    Dobutamine: 2–20 µg/kg/minute*
		    Ephedrine: 0.055–0.55 mg/kg bolus (small animals)*
		    0.022 mg/kg bolus (horse)*

Tachypnea	Pain Hypoxia Hypercapnia Hyperthermia Acidosis Drugs (i.e., doxapram) Airway obstruction	Correct underlying cause if possible
Apnea	Hypothermia Hyperventilation with 100% O_2 Drug effects (thiobarbiturates, ketamine) Deep anesthesia Aminoglycoside administration	Correct underlying cause if possible Assist ventilation until spontaneous ventilation returns

*These drugs may cause cardiac arrhythmias. Monitor electrocardiogram during administration.

Table 11–16
EMERGENCY DRUG DOSAGES AND DEFIBRILLATION SETTINGS USED FOR CARDIOPULMONARY RESUSCITATION

Drug	Concentration	Dosage	Indication	Comments
Epinephrine	1 mg/ml	0.2 mg/lb (SA) 0.0011–0.0055 mg/kg (LA)	Initiate heart beat Increase heart rate Increase contractility Improve blood flow during CPR	Dose may be repeated every 5 minutes
Atropine	0.5 mg/ml (SA) 15 mg/ml (LA)	0.044 mg/kg (SA) 0.011 mg/kg (LA)	Increase heart rate Treat ventricular asystole	
Lidocaine	20 mg/ml	2.2 mg/kg (dogs) 0.5 mg/kg (cats) 0.5 mg/kg (LA)	Treat ventricular arrhythmias	
Prednisone sodium succinate (Solu-delta) or	10 mg/ml 50 mg/ml	22 mg/kg (SA) 2.2 mg/kg (LA)	Shock and ischemia Stabilize cellular membranes Prevent cerebral edema	
Dexamethasone-SP	4 mg/ml	2.2–4.4 mg/kg		
Sodium bicarbonate	1 mEq/ml	0.5–1.0 mEq/kg per 5 minutes of arrest	Treat metabolic acidosis	Use after 10 minutes of arrest or with preexisting acidosis only
Calcium chloride	100 mg/ml	10 mg/kg (SA) 2.2 mg/kg (LA)	Prevent arrhythmias associated with hyperkalemia Treat hypokalemia	Has been incriminated in reperfusion injury
Hypertonic saline	70 mg/ml	4 ml/kg	Treat hypovolemic shock Restore vascular volume	Must be used with isotonic fluids
Furosemide	50 mg/ml	1.1 mg/kg	Treat pulmonary and cerebral edema	Monitor hydration status
Mannitol	200 mg/ml	0.55–1.1 mg/kg	Treat cerebral edema Protect brain against reperfusion injury	Monitor hydration status
Doxapram	20 mg/ml	1.1–4.4 mg/kg (SA) 0.22 mg/kg (LA)	Initiate breathing	Better to treat underlying problem
Direct-current defibrillation	Body Wt.: External: Internal:	<8 kg: 2 ws/kg / 0.5–2.0 ws/kg · 8–40 kg: 2–5 ws/kg / " · >40 kg: 5–10 ws/kg / "	Treatment of ventricular fibrillation	

SA = small animal; LA = large animal; ws = watt-second (Joules), which defines units of energy output produced by an electrical defibrillator.

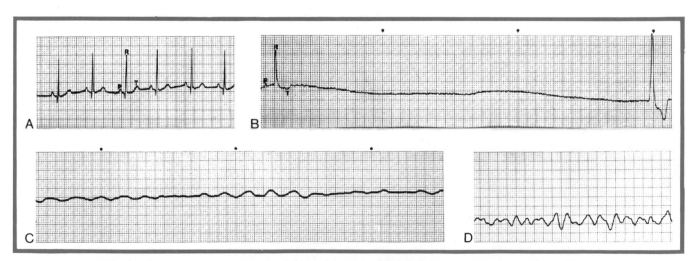

FIGURE 11–20. Representative electrocardiogram tracings of the different types of cardiac arrest. A, Electromechanical dissociation presents as a normal tracing, but no palpable pulse is associated with the electrical activity. B, Ventricular asystole presents as a flat tracing. Fine, C, and coarse, D, ventricular fibrillation present as wavy lines. It is important to distinguish between fine and coarse ventricular fibrillation because the latter is easier to convert to normal rhythm with defibrillation techniques. (From Tilley LP: Essentials of Canine and Feline Electrocardiography. 3rd ed. Philadelphia, Lea & Febiger, 1992. Reprinted with permission.)

Table 11-17
CLASSIFICATIONS OF CARDIAC ARREST AND SUGGESTED TREATMENT PROTOCOL

Arrhythmia	Treatment	Dosage
Ventricular asystole	Epinephrine	0.2 mg/kg IV or IT*
	Atropine	0.044 mg/kg IV or IT
	Solu-delta-cortef	22 mg/kg IV
	Sodium bicarbonate (if >10–15 minutes)	1.0 mEq/kg IV
Ventricular fibrillation	Precordial thump	(if defibrillator not available)
	Epinephrine	0.2 mg/kg IV or IT
	Defibrillate	(see Table 11–16)
	Defibrillate	(Double original dose)
	Lidocaine	2.2 mg/kg IV or IT (cats: 0.5 mg/kg)
	Sodium bicarbonate (if >10–15 minutes)	1.0 mEq/kg IV
Electromechanical dissociation	Epinephrine	0.2 mg/kg IV or IT
	Solu-delta-cortef *or*	22 mg/kg IV
	Dexamethasone SP	2.2 mg/kg IV
	Sodium bicarbonate	1.0 mEq/kg IV

*IT = intratracheal administration. double the recommended intravenous dose.

Cardiopulmonary arrest in the anesthetized patient may be successfully treated only if the anesthetist recognizes the arrest early through careful monitoring and acts rapidly and correctly to re-establish normal cardiac rhythm before permanent organ damage occurs.

References

Bednarski RM: Anesthetic equipment. In Muir WW, Hubbell JAE (editors): Equine Anesthesia: Monitoring and Emergency Therapy. St Louis, Mosby–Year Book, Inc., 1991, pp. 325–351.

Dorsch JA and Dorsch SE: The anesthesia machine. In Understanding Anesthesia Equipment. 2nd ed. Baltimore, Williams & Wilkins Co., 1984A, pp. 38–76.

Dorsch JA and Dorsch SE: Vaporizers. In Understanding Anesthesia Equipment. 2nd ed. Baltimore, The Williams & Wilkins Co., 1984B, pp. 77–135.

Dorsch JA and Dorsch SE: The breathing system. IV. In Understanding Anesthesia Equipment. 2nd ed. Baltimore, Williams & Wilkins Co., 1984C, pp. 210–246.

Dorsch JA and Dorsch SE: Controlling trace gas levels. In Understanding Anesthesia Equipment. 2nd ed. Baltimore, Williams & Wilkins Co., 1984D, pp. 247–288.

Hartsfield SM: Machines and breathing systems for administration of inhalation anesthetics. In Short CE (editor): Principles and Practice of Veterinary Anesthesia. Baltimore, Williams & Wilkins Co., 1987, pp. 395–418.

Haskins SC: Monitoring the anesthetized patient. In Short CE (editor): Principles and Practice of Veterinary Anesthesia. Baltimore, Williams & Wilkins Co., 1987, pp. 455–477.

Muir WW, Hubbell JAE and Skarda RT: Handbook of Veterinary Anesthesia. St. Louis, CV Mosby Co., 1989.

Paddleford RR: Anesthetic waste gases and your health. In Short CE (editor): Principles and Practice of Veterinary Anesthesia. Baltimore, Williams & Wilkins Co., 1987, pp. 607–620.

Shawley RV: Controlled ventilation and pulmonary function. In Short CE (editor): Principles and Practice of Veterinary Anesthesia. Baltimore, Williams & Wilkins Co., 1987, pp. 419–425.

Short CE: Anticholinergics. In Short CE (editor): Principles and Practice of Veterinary Anesthesia. Baltimore, Williams & Wilkins Co., 1987, pp. 8–15.

12

Instrumentation and Principles of Aseptic Technique

PETER SCHWARZ and CHARLES BLASS

INTRODUCTION

Surgical therapy is an exacting method of treatment. The operating room has a different "set of rules" to be followed in the handling of patients, instruments, equipment and supplies. Complete familiarity with instrumentation, surgical support equipment and aseptic technique must be mastered by all operating room personnel.

Surgical assistance by the veterinary technician, to varying degrees, will be required on most procedures performed by the veterinarian in both large-animal and small-animal practice. The veterinary technician must be prepared for both sterile and nonsterile support in a variety of procedures. Technicians will function in the surgical setting as scrub nurses, anesthetists, circulating nurses and surgical assistants. Oftentimes, the duties will encompass all of these functions.

INSTRUMENTATION

Almost all surgical instruments are made of stainless steel, which is rust resistant and retains a keen edge. There are basically two types of instrument finishes. One is a bright, highly polished mirror finish. This finish tends to reflect light and can hinder the vision of the surgeon; however, it does resist spotting and discoloration. The other commonly available finish is the satin or dull finish, which was developed to eliminate glare and lessen the surgeon's eye strain. It is less resistant to spotting and discoloration.

Tungsten carbide inserts are often added to the tips of stainless steel instruments that are used for cutting or gripping. These substances tend to prolong the life of the instrument because they are hard and resistant to wear. The inserts are attached to the stainless steel instrument and can be removed and replaced by the manufacturer.

The advancements in design of surgical instrumentation have played a significant role in the increased effectiveness of surgical treatment. Thousands of different instruments are available. Most veterinary hospitals and clinics develop surgical instrument packs for various procedures, such as a basic soft tissue surgical pack, emergency pack and basic orthopedic pack. The instruments found in these surgical packs are instruments commonly used and required to perform most surgical procedures performed by the veterinary surgeon. Specific instruments for special procedures are packed and prepared either individually or in special procedure packs. Large and bulky instruments are also generally packed and prepared separately. Tables 12–1 and 12–2 list the instruments most likely to be included in the basic surgical packs used in veterinary practice.

Instruments are designed for specific purposes: cutting, holding, clamping, retracting, and so on. Instruments should be handled gently. Avoid bouncing, dropping and weighing them down under heavier equipment.

Table 12–1

INSTRUMENTS FOR SMALL-ANIMAL STANDARD, EMERGENCY AND ORTHOPEDIC SETS AT COLORADO STATE UNIVERSITY

Standard Set	Emergency Set	Orthopedic Set
1 Ovariectomy hook	1 Mayo scissors (curved or straight)	1 Bone curette
1 Groove director	1 Needle holder	1 Large Kern bone-holding forceps
1 No. 3 scalpel handle	1 No. 3 scalpel handle	1 Small Kern bone-holding forceps
1 Thumb tissue forceps	1 Thumb tissue forceps	1 Rongeur
1 Brown-Adson tissue forceps	1 Brown-Adson tissue forceps	1 Periosteal elevator
1 Mayo scissors, straight	2 Allis forceps	1 Metal ruler
1 Mayo scissors, curved	2 Crile or Kelly forceps (1 curved, 1	2 Army-Navy retractors
1 Metzenbaum scissors (curved or straight)	straight)	1 Metal mallet
1 Needle holder (Snowden-Pencer)	4 Towel forceps	1 Nail set
2 Carmalt forceps (curved or straight)	6 Mosquito hemostats (3 curved, 3 straight)	1 Jacobs chuck and key
2 Crile forceps (1 curved, 1 straight)	1 No. 10 blade	1 Michel forcep
2 Allis forceps	1 Steam clock (sterilization indicator)	2 Gigli handles and 1 wire
8 Mosquito forceps (4 curved, 4 straight)	1 Towel	2 Volkmann rake retractors
12 Towel forceps	Sponges	1 Roll 18 ga. stainless steel wire
1 Wire suture scissors		1 Roll 20 ga. stainless steel wire
1 Sponge forceps (curved or straight)		1 Roll 22 ga. stainless steel wire
2 Lamp handles		Assorted pin set
1 Stainless steel bowl inverted with sponges		Kirschner wire
1 Steam clock (sterilization indicator)		6 .035 wires
2 Lap sponges		6 .045 wires
6 Towels		6 .062 wires
1 No. 10 blade		Steinmann pins
		6 $^5/_{64}''$ pins
		6 $^3/_{32}''$ pins
		6 $^7/_{64}''$ pins
		6 $^1/_8''$ pins
		6 $^9/_{64}''$ pins
		6 $^5/_{32}''$ pins
		6 $^3/_{16}''$ pins
		6 $^1/_4''$ pins
		1 Pkg Michel clips
		1 Steam clock (sterilization indicator)

Table 12–2
INSTRUMENTS FOR LARGE-ANIMAL STANDARD AND EMERGENCY SETS AT COLORADO STATE UNIVERSITY

Standard Set	Emergency Set
16 Towel forceps	4 Towel forceps
4 Curved mosquito hemostats	2 Curved mosquito hemostats
4 Straight mosquito hemostats	2 Straight mosquito hemostats
2 Curved Kelly or Crile forceps	2 Allis tissue forceps
2 Straight Kelly or Crile forceps	1 Curved Mayo scissors
2 Allis tissue forceps	1 Straight Mayo scissors
1 Curved Mayo scissors	2 Needle holders
1 Straight Mayo scissors	1 3 × 4 Thumb tissue forceps
1 S/S operating scissors	1 Brown-Adson tissue forceps
1 Curved Metzenbaum scissors	1 No. 3 scalpel handle
1 Straight Metzenbaum scissors	1 No. 4 scalpel handle
1 Bandage scissors	1 Towel
2 Needle holders	1 Steam clock (sterilization indicator)
2 Right-angle forceps	Sponges
1 Straight 15-cm Ochsner forceps	
1 Curved 15-cm Ochsner forceps	
1 No. 3 scalpel handle	
1 No. 4 scalpel handle	
3 3 × 4 thumb tissue forceps	
2 1 × 2 Adson tissue forceps	
1 Sponge forceps (curved or straight)	
1 Groove director	
1 Saline bowl	
2 Lamp handles	
4 Towels	
1 Steam clock (sterilization indicator)	
Sponges in inverted bowl	

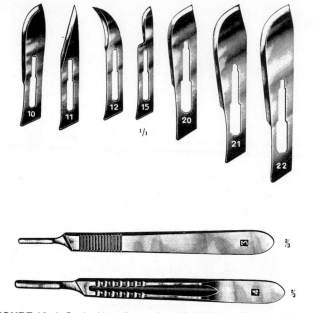

FIGURE 12–1. Scalpel handles and surgical blades. The No. 3 handle and the No. 10 blade are used most often in small animal surgery. The No. 4 handle and the No. 20 blade are used most often in large animals.

Needle Holders

Needle holders are forceps that are specifically designed for holding curved suture needles during suturing and for doing instrument ties. They should not be used for any other purpose (e.g., twisting or bending wire). *Mayo-Hegar* and *Olsen-Hegar needle holders* are two commonly used needle holders. The Olsen-Hegar is a needle holder and scissors combination. It may have an advantage for the veterinary surgeon who is doing surgery alone. Suture material can be placed and cut

General Surgical Instruments

Scalpel

The *scalpel* is the best instrument for dividing tissues with minimal trauma. Generally, scalpel handles with interchangeable, disposable blades are used (Fig. 12–1). The Bard-Parker No. 3 medium handle uses detachable blades Nos. 10, 11, 12 and 15 and seems to be the most applicable for small animal surgery. The No. 4 Bard-Parker handle is larger and uses detachable blades Nos. 20, 21, and 22. This handle is most commonly used for large animal surgery. Some veterinarians use a groove director when making incisions (Fig. 12–2). This instrument will protect underlying tissues when making an abdominal incision by providing a groove to cut on. Electroscalpels are sometimes used to cut tissue. They cut by the passage of electrical current through a small point of contact with the tissue (Fig. 12–3). Proper grounding is necessary. An incision made with a sharp scalpel will heal more rapidly than one made by an electroscalpel.

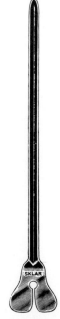

FIGURE 12–2. Groove director.

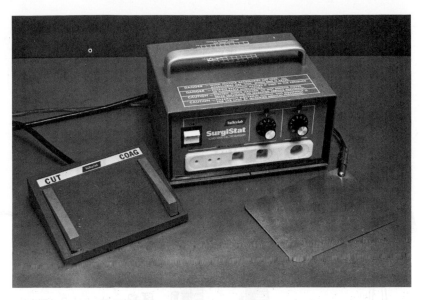

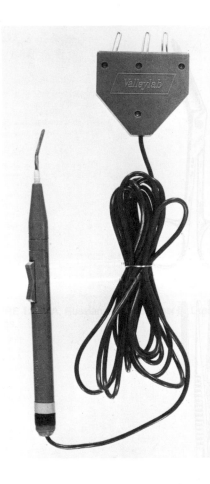

FIGURE 12–3. A, Electroscalpel. B, Electroscalpel foot switch, power source, and ground plate.

A

without requiring a separate suture scissors. The major disadvantage with this needle holder is accidental cutting of suture material during suture placement. Tungsten carbide inserts are available with the needle holder portion of both these instruments (Fig. 12–4A and B).

Scissors

Scissors are used for both sharp and blunt dissection and for cutting sutures and bandage materials. Dissecting scissors are made for accurate cutting and dissection of tissue. Many types of operating scissors are available. Operating scissors may vary by the type of blades (straight or curved), the type of points (blunt-blunt, blunt-sharp or sharp-sharp) and the cutting edge of the blades (plain or serrated) (Fig. 12–4C). *Mayo dissecting scissors* (Fig. 12–4D) are commonly used for cutting tough tissues, whereas *Metzenbaum scissors* (Fig. 12–4E) are used for more delicate tissues. Metzenbaum scissors are the instrument of choice for soft tissue dissection with minimal surgical trauma.

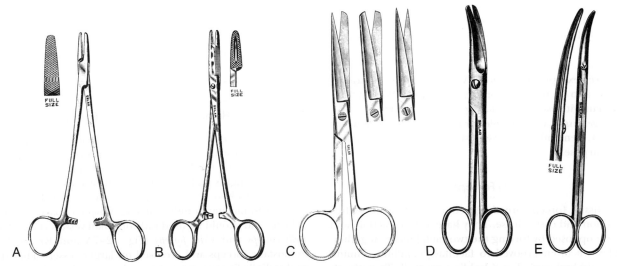

FIGURE 12–4. A and B, Needle holders: A, Mayo-Hegar; B, Olsen-Hegar. C, Operating scissors: sharp-blunt, blunt-blunt and sharp-sharp. D, Mayo dissecting scissors. E, Metzenbaum dissecting scissors.

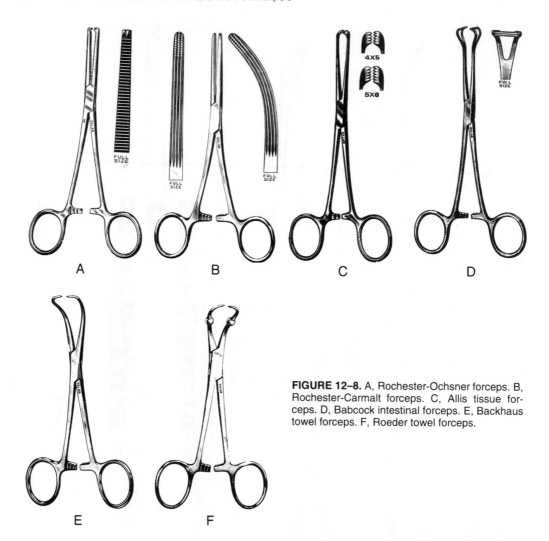

FIGURE 12–8. A, Rochester-Ochsner forceps. B, Rochester-Carmalt forceps. C, Allis tissue forceps. D, Babcock intestinal forceps. E, Backhaus towel forceps. F, Roeder towel forceps.

grooved in Crile forceps. *Rochester-Pean forceps* are still larger, transversely grooved forceps, which are useful for the control of large tissue bundles and vessels (Fig. 12–7C). *Rochester-Ochsner forceps* are similar forceps and have the addition of interdigitary teeth located at the end of the jaw (Fig. 12–8A). This modification helps prevent slippage of the forceps in tissue. *Rochester-Carmalt forceps* are large crushing forceps with longitudinal grooves to prevent tissue slippage. These forceps are used for cross-clamping tissues containing vessels. Cross grooves at the tip reduce tissue slippage when gripping with the tip (Fig. 12–8B). The Rochester-Carmalt forceps are commonly used for crushing the body of the uterus during an ovariohysterectomy (spay) operation.

When using hemostatic forceps, the smallest forceps that will accomplish the desired effect should be used. The tips of the forceps should be used to grasp only as much tissue as necessary. When clamping vessels and tissue stumps for ligation, the forceps should be applied with the concave surface facing upward. This will facilitate tying the ligature.

Allis tissue forceps are used for grasping tissues (Fig. 12–8C), as are *Babcock forceps* (Fig. 12–8D). These forceps are designed to grasp tissue with minimal trauma.

Towel forceps are used for attaching towels and drapes to each other and to the patient. These forceps have pointed tips that curve and join like ice tongs. *Backhaus towel clamps* (Fig. 12–8E and F) and *Roeder towel clamps* are two commonly used towel

clamps. The Roeder-type towel forceps has a metal bead or ball stop attached to the jaws. These prevent deep tissue penetration and also prevent the towels from slipping along the jaws of the forceps.

Retractors

Retractors are used to facilitate exposure of the operating field. Retractors may be hand-held or self-retaining. The ends of hand-held retractors may be hooked, curved, toothed, or spatula shaped (Fig. 12–9A–C). Hand-held retractors require a surgical assistant to maintain tension on the retracted tissues. The *Snook ovariohysterectomy hook* is a specialized type of hand-held retractor used to retrieve the horn of the uterus through the abdominal incision during ovariohysterectomy (Fig. 12–9D).

Self-retaining retractors are instruments that maintain tension on retracted tissues by various types of locking mechanisms. The locking mechanism on the handles holds the tips of the retractor at the desired point of tissue distraction. Self-retaining retractors offer the advantage of maintaining tissue separation once placed without the need of an assistant. *Gelpi retractors* (Fig. 12–10A) and *Weitlaner retractors* (Fig. 12–10B) are commonly used for muscle retraction. The *Balfour abdominal wall retractor* is used to retract the sides of an abdominal wall incision to maintain an unobstructed view of the abdomi-

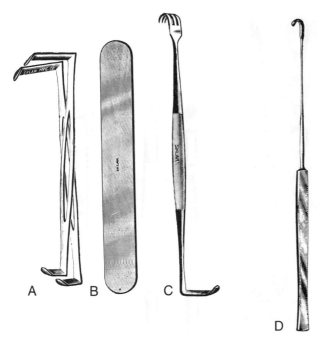

FIGURE 12–9. A through C, Hand-held retractors: A, US Army double-ended retractor; B, Malleable retractor; C, Senn double-ended retractor. D, Snook's ovariohysterectomy hook (spay hook).

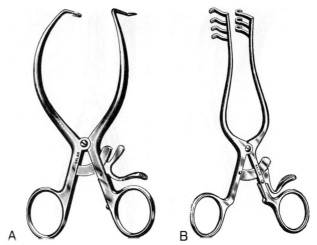

FIGURE 12–10. A, Gelpi self-retaining retractor. B, Weitlaner self-retaining retractor.

nal cavity (Fig. 12–11A). The two retracting blades on the side of the retractor maintain lateral distraction while the single end blade is usually placed under the xiphoid cartilage to allow cranial distraction as well as help position the lateral blades correctly along the incision line. The *Finochietto rib spreader* is used to retract a thoracic wall incision to maintain an unobstructed view of the surgical field within the chest (Fig. 12–11B). The ratchet end of the retractor is usually positioned at the dorsal end of the intercostal incision to keep it out of the way of the surgeon.

Orthopedic Instruments

Rongeurs

Rongeur forceps are used to cut and remove pieces of dense tissue (i.e., bone, cartilage, fibrous tissue). The opposing cutting jaws allow controlled removal of small pieces of dense tissue adjacent to delicate tissue (i.e., spinal cord). Rongeurs may be single- or double-action forceps (Fig. 12–12). Double-action rongeur forceps have a smoother cutting action and are mechanically stronger than the single-action forceps; therefore, they are the preferred instrument for cutting and removing large and dense tissues.

Bone-Holding Forceps

Bone-holding forceps are heavily constructed forceps designed to hold bone and bone fragments while they are manipulated into alignment and fixed into apposition with orthopedic implants (screws, pins, wires or plates) (Fig. 12–13).

Curettes

Curettes are used to scrape the surface of relatively dense tissue to remove loose or degenerate tissue (bone marrow, necrotic bone, cartilage flaps, abscess material). They are designed with a small cuplike structure at the end of a handle. The cup has a sharp cutting edge and comes in various sizes (Fig. 12–14A).

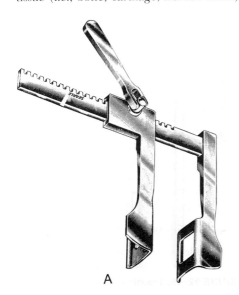

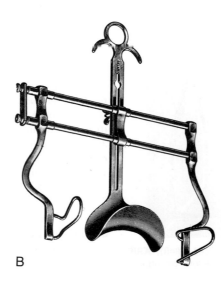

FIGURE 12–11. A, Finochietto rib spreader. B, Balfour self-retaining abdominal retractor.

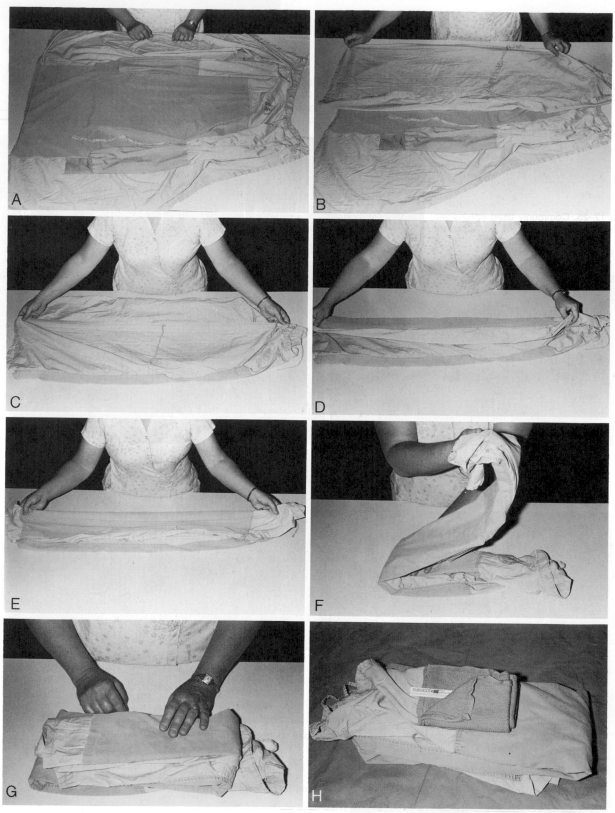

FIGURE 12–27. A, Method of folding a surgical gown. The gown is spread on a countertop with the outside of the gown facing up. B, The near edge of the gown is folded to the center. C, Next, the far edge of the gown is folded toward the center to meet the near edge. D, The gown is folded in half. E, The gown is folded in half again. F and G, The gown is folded lengthwise in accordian fashion into thirds. H, A hand towel and sterilization indicator are placed on top, and the gown is ready for wrapping.

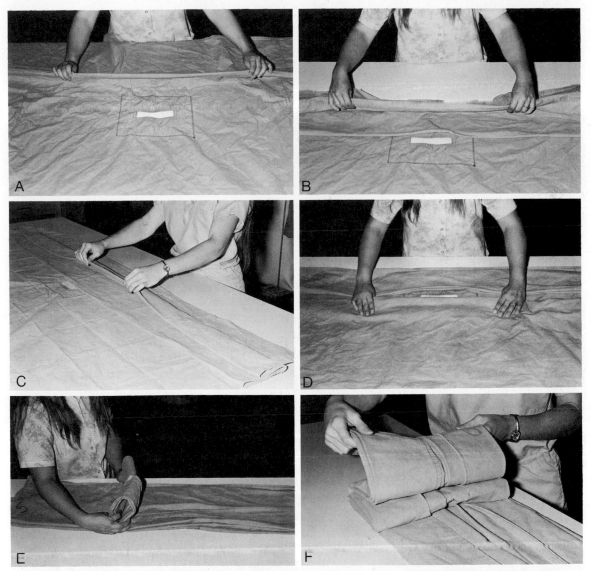

FIGURE 12-28. Drapes are folded in accordion fashion so that they are easily unfolded onto the patient. A–C, One side of the drape is folded to the center in accordian fashion. Each fold is approximately 15 cm wide. D, The opposite side is folded in a similar manner. E and F, Lengthwise, the drape is again folded to the center of the fenestration in accordian fashion. These folds are also about 15 cm in width.

Illustration continued on following page

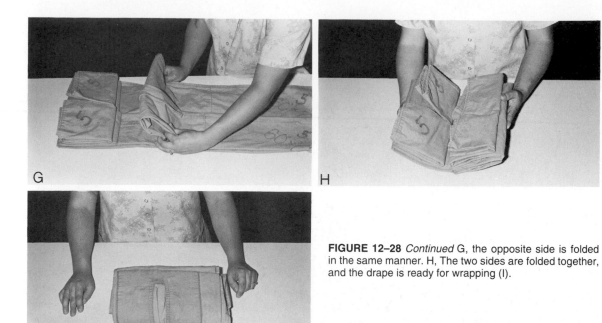

FIGURE 12–28 *Continued* G, the opposite side is folded in the same manner. H, The two sides are folded together, and the drape is ready for wrapping (I).

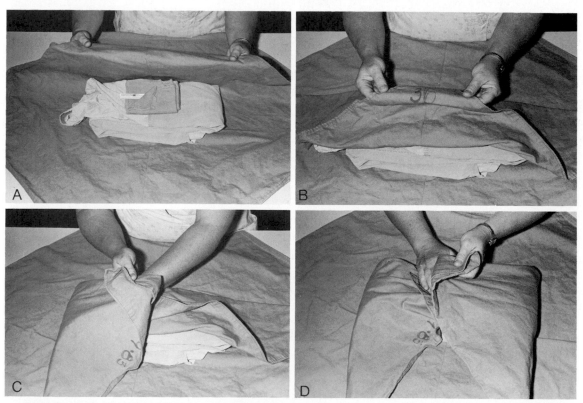

FIGURE 12–29. Wrapping of fenestrated drape and gown. A, The gown, along with a hand towel and sterilization indicator, is placed diagonally onto the nonfenestrated drapes. B–E, The corners are folded over the gown. F, Three corners of the second drape are folded in a similar manner.

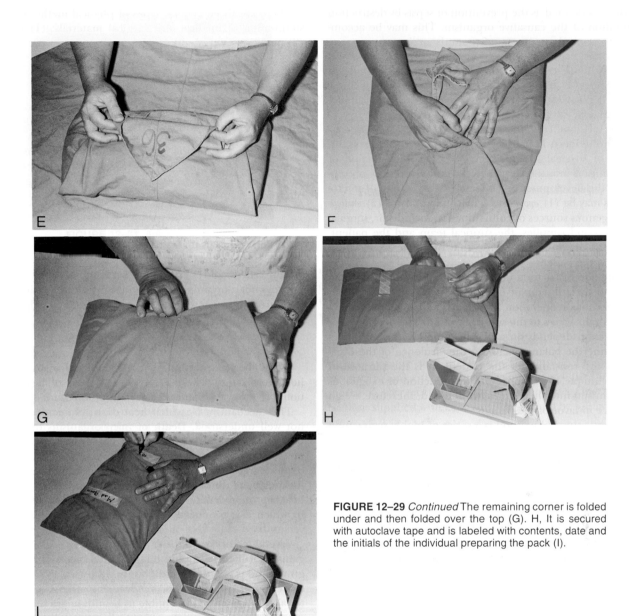

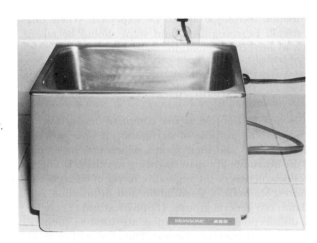

FIGURE 12–29 *Continued* The remaining corner is folded under and then folded over the top (G). H, It is secured with autoclave tape and is labeled with contents, date and the initials of the individual preparing the pack (I).

FIGURE 12–30. Ultrasonic cleaner.

pired air from the nose and mouth. Masks are effective filters for relatively short periods only and therefore should be changed between operations.

After the animal is positioned on the surgery table and caps and masks are in place, any final preparation of the surgical site is done, and the instrument packs, gown packs, drapes and surgical gloves are opened. After this, the surgical team is ready for the surgical scrub.

The purpose of the surgical scrub is to remove dirt and grease and, as much as possible, the bacterial flora from hands and arms. Several products are available for use as surgical scrubs (Betadine, Nolvasan, Hibiclens).

Prior to scrubbing, the cap and mask must be in place, and all jewelry should be removed from hands and arms. Once the scrub has started, the hands and arms should not touch unsterile objects. If this occurs, the scrub should be repeated from the beginning. There are two basic types of surgical scrubs, *timed* and *anatomical.* The timed scrub (5 to 10 minutes) is more commonly used. The anatomical scrub is based on the number of brush strokes used on each skin surface, rather than on time.

Several variations exist in scrubbing techniques. One very effective technique starts by lathering the hands and arms to a point 7.5 to 10 cm above the elbow for approximately 1 minute without using a brush. The hands and arms are rinsed in running water. The hands are always held above the level of the elbows so that water drains off the elbows instead of off the hands. Next, soap is applied to a sterile brush and a systematic scrub is begun. Each surface of the digits should be scrubbed, paying special attention to the fingernails (Fig. 12–37). The back, both sides and the palm of the hand should be scrubbed using a circular motion. Next, the wrist and forearm is scrubbed, working toward the elbow. After one hand and arm has been scrubbed, the brush is rinsed well and the scrub is repeated on the other hand and arm. After both hands and arms have been scrubbed, they are rinsed in running water, with the hands kept above the elbows (Fig. 12–38). The entire scrub process is then repeated again.

The initial scrub of the day should probably last about 10 minutes. For subsequent scrubbings between surgeries, 5 minutes is adequate unless gross contamination has occurred. For the anatomical method, five strokes on the surface of the hands and the arms are repeated four times.

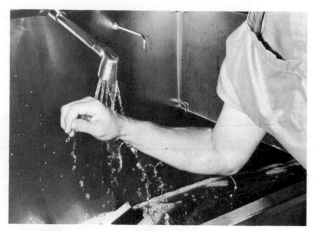

FIGURE 12–38. The hands, forearms and brush are thoroughly rinsed between scrubs. Keep hands above elbows.

Following the surgical scrub and drying of the hands and arms (Fig. 12–39), gown and gloves are donned. Gowns may be made of either cloth or paper. A properly folded gown is picked up by the inside at the shoulder seams without touching the outside of the gown. (A properly folded gown is accordion-folded from bottom to top inside out.) As the gown is picked up, it will unfold. Hands should be approximately at chest level, and the gown should be held out away from the body. Sometimes it is necessary to gently shake the gown to completely unfold it. After the sleeve openings are located, the arms are slid into the sleeves (Fig. 12–40). The method used for gloving determines whether the hands are extended through the cuffs of the gown at this point. The gown is then secured at the neck and waist by an assistant.

Two methods are available for gloving. *Closed gloving* (Fig. 12–41) has the advantage that it minimizes the chances of contaminating the gloves, since the outside of the gloves do not contact the skin. *Open gloving* (Fig. 12–42) is at a disadvantage because gloves are relatively easily contaminated by skin contact. Because closed gloving is not always possible (e.g.,

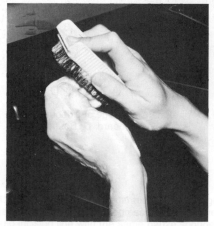

FIGURE 12–37. Each surface of every finger should be thoroughly scrubbed, paying special attention to the fingernails.

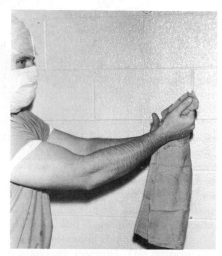

FIGURE 12–39. One hand and arm are dried at a time, using a double-thickness (folded longitudinally) towel. The hand is dried first, then the arm, using half the towel. The other hand and arm are dried in a similar manner, using the other half of the towel. The towel should be held so that it does not brush against the body.

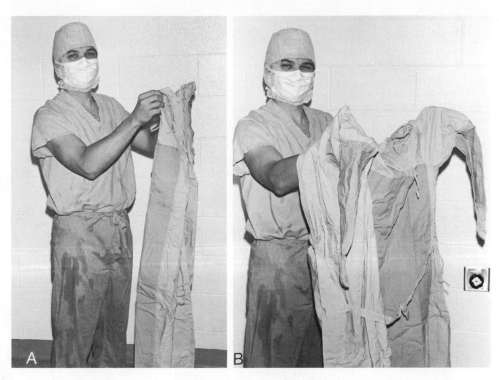

FIGURE 12–40. A, The gown is picked up at the shoulder seams, touching only the inside of the gown. The gown is unfolded and held away from the body at shoulder height. B, The arms are slid into the sleeves.

replacing gloves during surgery), it is necessary for one to be able to glove by the open method.

Operating Room Conduct

Basic Aseptic Techniques

All items are either sterile or unsterile. If there is any doubt, consider it unsterile. Only the outside of sterile wraps should be touched by ungloved hands, and sterile packs should always be opened away from the body. Sterile articles are handled only by sterile gloves or a sterile instrument. Any time a wrapper or sterile linen becomes moist, it should be considered unsterile. When removing materials from a sterile pack, lift them up and out. Do not drag them over the edge of the container. When solutions are poured into a sterile container, the solution container should not touch the sterile container, nor should solutions be poured from such a height that they splash (Fig. 12–43).

Correct Operating Table Conduct

The surgeon's efficiency is greatly increased by a competent surgical assistant. There should be no unnecessary talking unless initiated by the primary surgeon. Every effort should be made to keep the operating table neat and orderly and the instruments clean and free of blood. Soiled sponges should be removed from the sterile field as soon as they are used. Instruments are passed handle first, with a light slap. When an instrument is properly passed, the surgeon should not have to look away from the operative site to assure the instrument has been appropriately presented. Bleeding is controlled by blotting, not wiping. Learn to anticipate what is going to happen and be prepared. If it is necessary to change positions during surgery with another sterile individual, the individuals should pass back to back or front to front. The back of a sterile individual is considered nonsterile. Therefore, the back should never be directed toward the sterile field. It should be apparent that everything done in the operating room is for the purpose of minimizing microbial contamination, thereby minimizing postoperative infections and achieving maximal therapeutic benefit from the surgical procedure. The veterinary technician is a valuable member of the surgical team. By providing good assistance, one can ensure that the surgical procedure will be performed more efficiently and effectively.

POSTOPERATIVE CARE

The postoperative period is probably the most neglected area of care in veterinary medicine. The veterinary technician can become indispensable in providing quality postoperative care. Frequently, the technician is left alone to observe anesthetic recovery. The animal should be placed in a clean, well-ventilated environment for recovery. Supplemental heat should be provided (circulating warm water pad, blankets, straw) if the patient is excessively cold (less than 36°C). If the animal is still unconscious, it must be watched closely. If the animal is placed in a cage or stall, be sure the head is toward the door and slightly lower than the rest of the body. This makes observation easier and will help prevent any regurgitated material from being inhaled. Also, the animal's head and neck should be placed in a slightly extended position to prevent obstruction of the airway.

Once the animal has regained the ability to swallow (frequently manifested by chewing on the endotracheal tube), the endotracheal tube can be removed. The endotracheal tube should be untied to allow quick removal. Be sure to deflate the cuff if a cuffed endotracheal tube was used (Fig. 12–44). The airway should be checked frequently.

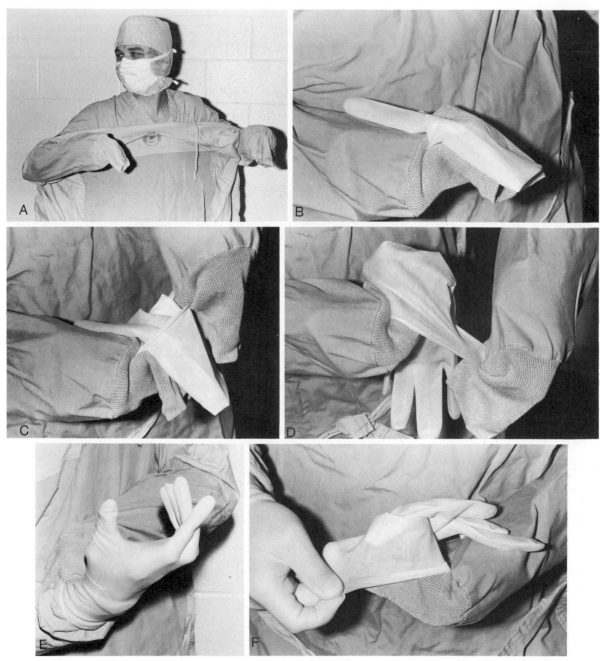

FIGURE 12–41. Closed gloving. A, When performing closed gloving, the hands are kept inside the sleeves while gloving takes place. B, The palm side of the glove is grasped at the cuff through the sleeve. C, The opposite side of the cuff is grasped in the other hand and D, pulled over the top side of the hand. E, The hand is slid completely into the glove. F, The opposite hand is gloved in a similar fashion. At no time should skin be visible while performing closed gloving.

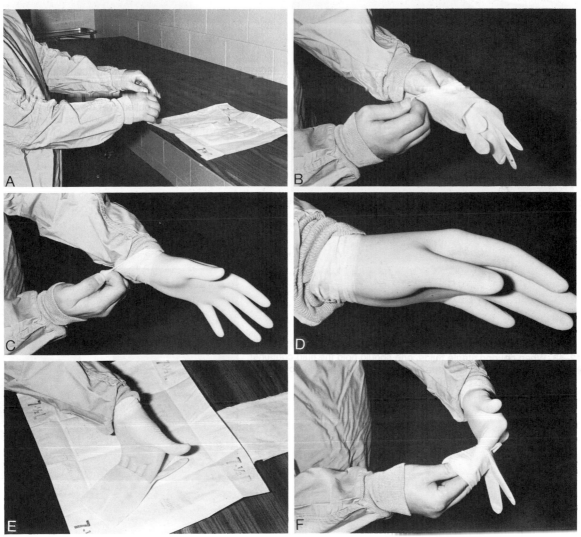

FIGURE 12–42. Open gloving. A, When performing open gloving, the hands are extended out of the sleeves while gowning. B, The palm side of the left glove is grasped at the fold by the right hand and is pulled onto the left hand. C and D, The left glove is pulled to the level of the sleeve and released. E, The gloved fingers of the left hand are then slid into the fold of the right glove. F, The fingers of the right hand are slid into the glove.

Illustration continued on following page

wound strength but will suppress early inflammation. Prolonged aspirin therapy may delay blood clotting. Chemotherapeutic drugs can have an adverse affect on wound healing, depending on their mechanism of action and the time of administration in relation to the time of injury. Radiation can have a profound adverse affect on wound healing, depending on dose and time of exposure in relation to time of injury.

WOUND CARE

Immediate Wound Care

The wound should be covered with a clean, dry bandage as soon as possible after injury to prevent further contamination and reduce hemorrhage. The bandage should remain in place until definitive treatment is initiated. Antibiotic ointments or powders act only as foreign bodies and delay wound healing and thus should not be applied.

Once the animal is stabilized and other, life-threatening injuries have been treated, the wound can be prepared for treatment. The bandage is removed, and the wound is packed with sterile gauze or filled with sterile water-soluble lubricant (K-Y jelly, Johnson & Johnson) or temporarily closed with sutures, towel clamps or Michel clips. This allows skin around the wound to be clipped and prepared for aseptic surgery without the introduction of hair into the wound. Hair from the edges of the wound can be removed by means of scissors dipped in mineral oil to prevent hair from falling into the wound. Once the skin is prepared, the K-Y jelly can be flushed out or the sponges removed from the wound.

Wound Lavage

Wound lavage is necessary to remove debris and loose particles and tissue from the wound. It also reduces the number of bacteria in the wound. If infection is suspected, a piece of tissue should be sampled for bacterial culture prior to lavage. Large volumes of warm, sterile normal saline are preferred for lavage. Antibiotics should not be added to the fluid. Soaps, detergents and antiseptic solutions should not be used, as they damage the tissue. The mechanical action of the lavage is the most important factor for successful lavage. Moderate pressure (7 psi) can be generated with a 35-cc syringe and 19-gauge needle; this method is more effective than pouring fluid over a wound. The syringe can be connected to a bag of fluid with a three-way stopcock to facilitate refilling of the syringe (Fig. 13–2). A pulsating, high-pressure (70 psi) stream can be generated by means of a Water Pik (Teledyne), which is even more effective in reducing bacterial population and removing necrotic tissue and foreign material from heavily contaminated wounds.

Wound Debridement

Wound debridement is necessary to remove all contaminated, devitalized or necrotic tissue and foreign material from the wound. This can be performed surgically by excising the affected tissue in layers, beginning at the surface and progressing to the wound depths. Alternatively, the entire wound can

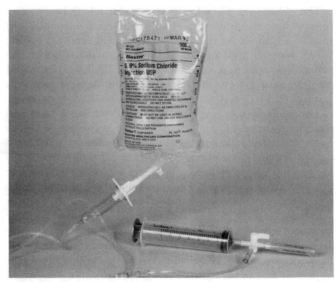

FIGURE 13–2. Connection of a 35-cc syringe and 19-gauge needle to a three-way stopcock and bag of sterile normal saline to facilitate copious lavage of a wound.

be excised *en bloc* if there is sufficient healthy tissue surrounding the wound and vital structures can be preserved. Enzymatic debridement with a commercial solution containing trypsin (Granulex, Beecham) can be used for wounds that are not suitable for surgical debridement. Enzymatic debridement is slower and may damage normal tissue.

Wound Closure

Selection of one of the four methods of wound closure depends on the nature of the wound. *Primary wound closure* results in healing by first intention. First-intention healing, known as appositional healing, is achieved by the suturing or grafting of a wound soon after injury. Primary wound closure is indicated in fresh, clean, sharply incised wounds with minimal trauma and minimal contamination that are seen within hours of injury. Wounds treated within 6 to 8 hours of injury are treated within the "golden period," that is, bacteria contaminating the wound have not multiplied to the critical number of 10^5 organisms per gram of tissue and the tissue has not become infected. Wounds treated after the golden period should not be closed, since infection is likely.

Delayed primary closure is primary closure of a wound 1 to 3 days after injury, before granulation tissue has appeared in the wound. It is indicated for mildly contaminated, minimally traumatized wounds that require some cleansing and debridement, or for relatively clean wounds seen 6 to 8 hours after injury. This method allows any local contamination or infection to be controlled before closure.

Healing by contraction and epithelialization is defined as second-intention healing and is indicated for dirty, contaminated, traumatized wounds when cleansing and debridement are necessary and when closure may be difficult. Adequate, loose skin surrounding the wound is necessary to allow contraction. Closure by second intention may not always be desirable because the new epithelium is fragile and easily abraded. In addition, contraction may impede normal function, depending on the location of the wound.

Secondary closure results in third-intention healing. The wound is sutured at least 3 to 5 days after injury. Granulation tissue will be present in the wound by the time of closure. The granulation tissue helps to control infection in the wound and fills in the tissue defect. Secondary closure is indicated when (1) the wound is severely contaminated or traumatized, (2) epithelialization and contraction will not completely close the wound or (3) second-intention healing is undesirable.

The decision whether to treat a wound primarily or to have it remain open initially and follow up with delayed closure, second-intention healing or secondary closure depends on the (1) time lapse since injury; wounds greater than 6 to 8 hours old should be kept open initially; (2) degree of contamination; wounds obviously contaminated should be kept open initially and thoroughly cleansed; (3) amount of tissue damage; wounds with substantial tissue damage have reduced host defenses, are more likely to become infected and consequently should remain open initially; (4) thoroughness of debridement; if the initial debridement was conservative, the wound should remain open until definitive debridement is performed; (5) blood supply to the wound; a wound with questionable blood supply should remain open until the extent of nonviable tissue is determined; (6) the animal's health; if the animal is unable to endure prolonged surgical debridement, the wound should be kept open and possibly undergo enzymatic debridement until the animal can withstand surgery; (7) closure without tension or dead space; if excessive tension or dead space is present, the wound should be allowed to remain open because dead space allows accumulation of fluid, separation of tissues and formation of seromas, which may predispose to infection and delay wound healing; and (8) location of the wound; certain locations may not be amenable to closure (such as a large wound on a limb).

WOUND BANDAGING

Bandaging promotes wound healing by protecting the wound from additional trauma and contamination, by preventing wound desiccation, by preventing hematoma and seroma formation by providing compression and obliterating dead space, and by immobilizing the wound to prevent cellular and capillary disruption. Bandaging minimizes postoperative edema around incisions and minimizes exuberant granulation tissue formation in open wounds on the lower limb region (below carpus or tarsus) of horses. In addition, the bandage can absorb wound exudate and debride the wound of foreign material and loose tissue that adheres to the bandage as it is removed. Covering a wound with a bandage promotes an acid environment at the wound surface by preventing carbon dioxide loss and absorbing ammonia produced by bacteria. An acid environment increases oxygen dissociation from hemoglobin and subsequently increases oxygen availability in the wound. The bandage also keeps the wound warm. Higher temperatures improve wound healing and facilitate oxygen dissociation.

A bandage usually consists of three layers: the primary or contact layer, the secondary or padded conforming layer and the tertiary or holding and protective layer. The primary bandage layer contacts the wound surface (if present) and may be adherent or nonadherent and occlusive or semiocclusive. Adherent bandages are indicated if some debridement is still necessary. Wounds discharging large amounts of exudate or containing embedded debris are often covered with an adherent, absorbent type of dressing such as a small stack of gauze pads, disposable baby diaper, cotton (such as combine), and the like, in what is called a *dry/dry bandage*, to absorb exudate and allow debris to adhere. The same absorbent material soaked with saline creates a *wet/dry bandage* to "rehydrate" and loosen dried exudate and debris from a wound, facilitating its removal. Nonadherent bandages are required when healthy granulation fills the wound to avoid disruption of this tissue during removal of the contact layer. Semiocclusive, nonadherent bandages are preferred, as they allow air to penetrate to the wound surface and exudate to escape from the wound surface. Occlusive bandages should not be used if wound exudate is present, as they keep the exudate at the wound surface, and this causes maceration of the wound and adjacent healthy tissue.

The secondary layer is an absorbent, padded, conforming layer of cast padding or roll cotton. The tertiary layer is the holding and protective layer, which uses some form of gauze and elastic or adhesive tape to hold the bandage in place.

Specific bandages and their indications for use in small animal practice are described below. The standard procedure for application of any bandage requires (1) application of anchoring tape strips (stirrups) to the distal portion of limb; (2) application of a primary bandage layer over the wound, if present; (3) application of the padded secondary layer over the stirrups; (4) application of the gauze tertiary layer; (5) application of the splint; (6) reflection and twisting of the stirrups to adhere to the gauze layer; and (7) application of the protective tertiary layer of tape. The middle two toes should always be exposed to allow assessment for color, warmth and swelling. A stockinette can be applied underneath the secondary layer to help prevent the bandage from slipping. Other modifications are acceptable.

WOUND BANDAGING IN SMALL ANIMALS

Casts

Fiberglass cast materials are currently used almost routinely because of their light weight, extreme rigidity, rapid setting time, and ventilation and waterproof properties. Casts are indicated for stabilization of certain fractures distal to the elbow or stifle, and for immobilization of limbs to protect ligament or tendon repairs. The cast material is applied instead of a tertiary layer; however, minimal padding is suggested to avoid cast loosening and movement (Fig. 13–3). It is advisable to monitor animals with casts at least weekly.

Bandages and Splints

The *Robert Jones bandage* is most commonly used for temporary immobilization of fractures distal to the elbow or stifle prior to surgery. It is a large bulky bandage that provides rigid stabilization owing to the extreme compression of the thick cotton secondary layer (Fig. 13–4). The Robert Jones bandage is not appropriate for fractures of the femur or humerus.

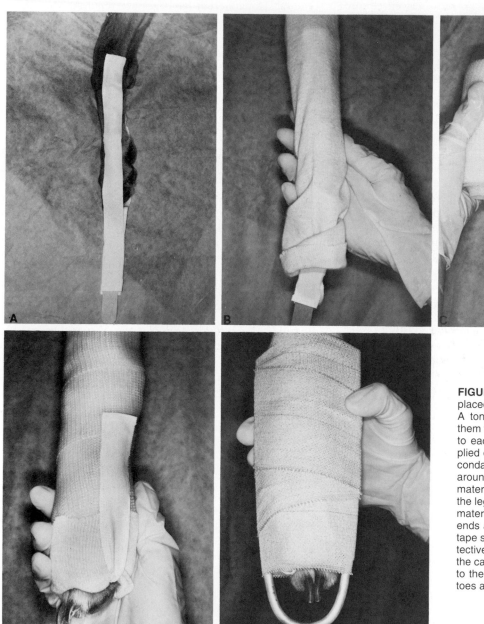

FIGURE 13–3. Cast. A, Tape stirrups are placed on the lateral aspects of the limb. A tongue depressor is placed between them to prevent adherence of the stirrups to each another. B, A stockinette is applied over the limb. A lightly padded, secondary layer is then applied firmly around the leg. C, The fiberglass cast material is applied firmly but not tightly to the leg, avoiding compression of the cast material with fingers. D, The stockinette ends are reflected over the cast and the tape stirrups reflected onto the cast. Protective tape is applied over the ends of the cast. E, A walking bar can be applied to the cast at this point. The middle two toes are exposed.

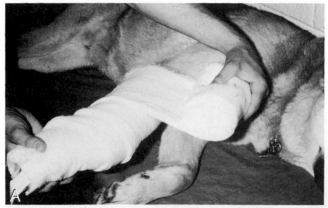

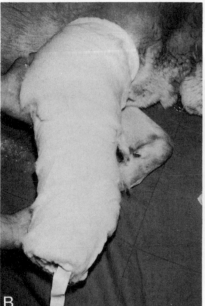

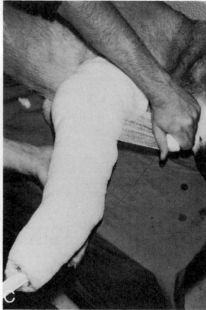

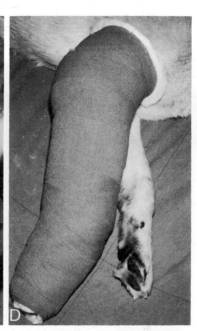

FIGURE 13–4. Robert Jones bandage. A, Tape stirrups are applied and the limb is wrapped in a secondary layer of roll cotton. B, A large amount of roll cotton is used to ensure good support. C, The roll cotton is compressed tightly with a gauze tertiary layer. D, Protective tape is then firmly applied. (Courtesy of Dr. John Berg.)

The *modified Robert Jones bandage* or simple padded bandage is a less bulky bandage and is used to reduce postoperative swelling of limbs (Fig. 13–5). It provides little or no splinting of the limbs. Less padding is used in the secondary layer, and cast padding is used instead of roll cotton.

A *chest* or *abdominal bandage* is applied in the standard three layers. These bandages should be applied firmly but without constricting the chest or abdomen (Fig. 13–6). If an abdominal bandage is used to control abdominal bleeding, the layers are applied more firmly. A rolled towel can be used to reinforce the bandage along the midline and is applied before application of the protective tape. The effectiveness of a compression bandage lasts for only 1 to 2 hours, and it should not remain in place longer than 4 hours.

Distal limb splints can be made with tongue depressors for very small animals, or with aluminum splints, cast material, or thermoplastics (Fig. 13–7). They are indicated for temporary immobilization or definitive stabilization of certain fractures of the distal radius and ulna, carpus, tarsus, meta-bones, and phalanges. They can also be used to support a traumatized distal limb. The limb should be well padded to avoid pressure spots. The splint should always be placed on the caudal aspect of the limb.

Slings

The *Ehmer sling* is used specifically to immobilize the hindlimb after reduction of craniodorsal coxofemoral luxation, and to prevent weight bearing after surgery on the pelvis. Correct application results in internal rotation and adduction of the coxofemoral joint (Fig. 13–8). Minimal padding is suggested, and the sling is usually applied with adhesive tape alone to prevent slippage.

The *90–90 flexion sling* is similar to the Ehmer sling, but the stifle and hock are placed in 90-degree flexion, and no attempt is made to adduct and internally rotate the coxofemoral joint (Fig. 13–9). The 90–90 flexion sling is used to prevent stifle joint stiffness and hyperextension caused by quadriceps muscle contracture after distal femoral fracture repair in young patients. It can also be used as a non–weight-bearing sling to protect other surgical procedures of the hindlimb.

The *Velpeau sling* holds the flexed forelimb against the chest and prevents movement in all joints (Fig. 13–10). It is used as a non–weight-bearing sling for the forelimb. The Velpeau sling is indicated after reduction of scapulohumeral joint luxation or to immobilize scapula fractures.

The *carpal flexion sling* is a non–weight-bearing forelimb sling

Text continued on page 289

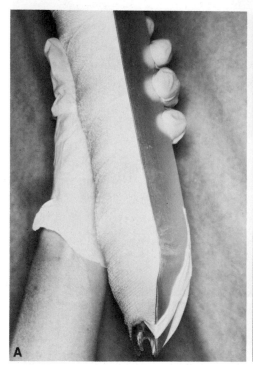 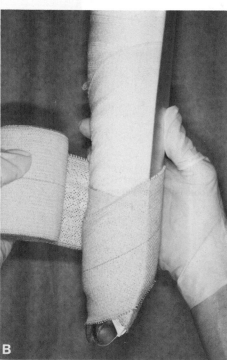

FIGURE 13–7. Splint. A, After application of a Modified Robert Jones or simple padded bandage (see Fig. 13–5), the splint is applied to the caudal aspect of the limb, and the stirrups are reflected onto the splint. B, Protective tape is then applied to hold the splint in place.

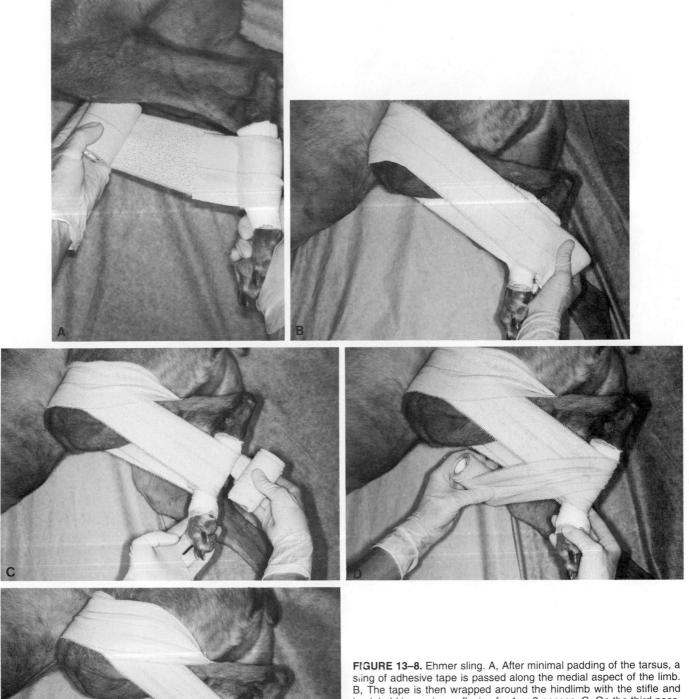

FIGURE 13–8. Ehmer sling. A, After minimal padding of the tarsus, a sling of adhesive tape is passed along the medial aspect of the limb. B, The tape is then wrapped around the hindlimb with the stifle and hock held in maximum flexion for 1 or 2 passes. C, On the third pass, the tape is brought over the flank and twisted behind the hock. D, The tape is then passed over the front of the metatarsus. E, This is repeated for 3 or 4 passes.

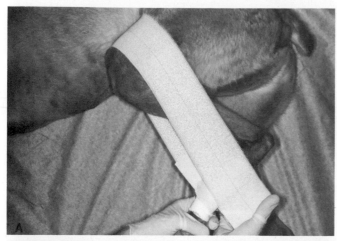

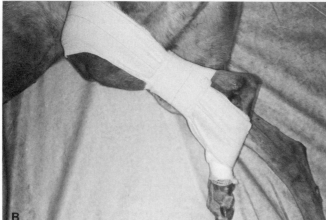

FIGURE 13–9. 90–90 flexion sling. After minimal padding of the tarsus, a sling of adhesive tape is passed along the medial aspect of the limb (see Fig. 13–8A). A, The tape is then wrapped around the hindlimb with the stifle and hock held in 90-degree flexion. B, A second layer of tape is passed horizontally around the tibia to hold the previous layer in place.

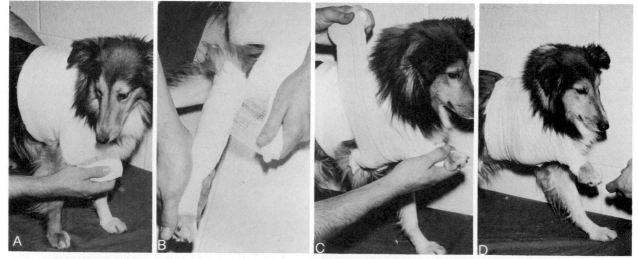

FIGURE 13–10. Velpeau sling. A, The chest wall and shoulder are covered with a lightly padded secondary layer and a gauze tertiary layer. B, The forelimb is bandaged similarly. C, D, The forelimb is flexed against the chest wall, avoiding extreme flexion of the elbow, and covered by a sling of protective tape. The foot is exposed. (Courtesy of Dr. John Berg.)

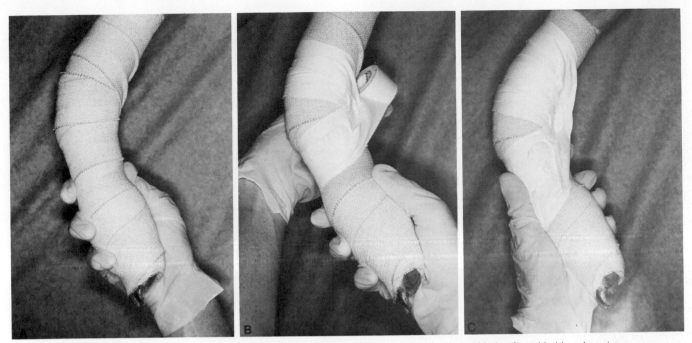

FIGURE 13–11. Carpal flexion sling. A, With the carpus in flexion, a minimally padded soft padded bandage is applied. B, Tape is then applied in a figure-of-eight fashion around the carpus to support the carpus. C, The tape begins in the middle of the carpus and extends distally and proximally, forming a web of tape behind the carpus.

(Fig. 13–11). The degree of carpal flexion can be reduced by partially cutting the criss-cross of tape formed at the caudal aspect of the carpus.

Hobbles can be applied to the hindlimbs to prevent excessive abduction of the limbs. They are specifically indicated after reduction of ventral coxofemoral luxation and to prevent excessive tension in the inguinal region. They can be used to prevent excessive activity after pelvic fracture repair or for nonsurgical, conservative management of pelvic fractures (Fig. 13–12).

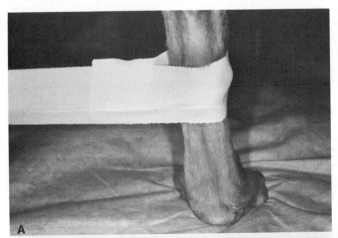

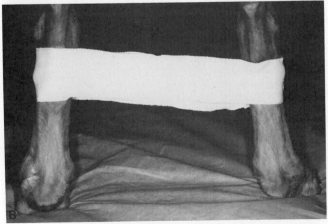

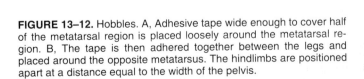

FIGURE 13–12. Hobbles. A, Adhesive tape wide enough to cover half of the metatarsal region is placed loosely around the metatarsal region. B, The tape is then adhered together between the legs and placed around the opposite metatarsus. The hindlimbs are positioned apart at a distance equal to the width of the pelvis.

Aftercare of Casts, Bandages, Splints and Slings

Close monitoring of animals with casts, bandages, splints or slings is extremely important and should be performed daily in the inpatient and at least weekly in the outpatient. Client education for the outpatient is essential. The toes should be monitored daily for warmth, color and swelling. Abnormal findings are indicative of a tight cast. Monitoring the bandage for a foul odor that would indicate tissue damage is necessary. Observing for areas of chafing from the cast is important. The animal should be restrained from chewing at the bandage (e.g., by means of an Elizabethan collar), and exercise restriction to short-leash walks is indicated. While the animal is outside, the bandage should be protected from dirt and moisture by application of a plastic bag or other waterproof material. The plastic covering should not remain on for more than 30 minutes, as it prevents the bandage from breathing, and the underlying tissue can become moist and macerated.

WOUND MANAGEMENT OF HORSES

Wound Care

Basic wound management is no different in large animals than in small companion animals. However, the size and nature of the animal as well as location of the injury may dictate the way a wound is approached. Thus some additional points will be briefly discussed.

When preparing a wound on a horse, K-Y jelly (Johnson & Johnson) or saline-soaked gauze can be used to fill the depths of the wound. Electric clippers are usually used to clip the hair from around the edges of the wound. However, if clippers are not available, the wound edges can be lathered with antiseptic scrub (Betadine Scrub, Triad Medical Products), and a straight-edge razor or No. 22 scalpel blade (Bard-Parker, Becton Dickinson AcuteCare) can be used to shave the hair (Fig. 13–13).

Various methods can be employed to lavage a wound, as described earlier in this chapter. Another available method of wound lavage is the Pulsavac Wound Debridement System

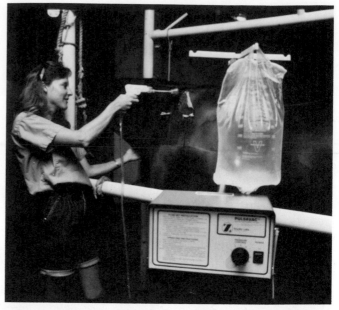

FIGURE 13–14. Pulsavac Debridement System applies a high-pressure (70 psi) stream of lavage solution to a wound, removing loose debris from the wound. (Courtesy of Dr. Michael A. Collier.)

(Zimmer, Snyder Laboratories) (Fig. 13–14), which is effective in removing debris from wounds. It is equipped with a hand-held spray nozzle that has a trigger to regulate fluid flow. The system can be attached to a vacuum to create suction, which facilitates removal of the lavage solution and debris when the coned head, at the end of the spray nozzle, is placed directly over the wound.

In most cases, local anesthesia with tranquilization or general anesthesia is needed before a wound can be properly treated. If tranquilization is used, local or regional anesthesia is necessary to debride and close the wound. Local infiltration is performed by injecting a local anesthetic, mepivacaine (Carbocaine-V 2 percent, Winthrop Veterinary, Sterling Animal Health Products) or lidocaine (AmVet Pharmaceuticals), approximately 1 cm from the wound edge, subcutaneously around the entire wound. A 22-gauge hypodermic needle is used in most situations and is reinserted repeatedly through the skin, each time at the end of the bleb formed by the preceding injection of local anesthetic (Fig. 13–15). In this

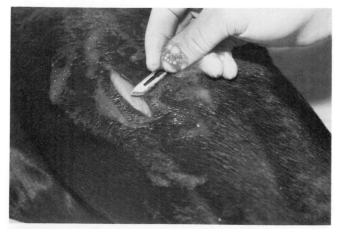

FIGURE 13–13. Once the hair has been lathered with antiseptic (Betadine) scrub, a No. 22 scalpel blade can be used to shave the hair away from the wound edge.

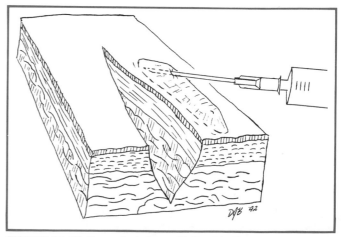

FIGURE 13–15. Proper technique of infiltration of a wound edge with a local anesthetic. The needle should enter through the skin at the point where the last injection ended.

BANDAGING AND CAST APPLICATION TECHNIQUES FOR HORSES

Introduction

Bandages and casts serve many purposes and can be named for the location and purpose they cover and serve respectively. Various materials are available for use in a bandage or cast, but the important aspect is their proper application and function. Development of good bandaging and cast application skills is important to ensure proper function of the bandage or cast. The application and purpose of the different types used on horses will be discussed.

Bandages

Lower Limb Wound Bandage

A *lower limb wound bandage* covers a wound on a limb distal to the carpus or tarsus. When the wound is traumatic in nature, after it has been cleaned and debrided, a topical medication is usually applied if it is left unsutured. Topical preparations usually are not applied to a surgical incision. A nonadhering dressing (Telfa pad, Kendall Corp.; Adaptic, Johnson & Johnson) is then placed directly over the wound. The wound dressing is secured to the limb with rolled conforming gauze (Kling, Johnson & Johnson). The conforming gauze is wrapped around the limb with *light* pressure, overlapping and without wrinkles to avoid pressure lines, which may cause skin sloughing if applied too tightly. It is wrapped proximal and distal to the wound approximately 2 to 4 cm (Fig. 13–17).

The padded layer is applied next. Combine cotton sheets cut from a roll, rolled cotton, layered cotton sheet, quilted leg wraps or a military field bandage can be used (Fig. 13–18). If cotton sheets are available, five are used, folded in half and neatly rolled. The fifth sheet is folded in the opposite direction of the other sheets to conceal the edges. The padded layer is secured to the limb with a roll of conforming gauze (brown gauze, J. R. Raynor; Kling, Johnson & Johnson). Pressure is applied when wrapping to compress and conform the padding to the limb. The outer shell of the bandage is finished using elastic wrap (Vetrap, Animal Care Products/3M; Ace bandage, Johnson & Johnson), adhesive elastic tape (Elastikon, Johnson & Johnson), or a flannel track wrap. The end of the Ace or track wrap is secured with white tape cut into strips or placed around the bandage in a "barber pole" fashion (Fig. 13–19). The "barber pole" method prevents a tourniquet effect from developing around the leg. Elastikon (Johnson & Johnson) is placed around the top and bottom of the bandage, with half of the tape sticking to the wrap and half to the skin, to prevent slippage and debris (such as bedding shavings) from getting down inside the bandage.

Lower Limb Support Bandage

This type of bandage is used to provide support of the soft tissues (such as ligaments and tendons) of the limb contralateral to the injured leg, which is bearing excessive weight because of decreased weight bearing on the injured limb. The bandage also minimizes static limb edema in a confined, inactive horse. A support bandage is placed on the lower limb, just

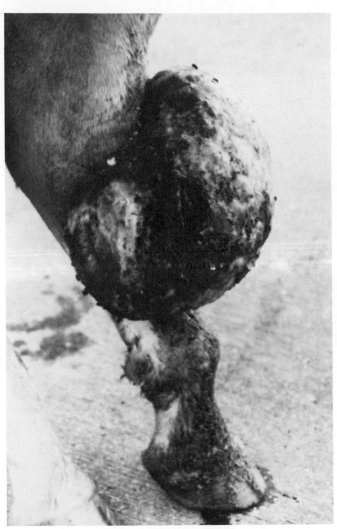

FIGURE 13–16. Excessive exuberant granulation tissue located on the dorsal aspect of the proximal metatarsus of a horse. (Courtesy of Dr. R. Stuart Shoemaker.)

way, the patient will not react to the succeeding injections. If the wound is located on the distal limb, a ring block or nerve block (such as a palmar nerve block) can be utilized to anesthetize the limb distal to the block.

The same considerations for wound closure in small companion animals apply to large animals as well. It is important to remember that open wounds on the distal aspect of the limb (below the carpus or tarsus) of the horse are notorious for developing exuberant granulation tissue. Exuberant granulation tissue, commonly referred to as "proud flesh," can form rapidly in horses. Various measures must be undertaken to keep exuberant granulation tissue in check, or it can become excessive (Fig. 13–16). Methods of controlling granulation tissue include immobilizing the limb (as with a cast), wound bandaging, surgical excision, caustic agents such as equal parts of copper sulfate and boric acid powder, cryotherapy, electrocautery, or topical corticosteroids. Regardless of the decision to allow a wound on the limb of large animals to heal by first or second intention, a bandage should be placed on the limb.

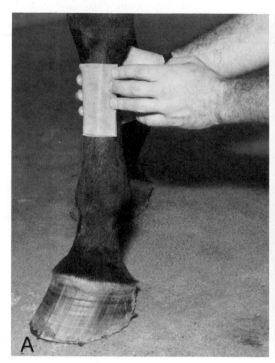
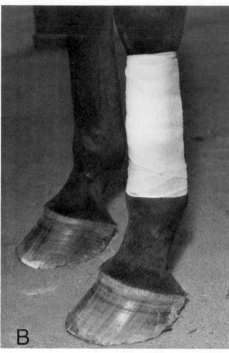

FIGURE 13–17. Application of wound dressing on the distal region of the limb of a horse. A, Nonadherent dressing applied directly over the wound. B, Conforming gauze (Kling) is used to maintain a nonadherent dressing over the wound.

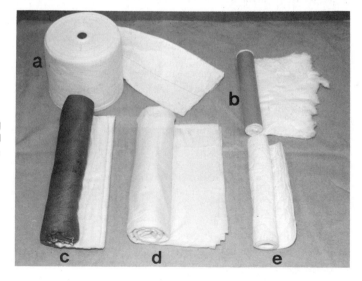

FIGURE 13–18. Various materials that can be used for the padded layer in a leg bandage for large animals. a, Cotton combine. b, Rolled cotton. c, Military field bandage. d, Cotton sheets. e, Quilted leg wraps.

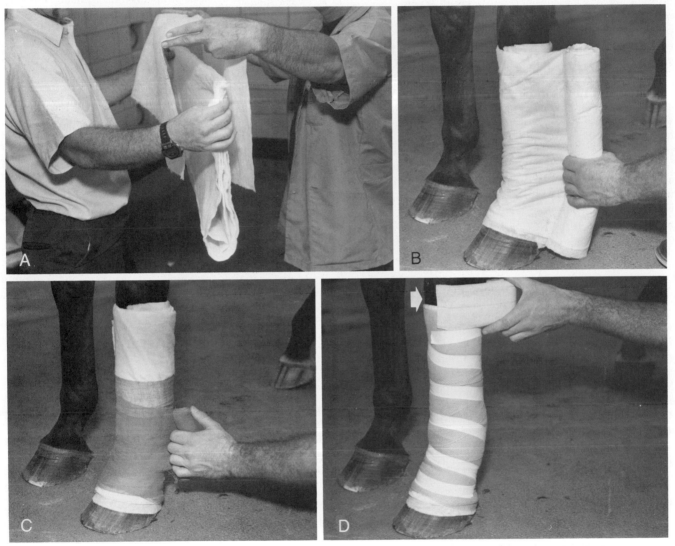

FIGURE 13–19. Application of the padded layer of a wound bandage. A, The wrap used is constructed by taking five cotton sheets and folding them in half with the fifth sheet folded opposite the other sheets to conceal the edges. This is then rolled. B, Cotton wrap is applied snugly around the limb. C, Conforming gauze is used to secure the padded layer to the limb. D, An elastic wrap is used to form the outer shell of the bandage. White tape is applied in a "barber pole" fashion to secure the wrap. Wide adhesive tape is used to provide a seal between the skin and bandage (arrow).

like the wound bandage described above except that the underlying wound dressing and inner conforming gauze layer are not utilized. It is also unnecessary to place wide adhesive elastic tape (Elastikon) around the top and bottom.

Carpal Bandage

This type of wound bandage is used primarily as a counterpressure bandage after an arthrotomy or arthroscopic surgery. However, it can be utilized to cover wounds of the carpus. Precautions must be considered to prevent ischemic necrosis of the skin over the accessory carpal bone. One method of protection is the use of a "doughnut" pad, made from a 2.5-cm thick piece of orthopedic felt (12 cm × 18 cm). An elliptical hole (2.5 cm × 5 cm) is cut out of the center of the pad, and then the hole is positioned over the accessory carpal bone and secured to the limb with a piece of tape lightly applied around the limb. A nonadherent dressing is placed over the wound or operative site, and the carpus is wrapped with conforming gauze. A figure-of-eight pattern can be used for wrapping. Because this is a high-motion region, an adhesive elastic tape is then used to form the outer shell of the bandage. The adhesive elastic tape is secured directly onto the skin, at the top and bottom of the wrap, to prevent slippage. A vertical cut is made in the bandage over the accessory carpal bandage to relieve the pressure on this area (Fig. 13–20). A support bandage can be placed on the lower part of the limb as an additional measure to prevent slippage.

Hock (Tarsal) Bandage

This bandage is used for the same purpose as the carpal bandage, but it is generally more difficult to apply. The bandage may be resented by some horses, who may try to dislodge it by kicking repeatedly with the affected limb. Several different methods may be used to apply a hock bandage. One application method is to use a piece of padding (such as cotton combine), which can be situated over the gastrocnemius tendon and point of the hock to prevent pressure necrosis, before securing the nonadhering wound dressing. *Very* light pressure is applied as the conforming gauze is placed over the point of the hock. A layer of padding can be placed around the hock and secured with conforming gauze. The bandage material and application used for the outer shell are the same as for the carpal bandage (Fig. 13–21). No pressure is applied as the point of the hock is covered. A support bandage can be placed on the lower part of the limb as an additional measure to prevent slippage.

Forelimb Full-length (Stack) Bandage

This type of bandage is used to cover a wound of the upper limb, to provide support of the limb or to provide padding under a full limb splint. A support bandage is first placed on the lower part of the limb. Then a wound or support bandage, depending on the circumstances, is "stacked" or placed directly above (proximal) the lower bandage to cover the upper part of the limb (Fig. 13–22). A "doughnut" pad can used under the bandage, and a vertical cut can be made in the bandage, over the accessory carpal bone, to prevent pressure necrosis of the skin over the prominence.

Robert Jones Bandage

This is a thick, bulky, full-length bandage designed to provide immobilization of a limb. It is usually used as a temporary measure of immobilization and support in emergency situations, such as long-bone fractures, in which the animal is going to be transported for surgical repair. Unfortunately, it is often not effective enough in immobilizing the limb. The bandage is devised by applying multiple layers (4 to 6) of rolled cotton or cotton sheets to the full length of the limb, in a stack bandage configuration, with elastic wrap (Vetrap, Animal Care Products/3M; Ace bandages, Johnson & Johnson) applied between layers of cotton. This increases the rigidity of the bandage. In large animals, a piece of rigid material (such as a metal bar or a wooden slat) is necessary to incorporate into the bandage for the entire length of the limb, on two sides, to help achieve a rigid, immobilizing bandage.

Foot Bandage

This bandage is used to retain a dressing on the hoof, primarily the sole, in the treatment of a subsolar abscess or puncture. When adequate drainage has been established in the sole, the area being treated is flushed with a mixture of equal parts of hydrogen peroxide and strong iodine (5 percent to 7 percent). The sole is then covered with cotton, which has been soaked with iodine. The entire foot is then wrapped with adhesive tape (Duct tape, 3M; Elastikon, Johnson & Johnson). The tape can be carried above the coronary band, but excessive pressure is avoided around this area (Fig. 13–23). A useful addition to this type of bandage is a protective boot (Medi-Boot, Tex-Sol Plastics, Inc.) placed over the bandage or a hard plastic sole pad placed underneath the tape to provide additional protection (Fig. 13–24).

Head Bandage

This type of bandage is used to cover wounds of the face, sinuses, mandible or eye. A piece of orthopedic stockinette (10 or 15 cm) is pulled over the horse's head and positioned just behind the commissures of the mouth back to the throat latch. Holes are then cut in the stockinette over the eyes and the ears. The ends of the stockinette are usually taped to the skin with elastic adhesive tape (Elastikon, Johnson & Johnson) (Fig. 13–25).

Abdominal Bandage

This bandage is used by some equine surgeons to provide additional support and to reduce or prevent ventral edema formation following abdominal surgery. A layered cotton pad constructed from cotton sheets, cotton combine or a military field bandage is placed over the ventral incision. Elastic adhesive tape (Elastikon, Johnson & Johnson) is then used to snugly encircle the entire abdomen and retain the pad in position along the entire length of the incision (Fig. 13–26).

Splints

A splint is an addition of a rigid material to a limb bandage to reinforce immobilization of a particular part of a limb.

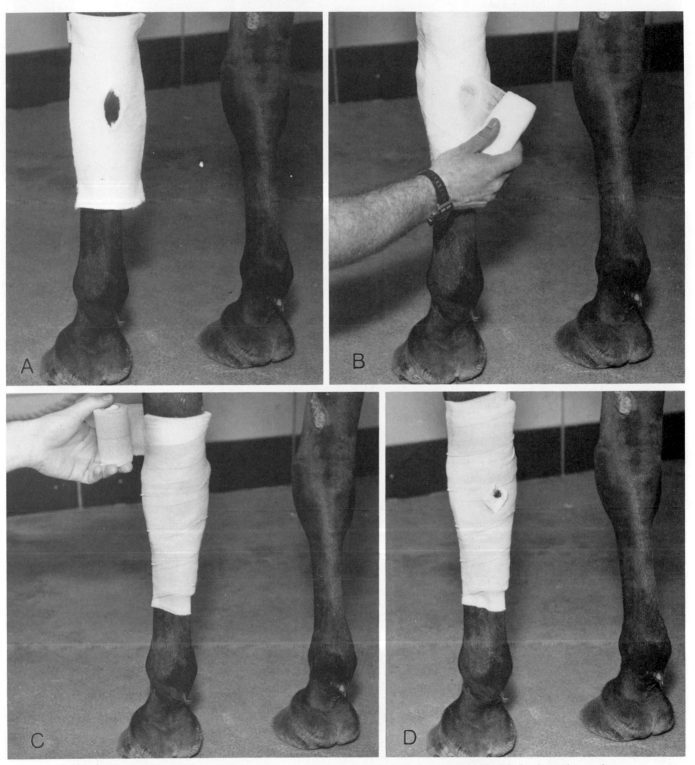

FIGURE 13–20. Equine carpal bandage. A, A "doughnut" pad, made from orthopedic felt, is situated over the accessory carpal bone. B, Nonadherent dressing is placed over operative site and the carpus is wrapped with conforming gauze in a figure-of-eight fashion. C, Wide adhesive tape is used to cover and secure bandage to the limb. D, A vertical cut is made in the bandage over the accessory carpal bandage to relieve pressure over this area.

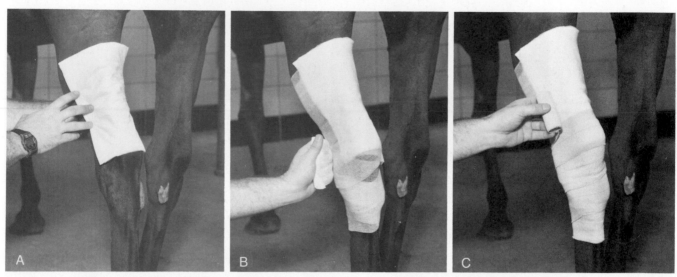

FIGURE 13–21. Equine hock bandage. A, Padding is situated over the gastrocnemius tendon and point of hock to prevent pressure necrosis when the tarsus is bandaged. B, Nonadherent dressing is applied over operative site and the tarsus wrapped with conforming gauze. C, Wide adhesive tape is used to cover and secure the bandage to the limb. No pressure is applied as the point of the hock is being covered.

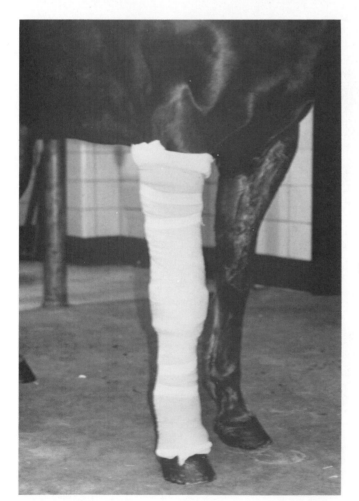

FIGURE 13–22. Forelimb full-length (stack) bandage.

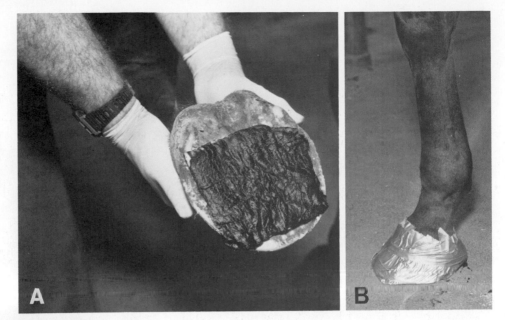

FIGURE 13–23. Technique for applying an equine foot bandage. A, Cotton soaked in medication is placed on the bottom of the sole. B, The foot is then wrapped with an adhesive tape (duct tape).

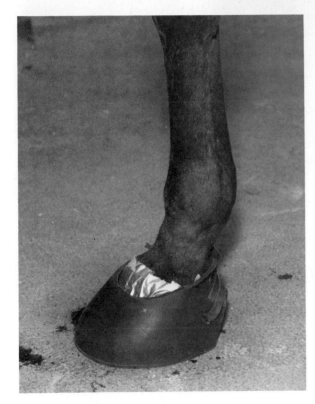

FIGURE 13–24. A boot can be placed over the foot wrap to provide additional protection.

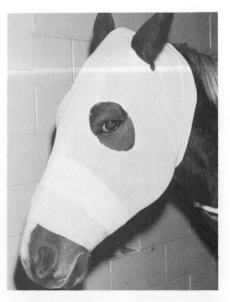

FIGURE 13–25. Head bandage made from orthopedic stockinette. (Courtesy of C. Wayne McIlwraith.)

297

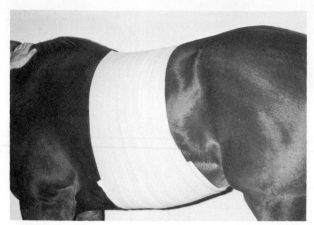

FIGURE 13–26. Abdominal bandage. (Courtesy of C. Wayne Mc-Ilwraith.)

Various materials can be used as the reinforcement including wooden slats, metal bars, low-temperature thermoplastics and casting material. However, the most common material used is polyvinyl chloride (PVC) pipe, because of its light weight and strength (Fig. 13–27). The pipe used is 10 cm in diameter and is split in half. It can be bent by heating with a cutting torch to conform to the fetlock angulation. The length and width of the splint varies with the size of the leg and the area being splinted. Depending on the amount of immobilization, splints can be placed the full length of the forelimb or from just below the carpus or tarsus all the way to the ground surface. In most situations, they are placed on the flexor surface of the limb. Splints are used in situations such as extensor or flexor tendon lacerations, flexure deformities in foals or needed limb support (as in radial nerve paresis).

A thick bandage is first placed on the limb. It should be long enough to cover the limb above as well as below the ends of the splint. This will prevent pressure sores from developing. Once the bandage is in place, the splint is secured to the limb with adhesive tape (Fig. 13–28). Splints should be reset frequently (at least twice a day) in foals.

Casts

A cast is the most frequently used external coaptation to manage various orthopedic injuries or problems when maximum support and immobilization are required. Casts are commonly used for lower limb problems; however, full-limb appli-

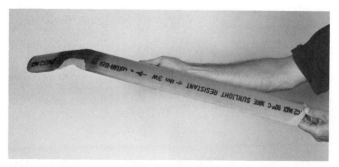

FIGURE 13–27. PVC pipe is commonly used to make limb splints for large animals.

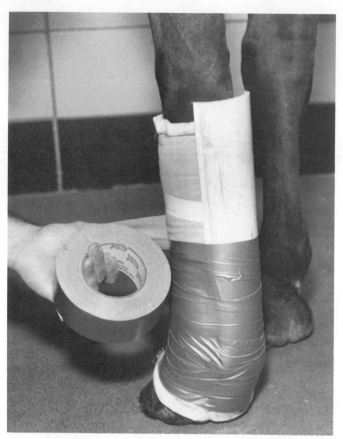

FIGURE 13–28. Application of a lower limb splint. A thick bandage is placed on the limb. The splint (PVC pipe) is positioned along the flexor surface and secured to the bandage with duct tape.

cation is sometimes indicated in large animals. Indications for use of a cast include lower limb fractures, adjunct to internal fixation, tendon laceration, support of the lower limb during recovery from orthopedic surgery, heel bulb lacerations, and luxations of the tarsus, fetlock or pastern.

For optimal effectiveness in immobilization, a cast must immobilize the joint proximal and distal to the injury. Full-limb casts must extend up to the elbow or stifle as far as possible. The most frequently used material today is fiberglass. Fiberglass (such as Delta-Lite, Johnson & Johnson) is appealing because it is lightweight, strong and relatively easy to apply. However, some veterinarians prefer to use a layer of the traditional plaster of Paris initially under the fiberglass. Plaster conforms well to the contour of the limb, reducing the risk of pressure sores.

Before cast application is begun, several things must be considered. It is important that a limb cast be applied properly or serious problems such as pressure necrosis can occur. Because of its importance, application of a limb cast will be described here in detail.

Before the procedure is begun, all the materials needed should be collected: orthopedic stockinette (3-inch), orthopedic felt, towel clamps, white tape (1-inch), wire (approximately 30 centimeters), ⅛-inch drill bit and hand drill, broom handle, hoof-trimming equipment, bandage scissors and cast material (Fig. 13–29). It is important that the cast is applied properly, especially if it is to remain on the limb for a prolonged period (4 to 6 weeks).

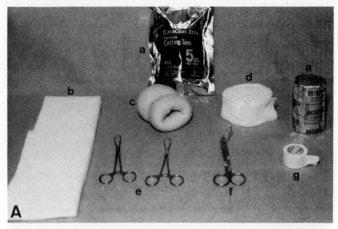

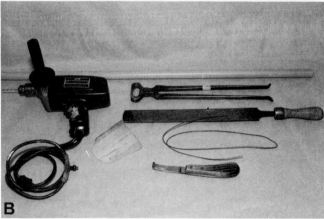

FIGURE 13–29. Materials needed to apply a limb cast on a large animal: A, a, Cast material. b, Orthopedic felt. c, Orthopedic stockinette (3-inch). d, Cast padding. e, Towel clamps. f, Bandage scissors. g, White tape (1-inch). B, Wire (approx. 30 cm), 1/8-inch drill bit and hand drill, wooden wedge block, broom handle and hoof-trimming equipment.

Generally, it is best to apply the cast with the horse under general anesthesia. The horse is positioned in lateral recumbency so that the limb to which the cast will be applied is uppermost. Debris is cleaned from the sole, the horseshoe removed and hoof trimmed. The limb is placed in an extended position perpendicular to the body. Effective support of the leg to maintain the limb in alignment is essential. Traction using wire looped through holes drilled in the hoof can be helpful in this matter. Two holes are drilled in the hoof wall, 5 cm apart near the toe, in the same direction as that in which a horseshoe nail is driven. The ends of the wire are twisted together to form a loop through which a broom handle is placed to apply traction (Fig. 13–30).

The frog can be packed with povidone-iodine (Betadine Solution, Purdue Frederick), especially if thrush is present. If a wound is present, a three-layer bandage consisting of a nonadhering dressing, conforming gauze and adhering elastic tape is used to cover it. The skin must be clean and dry. It can be powdered with talcum or boric acid to help keep the area dry under the cast. The limb is then covered with a double layer of stockinette. The length of the region to receive the cast is measured, and approximately 20 cm is added to this to determine the length of stockinette needed. One end is rolled outward and the other is rolled inward until they meet at the midpoint of the stockinette (Fig. 13–31).

The traction wire is threaded through the opening in the stockinette. The broom handle is placed through the wire loop and traction is applied. The outward roll is first unrolled up the leg. A twist is placed in the stockinette just beneath the toe, and the inward roll is unrolled up the leg (Fig. 13–32). Any wrinkles are smoothed out, and towel clamps are used to secure the stockinette to the medial and lateral aspect of the limb, above the area to which the cast will be applied.

A strip of orthopedic felt (5 to 7 cm wide) is placed around the leg at the most proximal limit of the cast. This is held in place with 1-inch white tape (Fig. 13–33). Additional padding on the leg should be avoided because this can become compressed, thus allowing the leg to move within the cast and cause sores. When a full-limb cast is used, a doughnut pad cut from orthopedic felt is placed over the accessory carpal bone of the forelimb. A thin strip of orthopedic felt is placed over the gastrocnemius tendon and point of hock of the hind limb to prevent the development of pressure sores.

Two layers of 3-inch plaster material is first carefully and snugly applied to the limb. To prevent pressure sores, it is important that these layers be applied without wrinkles. Application of the cast material is usually started at either the proximal or the distal aspect of the limb. We prefer to start distally (Fig. 13–34). A roll of plaster is started at the level of the fetlock and worked distally, then proximally. Approximately 1 cm of the orthopedic felt is left exposed above the top of the cast to prevent formation of a sore.

Next the fiberglass cast material is applied. Usually it is easier to begin with 3-inch material because it conforms to the limb better. The cast material is overlapped one third to one half. As the fiberglass casting material is worked toward the foot, the traction wires are cut, and an assistant holds the leg out at the upper limb region or by resting it on the palms of the hands placed under the metacarpus/metatarsus region. It is imperative to prevent finger imprints in the cast because they could cause a pressure sore to develop (Fig. 13–35).

More pressure is applied to the succeeding layers of fiberglass. This will allow them to laminate better. Generally, two layers of 3-inch fiberglass cast material are applied, followed by two or three layers of 4- or 5-inch fiberglass. At the time the last roll of cast material is applied, the stockinette is unclamped and the excess is cut off, leaving approximately 4 cm. This 4-cm excess is turned down over the top of the cast and incorporated in the last layer.

A wooden wedge block or a 3-inch roll of wet plaster cast material is placed underneath the heel and also incorporated with the last layer (Fig. 13–36). A heel wedge allows the horse to walk more easily while wearing a cast because it decreases the breakover force, reduces pressure on the dorsal proximal limits of the cast at the metacarpus or metatarsus, and allows more even axial weight bearing down through the cast.

It is best to wear gloves, especially when applying the fiberglass. To save time in identifying the end on a wetted plaster roll, unroll 2 to 3 inches of the plaster material and hold onto it while wetting the roll in a bucket of warm water (Fig. 13–37). The excess water is removed by shaking and squeezing the roll. Do not squeeze excessively or excessive plaster will be lost. Fiberglass material is held in a bucket of clean water until thoroughly wet, and the excess water is shaken out.

When application of the cast is completed, the outer layer is smoothed by running your hand cream-covered gloved hands up and down the cast. Hand cream provides a slick surface, which allows a smooth finish to be placed on the final layer.

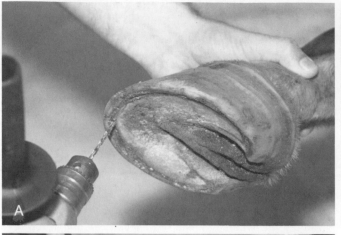

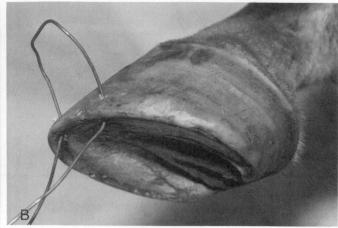

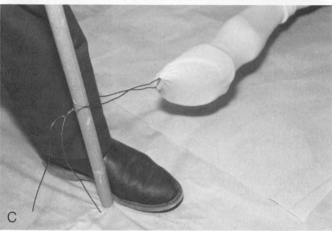

FIGURE 13–30. Traction can be applied to a limb prior to cast application by drilling two holes in the toe of the hoof (A), and threading a loop of wire through the holes (B), with a broom stick placed in the loop to apply traction (C).

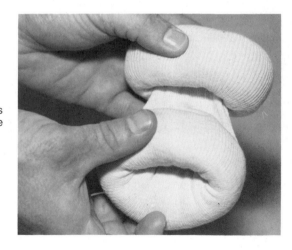

FIGURE 13–31. Orthopedic stockinette used under a cast is prerolled. One end is rolled outward and the other is rolled inward until they meet at the mid-point of the stockinette.

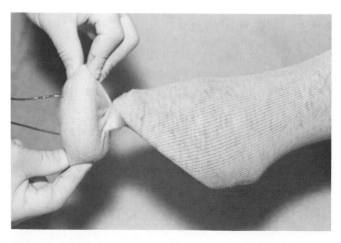

FIGURE 13–32. A twist is placed in the stockinette just beneath the toe and the inward roll is unrolled up the leg.

FIGURE 13–33. Prior to cast material application, orthopedic stocki-nette is secured with towel clamps to the medial and lateral aspect of the limb, above the area to receive the cast. A strip of orthopedic felt (5 to 7 cm wide) (arrow) is placed around the leg at the most proximal limit of cast. This is held in place with 1-inch white tape.

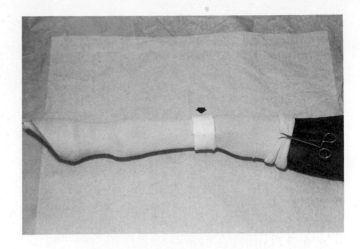

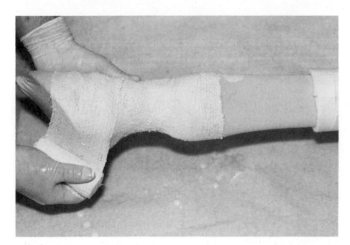

FIGURE 13–34. Application of the plaster of Paris.

FIGURE 13–35. As the fiberglass cast material is being applied, an assistant holds the leg out at the upper limb region by resting it on the palms of the hands under the metacarpus/metatarsus region. This method prevents finger impressions from being made in the uncured cast material.

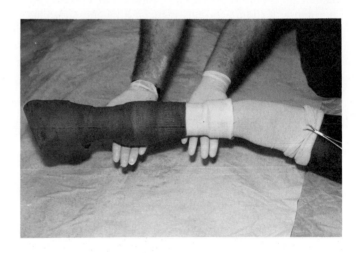

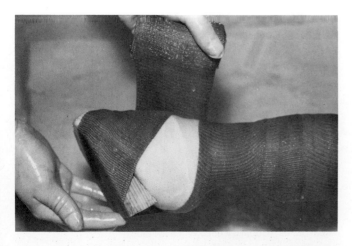

FIGURE 13–36. A wooden wedge block is placed underneath the heel and incorporated with the last layer of cast material.

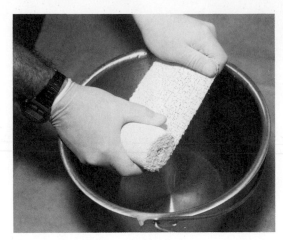

FIGURE 13–37. The end of the plaster cast material is held away from the roll while it is being wetted.

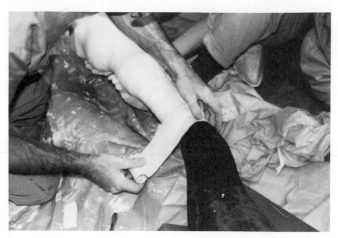

FIGURE 13–39. Elastic adhesive tape is placed on top of the cast to form a seal between the skin and cast to prevent debris from getting down inside the cast.

The hand cream should only be used following the completion of the cast, since it may interfere with curing and bonding of the deeper layers. The bottom of the cast is protected from wear by capping it with hard acrylic (Technovit, Jorgensen Laboratories) (Fig. 13–38). An elastic adhesive tape is placed around the top of the cast and attached to the skin or a piece of stockinette pulled over the top and taped to the cast and the limb above the cast to prevent debris (wood shavings) from getting down inside the cast (Fig. 13–39).

Stall confinement is mandatory after cast application. The patient must be monitored daily. Indications for cast change or removal include breakage, increased lameness, swelling or exudates coming out of the top of the cast. Horses vary in their reaction and tolerance to a cast. If there is any doubt, a cast should be removed and the limb evaluated.

Tube Casts

In most cases, a cast completely encloses the foot. However, casts are modified for other purposes as well. *Tube* or *sleeve casts* are a special type of cast used in foals for the treatment of angular limb deformities associated with defective ossification in the carpus or tarsus (Fig. 13–40). By not incorporating the foot, these casts allow continued use of flexor tendons and prevent laxity that may develop with full-limb casts in foals.

To apply the cast, the foal is anesthetized or heavily sedated and placed in lateral recumbency. A double layer of stockinette (2-inch diameter) is placed over the entire limb. A strip (3 to 5 cm wide) of orthopedic felt is placed around the limb a few centimeters distal to the olecranon and at the level of the fetlock. The limb is positioned as straight as possible, and a layer of plaster of Paris followed by two or three layers of fiberglass (3-inch) is applied to the limb to the level of the orthopedic felt pads. The ends of the stockinette are folded over and incorporated into the last layer of cast.

Cast Removal

Removal of a cast is best performed with the animal standing. During cast removal there is a risk of reinjury to the limb in the animal trying to recover from anesthesia. However, general anesthesia is used if the cast is being changed. The cast is split on the medial and lateral surface, and the cut is continued

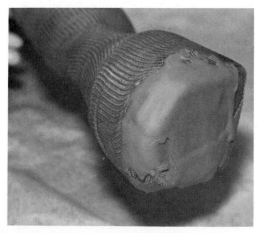

FIGURE 13–38. The bottom of the cast is protected from wearing by capping it with hard acrylic (Technovit).

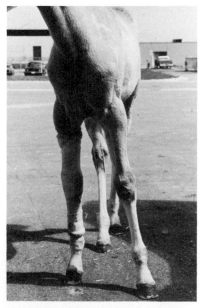

FIGURE 13–40. Tube cast on a foal with defective ossification of the carpal bones. (Courtesy of C. W. McIlwraith.)

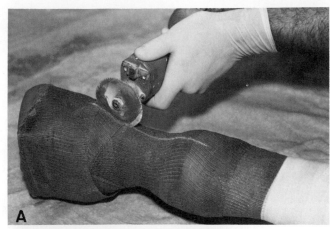

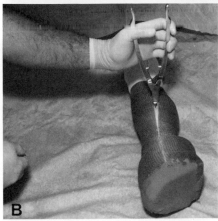

FIGURE 13–41. Removal of a limb cast from a horse. A, The cast is split on the medial and lateral surface and the cut continued under the foot with a Stryker saw. B, Once the cast is completely cut, the two halves are separated with cast spreaders.

under the foot with a Stryker saw (Fig. 13–41). With this approach, injury to the flexor and extensor tendons can be avoided. When cutting over bony prominences, one should be careful to avoid lacerating the skin. Once the cast is completely cut, the two halves are separated with cast spreaders. A support wrap is then placed on the limb.

BANDAGING AND CAST APPLICATION TECHNIQUES FOR CATTLE

Limb Bandaging and Cast Application

The principles applied to these procedures are the same in cattle as in horses, but there are specific techniques related to cattle. Cattle often are not so cooperative as horses, and more restraint is required.

With cattle, a cast can be applied directly over the dewclaws without causing major problems. Sores from motion of the cast can occur in this area because of the inability to closely fit the cast. This can be remedied by placing a pad of orthopedic felt, with holes cut out for the dewclaws, between the dewclaws (Fig. 13–42).

Application of a Claw Block

A wooden block is applied to an unaffected claw for various reasons: to alleviate weight bearing on adjacent claw if it is

fractured or injured, or to protect an operated area by raising it higher off the ground after amputation of an adjacent claw. The block is usually made from a piece of wood 5 cm thick and cut to the shape of the sole surface of the claw. Grooves are cut in the ground surface for traction (Fig. 13–43).

The claw is first trimmed and debris removed by means of an electric sander or rasp. This is an important key step for effective bonding of the acrylic to the claw. The block is then bonded to the horny surface of the claw with acrylic cement, such as Technovit (Jorgensen Laboratories) (Fig. 13–44).

Modified Thomas Splint

Despite advancements in external and internal skeletal fixation, modified Thomas splints are still often used in cattle and small ruminants as a means of external skeletal fixation. The modified Thomas splint is usually used in combination with internal fixation or a cast. The indications for its use include fractures of the tibia or radius, or ligamentous injuries of the stifle. Pressure sores of the inguinal or axillary region are a problem when a Thomas splint is used, despite padding of the metal ring.

Application of a modified Thomas splint in large ruminants does require special equipment, such as a conduit bender, to bend the round rod iron used to construct the splint. The design of the splint varies somewhat among clinicians, but the purpose is the same.

The animal is first placed in lateral recumbency with the affected leg uppermost. A template to fit the individual animal, devised from a nasogastric tube or other similar flexible tub-

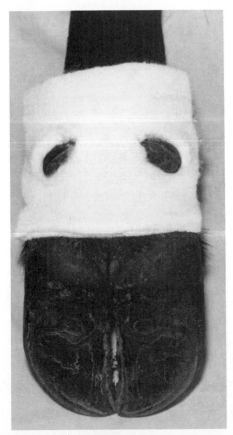

FIGURE 13–42. A piece of orthopedic felt, with holes cut out, can be placed between the dewclaws to reduce pressure sores and motion under a cast.

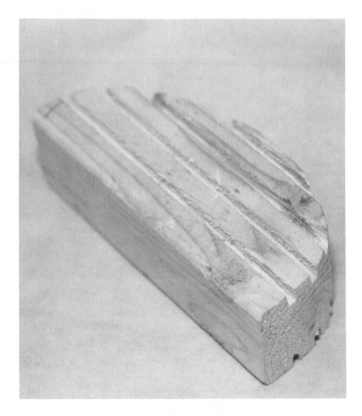

FIGURE 13–43. A claw block made from wood. Grooves are cut in the block to improve traction and bonding.

FIGURE 13–44. A wooden block cemented to the unaffected claw with acrylic.

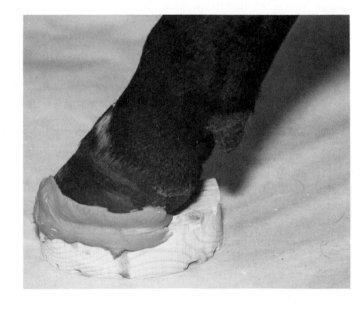

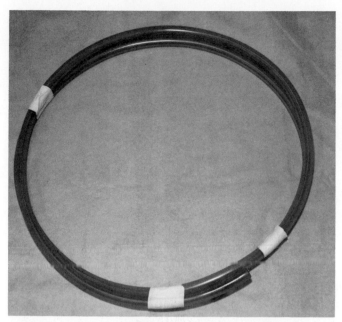

FIGURE 13–45. A nasogastric tube can be used as a template to construct the ring of a modified Thomas splint that will encircle the proximal part of the leg.

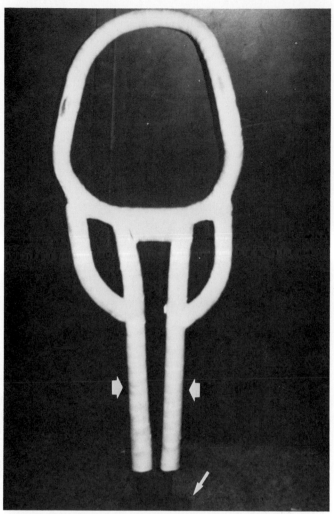

FIGURE 13–46. A modified Thomas splint. Extensions of the splint (large arrows) come off the ventral aspect of the ring and are positioned medial to the leg. A plate with threaded rods is constructed to fit under the animal's foot (small arrow). (Courtesy of Dr. Dwight F. Wolfe.)

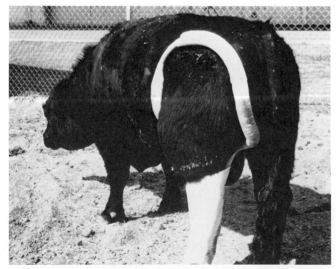

FIGURE 13–47. The limb and modified Thomas splint are covered with layers of cast material and thereby incorporated together to stabilize the limb. (Courtesy of Dr. Dwight F. Wolfe.)

ing, is used to construct the ring that will encircle the proximal part of the leg (Fig. 13–45). The ring should be large enough not to impinge on any bony prominences. The rod iron is bent in a ring the same size as the template. The variation in design occurs with the extensions that come off the ring to support the animal's limb.

One design has the extensions coming off cranially and caudally to the leg. The extensions of the splint must be shaped to conform to the angles of the hock and stifle. These extensions are also bent away (lateral) from the flat plane of the ring to allow the ventral part of the ring to fit into the axillary or inguinal region. Another design has the extensions coming off the ventral aspect of the ring (Fig. 13–46). The ring is then bent so that the extensions are positioned medial to the limb, and to fit the contour of the upper limb (Fig. 13–47).

A foot plate is constructed with two threaded rods attached to the extensions of the splint (Fig. 13–46). A piece of rod iron can be used instead and bent in a "U" shape and is positioned under the foot and connected to the ends of the extensions of the splint. Some splints are devised with extensions that are threaded so that the length of the splint can be adjusted. The ring is lightly padded with cotton. Holes are drilled into the toes of the hoof wall and wired to the bottom of the splint. A slight amount of traction should be applied to the limb as the splint is applied. Traction should be minimal within the splint, so as not to create excessive pressure in the axillary or inguinal regions, which could interfere with venous drainage or distract the fracture fragments.

Once the splint is in position, the limb and splint are then covered with layers of cast material, and thereby incorporated together (Fig. 13–47). Cast material should first be placed around the carpus or tarsus to give these areas initial support from bowing medially. The cast material should be applied as proximal as possible.

Recommended Reading

Small Animal

Knecht CD, Allen AR, Williams DJ, Johnson JH: Fundamental Techniques in Veterinary Surgery. 3rd ed. Philadelphia, WB Saunders Co., 1987.

Swaim SF: Surgery of Traumatized Skin: Management and Reconstruction in the Dog and Cat. Philadelphia, WB Saunders Co., 1980.

Swaim SF and Henderson RA: Small Animal Wound Management. Philadelphia, Lea & Febiger, 1990.

Large Animal

Adams SB and Fessler JF: Treatment of radial-ulnar and tibial fractures in cattle, using a modified Thomas splint-cast combination. J Am Vet Assoc 183:430–433, 1983.

Fiberglass Casting Techniques. Product information pamphlet. New Jersey, Pitman-Moore, 1984.

Lindsay WA: Wound treatment in horses: Healing by third intention. Vet Med 83:506–514, 1988.

Peyton LC: Wound healing in the horse. Part II. Approach to the treatment of traumatic wounds. The Compendium 9:191–202, 1987.

Stashak TS: Bandaging and casting techniques. In Stashak TS (editor): Equine Wound Management. Philadelphia, Lea & Febiger, 1991, pp 258–272.

Turner AS: Large animal orthopedics. In Stashak TS (editor): The Practice of Large Animal Surgery. Philadelphia, WB Saunders Co., 1984, pp 768–780.

14

Surgical Assistance and Suture Material

ERICK L. EGGER

ROLE OF THE VETERINARY TECHNICIAN IN SURGICAL ASSISTANCE

The purpose of surgery in veterinary medicine is primarily that of service. In cases of clinical disease or injury, surgery is used to relieve suffering and improve the quality of life for the animal patient and consequently the owner. Veterinary surgery is also performed to maintain or increase the economical value of animals that are used for food, breeding, show or competitive purposes. The veterinary technician's role is to assist in providing this specialized service to the animal and owner. The technician accomplishes this by both helping the surgeon and protecting the patient. Surgical assistance includes improving the surgeon's visualization by providing retraction and hemostasis in the surgical field, being familiar with the technique objectives and manipulating the instrumentation and tissues into position for completion of the surgical task. The second charge of the technician is to protect the patient from hazards of surgery, such as infection, by maintaining an aseptic surgical field and expediting surgical completion by proper instrument and suture readiness. Since the surgeon is often concentrating on the surgical procedure, the technician must also be constantly aware of the patient's anesthetic and cardiovascular status while assisting.

PROPER TISSUE HANDLING TECHNIQUES

Each of the various body tissue systems has specific attributes that require consideration when being surgically approached.

If the technician understands the general surgical principles of each system, the appropriate actions and measures to be taken in each specific case will be apparent.

Skin

The preparation of the patient's skin for surgery has been described (Chapter 12). One must remember that preparation results in an *aseptic* but not *sterile* skin. This means that the number of bacteria have been reduced below the number required to overwhelm the body's defense mechanism. However, with a depressed immune system or prolonged surgery, these resident bacteria can start to multiply and result in infection. Therefore, the surgeon and assistant should avoid unnecessary direct handling of the skin with the gloves or instruments that will be used in the deeper incision. These items could then carry organisms into the deeper tissues. For lengthy or complicated procedures, a sterile plastic drape (Barrier, Johnson and Johnson) that directly adheres to the skin surface may be used (Fig. 14–1). A spray adhesive may be applied to the skin to augment the plastic's ability to remain in place throughout the surgery. The incision is made directly through the plastic drape. Alternatively, sterile towels or drapes may be applied to the margins of the skin incision to protect the deeper incision (Fig. 14–2). These towels may be attached with additional towel clamps spaced every 5 to 10 cm along the incision (Fig. 14–3) or by suturing the rolled edge of the towel or drape to the subcutaneous tissue with a simple continuous pattern of a strong, inexpensive suture material. For orthopedic surgery, the limb is often enclosed in a sterile stockinette to allow movement and manipulation and to limit exposed

thoracic viscera is made to rule out organ rupture or vascular compromise.

Diaphragmatic hernia repair requires working in a deep cavity. Gentle retraction of viscera to expose the defect is necessary throughout the procedure to preclude damage to abdominal organs. The diaphragmatic defect is sutured with a nonabsorbable suture material in a simple continuous suture pattern. This will effect an airtight and watertight seal. The completed suture line is inspected for leaks by filling the abdominal cavity with warm, sterile physiologic saline solution. The lungs are then inflated, and the incision is inspected for bubbles. Air is evacuated from the chest by thoracocentesis through the diaphragm. The celiotomy is closed in a routine fashion.

Postoperative Considerations. The patient should be monitored carefully for signs of respiratory distress. If dyspnea occurs, the chest should be evacuated with a hypodermic needle, three-way stopcock and a large syringe. A rapid return to normal negative thoracic pressure and normal lung capacity should occur.

In some patients, an indwelling chest tube is placed for the first 1 to 2 days postoperatively. In these cases, periodic aspiration using positional changes (right lateral recumbency, left lateral recumbency, standing on hindlegs, standing on front legs) will afford maximal removal of air and fluid. During the drain management period, it is of utmost importance to keep the patient from chewing a hole in the drain or removing it from the chest cavity. Removal can result in acute death. It is also imperative to keep all connections on the chest drain airtight. Leaks will result in a pneumothorax, respiratory difficulty and possibly death. Proper management of a chest drain requires full-time patient monitoring.

A chart quantitating the amount of air and fluid removed during a given period of time (12 to 24 hours) will help to determine when the drain should be removed. Generally, the drain can safely be removed as the amount of air and fluid decreases toward zero.

Mammary Neoplasia

General Considerations. Mammary cancer is the most frequently occurring neoplasm in the female dog, and mammary gland neoplasms are the third most frequently found tumors in the female cat.

In dogs there is a significantly higher incidence of mammary gland tumors in nonspayed females or females that are spayed at an age older than $2\frac{1}{2}$ years. Spaying prior to the first estrus cycle provides a definite protective factor.

In the initial stages, the tumor will usually appear as a hard lump in any of the glands of the mammary chain. Long-standing or fast-growing tumors may present a sizeable mass with ulceration and drainage. Early diagnosis and therapy will ultimately give the best possible prognosis for mammary gland cancer.

Before surgery can be considered, an examination for possible metastasis (spread) of the tumor is done. Malignant tumors will generally metastasize to the lymph nodes and lungs. Biopsy of regional lymph nodes and chest radiographs may detect metastases. About 50 percent of mammary tumors in the dog are malignant, and about 80 to 90 percent of mammary tumors in cats are malignant.

Surgery is currently considered the most effective therapy.

Early surgery can cure up to 50 percent of canine mammary gland cancer. The primary objective of surgical treatment is complete removal of the tumor tissue.

Technique. The skin is clipped widely to include all affected mammary glands. The patient is placed in dorsal recumbency, and a standard skin preparation is performed. An elliptical incision is made, attempting to include a 1-cm margin around the tumor. The skin, mammary gland and tumor are gently undermined and removed. The skin incision is often gaping after tumor excision, requiring a meticulous subcutaneous closure. Subcutaneous tissues are closed with a simple interrupted pattern using absorbable suture material. The skin is closed in a routine fashion. The excised mammary masses are placed in formalin and sent to a laboratory for histopathological evaluation.

Postoperative Considerations. Major complications that can occur postoperatively are generally related to the tension placed on the skin to adequately close the wound. Dehiscence is not common, but the incision should be examined daily for evidence of separation. Bruising along the incision edges is common and is no cause for alarm. Immediate postoperative hemorrhage can occur. In the event of oozing blood, an abdominal bandage should be applied with gentle pressure. This will help ensure hemostasis and is also comfortable for the patient. The incisions are often very long and must be kept clean and dry at all times. Dogs that prefer to lie on the incision should be well padded or bandaged. If the patient irritates the incision by licking, an Elizabethan collar should be applied until suture removal.

NEUROLOGICAL PATIENT CARE

General Considerations. The most common neurological disorder in the dog is spontaneous intervertebral disk disease. Disks are normally found between vertebral bodies in the spine and act as shock absorbers during spinal movements. With time, the disks can undergo degeneration and calcification. When this occurs, the normal shock absorber–like effect is impaired, and extrusion (rupture) of the disk material into the spinal canal can occur. This puts pressure on the spinal cord and can cause an array of neurological deficits and/or pain.

The most common neurosurgical procedure performed in small-animal practice is *intervertebral disk fenestration*. In this procedure, each of the disks that are calcified or that may become calcified are removed (scraped) from the intervertebral space. This procedure is performed to *prevent* rupture of the disk material into the spinal canal. Dogs may develop spontaneous intervertebral disk extrusions in the cervical spine (neck) or the thoracolumbar spine (lower back). If the disk has already ruptured, a "decompressive" procedure must be performed. The most common decompressive procedures are the ventral slot (for cervical disk rupture) and hemilaminectomy or dorsal laminectomy (for thoracolumbar disk rupture). The most commonly affected breed is the dachshund, but the beagle, Pekingese, poodle and terrier breeds are also frequently presented with disk herniation.

The pre- and postoperative care of neurological patients is dependent on their neurological status. Patients that have the ability to walk (ambulatory status) on presentation can be managed much like any other animal in the hospital, except that they must be handled with care so as not to exacerbate their

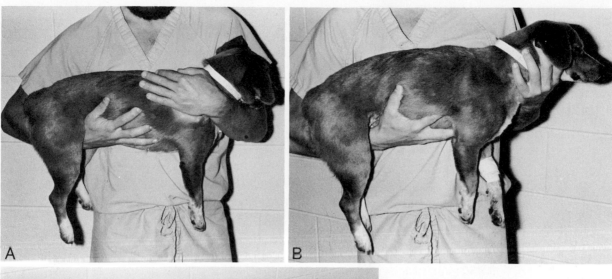

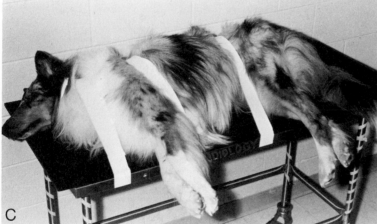

FIGURE 15–12. Proper technique for transporting an anesthetized patient with a spinal problem. A, Thoracolumbar support; B, cervical support; C, patient secured to rigid platform.

cervical or thoracolumbar disk herniation. Patients that have motor weakness (inability to walk normally) or paralysis (inability to walk) on presentation demand frequent attention and careful pre- and postoperative care.

Surgical Technique. When a patient with a herniated cervical or thoracolumbar disk is anesthetized, the normal protective abilities of muscle support and conscious perception of pain are removed. It then becomes the responsibility of the veterinary technician, anesthesiologist and surgeon to protect the patient from further neurological deficits by handling the spine with extreme care. It is important to keep the neck and back as straight as possible when moving the patient from one location to another. This needed support can be achieved in various ways. The patient can be taped to a rigid, flat surface or can be cradled in the arm, being careful to completely support the affected area (Fig. 15–12). The means of transportation may often be dictated by the size of the patient, but, generally speaking, a rigid, flat surface is the preferred method.

Patients undergoing cervical disk surgery are placed in dorsal recumbency with the head and neck in slight extension (Fig. 15–13). The ventral aspect of the neck is widely clipped from the manubrium sterni to the cranial aspect of the larynx. A standard skin preparation is performed. A ventral midline incision is made through the skin and muscles to expose the intervertebral spaces. A dental tartar scraper, curved needle,

fenestration hook or curette can be used to remove the disk material from the interspace. The fenestration technique is carried out from the C2 to C3 disk space to the C6 to C7 disk space. If decompression is needed, an oblong slot is made through the vertebral bodies into the spinal canal using a pneumatic or electric-powered burr. The disk material is then carefully removed from the spinal canal. The surgical wound is closed in layers with a continuous suture pattern using an absorbable suture. The skin is closed in a routine fashion.

Patients undergoing thoracolumbar disk surgery are placed

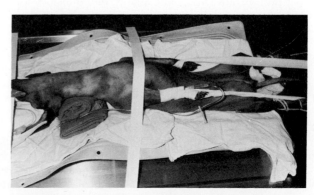

FIGURE 15–13. Proper positioning for cervical disk surgery.

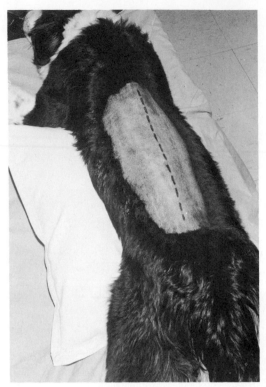

FIGURE 15–14. Proper positioning for thoracolumbar disk surgery.

in ventral recumbency (Fig. 15–14). The back is widely clipped from the midthoracic region to the pelvis. A standard skin preparation is performed. A skin incision is made from T11 to L6. Careful dissection between epaxial muscles (muscles of the back) allows palpation and limited visualization of the disk spaces. Each space between T10 and L5 is curetted with a technique similar to that described for cervical disk fenestration. If decompression is needed, a portion of the bony lamina covering the spinal cord is removed with a pneumatic or electric powered burr and/or bone rongeurs. The ruptured disk material is then carefully removed from the spinal canal. The muscles, subcutaneous tissue and skin are closed in a routine fashion.

Postoperative Considerations. Postoperative management for the nonambulatory patient is demanding. These patients are subject to decubital ulcers (bed sores or pressure sores), urinary bladder infections, joint stiffness, muscle atrophy (muscle wasting), pneumonia and gastrointestinal ulceration. Preventing these conditions from occurring is the main objective of proper postoperative management and should include the following:

1. Passive range-of-motion exercises and whirlpool baths to encourage joint motion and muscular activity

2. Urinary bladder expression four to five times a day to keep the urinary bladder empty, thus lowering the incidence of infections secondary to large residual volumes

3. Turning the patient frequently to reduce the incidence of pneumonia

4. Keeping the patient well padded to prevent the formation of decubital sores

5. Using an elevated, perforated, rubber-coated rack to keep the patient from urinating and defecating on itself (Fig. 15–15)

6. Observation of the stool for evidence of fresh blood (bright red on feces) or digested blood (dark, tarry feces), which may be an indicator of colonic or gastric ulceration, respectively; this may be observed following cortisone therapy

7. Observation for vomiting, especially if the vomitus contains coffee ground-like material, indicative of gastric bleeding

As can be seen from the list, the veterinary technician and veterinarian must work diligently and continuously to properly manage the nonambulatory neurological patient back to health.

ORTHOPEDIC SURGERY

Long Bone Fractures

Preoperative Considerations. When a patient is presented at the veterinary hospital with a fracture, several steps must be taken to ready the patient for a permanent repair. First, the patient must be stabilized with respect to all other body systems (treated for shock, chest injuries, abdominal injuries). Second, any open wounds associated with the fracture should be managed, and, third, the fracture must be immobilized by means of a bandage, cast or sling. Once these three things have been achieved, fracture repair can be safely considered. Most long bone fractures are not life threatening and do not require emergency surgery.

Operative Considerations. An extensive clip is required on all limb preparations. The surgeon and assistant will manipulate the limb during reduction and repair. For this reason, the limb is clipped from the level of the metacarpus or metatarsus to the scapula or pelvis, respectively, including the medial and lateral aspects of the extremity. This may vary slightly, depending on the particular bone that is fractured, but the general rule should be a wide and thorough clip. The remaining hair at the tip of the paw is covered with a rubber glove and is taped to the clipped skin (Fig. 15–16).

Positioning. Patient positioning depends on the specific bone that is fractured. Generally, the following positions are recommended for each fracture:

1. Femur: lateral recumbency, affected side uppermost
2. Tibia-fibula: lateral recumbency, affected leg down
3. Humerus: lateral recumbency, affected leg uppermost

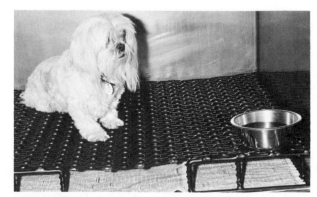

FIGURE 15–15. Spinal trauma patient on an elevated rack. The rack protects the patient from being soiled with urine and feces and helps prevent decubital sores.

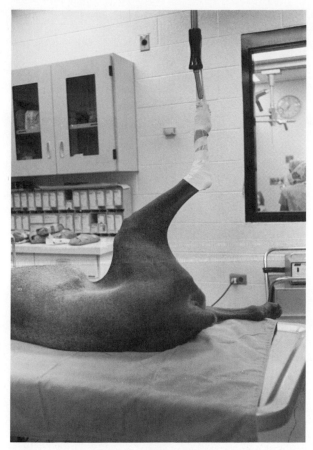

FIGURE 15–16. Properly prepared extremity must include a thorough clip of the medial and lateral aspects, as well as proper covering of the paw.

4. Radius-ulna: dorsal recumbency, affected leg craniad
5. Pelvis: lateral recumbency, affected leg uppermost

With so much skin exposed, skin preparation is time-consuming, but it must be meticulous. The surgeon eventually covers the extremity with a sterile stockinette, but this should not preclude an adequate skin preparation.

Surgical Assistance. Orthopedic procedures are often very difficult and time-consuming, and may demand the help of an assistant. Often, the veterinary technician is called upon to participate as a surgical assistant and, therefore, should have a general understanding of orthopedic tissue handling.

Several basic maneuvers commonly needed by the surgeon are often performed by the veterinary technician. They include retraction, muscle fatigue, alignment and reduction, and suction of the field. Proper techniques for each will be discussed separately.

Retraction. Care should be taken to preserve the soft tissues in the operative field. It will be necessary to have functional muscle groups remaining when the bone is repaired. Retraction should be firm but not so traumatic as to bruise or tear the muscle.

Muscle Fatigue. Large-breed dogs, or fractures that are 3 to 5 days old may be difficult to reduce because of heavy muscle mass or severe muscle contraction, respectively. In such cases, constant steady traction on the muscle groups will cause them to fatigue and relax, thus facilitating reduction.

Alignment and Reduction. In order to repair fractured bones, the ends must be reduced and aligned. It is often necessary for an assistant to hold reduction during the fixation of the fracture. For rapid bone healing to occur, the fractured bone must be held in rigid fixation. Pins, wires, screws and plates of stainless steel may be used to achieve the necessary fixation.

Suction. Whenever a fracture occurs, bleeding into the fracture site can be massive. Some continuous oozing occurs during fixation. A clean surgical field is of the utmost importance in facilitating early and accurate reduction and fixation.

Postoperative Considerations. Some postoperative orthopedic patients may require external coaptation. The patients should be managed as described in Chapter 13. Other patients may require range-of-motion exercises, but the majority require limited activity. It is important to realize the relatively unsure gait of a three-legged dog or cat, and, when exercising them, one must be certain to keep them away from slippery surfaces (vinyl or wet floors). Cement, grass, gravel or dirt provides a much more sure-footed environment. Physical therapy should become part of most fracture patients' rehabilitation therapy. Flexing and extending the affected limb along with muscle massage will improve blood flow and muscle tone as well as reduce muscle contraction (Fig. 15–17). Therapy should be done for a period of 5 minutes each time, repeated two to three times per day. A demonstration by the technician of the proper technique will aid the client in understanding the therapy.

Joints

Preoperative Considerations. The majority of orthopedic procedures involving the joints are elective and rarely need emergency care. The preoperative management includes limiting the patient's activity. External coaptation is rarely necessary. The indications for joint surgery involve dislocations, ligament ruptures, infections, fractures involving the joint surfaces, joint capsule biopsy and osteochondrosis (lytic lesions of the articular cartilage).

Operative Considerations. An extensive clip, as for fractures, should also be done for joint surgery. Positions will vary depending upon the joint involved. Generally, the following positions are recommended for each joint:

1. Hip: lateral recumbency, affected leg uppermost
2. Stifle: lateral recumbency, affected leg uppermost or dorsal recumbency (can be used for unilateral or bilateral stifle surgery—surgeon's preference)
3. Shoulder: lateral recumbency, affected leg uppermost
4. Tarsus: lateral recumbency, affected leg uppermost
5. Elbow: lateral recumbency, affected leg uppermost
6. Carpus: lateral recumbency, affected leg uppermost

Intraoperative assistance in joint surgery is similar to that necessary in fracture repair. Some special precautions should be taken while joints are exposed.

Retraction. Care should be taken *not* to place retractors in direct contact with the articular cartilage. Cartilage has a relatively poor response to trauma. When exposure of the joint is necessary, sharp retraction of the joint capsule will decrease trauma.

Flush. The cartilage should be frequently flushed with saline to keep it from drying out during the procedure. This is true of all tissues, but especially the articular cartilage because of its poor regenerative ability.

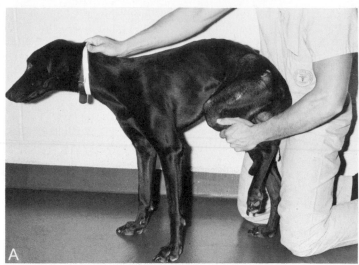
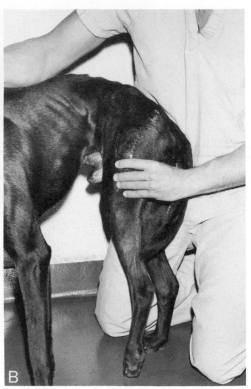

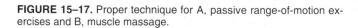

FIGURE 15–17. Proper technique for A, passive range-of-motion exercises and B, muscle massage.

Postoperative Considerations. Postoperative care of patients undergoing joint surgery can be variable, depending on the surgical procedure, the joint involved and the surgeon's preference. Generally, the joint is immobilized for 1 week to 2 weeks, is gradually exercised with passive range-of-motion exercises for 7 to 10 days, then is gradually (1 week to 2 weeks) worked back to normal activity.

CLIENT EDUCATION

When a patient is discharged from the professional care available in a veterinary hospital, it becomes the responsibility of the hospital staff to ensure that the same type of care be given at home. This requires that time be spent with the client and the pet to educate the client on appropriate treatment techniques. There are several methods of client education in surgical cases, the degree of difficulty of which is often associated with the type of surgical procedure performed (e.g., ovariohysterectomy versus disk fenestration).

Whenever a patient is sent home with a sutured skin incision, the client must be instructed to observe the incision daily for evidence of swelling, redness or drainage and to feel the incision for heat. The client should also watch the animal for aggressive licking, removal of skin sutures or both.

If a patient is sent home with a bandage, a written discharge form should be given to the client describing in detail the proper management necessary to prevent complications.

In orthopedic cases, as well as in many elective soft tissue surgery cases, the owner should be instructed specifically on what kind of limited activity should be enforced. If passive range-of-motion exercises are expected, the client should be given both verbal and written instruction in providing the cor-

rect care. A demonstration by the technician of the correct method of therapy is helpful.

In many instances, such as complicated orthopedic and neurological discharges, a written handout explaining in detail the care necessary is very informative and gives a handy reference for the client to refer to if a problem arises.

The use of visual aids, such as a skeleton or overlay books that illustrate anatomy, can be effective in helping the client understand the scope of the problem. Clients are generally willing and capable of handling the postoperative patient, and with a little help from the veterinary hospital staff, a predictably successful end result can be expected to occur.

VETERINARY DENTISTRY

Veterinary dentistry has been practiced for decades. It has only been over the past ten years, however, that the significance of dental problems in companion animals has been acknowledged and treated by methods other than tooth extraction. With the resources available to perform endodontic, periodontic, orthodontic, and restorative procedures, extraction may not be the only option for a diseased tooth. An understanding of the different types of dental problems and how they should be treated is important so that the client can be informed of the treatment options available.

This section provides a detailed discussion of periodontal disease and its prevention. Also included will be an overview of the specialty branches of veterinary dentistry. Since veterinary technicians often perform dental scaling and polishing procedures, it is important that they have detailed knowledge of the necessary equipment and its proper use and care. Suggested readings can be found at the end of this chapter for more detailed discussions of each specialty area.

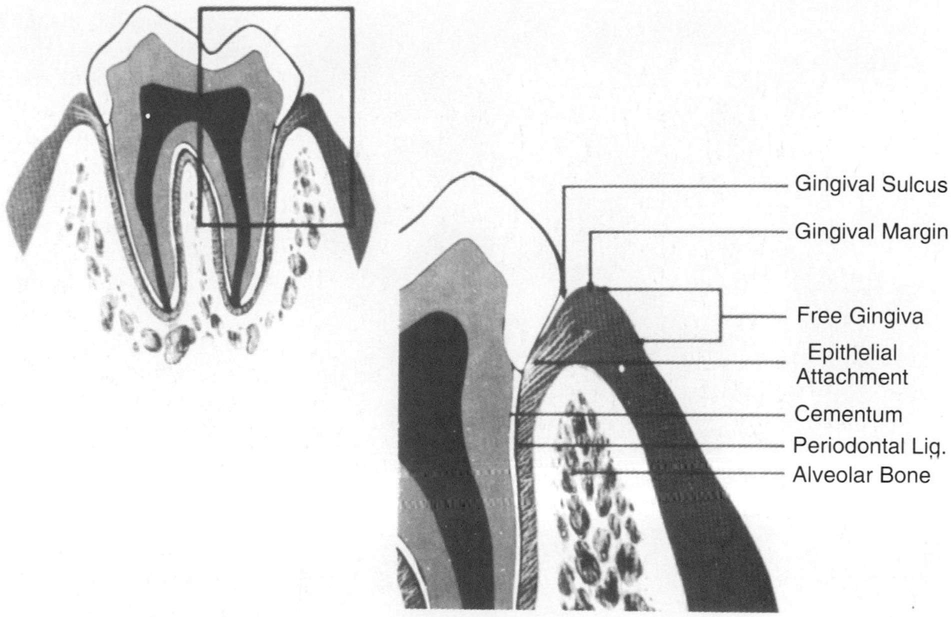

FIGURE 15–18. Structures collectively referred to as the periodontium. Notice how the tooth is suspended in the socket by the periodontal ligament. (From MJ Bojrab and M Tholen: Small Animal Oral Medicine and Surgery. Philadelphia, Lea & Febiger, 1990. Reprinted with permission.)

Gingival Sulcus

Gingival Margin

Free Gingiva

Epithelial Attachment

Cementum

Periodontal Lig.

Alveolar Bone

Periodontics and Periodontal Disease

Periodontics is the branch of dentistry concerned with the study and treatment of the periodontium. The periodontium is composed of the supporting structures of the tooth. These supporting structures are the gingiva, periodontal ligament, alveolar and supporting bone (tooth socket) and the cementum of the tooth root (Fig. 15–18). Healthy gingiva has a sharp, tapered edge (margin) that lies closely against the crown of the tooth (Fig. 15–19). The free gingiva forms a moat around the tooth called the gingival sulcus. The epithelial attachment of the gingiva to the cementum of the tooth root forms the bottom extent of the gingival sulcus. The depth of this sulcus ranges from 1 to 3 mm in a healthy mouth of a dog or cat. The sulcus depth will increase as the periodontium is destroyed. Depths greater than 4 mm in the dog or cat are called periodontal pockets and usually indicate periodontal disease.

Periodontal disease (periodontitis) means inflammation of the structures around the tooth (Gr. *perio* = around + Gr. *odous* = tooth + Gr. *itis* = inflammation). It is the most common disease of animals and humans and is caused by plaque. Approximately 85 percent of dogs and cats 6 years of age and older have periodontal disease.

Plaque is a white slippery film that collects around the gingival sulcus of the tooth. Plaque is composed of bacteria, food debris, exfoliated cells, and salivary glycoproteins. Over time, plaque will mineralize on the teeth to form dental calculus, a brown or yellow deposit (Fig. 15–20). As the plaque collects around the tooth, it damages the gingival tissues by releasing bacterial endotoxins. The animal's immune system further damages these tissues through the release of harmful by-products released from white blood cells as they attempt to destroy the bacteria. In the early stages, the gingiva becomes inflamed and bleeds easily. This stage is called gingivitis (Fig. 15–20). As the disease progresses, the periodontium is affected, and this stage is called periodontal disease (Fig. 15–21).

Periodontal disease is difficult to control once it has developed. For this reason, great emphasis must be placed on its prevention. Although many diseases can contribute to the se-

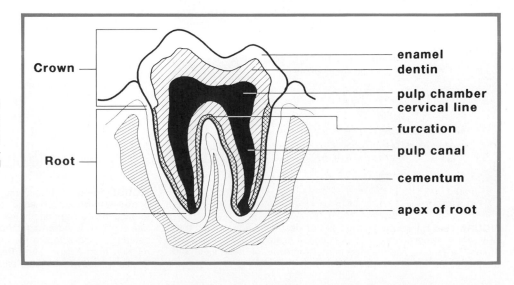

FIGURE 15–19. Typical external and internal gross anatomy of a tooth. The model is a premolar. (From MJ Bojrab and M Tholen: Small Animal Oral Medicine and Surgery. Philadelphia, Lea & Febiger, 1990. Reprinted with permission.)

Crown

Root

enamel

dentin

pulp chamber

cervical line

furcation

pulp canal

cementum

apex of root

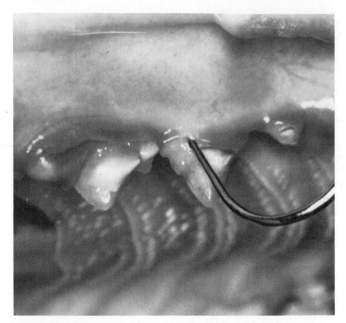

FIGURE 15–20. The calculous deposits on these teeth have caused the gingiva to become inflamed (gingivitis). A dental explorer is used to detect subgingival (under the gingiva) calculus or dental abnormalities.

verity of periodontal disease, there is only one primary cause: plaque. The key to prevention of periodontal disease is to minimize plaque accumulation by means of proper diet, routine professional dental scaling and polishing, and daily teeth brushing or mouth rinsing.

When periodontal disease is already present, destruction of the periodontal tissues has begun and will continue if not treated. Once the periodontal ligaments are destroyed, they are extremely difficult to replace. As the tooth begins to lose

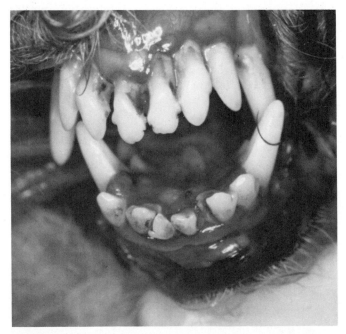

FIGURE 15–21. Periodontal disease has destroyed a significant portion of the alveolar bone and periodontal ligament of these incisor teeth. The gingiva has receded from the crowns of these teeth and the tooth roots are now exposed.

its periodontal tissue, it becomes more susceptible to plaque accumulation in the deep periodontal pockets that form around the tooth root(s). When the tooth loses a significant portion of its periodontium, it becomes mobile (loose) and will eventually fall out. This is nature's way of clearing the infection from the body. The infection, however, is usually present for months to years before the tooth is eventually lost. During this time, the bacteria can gain entrance to the animal's blood stream and become systemic spreading to numerous organs such as the liver, kidney and heart.

For patients with periodontal disease, the treatment goal is to remove the plaque from the teeth and to minimize plaque reattachment. Treatments to minimize plaque accumulation include those listed for prevention of periodontal disease, as well as periodontal surgery when deep periodontal pockets have formed around tooth roots.

Periodontal surgery entails incising and elevating the gingival tissue so that the involved tooth roots can be exposed and cleaned of all calculus and diseased tooth root cementum. The removal of calculus and necrotic cementum from the tooth roots is called root planing (Fig. 15–22). The gingiva covering these roots must be debrided of foreign debris and granulation tissue. This procedure is called subgingival curettage, and the instruments used to perform these procedures are the curettes. The gingival tissue is sutured after the procedure is completed. The gingival flap can be apically (toward the root tip) repositioned to decrease the depth of the periodontal pockets. Subgingival curettage and root planing can be done without incising and elevating the gingival tissue as long as there is sufficient access to the roots and gingival epithelium to thoroughly debride the area.

Loose teeth can be stabilized by splinting them to adjacent teeth in order to prevent their loss while the periodontium is healing. A thorough dental prophylaxis with radiographs, root planing and subgingival curettage must be performed prior to splinting the loose teeth. Splinting is performed only if the pet owner is willing to provide dental home care and have the teeth professionally cleaned as needed. If the splints and teeth are not properly cleaned by the owner, the splints will retain foreign debris and worsen the condition. Pets with advanced

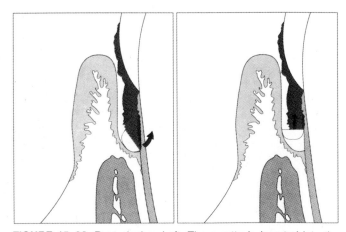

FIGURE 15–22. Root planing. Left, The curette is inserted into the pocket with its curved edge against the epithelium. It is turned to engage the cutting edge in the necrotic cementum and debris. Right, The curette is withdrawn, removing the subgingival debris and necrotic cementum and scraping the pocket epithelium. (Reprinted with permission from Emily P and Penman S: Handbook of Small Animal Dentistry. Copyright 1990, Pergamon Press Ltd.)

periodontal disease may require professional dental cleaning every 3 to 4 months.

Proper Diet

Dry pet food is the diet of choice for minimizing the rate of plaque accumulation on the dentition. The semimoist and canned pet foods are tacky and tend to stick to the teeth. This accelerates plaque accumulation.

Proper chew toys should be encouraged. Rawhide bones and chews are excellent for exercising the teeth and periodontium, maintaining a healthy mouth. Some pets have a desire to chew on hard objects such as rocks. Hard objects can damage the teeth and should be removed from the pet's environment when possible.

Dental Scaling and Polishing

Prior to beginning the dental prophylaxis procedure, the dental treatment area should be prepared. The proper instruments should be out for easy access, and they should be clean and sharp. The patient should be examined by the veterinarian prior to anesthesia for evidence of bacterial infection of the gingiva. When oral infection is present, preoperative antibiotics should be given to prevent the systemic spread of oral bacteria to internal organs. Patients with periodontal disease should begin antibiotic treatment at least 3 days prior to the dental cleaning procedure.

The patient is anesthetized and a cuffed endotracheal tube is used to prevent water and foreign debris from entering the trachea. The patient should be placed on a slight incline (nose downward) to allow water to run out of the mouth while mechanical scalers are used with irrigation (Fig. 15–23). A gauze square can be placed in the back of the pharynx to keep debris from entering the trachea and esophagus, but it must be removed at the end of the dental procedure.

Once the anesthetized patient is prepared, the technician should don the proper attire and begin the dental prophylaxis. Proper attire consists of a mask, gloves, eye protection (glasses or a shield), cap and lab coat. It is important to wear these protective coverings because large numbers of bacteria are aerosolized during the mechanical scaling procedure, and these could be inhaled or could saturate clothing, leading to contamination of other areas in the hospital.

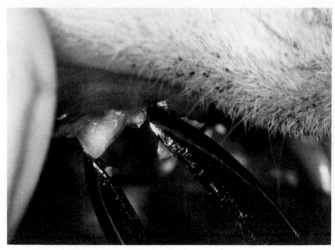

FIGURE 15–24. Large pieces of calculus can be removed quickly with forceps. Care should be taken not to place excessive pressure on the tooth, especially cusp tips, to avoid fracturing the tooth.

The dental prophylaxis begins with a thorough examination of the oral cavity. Clinical findings should be recorded at either the beginning or the end of the procedure. Important findings to include are areas of ulceration, missing teeth, loose teeth, periodontal pockets, receded gingiva, degree of periodontal disease, fractured teeth and so forth.

Large pieces of calculus can be removed quickly with calculus-removing forceps (Fig. 15–24). If the patient has minimal amounts of calculus present, the calculus can be removed with hand scaling instruments alone. Electric and air-driven mechanical scalers can be used on patients with significant amounts of calculus present (most patients!) because they remove calculus rapidly (Fig. 15–25). Since the mechanical vibrations of the tips of these scalers dislodge the calculus, minimal pressure is used when operating these instruments. Most of these instruments generate heat owing to the rapid vibrations, so it is imperative to use irrigation to cool the working tips of these instruments (exceptions are piezo ultrasonic scalers and

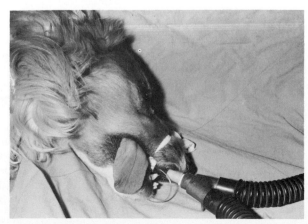

FIGURE 15–23. Proper patient positioning for dental scaling and polishing. Note that the head is placed in a downward position.

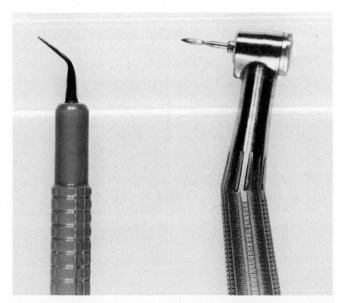

FIGURE 15–25. The working ends of two mechanical scalers are shown here. On the left is an ultrasonic scaler and on the right a highspeed handpiece with a Rotopro flame burr (Ellman).

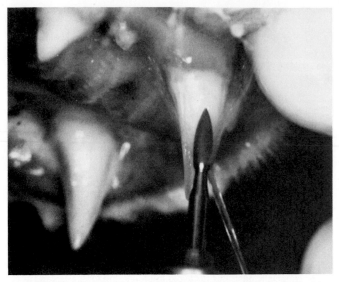

FIGURE 15–26. The Rotopro flame burr (Ellman) is cooled with a stream of water as it removes calculus from the teeth. The stream of water flushes the calculus off the tooth and away from the gingival sulcus.

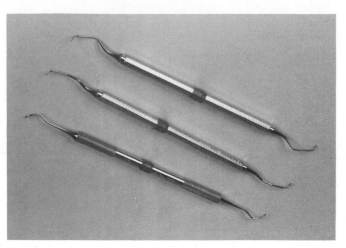

FIGURE 15–28. Curettes can be used subgingivally (below the gingival margin) to scale tooth roots and debride the gingival sulcus. Note the rounded toe and curvature of the instrument. Curettes can be purchased with different angles to the shank to improve access to the tooth roots.

subsonic scalers) so that the pulp tissue does not receive thermal damage (Fig. 15–26). When using mechanical scalers, the instrument must be kept moving on the tooth surface and should not be on the tooth for more than 10 to 15 seconds. If the scaling of a tooth is not completed in this time, the adjacent tooth can be scaled while the first tooth cools. Once cool, the first tooth can be scaled again.

Most dental prophylaxis procedures require the use of mechanical and hand scalers. Hand scalers can be used to reach those areas that are inaccessible to the mechanical scaler. Curettes and scalers should be held in a modified pen grasp. Supragingival scalers are to be used only on the crown of the tooth, which is above the gingiva. They are larger than the curettes and often have a sharp tip that could injure the gingival sulcus if used subgingivally. An example of a supragingival scaler is the jacquette (Fig. 15–27). Curettes are used above the gingiva (supragingival) and below the gingiva (subgingival) to remove plaque and calculus. Curettes have a rounded toe and back to prevent damage to the gingival tissue (Fig. 15–28).

To remove subgingival calculus from the gingival sulcus, the curette is placed to the bottom of the gingival sulcus with its curved smooth back toward the gingival epithelium. Once it is seated at the bottom of the sulcus, the cutting edge is turned to engage the calculus on the tooth root. The curette is then pulled toward the crown to dislodge the calculus and remove it from the sulcus, as illustrated for root planing (see Fig. 15–22). This pull stroke is repeated until all the calculus has been removed from the tooth. Proper instrument positioning takes practice and concentration. It is important to master this technique to ensure that the gingival tissue is not damaged by the instruments and the subgingival calculus is completely removed.

After the teeth have been properly scaled, they must be polished. This step is performed to smooth the microscopic pits and scratches on the tooth surface created by the scaling procedure. If this step is skipped, the plaque will rapidly return because of increased surface area created by the scratches. Polishing is achieved using a slow speed handpiece with a prophy cup attached and filled with prophy paste. Enough pressure should be applied to just flare the edge of the prophy cup. Flaring the edge will allow it to be gently inserted into the gingival sulcus to polish subgingivally (Fig. 15–29).

All surfaces of the tooth crown should be polished. The rotational speed should be kept slow (4000 rpm or less) and the polisher should be constantly moved on the tooth surface to prevent thermal damage to the tooth and gingiva. The tooth should not be polished for more than 5 seconds or thermal damage could result. If the polishing is not completed in 5 seconds, another tooth should be polished, and the unfinished tooth can be polished once it has been given time to cool.

Ample prophy paste should be kept in the prophy cup to help prevent excessive heat generation and to smooth the tooth surface. Several polishing pastes are available. For routine dental prophylaxis the fluoride-containing pastes are preferred. Fluoride strengthens enamel, decreases tooth sensitivity, has antimicrobial properties and decreases the rate of plaque reattachment.

The oral cavity is rinsed of prophy paste and calculus after all surfaces of the teeth have been polished. The gingival sul-

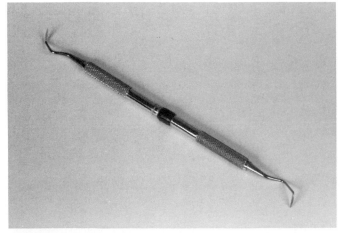

FIGURE 15–27. Supragingival scalers are used to scale the crowns of the teeth. A jacquette scaler is shown here.

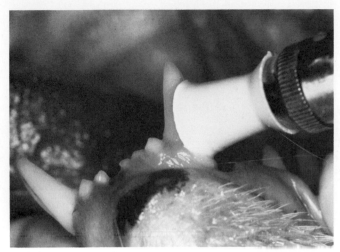

FIGURE 15–29. Polishing the teeth after scaling is extremely important to prevent rapid plaque accumulation after the teeth have been cleaned. The flared edge of the prophy cup can be placed into the gingival sulcus to polish subgingival enamel.

cus must be irrigated to remove debris and bacteria. Irrigating systems or syringes can be purchased or a blunt 18-gauge needle on a syringe can be used. A dilute 0.1 percent chlorhexidine solution is an excellent irrigation agent, but other solutions can be used such as physiologic saline, 3 percent hydrogen peroxide, or zinc ascorbate.

The teeth are checked for any abnormalities and remaining plaque after they have been scaled and polished. Plaque disclosing solutions, such as Reveal (Henry Schein Inc.), are available to enhance visualization of areas of plaque retention. Drying the teeth with air will further enhance visualization of any remaining plaque. Dental explorers are used to detect calculus or tooth abnormalities below the gingival margin, which cannot be visualized (see Fig. 15–20).

Periodontal probes are used to check for periodontal pockets around the teeth. The probe is graded in millimeters to allow measurement of sulcus and pocket depth (Fig. 15–30). Multiple sites along each tooth should be probed and these values recorded (Fig. 15–31). Any problems noted during the

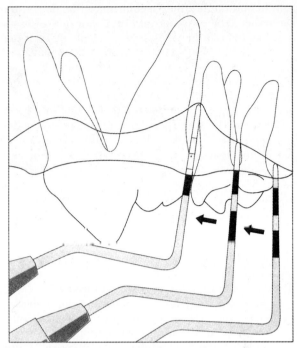

FIGURE 15–31. Multiple sites on a tooth should be probed to detect any deep pockets present. (Reprinted with permission from Emily P and Penman S: Handbook of Small Animal Dentistry. Copyright 1990, Pergamon Press Ltd.)

dental prophylaxis should be brought to the attention of the veterinarian and dental radiographs should be taken if indicated.

All tooth extractions should be performed by the veterinarian. Multirooted teeth may require sectioning prior to extraction. Gingival tissue may need to be reflected and buccal cortical bone removed in order to extract teeth with large roots and a healthy periodontium. Complications associated with extractions include hemorrhage, damage to surrounding soft tissue or the orbital cavity from sharp elevators, and fracture of the alveolar bone, mandible or maxilla, especially when the animal has significant bone loss from chronic periodontal disease.

Proper elevation of the root prior to removal with forceps helps to prevent fracture of the tooth root. If the root does fracture, the retained root tip should be removed to prevent infection of the alveolar socket. After scaling, polishing and sulcus irrigation have been performed and all problems have been addressed, a fluoride gel can be applied to the teeth and the animal can be allowed to recover from anesthesia.

Dental Home Care

The final stage of dental prophylaxis is client education on dental home care treatment along with the dispensing of dental home care products. There are many products available to encourage good compliance and meet individual needs.

When the owner comes to pick up the pet, he or she should be taken into an examination room, where the technician can demonstrate the proper brushing technique on a dental model. The owner should be instructed to start slowly with the pet and to use ample praise. The owner should then be asked to repeat the brushing procedure to ensure correct technique. If the pet is amenable to demonstration, it can then be

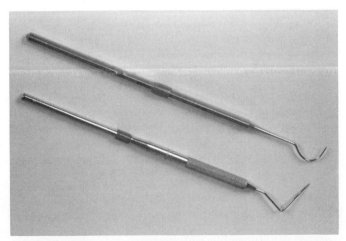

FIGURE 15–30. Dental explorer (top) and graduated periodontal probe (bottom). The periodontal probe is marked in millimeter increments to measure periodontal pocket depth. The dental explorer has a fine tip and is used to detect subgingival calculus and tooth abnormalities.

brought in and the brushing technique can be demonstrated for the owner. The owner should be shown how to properly grasp the muzzle so that the pet is not injured. Daily dental home care is the best way to prevent the accumulation of plaque. For owners with busy schedules, however, an every other day or twice weekly home care session is a more realistic goal and will still provide benefits to the pet.

The owner should be informed of any dental problems the pet may have as well as the date on which the pet's next dental prophylaxis will be due. As a general rule, pets with healthy mouths or mild-to-moderate gingivitis will benefit from annual dental prophylaxis. Those with early periodontal disease will probably require a dental prophylaxis every 6 to 8 months, and those with moderate-to-severe periodontal disease may require a dental prophylaxis every 3 to 4 months.

The key to success with dental home care is finding a product that works well for the owner and is acceptable for the pet. There are many different types of toothbrushes available. Dog and cat toothbrushes can be purchased, or the owner can buy a child's or pediatric soft-bristled toothbrush. Many pets will not tolerate a toothbrush and may respond better if the owner uses a sponge-type swab or a gauze pad wrapped around the owner's finger. If this is unacceptable to the pet, or if the owner risks being bitten, a mouth rinse or spray can be used.

Pet toothpaste formulas are well tolerated by most pets because they like the malt, poultry, or beef flavoring that has been added. Human toothpaste should not be used on pets. The flavors of the veterinary chlorhexidine and zinc ascorbate oral rinses and spray products are not as well liked by pets. However, they are excellent for keeping oral bacterial levels under control and for healing damaged gingival tissue. They can be applied more quickly than pastes and are easier to use on animals that will not tolerate much handling. With patience, praise and guidance, the owner should be able to find a dental home care treatment that will work for his or her pet.

Dental Radiography

Dental radiography is an important tool in the diagnostic and prognostic evaluation of oral disorders in veterinary medicine. As advances have been made in veterinary dentistry, there has been a demand for high-quality dental radiographs to evaluate teeth and oral structures more accurately. The use of dental radiograph machines and intraoral dental film in veterinary medicine has increased dramatically during this time.

Traditionally, radiographs of the teeth, mandible and maxilla were taken to evaluate disorders such as oral masses, fractured jaws and teeth, and facial pain and swelling. Many veterinarians are now using this diagnostic aid to assess problems such as discolored teeth, idiopathic feline dental resorptive lesions and periodontal disease and to aid in the treatment of endodontically compromised teeth, dental restorations and difficult extractions.

Dental radiographs can be taken with the film placed in the mouth (intraoral technique) or outside the mouth (extraoral technique). Intraoral dental film is a non-screened flexible film (Fig. 15–32). Regular screened or non-screened x-ray film can be used for extraoral radiographic views (Chapter 7). Non-screened x-ray films provide greater detail than the screened films but require increased exposure times.

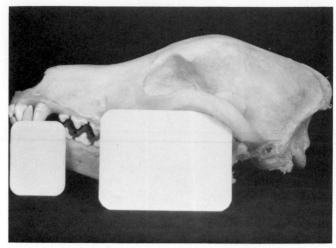

FIGURE 15–32. Intraoral dental film.

There are several advantages of the intraoral radiographic technique over the extraoral technique. Perhaps the greatest advantage of the intraoral technique is the ability to minimize the superimposition of teeth and surrounding structures on the area of study. Intraoral dental film can be purchased in small enough sizes to fit in the mouth next to the tooth or teeth to be studied. The closer the x-ray film is to the subject of interest (the tooth), the better the detail. The anode of the dental radiograph machine can be moved and angled to radiograph the tooth of interest and be placed close enough to the tooth to eliminate the opposite dental arcade.

When using the extraoral technique, there is usually some degree of superimpositioning of teeth from the other arcades that are in the path of the primary beam. The teeth in the opposite arch may obstruct the view of the teeth of interest, and dental abnormalities could be missed.

The film focal distance (FFD) for the dental radiograph machine is 16 inches or less, in contrast to the standard radiograph machines for which a FFD of 36 to 40 inches is commonly used. The shorter FFD of the dental radiograph machine allows closer placement of the anode to the tooth, eliminating the opposite dental arcade or surrounding soft tissue or bone from the path of the primary beam. The shorter FFD also minimizes harmful scatter radiation, as does the small cone size and lead lining, which many of the dental radiograph cones contain.

Intraoral radiographs require less movement of the patient than the extraoral radiographic technique. The extraoral views require the patient to be placed in many different positions so that the skull is angled in order for the primary beam to avoid the surrounding oral structures. This proper positioning takes time and skill. Intraoral dental film can be placed in the mouth, and the radiograph anode can be moved instead of the patient. The patient is placed in dorsal recumbency to radiograph the mandible and in ventral recumbency to radiograph the maxilla. A complete evaluation of all four oral quadrants requires at least six views.

Intraoral dental film can be processed by hand or "piggy backed" to a regular film with electrical tape and automatically processed. Extraoral non-screened x-ray film may not be compatible with the automatic processor's developer and might require hand developing. The extraoral non-screened x-ray

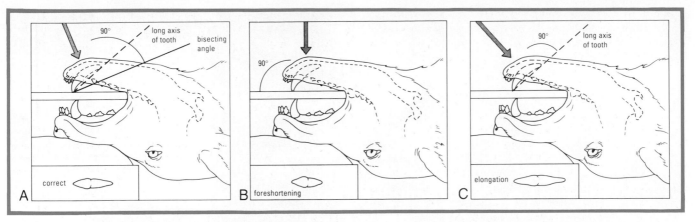

FIGURE 15–33. A, Bisecting angle technique, producing an accurate image of the tooth. B, Directing the x-ray beam at right angles to the film, shortening the tooth's image. C, Directing the x-ray beam at right angles to the long axis of the tooth, elongating the tooth's image. (Reprinted with permission from Emily P and Penman S: Handbook of Small Animal Dentistry. Copyright 1990, Pergamon Press Ltd.)

film is considerably more expensive than the smaller intraoral dental film. If rapid developer and fixative are used, intraoral dental film can be hand developed in 1 minute, which is helpful in minimizing anesthesia time.

To use the intraoral radiographic technique, one must master the bisecting angle technique. This method minimizes distortion of teeth caused by angling the radiographic anode and the inability to place the film parallel to the maxillary teeth and the mandibular canines and incisors. The reader is referred to the suggested reading section for a detailed discussion and illustration of this technique. By directing the radiographic anode perpendicular to a line that bisects the angle created by the plane of the tooth and the intraoral film, an image with minimal distortion can be made on the x-ray film, preventing foreshortening or elongation of tooth roots (Fig. 15–33).

Endodontics

Endodontics deals with the study and treatment of the inside of the tooth (pulp) and periapical tissues. The periapical tissue is located around the tip (apex) of the tooth root. The tooth pulp consists of nerves, blood vessels, lymphatics, and connective tissue. The pulp tissue is found in the pulp chamber (crown) and pulp canal (root) of the tooth and enters the tooth through numerous small openings in the apex of the tooth root called the apical delta.

The dental pulp is important to the development of the tooth in a young animal. It supplies the nutrients needed by the odontoblasts to deposit dentin. This makes the tooth walls thicker, so the tooth is stronger. Once the dog or cat is past 10 to 18 months of age, the majority of the dentin has been deposited, the tooth walls are fairly thick and the root apex should be closed. As the animal continues to age, the pulp chamber and canal will become smaller because the odontoblasts will continue to deposit dentin (Fig. 15–34).

Treatment for teeth with endodontic disease depends on the age of the animal, duration of endodontic disease and anatomy of the tooth. Conventional root canal therapy is usually performed on dogs and cats 18 months of age and older. Treatment involves removing the pulp tissue from the tooth with small files or reamers, disinfecting the root canal and filling the canal (obturation) with an appropriate material to seal the apex from the periapical tissues. Radiographs are necessary to ensure that a proper apical seal has been achieved.

Among the most common causes of endodontic disease in dogs and cats are pulp exposure from fracture of a tooth and attrition (wear) of the tooth. Many dogs will cause severe attrition of their teeth by chewing on hard objects such as rocks or fences. The teeth most commonly fractured are the canines and the maxillary fourth premolar (carnassial) teeth (Fig. 15–35). Attrition usually occurs on the incisors and canines but can be seen on the premolars and molars as well. If the attrition occurs slowly, the odontoblasts will deposit secondary dentin over the pulp tissue to prevent pulp exposure as enamel and dentin is lost. The pulp tissue may be visualized through the secondary dentin as a brown or red dot (Fig. 15–36). A dental explorer should be run over the tooth surface to make sure the pulp tissue is not exposed. When the pulp tissue is exposed, the tip of the dental explorer will drop down into the pulp chamber as it crosses the surface of the tooth.

In fresh fractures the tooth may be bleeding from the center. These fractures are most painful during the first 72 hours. If the tooth is treated within the first 48 hours, a vital pulpotomy procedure can usually be performed. This involves removing the coronal pulp tissue (the pulp tissue in the tooth root remains), covering the pulp tissue with calcium hydroxide and sealing the coronal exposure site with appropriate dental restorative materials.

All teeth with exposed pulp tissue should be treated either by endodontic treatment (root canal, pulp capping, pulpotomy) or by extraction. If left untreated, infection from the exposure site will spread to the periapical tissues, and a periapical abscess will develop. This condition is seen fairly frequently in dogs with maxillary carnassial tooth abscesses. The owner will notice swelling or a draining tract just below the dog's eye and treatment is usually sought (Fig. 15–37). Surprisingly, only about 20 percent of periapical abscesses will fistulize to the skin, which means that unless the teeth of these pets are being examined for endodontic disease, many abscesses go untreated. These abscesses are painful and are a source of infection, which can spread to other teeth and the blood stream.

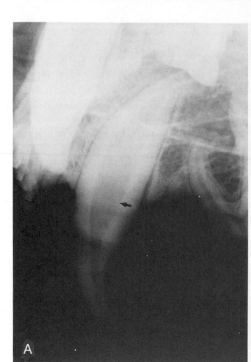

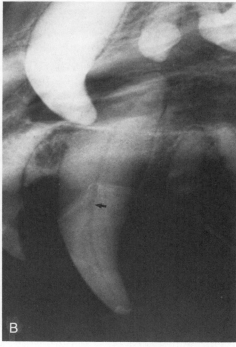

FIGURE 15–34. A, Notice the large pulp chamber and canal in this young cougar's canine tooth (arrow). B, As the animal ages, dentin is deposited and the pulp chamber and canal become narrow (arrow).

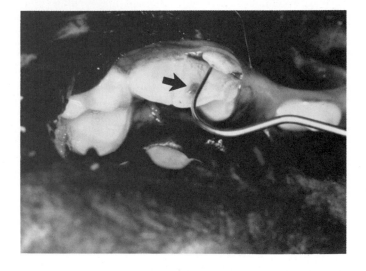

FIGURE 15–35. Slab fractures of the maxillary fourth premolar teeth are a common problem in dogs. This fracture extends subgingivally and the pulp tissue has been exposed (arrow).

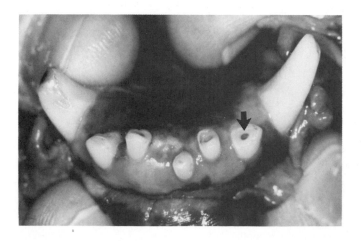

FIGURE 15–36. Severe attrition of the incisor and canine teeth. The brown or red dots (arrow) in the center of these teeth are the pulp tissues below the less opaque secondary dentin.

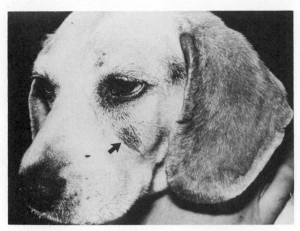

FIGURE 15–37. Patient with a maxillary tooth abscess.

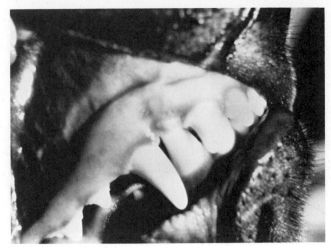

FIGURE 15–39. Lingually displaced mandibular canine tooth. The mandibular canine is displaced toward the tongue and is striking the gingival tissue.

Other signs of endodontic disease include discolored teeth and painful teeth. Diagnosing a painful tooth in an animal can be difficult, but when there is a question, a dental radiograph can be taken to assess the periapical area for signs of disease.

Orthodontics

Orthodontics is concerned with the correction and prevention of irregularities and malocclusion of the teeth. The primary reason for performing orthodontic correction of mal-aligned teeth in veterinary medicine is to alleviate a painful malocclusion or a malocclusion that will lead to endodontic or periodontal disease. When genetic malocclusions are suspected, the owner should be counseled on the problem in order to prevent breeding of these animals and the propagation of inferior genes.

Interceptive orthodontics involves the extraction of retained deciduous teeth, which will usually cause displacement of the permanent dentition (Fig. 15–38). This treatment can be extremely beneficial, and many abnormally erupting permanent teeth will correct spontaneously after extraction of the retained deciduous teeth. The most important factor determining success with this treatment is early detection of the problem. Many

companion animals have completed their vaccination series by the time they reach this mixed dentition stage and will not be seen again until 6 months of age if the owner has elected to neuter the pet. To prevent this condition from going undetected, the owner should be instructed to monitor the dentition closely to ensure that the deciduous tooth is shed prior to the emergence of the permanent tooth. Dental models can be used to show the owner the difference between deciduous teeth and permanent teeth. Dental recheck examinations can be scheduled so that a dental problem does not go undetected.

Some of the most common dental malocclusions seen are lingually displaced mandibular canine teeth (Fig. 15–39), mesially displaced maxillary canine teeth (Fig. 15–40), and even or level bites (Fig. 15–41). These malocclusions can be corrected with orthodontics in most cases, but the owner must be willing to invest the time to clean the oral appliance and return for rechecks as needed. Orthodontic treatment generally costs more than tooth extraction and involves more anesthetic procedures, but it is less invasive than extraction. Orthodontics can be an important treatment option when considering alternatives to extraction of large teeth such as the canines or

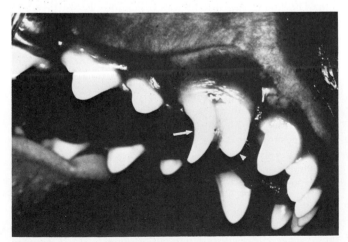

FIGURE 15–38. A retained deciduous maxillary canine tooth (arrow) has displaced the permanent canine tooth mesially (toward the nose) (arrow head). This abnormal tooth alignment can lead to periodontal disease and interference with other teeth or oral soft tissues.

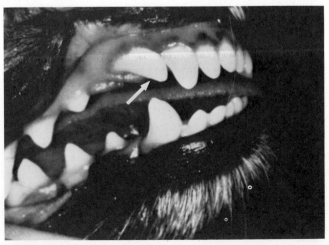

FIGURE 15–40. Mesially displaced maxillary canine tooth. The maxillary canine tooth is displaced mesially (arrow) and is striking the mandibular canine tooth when the mouth is closed.

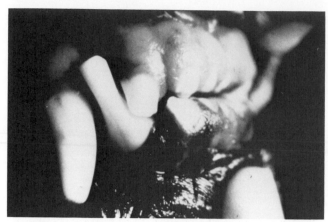

FIGURE 15–41. This dog has severe attrition of the incisor teeth secondary to an even or level bite.

multiple teeth such as the six incisors in a dog with an even bite. Many of the cases that present with the malocclusions listed above can be corrected rapidly with orthodontic treatment.

Odontoplasty or pulp capping is another option for animals with malocclusions, particularly severe malocclusions. These procedures entail shortening the tooth to remove the interference it is causing with another tooth or surrounding soft tissue. This method is less invasive than extraction, removes the animal's source of discomfort and achieves results more quickly than does orthodontics. However, it does permanently alter the appearance of the tooth (Fig. 15–42).

Restorative Dentistry

The goal of restorative dentistry is to restore a tooth, as closely as possible, to its natural structure and function. No

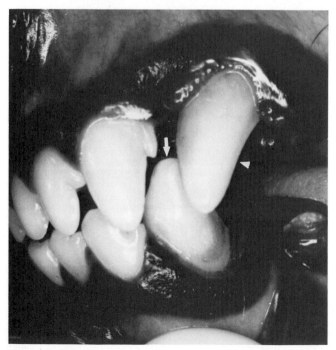

FIGURE 15–42. The mandibular canine tooth (arrow) has been shortened to prevent it from impinging on the palate. Note that the maxillary canine tooth (arrow head) is displaced mesially, preventing the mandibular canine tooth from returning to its normal position.

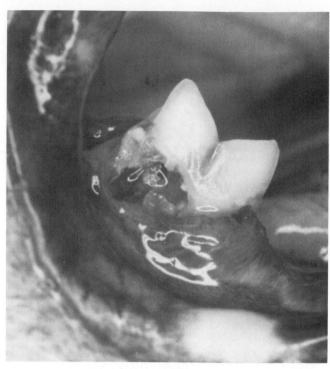

FIGURE 15–43. Feline dental resorptive lesion. The large erosion on this tooth involves the distal root and cervical portion of the tooth crown.

restorative material is as strong as the original tooth structure, so an attempt is always made to preserve as much of the original tooth as possible. Indications for restorative dentistry include teeth with dental caries (cavities), idiopathic feline dental resorptive lesions, fractured teeth and endodontically treated teeth.

Dental caries rarely occurs in the dog and cat. When present, the carious tooth structure must be completely removed and the defect restored. If left untreated, the caries will dissolve the enamel and dentin and gain access to the pulp tissue. The tooth will eventually be destroyed.

A common problem of feline dentition is the development of idiopathic feline dental resorptive lesions (Fig. 15–43). It is estimated that 20 percent of cats are affected with this problem. The lesions are usually found at the neck of the tooth (the junction of the enamel of the crown and the cementum of the tooth root), which is often hidden by the free gingival tissue. Cats must be examined closely for these lesions. Often the gingival tissue over these lesions is inflamed. A dental explorer must be used to check for irregularities below the gingiva. Early detection and restoration of these lesions usually prevents the continued resorption of the tooth. Many of these teeth are identified in the advanced stages of the disease with pulp exposure and root resorption. When the resorption has progressed this far, the tooth cannot be saved and should be extracted.

Fractured teeth are frequently restored to return function and maintain periodontal health. The tooth has a natural design to allow self-cleaning and deflection of food away from the gingival sulcus. When the teeth lose this proper contour they can become predisposed to periodontal disease. Fractured teeth can be restored with restorative materials alone or in combination with retention pins and/or posts. Pins and posts do not add strength to the restoration but aid in retaining the restoration.

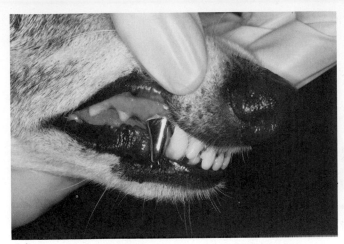

FIGURE 15-44. A nonprecious metal crown has been cemented to the maxillary canine tooth after the tooth was traumatically fractured and received endodontic treatment.

Another option available for restoring a tooth with loss of coronal structure is to cover the crown of the tooth with a prosthetic crown. The silver-colored metal crowns, which are made of nonprecious metals, are the most common type used because of their greater strength and decreased cost when compared with gold or porcelain crowns. The teeth most commonly crowned in dogs are the canines and maxillary fourth premolars (Fig. 15-44). In the cat, the canine is the most commonly crowned tooth.

Veterinary dentistry is a specialty field in veterinary medicine. Advanced procedures require a strong background knowledge of the materials used, the anatomy and physiology of the teeth and periodontium, and the principles applied to each procedure. It is important for the general practitioner and veterinary technician to be able to identify dental abnormalities and to be able to recommend treatment alternatives to the owner. The pet can then be referred for advanced dental procedures if the owner wishes to pursue treatment.

Recommended Reading

Bojrab MJ and Tholen M: Small Animal Oral Medicine and Surgery. Philadelphia, Lea & Febiger, 1990.

Holmstrom SE, Frost P and Gammon RL: Veterinary Dental Techniques. Philadelphia, WB Saunders Company, 1992.

Seim HB III, Creed JE and Smith KW: Restraint techniques for prevention of self-trauma. *In* Bojrab MJ (editor): Current Techniques in Small Animal Surgery. 3rd ed. Philadelphia, Lea & Febiger, 1990.

16

Equine Medical and Surgical Nursing

GEORGE S. MARTIN and A. SIMON TURNER

EQUINE PRACTICE OVERVIEW

The general role of veterinary technicians in equine practice is that of an important team member in providing quality veterinary care. While the size of the team and specific tasks may vary among practices, the general goal is the same. The goal is to provide high-quality veterinary care to equine patients, which will improve or maintain the pleasure or utility derived from the animal by the owners, at a fee that provides a profit to the practice. Thus, as a member of this team, your purpose is to help provide efficient delivery of veterinary care.

The growth of the equine industry has been phenomenal over the last few years. There are now more horses in North America than at any other time. Like dogs and cats, horses have great sentimental attachment and for the most part can be considered companion animals. However, many horses are moneymaking prospects, such as show horses, race horses and breeding stock. In some areas of North America, there are some counties with large populations of religious people (e.g., Amish, Mennonite) whose beliefs do not permit modern machinery. These people are largely dependent upon the horse for day to day farm use.

Generally speaking, horse owners will spend more money on their animal if necessary when compared with the dog and cat owner. For example, if a horse is worth $75,000 as a breeding stallion, a bill of $2,000 to $3,000 to save the animal's life is not unreasonable, whereas a similar amount for a small animal would often be out of the question. Furthermore, the costs associated with providing care to large animals are considerably greater.

Horse owners and horse traders have a *language* of their own that has been passed on for generations. This language in many cases does not describe the particular condition and is confusing to someone who has not been raised with horses. Examples are spavin, thoroughpin, sweeny, windpuffs, curb and so on. These terms must be learned as part of the overall language in equine practice. The veterinary technician must spend considerable time around horse people, horse shows or racetracks to pick up this language.

Many treatments in the equine industry are also "hand-me-downs" based on years of tradition. Such treatments are often based on home remedies and have extremely doubtful scientific merit. One classic example is the practice of pin-firing, whereby a hot steel iron is inserted into the locally anesthesized skin over a particular diseased joint. The practice is still performed by some veterinarians and in my opinion is of questionable scientific value. Economics play a large role in the equine industry, especially in racetrack practice. The veterinary technician may observe procedures performed on a horse that are of doubtful scientific value but may be the most economical for that particular horse. An example would be the injection of a corticosteroid into an arthritic joint, rather than rest or surgery or both; rest and surgery have more scientific merit but may be uneconomical for the owner.

CARE OF THE HOSPITALIZED HORSE

Signs of Illness in the Horse

Apart from the observation of the lack of "twinkle in the eye," the veterinary technician must play an integral part in the daily physical examination of a hospitalized horse in conjunction with the veterinarian. The horse's normal rectal temperature is 36° to 38.5°C. The technician must be careful when taking the horse's temperature . . . and take proper safety precautions to protect one's self from injury. Some horses will resent this by kicking, and the horse should be approached from its left side, standing as close to it as possible. The handler should slowly work his way to the back of the horse, carefully raise the tail and insert a lubricated thermometer into the rectum. Some horses will resent this by clamping their tail down. The handler should not get directly behind the horse for obvious reasons. A kick from a horse can cause considerable injury or even death. When a horse kicks, it is usually extremely fast and accurate, since this is its main form of defense. The thermometer should be attached to a string and an alligator clip so that it can be attached to the tail hairs. This will prevent the thermometer from being aspirated into the rectum and prevent it from dropping to the floor during a bowel movement.

The most common cause of a temperature rise in a horse is an infectious process somewhere within the animal. The temperature of foals is normally a degree or so higher than that of adults and may increase with excitement. When taking the temperature in foals, assistance is usually required to restrain the animal in order to prevent undue excitement. The pulse of a horse is taken from the maxillary artery, at the point at which the artery curves around the jaw (Fig. 16–1). The heart rate is taken with a stethoscope over the left lateral thoracic region, just behind the elbow. In the adult horse, the normal heart rate is 28 to 42 beats per minute. Care must be taken not to count the two major heart sounds. The best way to take the respiratory rate is to place the hand over the nostrils and count the number of breaths per minute. The normal respiratory rate is 8 to 15 breaths per minute. All such data should be recorded for the veterinarian in the medical record. In addition, any change in appetite, consistency of feces or amount of

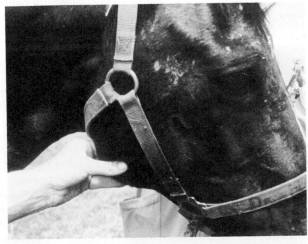

FIGURE 16–1. Taking the pulse of a horse at the maxillary artery.

feces should be noted. Other observations should also be noted, such as signs of abdominal pain, and they are discussed in detail further on. It is the technician's job as well to attend to bandages or casts and various wounds at the discretion of the veterinarian. This is discussed in Chapter 13.

Day to Day Care of the Hospitalized Horse

It is not the purpose of this chapter to discuss all aspects of horse husbandry. Instead, we will concentrate on the day to day care of the horse once it is hospitalized. The horse's stall should be large enough to permit the animal to move around freely. This may require turning into a larger corral for exercise or for orthopedic rehabilitation. There should be no obstacles or hazards, such as sharp objects, in the stall so that the horse does not injure itself. Naturally, clean, dry bedding is essential, and the stall should be "mucked-out" (cleaned) at least once a day. There should be no drafts or breezes, and dust should be minimized. Moldy bedding should never be used because this predisposes to certain conditions of the respiratory tract, in particular chronic obstructive pulmonary disease (COPD). Many cases of COPD (or heaves, as it was once called) can be managed merely by eliminating the dust in the horse's stall. The horse should be provided with clean, fresh water, and in some cases the water consumption should be monitored. The horse should also receive adequate nutrition (see Chapter 21 for more information). The horse should be housed away from others with contagious diseases, especially if upper respiratory tract infections are present, which are spread by aerosol; a horse with such an infection can rapidly spread this disease through most hospital facilities. The stall should have adequate footing. The stall floor should be kept dry because this will decrease the incidence of "thrush."

The horse's feet should be picked up daily and checked not only for thrush but also for foreign bodies, such as nails and stones. Thrush is a disease of poor management and is caused by excessive moisture combined with inadequate foot care. Conversely, if the horse's feet are *too dry*, a commercially available hoof dressing may have to be applied to the feet. Dry feet are more common in the western states of North America. The technician must be familiar with the techniques of how to pick up the horse's feet and examine them without endangering himself. Hospitalized horses, if shod, should have attention paid to their shoes. If the shoes are too loose, they should be replaced, but this will require close collaboration with the local farrier. If horses are to be hospitalized for a considerable time, the shoes may need to be reset (shoes removed, the feet trimmed and new shoes applied) every 6 to 8 weeks. The veterinary technician must become familiar with each patient in the hospital, and it will soon be obvious that there is much individual variation between horses. What may appear to be a depression in an excitable thoroughbred may be normal for one of the draft breeds.

Treatment of the Sick Horse

The administration of drugs is discussed in Chapter 8, but some problems associated with drug administration specific to the horse should be reviewed here. First, the volume of material injected, especially for intramuscular injection, should be no more than 15 to 20 ml, because large volumes can cause localized swelling. It is absolutely essential that irritating solutions not be injected intramuscularly, because this can cause abscess formation and tissue death. Phlebitis is an inflammatory reaction around a vein and is seen in horses especially around the jugular vein. This is an extremely serious condition in horses and can on occasion lead to the animal's death. The cause of phlebitis is inadvertent perivascular (given outside the vein) administration of irritating substances. The substances most commonly incriminated as causing phlebitis in horses are the following: phenylbutazone, thiamylal or thiopental sodium (intravenous anesthetics), chloral hydrate (sedative and intravenous anesthetic) and bromsulphalein (BSP). The best assurance that substances will not be administered perivascularly and cause phlebitis is the proper *placement of a commercially available catheter*. The technique of catheter insertion is discussed in Chapter 8. Intra-arterial administration of anything but normal physiological solutions can lead to the death of the animal and should be avoided at all costs. Another problem associated with drug reaction is anaphylaxis, which is an allergic reaction but fortunately is uncommon. Occasionally, horses will react to intramuscular procaine penicillin. The horse will become anxious, will start sweating and pacing the stall and will appear frightened. This has often been interpreted as inadvertent injection of some of the solution into a vein, which is best avoided by aspiration of the syringe prior to injection. True allergic reaction should be noted in the medical record.

Oral Administration

Some medications, provided in tablet form from the manufacturer, are administered most easily by mouth in crushed form. Oral phenylbutazone (anti-inflammatory) and oral trimethoprim-sulfamethoxazole (antibiotic), two widely used medications, are administered in this manner. A mortar and pestle are used to crush the tablets into powder. A 60-cc syringe is prepared by removing its tip end with a rasp. The plunger is pulled fully back and 10 to 20 cc of molasses or Karo syrup is poured into the empty syringe barrel. The medication is then added and the remainder of the barrel volume is filled with molasses or Karo syrup. A disposable wooden applicator works well to stir the mixture. Administration to the patient involves putting the syringe into the horse's mouth through the interdental space and depositing the mixture on top of the tongue. Seldom do patients fail to swallow most of the doze administered, and generally this technique is not stressful to a sick patient.

Nasogastric Administration

Another efficient way of administering substances into the gastrointestinal tract of the horse is through a stomach tube. The stomach tube is passed through the nose into the esophagus and then into the stomach. This procedure should be performed either by a veterinarian or under the direct supervision of a veterinarian. The stomach tube has many uses, the most common being the administration of vermifuges. It can also be used to relieve gas accumulation (e.g., during an attack of colic or during postoperative colic management). The stomach tube is also useful for feeding when a horse has a painful

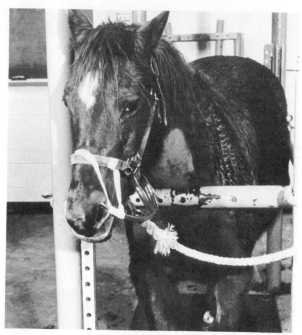

FIGURE 16–2. A stomach tube can be maintained in place on a semipermanent basis by taping it to the horse's halter.

condition of the mouth or is unable to grasp food as in a fracture of the mandible. The stomach tube can be left in place on a semipermanent basis by taping it to a halter (Fig. 16–2). This will allow the horse to be fed frequently without the trauma of repeatedly passing the stomach tube. A number of problems can arise if a stomach tube is passed inadvertently into another organ. The most serious problem is passage of the tube into the trachea and then into the lungs. If any substance is administered into the tube, it can obviously lead to severe pneumonia and death of the animal. Another problem not infrequently observed in stomach tube passage is epistaxis (nosebleed).

Care of the Recumbent Horse

Many conditions can cause a horse to become recumbent and, regardless of the causes, the recumbent horse will require an enormous amount of nursing, medical treatment and tender loving care. The causes of recumbency in horses include various neurological conditions, colic, fractures and severe laminitis. Because of the weight of the patient, pressure sores develop easily and must be cared for on a day to day basis. It is better to keep pressure sores dry rather than to use moist ointments. The most important part of caring for the recumbent horse is to ensure adequate bedding and padding.

Several university veterinary teaching hospitals prefer an inflatable water bed or water mattress for the recumbent horse because it conforms well to all areas of the horse's body and provides even pressure. Other methods include air mattresses and foam pads. No matter how heavily a stall is bedded with straw, the horse eventually ends up getting severe pressure sores, especially over the tuber coxae or hip region. The recumbent horse must be turned frequently, and this will require several assistants and should be done without endangering personnel. If the horse is paddling or making efforts to stand, the lower limbs should be bandaged and, of course, any shoes or sharp protruding nails should be removed. To protect the eyes and face from trauma, a commercially available face pad can be used. One problem frequently seen in the recumbent horse is corneal ulceration, which must be avoided. Slings sound like useful objects for the recumbent horse, and many owners are impressed by their theoretical advantages; however, from a practical standpoint, slings are difficult to manage in horses and do not provide simple answers. Not all horses tolerate slings, and some tend to slump in them or fight them and become entangled. Pressure sores are also a problem with slings. Generally, nursing care for recumbent horses is a substantial challenge, but in selected cases, quality nursing care is often the key to a successful outcome. Providing care to recumbent horses requires commitment from the owners and veterinary team, and each case may require daily assessment of the quality of life for the patient.

SPECIFIC MEDICAL CONDITIONS IN HORSES

In this section, the salient aspects of common medical conditions encountered in horses will be discussed. The intent is not to have the technician become an expert diagnostician, but rather to provide some background knowledge and an understanding of the rationale behind nursing and support care required in each disease. The technician is referred to Colahan et al. (1991) for additional background information. Chapter 31 provides a complete overview of equine preventive health programs and vaccination recommendations.

Conditions of the Upper Respiratory Tract

Influenza (Flu)

Influenza is a highly contagious infection of the upper respiratory tract. It is caused by either of two related viruses. The virus attacks the lining of the respiratory tract, producing a cough, fever, loss of appetite and nasal discharge. Influenza is frequently complicated by secondary bacterial invasion. It is spread by a droplet infection, and young horses are most susceptible. Outbreaks frequently occur when an infected horse comes into contact with healthy animals as would occur at a horse show or even a large equine hospital. The disease is controlled by annual vaccination (in the spring). Although there are many other causes of respiratory infections in horses that can cause a similar-appearing disease, annual influenza vaccination is recommended. Treatment of influenza is discussed further on.

Viral Rhinopneumonitis

Viral rhinopneumonitis, like influenza, is also a highly contagious upper respiratory tract infection caused by a virus. Rhinopneumonitis is characterized by cough, fever, loss of appetite and nasal discharge. It is also spread by aerosol. The virus that causes the disease can also invade the reproductive tract, causing abortion of foals or birth of a weak foal. With the high stud fees that are now demanded in many areas, this can be a considerable financial loss to a particular farm or owner.

A vaccine is available for viral rhinopneumonitis; however, it provides a short duration of immunity and usually has to be repeated several times in 1 year.

Viral Arteritis

As the name implies, viral arteritis is a virus causing inflammation of the arteries. It is relatively uncommon, and outbreaks are sporadic when compared with influenza and rhinopneumonitis. The signs include fever, depression, muscular weakness, congestion of nasal mucosa, nasal discharge and coughing. Other body systems can also be affected (such as the gastrointestinal tract, producing colic or diarrhea). A modified live virus vaccine is available for the prevention of viral abortion and respiratory infection due to equine viral arteritis. Treatment of the disease is largely symptomatic.

Strangles

Strangles is an upper respiratory infection caused by the bacterium *Streptococcus equi*. It has been recognized in horses for many years and is spread by contact with secretions of infected horses. The typical form of the disease is an inflammation of the upper respiratory tract with fever, depression, loss of appetite and nasal discharge. The condition infects local lymph glands (nodes) under the neck and throat region, which become swollen and painful and may rupture 10 to 14 days after onset of signs. The bacteria are resistant in the environment and may live away from the horse for some time, resulting in recurring problems; that is, a farm may have a strangles problem year after year after year. The course described is typical for most cases of strangles, but more serious problems may arise.

The lymph nodes behind the guttural pouch may rupture into the pouch, producing a pouch full of pus. This condition is known as *guttural pouch empyema*. Bacteria may also localize in other parts of the body and produce abscesses within the abdominal cavity. Such abscesses may be the cause of chronic weight loss in the horse. Another bacterium, *Streptococcus zooepidemicus*, can cause an upper respiratory tract infection similar to strangles. *Streptococcus zooepidemicus* can also be responsible for guttural pouch empyema and abscesses of the internal organs. It is also seen as a secondary invader in various viral diseases.

Treatment of Respiratory Conditions

Nursing is important in the management of respiratory infections. First and foremost, the animal must not be subjected to stressful incidents, such as transport, severe exercise, exposure to cold drafts or poor nutrition. These problems should be corrected as part of management of an upper respiratory infection. The animal should be kept isolated in a well-ventilated stall. Mold and dust in the stall should be reduced, and the animal should be provided with fresh water. The veterinarian may require that antibiotics be administered or the disease may be allowed just simply to run its course. Antibiotics are useful against the secondary bacterial invaders of viral respiratory conditions. Other things that a veterinarian may administer are cough suppressants and decongestants. Nebulization (inhalation therapy) may also be used.

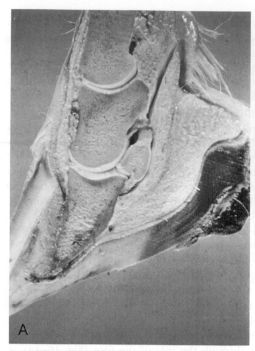

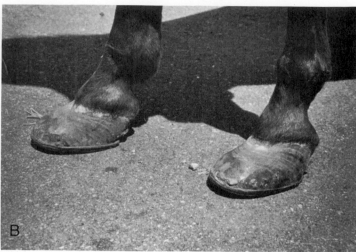

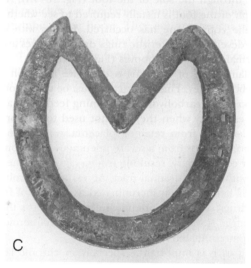

FIGURE 16–4. A, Cross section of a horse's hoof that was destroyed because of chronic laminitis. The distal phalanx has "rotated" and is protruding through the sole. B, A horse with chronic laminitis, showing characteristic rings in hoof wall. C, "Heart bar" shoe used for certain cases of laminitis.

analgesic. The most popular is a nonsteroidal anti-inflammatory drug, such as phenylbutazone. The chance of a horse with laminitis (especially when there is rotation of the distal phalanx) returning to strenuous activity is poor. The changes in the feet are usually irreversible. Some animals can be salvaged for breeding purposes.

Diarrhea

Diarrhea is an increase in the water content of the stool. It is seen primarily in foals but can also affect adult horses. Diarrhea in the horse results from a variety of causes, but the same basic change in the overall physiology exists whatever the cause. If not attended to, diarrhea can be a life-threatening situation. Affected animals will become dehydrated, have excess acid in the blood (metabolic acidosis) and suffer electrolyte imbalances. This can take a fatal course and cause death, especially in foals. Chronic cases of diarrhea can cause weight loss and failure to thrive.

The main causes of diarrhea in horses are various viruses (e.g., rotaviruses), bacteria (e.g., *Salmonella* spp.) or occasionally parasites (e.g., roundworms). Frequently, bacteria invade the intestinal tract *after* viruses. Diarrhea may also have noninfectious causes, the most common being *foal heat diarrhea*. The actual cause of foal heat diarrhea is unknown. It is a diarrhea that develops in foals at 6 to 14 days of age and corresponds to the mare's first heat cycle after the birth of the foal, hence the name "foal heat" diarrhea. Diarrhea in nursing foals can result from excess ingestion of milk. However, a sudden change in diet also can lead to diarrhea.

Salmonellosis is caused by a bacterium and may be responsible for diarrhea in foals and adult horses. It can also cause a severe and sometimes fatal diarrhea in humans; hence, strict sanitary measures (disinfection, isolation, handwashing) are mandatory when working with a potential *Salmonella*-infected horse. *Salmonella* diarrhea is sometimes seen in horses that have been recently "stressed." Such stresses include transport over a long distance, recent surgery that has required a general anesthetic or any severe systemic disease. The horse becomes depressed for 1 to 2 days after the stressful incident, with fever and inappetence followed by a profuse, musty-smelling diarrhea. Several cultures of the feces need to be performed to diagnose salmonellosis.

Treatment of Diarrhea. The most important thing for the veterinary technician to realize is that the agent causing the disease may be a hazard to human health, especially *Salmonella.* This is cause for caution and for taking specific precautions. Such precautions include the use of gloves when working around the horse (plastic obstetrical sleeves), foot baths placed outside the stall with the appropriate disinfecting agents and the use of separate thermometers for each horse. The patient should be isolated from other horses. Protective clothing should be worn; one should not wear street clothes. Overboots, Wellington boots and so on are also required. Hands must always be washed before proceeding to the next case.

Treatment is directed on several fronts and is obviously left to the discretion of the veterinarian. Such treatment will include various intestinal drugs, antibiotics and orally administered charcoal. One of the main thrusts of treatment is coping with the dehydration that can occur. If dehydration is mild, the veterinarian may elect to administer fluids through a stomach tube. If, however, the dehydration is severe, as measured by the packed cell volume (PCV) and total protein from the blood, the veterinarian may elect to administer intravenous fluids. Usually, intravenous fluids are required for some days. Therefore, meticulous care of indwelling catheters is absolutely mandatory. Such catheters should be anchored or sutured to the skin so that they cannot become dislodged. They should also be aseptically placed. The veterinary technician may be needed to watch the fluids in the containers supplying the intravenous therapy and may be required to change them frequently. In addition, dehydration will be monitored by PCV and total protein measurements at appropriate times. Usually, some sort of flow sheet is required so that the veterinarian can check the progress of the horse at a glance.

Diseases of Teeth

A horse's teeth require constant attention throughout its life. The most common procedure performed by veterinarians is rasping or *floating.* This is usually done every 6 months or more often, if indicated. The veterinarian will rasp the sharp edges from the teeth. Such sharp edges occur on the medial (lingual) side of the lower arcade and lateral (buccal) side of the upper arcade. If not removed, such points will cause laceration of the gum, pain, poor mastication of feed and formation of small wads of feed (quidding). Usually, the veterinary technician is required to set out the necessary equipment, such as floats and mouth gags for floating the teeth. Some horses require tranquilization for this procedure to be performed. Frequently, radiographs are required as part of the dental examination, especially if sinusitis or a diseased tooth is suspected. Sometimes excessively long teeth or a row of teeth that have become uneven require more radical rasping under general anesthesia.

Other Problems with Teeth

Tooth Removal. Tooth removal is sometimes required if the teeth have become abscessed or split. Abscessed teeth may be accompanied by a concurrent secondary sinusitis. Tooth removal in horses is almost always done under general anesthesia, in lateral recumbency with the affected tooth uppermost. Instruments required for these types of procedures are a mouth speculum, molar forceps, mallet or hammer, straight and curved dental punches as well as some type of dressing to place in the tooth socket once the tooth has been removed. It is rarely possible to pull a tooth directly out of the socket as it is done in humans. Usually teeth are *repelled.* A hole (trephine hole) is made over the tooth root, and it is punched into the mouth with a metal punch placed on the root of the tooth. The veterinary surgeon will have one hand in the mouth and one positioning the punch on the appropriate tooth; an assistant (e.g., veterinary technician) may then be required to hammer the punch to push the tooth into the mouth, thereby removing it.

Removal of deciduous teeth that have not dislodged off the permanent teeth (caps) is often required in 2-year-old and 3-year-old horses.

Removal of Wolf Teeth. The wolf tooth is a vestige of the first premolar, and some owners request its removal. This procedure is usually done in the standing horse, with or without tranquilizers, and a special instrument to gouge out the wolf tooth is required.

Colic

Owing to the anatomy and physiology of the equine digestive tract and the fact that all horses suffer from varying degrees of bloodworm (*Strongylus vulgaris*) infestation, the horse is more prone to colic than are most animals. It is one of the most important diseases of the horse and is one area in which the veterinary technician plays a vital role in assisting in the treatment, both surgically and medically. The veterinary technician is intimately involved in the aftercare of such cases, especially monitoring the horse's progress following surgery.

Colic is *not* a disease itself but is a clinical sign. Colic means abdominal pain, and there are many causes of abdominal pain in horses. The classic cause of colic is an obstruction to flow of ingesta through the intestinal tract, causing a distention of the intestine and stretching of the wall. This stretching is painful and causes the horse to exhibit a variety of behavioral abnormalities, which will be discussed further on. Not all colic is caused by blockage of intestine. A mare that is about to foal, for example, will show similar signs resulting from painful contraction of the uterus. A horse with an obstruction of the urinary tract (e.g., a urinary stone [calculus]) may also show signs of colic. It is important that the veterinary technician recognize the signs of colic, though the diagnosis of the actual cause of colic is left to the veterinarian. Signs of colic are variable; however, certain signs are common to most. Mild signs include inappetence, stretching more frequently than normal, yawning and looking at the flank. Other signs include playing with water or frequent urination. More obvious signs include pawing the ground, stamping the feet, walking the stall, kicking the abdomen and violent rolling. Some horses will actually sit like a dog to relieve the pain. In addition, the horse will usually sweat, and there will be an increased heart rate and respiratory rate. Mucous membranes of the gum, eyes and vulva become congested.

The causes of intestinal colic include volvulus (twisting of the intestine), impactions of foreign bodies or ingesta, *Strongy-*

PROCEDURE: Arthroscopy-carpal

SKIN PREP: Standard

          Bilateral-1 towel pack
               2 sponge packs

POSITION OF PATIENT: _____ Dorsal _____

DRAPES: Arthroscopy drape, 18x20 barrier

SUTURES AND NEEDLES	INSTRUMENTS AND EQUIPMENT
2-0 nylon	Arthroscopy standard
	Arthroscopy instruments
X-Ray cassettes	Arthroscopy camera and cables
X-Ray machine	Cidex pan
X-Ray gowns	Cidex
X-Ray labels	Sterile water (4)
	Room temp ECF
	Sterile IV set
DRESSINGS:	Sterile IV extension
1 3x8 telfa	Sterile bulb pump
1–4"sterile kling	No. 15 blade
1 cotton roll	18 g 1½" needle
1 6" kling	20 cc syringe
1 4" vetwrap	Camera bag
1–3" elasticon	Sterile rubber band
	MTC
	Light source and video

CLINICIAN'S VARIATIONS OVER:

FIGURE 16–12. The card system used at Colorado State University to enable the technician to set out the requirements of the individual surgeon.

Arthroscopic Surgery

Since the first edition of this book, one area of veterinary surgical nursing that has emerged is that involving arthroscopic surgery. Arthroscopic surgery has been one of the most significant advances in equine surgery in the past decade, and it is important that the veterinary technician be familiar with arthroscopy and the nursing techniques.

Bone fragments that were previously removed by completely opening the joint are now removed through much smaller incisions. The surgeon looks into the joint through the arthroscope, which is a small (4.0 mm) telescopic device that is placed into the joint through a stab incision. The surgeon views the fragment of bone through the arthroscope, and through a separate stab incision a pair of forceps or similar instrument is inserted and the chip removed. The surgery has now become routine in most equine surgical facilities.

A well-organized nursing staff is essential for the surgeon performing the arthroscopy. The technician will have to learn a *completely new group of instruments*, previously unknown to veterinary surgeons. Outlined below are some details that technicians involved with arthroscopic surgery should know. These details are based on how cases are managed at Colorado State University.

Selection of Equipment

The surgeon will have a set of specially selected arthroscopy instruments suitable for that particular procedure. The instruments may vary depending on the joint involved, but, generally speaking, there will be a *standard set of instruments* useful in all joints. These instruments, owing to their delicate construction and expense, are kept in some type of protective muslin "pouch." They are stored in these pouches *unsterilized*. Because of the expense of these instruments, rather than having four or five instrument sets sterilized, one set is sterilized with cold sterilization solution (discussed below) after each use. Additional items necessary will be a sterile (18-gauge usually) needle and syringe used to distend the joint prior to entry. During arthroscopic surgery, the joint is kept distended with sterile physiological solution. To deliver this solution a sterile intravenous set and appropriate extensions will be required.

A standard set of arthroscopic instruments may also contain some additional items such as Brown-Adson thumb forceps, a needle holder, several hemostats, scalpel handle, a dozen or so towel clamps and a saline bowl. These instruments are packed into a stainless steel pan, later to be used to rinse the disinfecting solution off the arthroscopy instruments. One of the most important, and most expensive, instruments is the arthroscope

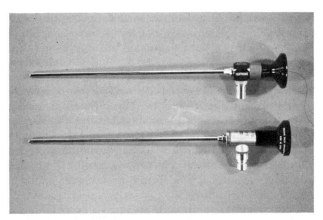

FIGURE 16–13. The arthroscope (two different sizes are shown) is a delicate instrument and must be handled carefully.

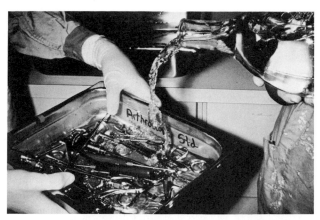

FIGURE 16–14. Following the appropriate time in the sterilizing solution (such as Cidex, Surgikos), the instruments are rinsed with sterile water. Note that the surgeon has double-gloved.

itself. It should be treated carefully to avoid expensive repairs (Fig. 16–13).

Many universities and private practices are now performing arthroscopic surgery with the aid of a video camera so that the entire procedure can be viewed on a television screen. This causes less strain for the surgeon's eye and makes the procedure more interesting for the surgeon's assistant and technical staff. To provide the intense light that is required to view inside the horse's joint, a fiberoptic light source and light cable (that attaches to the arthroscope itself) will be required. It is, therefore, essential for the technician to become acquainted with the functioning of this new electrical equipment, as well as the proper care, cleaning and disinfecting of the instruments themselves.

Positioning and Draping of the Arthroscopy Patient

The technician will be responsible for the correct positioning and padding of the patient and, therefore, must know what position the surgeon wants the horse for the particular joint(s) being operated on. We do virtually all arthroscopic surgery (except shoulders and elbow joints) in dorsal recumbency. The appropriate draping system must be available. We use a commercially available disposable draping system designed specifically for arthroscopic surgery.

Instrument Disinfection

The specialized arthroscopy instruments are disinfected with a cold sterilization solution. We use activated dialdehyde (Cidex, Surgikos) to soak the instruments, arthroscope and light cables for a minimum of 10 minutes. One should check the label from the manufacturer for the exact time required for disinfecting. To avoid delays, the instruments can be placed in the sterilizing solution at the start of anesthesia. This will also ensure ample sterilizing time. Before using the instruments, the surgeon will transfer them into an empty sterile tray. The instruments are then rinsed with sterile water to remove the activated dialdehyde solution (Fig. 16–14).

Preparation of the Surgical Site

We try to clip the affected limb the day before surgery. If the horse does not allow this, it is done just prior to surgery when

the animal is recumbent. Following the appropriate positioning of the horse, the surgical sites (called portals) are shaved, and a routine surgical preparation is performed. The surgical sites are then dried and sprayed with a sterile adhesive that will allow the sterile plastic adhesive drape to adhere to the limb.

Intraoperative Nursing

After the patient has been draped and the instrument has been retrieved from the sterilizing solution, the technician will be responsible for attaching the fiberoptic cable to its light source. If an older camera is being used, the camera must be passed carefully through the commercially available plastic sleeve, allowing the surgeon to touch the camera without breaking aseptic technique. Newer cameras may be cold-sterilized in activated aldehyde with the arthroscope. In addition, the system that delivers the fluids that will distend the joint during surgery is connected to the appropriate fluid source (Fig. 16–15). (Throughout these procedures the technician must see that there is no break in sterile technique.) When the system is connected to the fluid source, the surgeon must

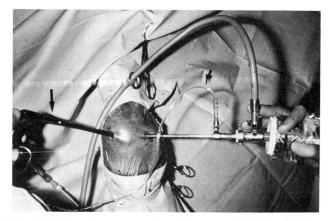

FIGURE 16–15. Arthroscopic surgery in progress. The camera (in the surgeon's hand) is attached to the end of the arthroscope. Note the following: plastic sleeve covering the camera to maintain sterility, flexible fiberoptic cable to provide the light to see into the joint, the tubing delivering a sterile physiological solution into the joint to maintain distention (small arrow), and instrument held in surgeon's other hand to grasp osteochondral fragments (large arrow).

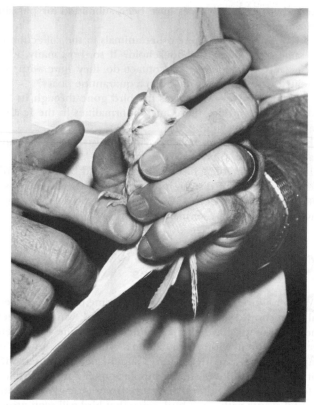

FIGURE 18–3. Restraint techniques similar to those used in the Amazon parrot (see Fig. 18–2) can be used for a budgerigar.

The bird cannot bite the catcher if it is chewing on the cage. Once the head is secured, the body is wrapped in the towel, the feet are held and the bird is held against the holder's body to control the wings. The towel or drape may then be slowly removed from the patient's head for examination, keeping the towel around the wings to secure them from flapping (Fig. 18–3).

Restraint Techniques for Passerine Species

Canaries and finches are the most common passerine species seen in veterinary offices. These birds are easily stressed under normal conditions but are extremely sensitive when they are ill. Catching the patient for an examination must be done quickly and efficiently. To catch the passerine patient, all lights should be turned off and the cage door slowly lifted. Grab the patient with one hand and then turn on the lights. To hold the bird for examination, let the bird's head rest between the middle and index fingers while lying on its back. Do not put pressure on the breast or the patient may suffocate (Fig. 18–4).

Restraint Techniques for Raptorial Species

Birds of prey use their anatomical weapons in a different way. For them, it is of utmost importance to secure the talons. Although many raptors will bite, their jaws are not tremendously strong, and they do little damage with the beak. The mouth is soft except close to the very point of the beak, which

the birds use for tearing flesh. The wings should also be considered a weapon and should be properly secured. Equipment needed for restraining raptors includes towels or drapes, gloves of appropriate size and thickness, and hoods. To approach a bird of prey using gloves, the handler should be bent down low and approach quietly. Dimming the lights may be a disadvantage for examining a species that hunts at night. The handler should present as little threat as possible to the raptor. As the handler places one hand in front of his face, the second hand should be brought in low—toward the bird's feet. The upper hand should be held between the handler's face and the bird and may be used to distract the bird. The lower hand should quickly grasp the feet, trying to place the index finger between the bird's feet. The bird is then smoothly and quickly pulled up out of the cage or off the floor so that it does not beat its wings on any surfaces in the room. It is important to hold the bird away from objects, such as the examining table or cage. The bird can then be brought into a cradle position, the wings secured between the handler's arm and body, and hooded (Fig. 18–5). If hoods are not available, a towel may be draped over the bird's head; reducing visual and auditory stimuli will help to calm the bird significantly. An alternative approach to secure a bird of prey may be done with a towel or drape. Again, the handler approaches quietly and bent low, with the towel or drape spread in front with both hands. The handler moves in slowly until close enough to almost reach the bird, and then quickly—with the drape or towel used as a large glove—the bird is completely covered, with the handler's hands resting roughly on the bird's shoulders. It is important to avoid simply throwing the drape or towel, as the bird will be able to dodge it or move from under it. The bird is then pressed through the towel with enough pressure to make the bird push upward, using its legs on the ground. The technician's hands are then worked downward, alongside the wings, toward the legs, and the legs are grasped at the tarsometatarsus. Now, with the bird still on the ground, its body covered by the towel and its feet secured, the bird is lifted up to the handler's body with the back adjacent to the handler's abdomen. The towel over the head may then be replaced by a hood. It is important never to release the feet of a bird of prey until someone else has secured them. When examining a bird of prey, one should use 1-inch white cloth tape to secure the

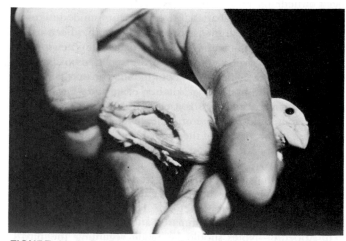

FIGURE 18–4. Proper technique for restraining a passerine for a physical exam.

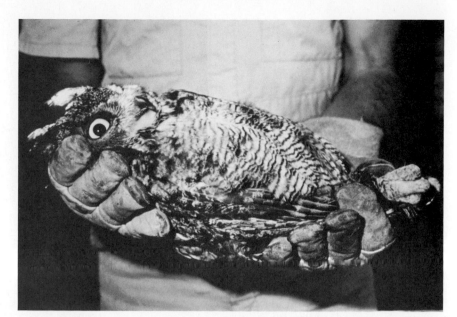

FIGURE 18–5. Restraint, using gloves, of a great-horned owl. Emphasis is on restraint of the talons.

talons. A 4- to 5-inch piece of tape wrapped around the closed foot will prevent accidents when these strong birds are being handled. If taloned, the legs must be fully extended before the talons can be removed. Birds of prey under the control of a falconer are a different story, since the falconer is often adept at restraining the bird for a physical examination (Fig. 18–6).

Sample Collection and Diagnostic Procedures Commonly Used in Birds

Diagnostic plans in avian species are no different from the clinical approach to other domestic pets. Evaluation of the

stool is an important first step. The technician should become familiar with normal stool in order to determine differences between polyuria (excessive urine output) and diarrhea (change in the fecal consistency and amount) (Fig. 18–7). Fecal parasites may be detected on fresh smears with saline and a cover slip. This is the best method to check for protozoa, such as *Giardia*. Fecal flotations will bring some parasite ova to the surface, such as ascarids and *Capillaria*. Fecal sedimentation is an important procedure for the diagnosis of flukes, which are common in imported cockatoos and raptors. Fecal specimens that are Gram-stained are useful to determine the bacterial flora of the digestive tract. Most cage bird species have predominantly gram-positive organisms inhabiting the digestive system. Fecal Gram stains are only a preliminary diagnostic test and should be followed up with bacterial culture.

Cloacal Swab. A cloacal swab is often done on psittacine species to determine the bacterial flora of the lower gastrointestinal (GI) tract. A cotton swab is moistened, inserted into the cloaca and gently rotated. Cloacal swabs are useful for cytological evaluations, looking for inflammatory cells, such as

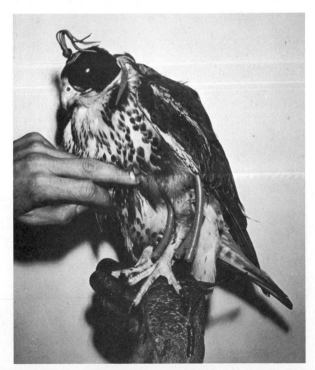

FIGURE 18–6. A falconer restrains a prairie falcon with hood and jesses for examination of an external fixator applied to a tibiotarsal fracture.

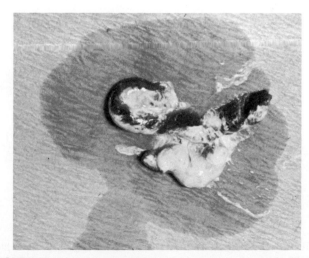

FIGURE 18–7. Normal psittacine stool. Note the dark solid feces, the white, solid urates and the liquid urine.

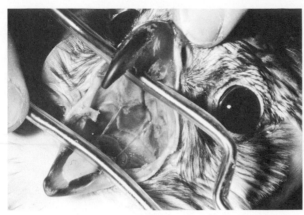

FIGURE 18–8. Oral examination demonstrating location of the glottis at the base of the tongue, and the choanal slit of the palates in a gyr falcon.

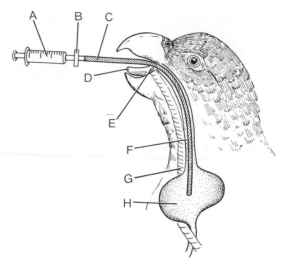

FIGURE 18–10. Proper tube placement for a crop wash or tube feeding a bird. The bird's neck should be gently stretched. A, Syringe; B, adapter if necessary; C, tube; D, tongue; E, tracheal opening; F, proximal esophagus; G, trachea; H, crop.

heterophils. They may also be used for culture and sensitivity tests and *Chlamydia* or viral isolation.

Oral Examination and Crop Wash. The technician should become adept at assisting in the performance of oral examination and crop wash by the veterinarian. Good restraint technique is essential. An avian beak speculum is placed in the bird's mouth parallel to the commissure and then rotated to open the mouth (Fig. 18–8). A choanal culture should be taken when birds are exhibiting upper respiratory signs. The culturette is placed in the rostral area of the choana to prevent cross contamination with the oral cavity (Fig. 18–9).

Another important diagnostic technique is the crop wash. The crop wash permits examination of the upper GI tract. A sterile or clean tube is passed through the mouth into the crop, or into the esophagus in those birds that do not have a crop. A syringe of sterile saline is connected to the tube, and a simple flush is performed (Fig. 18–10). Tubes may be made of plastic, rubber or metal, with a ball tip (Fig. 18–11). The crop wash is important for direct microscopic examination to check for protozoans, such as *Trichomonas* or yeast (*Candida albicans*), using a wet mount technique. Slides may be prepared for cytological examinations with Diff-Quick stains or Wright's stain, looking for inflammatory cells such as heterophils. A Gram stain is often done on crop wash samples from psittacine

species, or the sample may be submitted for culture and sensitivity (see Color Plate 1, Part I in Chapter 4). A culturette may be passed into a bird's crop for culture and sensitivity diagnostics. Care must be taken so that the patient does not bite the culturette and swallow it. Young psittacine species readily accept culturettes into the crop through normal feeding responses.

Passing a tube into the crop of the psittacine bird is an important technique to learn, because tube feeding is often necessary. The one rule of thumb to remember when using a tube for either feeding or a crop wash is to try to pick a tube with a diameter larger than the glottis. The glottis of the bird is located at the base of the tongue and is easy to visualize (Fig. 18–8). The tube may be passed into the crop easily by positioning the tube in the side of the bird's mouth (Fig. 18–8). The tube is easily palpated through the wall of the crop and the skin. While doing a crop wash or tube feeding, the handler should watch the back of the bird's mouth to ensure that food or water does not begin to accumulate. If the crop is overfilled, the bird may aspirate. If the crop overfills, put the bird down and let it attempt to clear its airway. The bird itself has a better

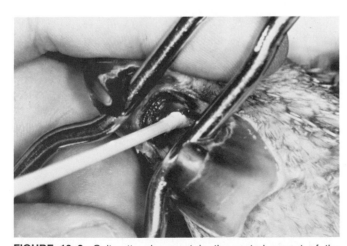

FIGURE 18–9. Culturette placement in the rostral aspect of the choana.

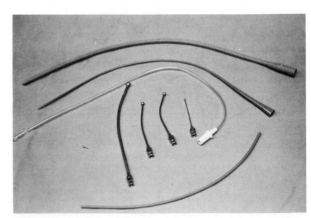

FIGURE 18–11. Various tubes used for tube feeding and crop washes.

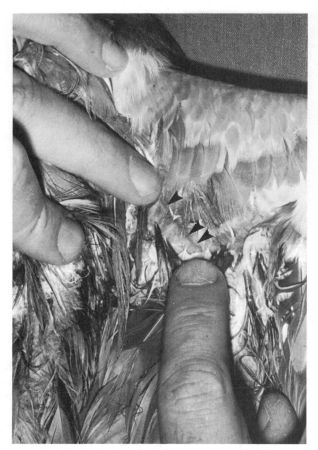

FIGURE 18–12. Location of the cutaneous ulnar vein (black arrows). Medial view with index finger on the elbow.

chance of clearing its airway than does the technician or veterinarian using Q-tips. Never handle a bird after placing oral medication into the crop or filling the crop unless the bird is experiencing respiratory difficulty.

Bloodwork. Bloodwork is an important part of the diagnostic examination in avian species. Venipuncture sites include the cutaneous ulnar vein, the right jugular vein, the medial metatarsal vein and toenail clipping. Each has its own advantages

and disadvantages, and the veterinarian and technician will tend to develop their own sites of preference, but the right jugular vein is the recommended site.

The right jugular vein is large and easily found in most birds on the right dorsolateral aspect of the neck. However, it is highly mobile and therefore difficult to immobilize. In most birds the right jugular vein is located in a featherless tract lateral to the trachea. With minimal practice and proper restraint, it becomes an easy procedure. An avian restraint board is recommended for blood collections from larger psittacine patients. Small psittacine and passerine patients can be hand-held when blood is being drawn for diagnostic tests.

In general, the cutaneous ulnar vein is accessible but difficult to completely immobilize in the psittacine patient, owing to the tremendous strength of the pectoral muscles (Fig. 18–12).

The medial metatarsal vein is easy to immobilize and secure, even on an awake and fractious patient. However, if large volumes of blood are to be collected, the medial metatarsal vein may not be a good choice (Fig. 18–13).

Toenail clipping is available but is painful to the patient and often causes limping for several days following the procedure. It may result in a poor blood flow, low yield and invalid results.

The blood may be collected in syringes, microhematocrit tubes or blood collection tubes from the hub of the needle. A 3-cc syringe with a 26-gauge needle should be used in most avian patients. In extremely small psittacine and passerine patients a 1-cc syringe with a 30-gauge needle may be utilized. The technician should learn to proficiently perform a complete blood count (CBC) on avian blood.

Radiography. Radiography is an important diagnostic tool in avian patients. Typically, lateral and ventrodorsal views of the whole body or selected extremities may be taken (Fig. 18–14). Technique charts must be developed based on the equipment available. Contrast films may be made with standard contrast agents, including barium sulfate. Because good positioning and absence of motion are important to high-quality radiographs, it is generally recommended that all avian patients be sedated or anesthetized, except those who may be too ill (Fig. 18–15). Proper positioning is important and an avian restraint board is essential. Other diagnostic procedures, such as laparoscopy, endoscopy, tracheal or air sac washes, biopsies and

FIGURE 18–13. IV injection using the medial metatarsal vein of an Amazon parrot just above the hock joint.

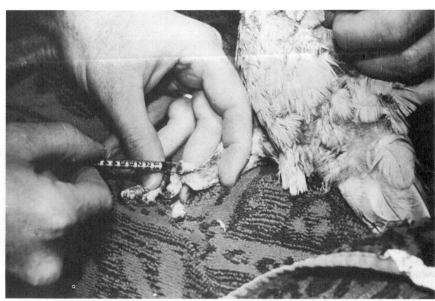

Sample Collection and Diagnostic Procedures

Diagnostic approaches in reptiles are often similar to those of other small animal species.

Colonic Wash. Fecal samples may be collected and examined for GI parasites. A fresh sample should be examined under a wet mount, and fecal flotation and sedimentation should also be done. If a fecal sample is not available at the time of the examination, specimens may be collected by performing a colonic wash. This is done by passing a lubricated tube or catheter through the cloaca into the colon. A syringe of sterile saline is attached, and a typical flush is performed (Fig. 18–22). Samples may then be examined for parasites or parasite eggs or prepared for cytology or culture and sensitivity tests.

Stomach Wash. To examine the upper GI tract, a stomach wash is often performed. This procedure is well tolerated by most reptiles and is a quick and easy procedure in the clinic. A soft rubber catheter is advanced through the mouth into the stomach. A syringe containing sterile isotonic saline is attached to the catheter, and a simple flush is performed (see Fig. 18–19). Samples obtained are used for direct microscopic examination for parasites, to prepare slides for cytology, or to perform Gram's stains or culture and sensitivities.

Urine Samples. Urine samples may be collected from those species that produce a large volume of urine. Many turtles and lizards have urinary bladders. All reptiles have a cloaca into which the reproductive, GI and urinary tracts empty. A routine urinalysis (UA) may be performed on fresh urine samples. A cystocentesis may be performed on turtles, advancing a needle cranial to the hind limb. Turtles will typically void when stressed, thus simply handling them may yield a urine sample.

Blood Samples. Blood collection in reptiles varies considerably, depending on the species. Venipuncture techniques in snakes depend on the experience of the handler. Sites that are often used include the caudal or coccygeal vein of the tail, cardiac puncture, the ventral abdominal vein or palatine vessels. For any site, good restraint is necessary. For lizards, the caudal tail vein is often the most accessible; however, cardiac puncture, the ventral abdominal vein and a toenail clip may also be used (Figs. 18–23 and 18–24). In turtles, large jugular veins are present and are easily used for venipuncture sites (Fig. 18–25). Additionally, toenails may be clipped, or blood may be drawn from the occipital sinus. In large crocodilians, the occipital sinus or the caudal vein of the tail may be used. The site chosen will depend on the veterinarian and the technician and their experience with that species.

Radiography. Radiography is often useful to aid in the diagnosis of reptile patients. For many species, radiographs may be taken on unsedated animals by restraining them in shallow boxes, in acrylic tubes or in canvas bags. It is important to remember to take at least two views. With turtles, a third view—a frontal view—should also be taken. Contrast studies may be done, and barium sulfate is easily administered. However, GI transit times are long, and it may take a week to complete a GI barium study. Various other diagnostic procedures may be used, according to the preference of the veterinarian. The technician's knowledge of restraint techniques and reptile behavior will aid in any immobilization process.

Husbandry in the Hospital. Reptiles are easily provided for in a hospital setting. It is important to remember that tempera-

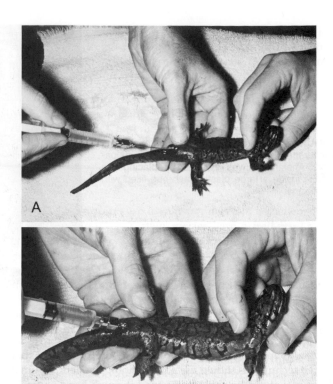

FIGURE 18–22. Colonic wash in a tiger salamander using A, a metal ball-tipped gauge needle and B, a syringe of warm, sterile saline.

ture and humidity are important, since these animals are poikilothermic—dependent upon their environment to regulate their body temperature. A temperature *gradient* should be provided whenever possible, with a thermostat at each end of the cage resulting in a cooler and a warmer end. For most species, temperatures should not exceed 32°C (90°F) nor dip below 24°C (75°F). For many species, a variety of aquaria are sufficient for short-term hospitalization. Any substrate used should be one that is easily cleaned and disinfected or disposable, such as newspaper or artificial turf. It is important to house reptiles separately from psittacine birds, in particular, to avoid contamination of birds from the normal gram-negative flora of most reptiles. Cages should be provided with hide boxes or areas of seclusion, as well as perching for some species such as iguanas and some snakes.

Tube feeding is an important technique for the veterinary technician to become adept at when handling reptiles. Tube feeding is easily accomplished, even by those without much experience with reptiles. A tube of a diameter larger than the diameter of the glottis should be chosen, well lubricated and then passed the distance necessary to place it in the stomach. The glottis of reptiles is adjacent to the base of the tongue and is easily avoided. The glottis of snakes may actually be extended by the animal outside the mouth to accommodate large prey items. The tube is gently passed all the way to the stomach and food injected. Fluids may also be administered by this route. For carnivorous species that are anorectic, supplemental tube feeding may be accomplished by using a blended formula of a high-quality cat food. For species such as herbivorous iguanas,

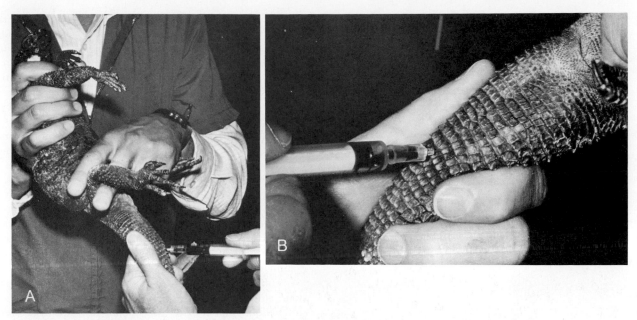

FIGURE 18–23. A and B, Restraint of a giant chuckwalla for venipuncture using the tail vein.

a soy-based dog food or monkey chow may be blended and used.

Injections in reptiles are usually performed on the cranial half of the animal's body. This is due to the renal portal system that routes blood from the caudal third of the body through a capillary network into the kidneys before returning it to general circulation. It is important to remember not to give nephrotoxic drugs in the caudal third of the reptile's body. Injection sites are easily found in all reptile species, either in the forelimbs or in the epaxial musculature of the snake. Oral medications are easily given by using a stomach tube. Once again, liquids are preferred over tablets, which are not consistently absorbed.

Dietary requirements vary tremendously from species to species and may be an important factor in disease of the patient. Dietary deficiencies are not commonly seen in snakes, which eat a whole-animal diet. However, a variety of dietary deficiencies are commonly seen in lizards, turtles and crocodilians. One of the most common is metabolic bone disease. Metabolic bone disease is caused by inappropriately low calcium intake, low vitamin D_3 intake or excessive phosphorus intake (Fig. 18–26). This may be prevented by suitable diets and exposing the animal to ultraviolet light, either naturally or artificially. It is essential that reptiles, especially lizards, have full-spectrum light available during normal daylight hours. Sunlight through glass is insufficient in preventing nutritional deficiencies. The animal with metabolic bone disease must be treated very gently, as the bones are subject to pathological fractures. Vitamin A deficiency is commonly seen in turtles and tortoises and usually manifests itself by overgrown beak, palpebral edema and conjunctivitis. This underscores the importance of researching the dietary history of the reptile patient thoroughly.

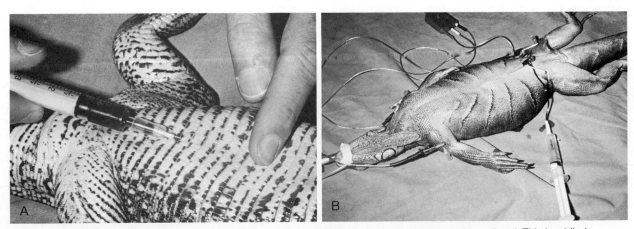

FIGURE 18–24. A, Venipuncture from the ventral abdominal vein from an anesthetized tegu lizard. This is a blind technique. B, IV catheter placed in ventral abdominal vein and ECG lead placement in an anesthetized common iguana.

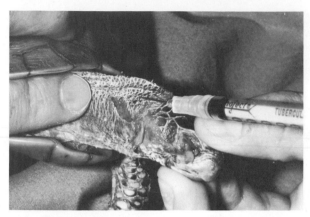

FIGURE 18–25. Jugular venipuncture in a box turtle. The jugular veins are located dorsally in the 10 and 2 o'clock positions.

Zoonoses and Common Clinical Problems

The technician should be aware of some common zoonotic infections and clinical problems.

Most reptiles carry a variety of gram-negative enteric bacteria. This may include such species as *Salmonella* species, *Arizona* species, *Klebsiella* species and *Providentia* species. Many of these may cause infection in people as well as in other animals. It is therefore important to keep the reptile separate and to maintain a high standard of sanitation when working with these animals.

Bites from reptiles should be treated as potentially severe infections. Wounds should be thoroughly scrubbed out, and medical attention should be sought.

FERRETS

Ferrets have been gaining in popularity over the past decade. Elective surgery (ovarohysterectomies and neutering) is common in these animals. As ferrets are seen with increasing frequency in veterinarians' offices, it is imperative that technicians become familiar with these pets.

Restraining a ferret is sometimes difficult. Ferrets belong to the family group that includes weasels, and as such, are quick,

agile animals and possess a sharp set of teeth. The ferret's primary weapons are its teeth, and when threatened, it will not hesitate to bite. Ferrets that are hand raised with lots of human contact, however, do make docile pets in the right circumstances. As with all animals in the veterinary clinic, proper precautions should be taken when restraining ferrets.

Primary restraint for a ferret is to secure the head and forelegs by gripping the animal with one hand behind the neck and around the shoulders (Fig. 18–27). The other hand is used to support the bottom of the animal. For the highly aggressive ferret, a towel or drape may be placed over the animal to occlude its vision and the animal's head, neck and shoulders grasped through the drape or towel. The handler may want to use gloves. Remember, it is not good for any pet animal to associate negative experiences with gloved hands. Once the animal is restrained in this method, the handler may alter the grip on the head to perform a thorough physical examination and other diagnostic techniques.

For obtaining sample collections of blood, physical restraint alone is not often adequate. Blood samples are drawn from either the jugular vein or the cephalic vein. To draw samples of blood from either of these sites, the animal's head must be securely restrained and grasped around the neck with thumb and fingers resting on the mandibles. To position an animal for jugular venipuncture, it is often best to stretch the animal out, using the other hand grasping the hind limbs. The ferret's thick skin and subcutaneous fat make blood collection from the jugular vein difficult. To draw adequate blood samples,

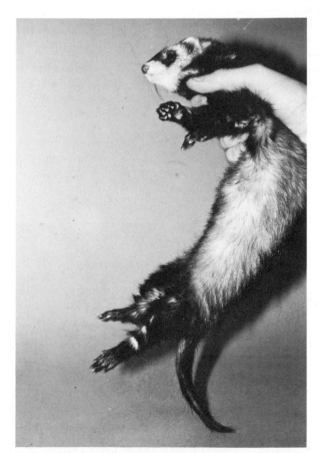

FIGURE 18–27. Proper restraint of a ferret securing the head and forelegs. The other hand should be placed beneath to support the bottom of the animal.

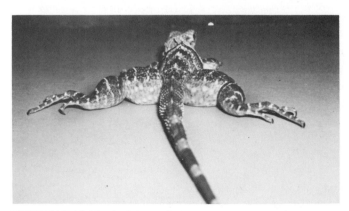

FIGURE 18–26. Metabolic bone disease in a lizard due to an improper diet.

however, anesthesia or sedation is commonly employed (Fig. 18–28). Ketamine hydrochloride or gas anesthetic agents such as halothane or isoflurane may be used. When using gas anesthetics in ferrets, it is easiest to place them in an induction chamber, such as a Plexiglas box, to which the anesthetic machine is then attached. The animal may be removed from this chamber as soon as it loses the ability to right itself. Anesthesia may then be continued with the use of a face mask. Sample collection on the anesthetized animal is much easier and less stressful to the animal. Urine may be obtained by cystocentesis since the bladder is easily palpated. If desired, for prolonged anesthesia, ferrets are easily intubated with small standard endotracheal tubes or Cole tubes.

Strategies for treating ferrets in the clinic revolve around the handler's ability to restrain the animal and perform the treatment in the most efficient and quickest manner possible. For giving drugs, dairy products and sweets are useful in bribing animals and in hiding medications. Most ferrets will do almost anything for yogurt or ice cream. Liquid medications are much easier to administer than pills.

A potentially fatal common clinical problem of the ferret is estrogen toxicity in females due to prolonged estrus. Female ferrets are induced ovulators and occasionally will not cycle out of heat unless bred. These animals then become severely anemic and thrombocytopenic owing to the toxic effects of estrogen on the bone marrow. Ferrets often present with signs of lethargy, dyspnea, petechial hemorrhages, vomiting and diarrhea. This is best treated by prevention and client education. Female ferrets not intended for breeding should be spayed. Ferrets are susceptible to human influenza, and therefore clients should be counseled that when members of the family have influenza the ferret should not be handled. Human influenza in a ferret must be differentiated from canine distemper and bacterial pneumonia, to which ferrets are also susceptible. Both present with similar signs of respiratory disease: nasal and ocular discharges, coughing and sneezing. The ferret with influenza will, in most cases, get over the infection on its own in 5 to 10 days. Topical antihistamines and decongestants may be of benefit. The nonvaccinated ferret will not survive a canine distemper infection, and signs usually progress to severe dyspnea, anorexia and sometimes involvement of the central nervous system.

Ferrets are also fond of chewing on things, preferably soft rubbery objects, and, as such, should be watched closely for foreign body ingestion. A ferret that presents with signs of anorexia should be considered as having a potential GI obstruction. There are also many reports of various neoplastic diseases in ferrets, including insulinomas, osteomas, lymphosarcomas and fibrosarcomas. If a ferret presents depressed or moribund, a blood serum glucose should be taken.

Ferrets should be vaccinated for canine distemper with a chick embryo cell line product. Under no circumstances should a canine distemper vaccine of ferret cell origin be used. The animal should be revaccinated according to the schedule employed for dogs. Ferrets are not susceptible to feline panleukopenia and therefore need not be vaccinated. Other preventive medicine measures regarding ferrets include good dental care and surveillance for GI parasites. Ferrets are strict carnivores and, as such, should be fed a strict carnivore diet. Purina Company does make a ferret chow. If this is not available, a high quality cat food may be used. Although this may be slightly low in protein requirements for the pregnant or lactating ferret, few problems have been reported in ferrets on high-quality cat food diets.

The zoonotic disease of primary importance in ferrets is rabies. Although ferrets are potential carriers, their indoor lifestyle makes exposure very unlikely. Only one case of a rabid ferret's biting a human has been documented, and this was an animal that had escaped from its owner. There is a rabies vaccine, currently available, approved for ferrets. Ferrets should be vaccinated for rabies, using only the ferret-approved vaccine.

RABBITS

The rabbit is not a rodent, but a lagomorph of the family Leporidae. Rabbits may be housed indoors or outdoors and may be fed one of many commercial pelleted feeds. Rabbits come in many sizes, ranging from the Flemish Giant, 6 to 7.5 kg, to the Dutch and Polish breeds, 1 to 2 kg. If proper husbandry practices are maintained, a pet rabbit should live a long, healthy life (5 to 6 years). Rabbits are sensitive to extreme hot and cold conditions.

Rabbit restraint is important (Fig. 18–29). The most common cause of spinal fracture or dislocation is improper restraint. A rabbit should *never* be picked up, carried or restrained by the ears. To carry a rabbit short distances, grasp the nape skin with one hand while supporting the rear legs with the other (Fig. 18–30). When walking long distances the handler should conceal the head in the bend of the elbow while supporting the body with the forearm and grasping the flank with the opposite hand (Fig. 18–31). Small plastic pet carriers should be used when carrying rabbits long distances.

Rabbits defend themselves by using their long incisors to bite and by kicking with the hind legs. To sex the rabbit, stretching the perineum while the animal is in dorsal recumbency will reveal the anogenital area. Males have a round urethral opening; females have a slit opening.

The rabbit that is a candidate for anesthesia should have food withheld for 8 to 12 hours and be free from respiratory disease. Some strains of rabbits have atropinesterase, which inactivates atropine. Atropine may be given subcutaneously as a preanesthetic to decrease salivation. If a rabbit has atropinesterase, it may be necessary to increase the dose of atropine.

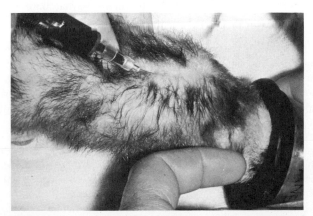

FIGURE 18–28. Jugular venipuncture of an anesthetized ferret with its head in an anesthetic mask to the right.

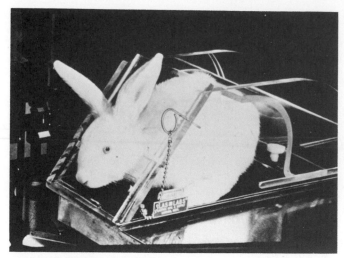

FIGURE 18–29. Rabbit in special restraint box.

Rabbits are seldom intubated during anesthesia because they rarely regurgitate and are difficult to intubate. Recommended endotracheal tubes in rabbits have inside diameters of 2.0 to 4.0 mm. A medium laryngoscope will aid in passing the tube into the rabbit's glottis to near the thoracic inlet. Do not use topical anesthetic in rabbits to prevent laryngospasm.

Injectable anesthetic agents used in rabbits include ketamine, xylazine, and acepromazine; isoflurane is the inhalation anesthetic of choice. The movement of the nictitating membrane over approximately one third of the cornea, a respiratory rate of 18 to 24 respirations per minute, abdominal musculature relaxation and the loss of the ear, mouth, toe pinch and palpebral reflexes indicate a suitable plane of surgical anesthesia in the rabbit.

By placing a rabbit in dorsal recumbency and gently stroking its ventrum, one causes hypnosis to occur. Hypnosis is a good restraint for injections and radiographic procedures.

To give intravenous injections to rabbits, the dorsal surface of the ear should be shaved to expose the marginal ear vein. Visibility of this vein will increase if alcohol is rubbed on the area. The marginal ear vein or central artery can also be used for bleeding. Cardiac puncture for blood collection should be used only under strict professional supervision and only as a last resort in the clinical setting.

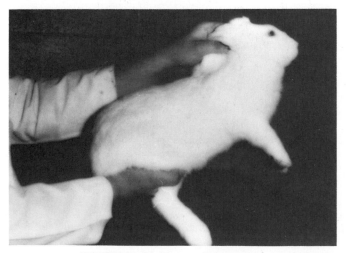

FIGURE 18–30. Proper rabbit restraint.

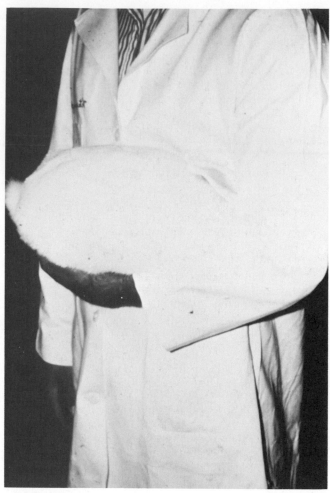

FIGURE 18–31. Technique for carrying a rabbit over short distances.

Rabbits are affected by a number of infectious and parasitic organisms. A pet rabbit may be presented for hair loss due to self-trauma, nutritional deficiencies, bacterial dermatitis (*Pasteurella multocida*, *Pseudomonas aeruginosa*, *Staphylococcus aureus* and *Fusobacterium*) or parasites (ear mite *Psoroptes cuniculi* [Figs. 18–32 and 18–33], fur mite *Cheyletiella parasitovorax* and rabbit lice *Haemodipsus ventricosus*). Ulcerative lesions on the ventral surface of the rear hocks is usually due to poor husbandry or environmental pressures. Fungal organisms that have been noted to cause dermatopathies in rabbits are *Microsporum gypseum* and *Trichophyton mentagrophytes*.

An anorexic pet should be examined for malocclusion, hair balls, trauma, dietary change, stress or poor feed. Heat stress (stroke) is common when adequate cooling is not provided in the summer. Diarrhea may be caused by colibacillosis, rotavirus infections, *Clostridium* infections, mucoid enteropathy, antibiotic intake and Tyzzer's disease (*Bacillus piliformis*).

One of the main disease problems in rabbits is *Pasteurella multocida* infection (snuffles). Clinical signs include nasal discharge, torticollis, abscesses, conjunctivitis and respiratory distress. Venereal spirochetosis should always be considered when rabbits are exhibiting infertility. *Eimeria steadia* is a hepatic coccidium that may affect attitude and eating habits.

Rabbits are territorial and fight when sexual maturity is reached or a male is placed in a female's cage for breeding.

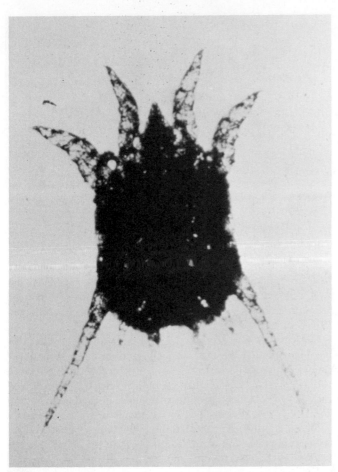

FIGURE 18–32. Microscopic view of *Psoroptes cuniculi,* the rabbit ear mite.

Neutering or ovariohysterectomy is recommended to prevent unwanted offspring.

RODENTS

Rodent species commonly presented to the veterinary hospital include guinea pigs, hamsters, gerbils and, to a lesser extent, mice and rats. Although all of the animals listed above are rodents, each species has particular anatomical characteristics, dietary requirements and diseases.

Antibiotics in Rodents

Care must be taken when prescribing antibiotics to rodents. Guinea pigs, rabbits and hamsters are extremely sensitive to penicillin antibiotics, which may cause severe intestinal flora changes. Penicillins, streptomycin and dihydrostreptomycin are drugs that may cause this problem. Tetracyclines work well in cases that require antibiotic therapy.

Anesthetics in Rodents

Ketamine HCl, pentobarbital sodium and thiamylal sodium are injectable anesthetics that may be used in rodents. Isoflur-

ane is an acceptable gas anesthetic that provides quick induction and recovery while providing an adequate plane of anesthesia. Chapter 11 discusses anesthesiology.

Antiparasitic Agents in Rodents

Carbaryl powder, dichlorvos and ivermectin can be used safely to treat ectoparasites. Dichlorvos, thiabendazole and ivermectin are adequate to treat internal parasites. See Chapter 5 for additional information on parasitology.

Guinea Pig

The cavy or guinea pig is a rodent related to porcupines and chinchillas. Guinea pigs have a long gestation that leads to the birth of large precocious young.

The most common guinea pig species kept as pets are the English or American, Abyssinian and Peruvian long hair (Figs. 18–34 and 18–35).

The guinea pig has open-rooted teeth that may become maloccluded. The overgrown teeth will irritate the gingiva, causing excessive salivation (Fig. 18–36).

Although the female has only two vaginal mammary glands, it can successfully raise litters of three or more offspring.

A female that is bred past 7 or 8 months of age may have trouble separating the pubic symphysis. Fat pads may also occlude the pelvic canal, complicating parturition. These problems usually lead to dystocia and/or death. If the sow is experiencing dystocia, a cesarean retrieval of the young often yields excellent results. Food preferences are established within a few days following birth for the young. Hand-rearing of the young requires regular stimulation of defecation and urination as with most neonatal mammals. Females usually allow foster nursing of other young.

The pet cavy should be lifted with one hand supporting the dorsal thorax region and one hand under the hind quarters (Fig. 18–37). They rarely become excited or bite. Through their gentle nature, guinea pigs become conditioned to their surroundings and may have an adverse response to change. If

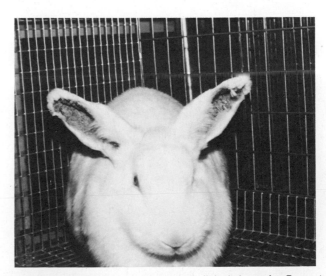

FIGURE 18–33. Rabbit exhibiting typical clinical signs of a *Psoroptes cuniculi* infestation.

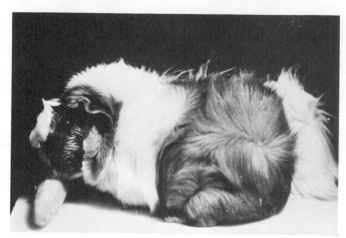

FIGURE 18–34. An Abyssinian guinea pig.

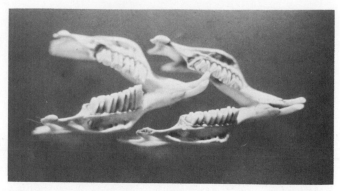

FIGURE 18–36. Examples of elongated premolars and molars in a maloccluded guinea pig.

a group is contained in an enclosure, subordinate animals may be traumatized (as by hair loss and bite wounds).

Foot pad dermatitis ulcers may develop on animals placed on wire. Metal, plastic and glass make excellent habit cages. Substrate may be paper (shredded), wood shavings or hay. Chewing their substrate is a vice commonly associated with an animal developing submandibular abscesses (Fig. 18–38). Hard fibrous splinters penetrate the oral mucosa, inoculating the tissue with bacteria (usually *Streptococcus zooepidemicus*) that develop into abscesses. Changes in the substrate may be indicated to stop this problem, although it may be difficult to find an adequate alternative substrate, which must have absorptive qualities for the opaque, pale yellow crystalline urine.

The feed and water are best placed in bowls that cannot be chewed (such as stainless steel and ceramic crocks). A vitamin C supplementation may be added to the water, such as Tang (General Foods Corp., White Plains, NY). The food should be a freshly milled complete guinea pig ration. Storage in a freezer or refrigerator will extend the life of the food. All food and water containers should be placed above the substrate to prevent soiling.

Unlike other pet rodents, guinea pigs require dietary vita-min C supplementation. Vitamin C is highly unstable in the feed, especially when exposed to heat. Old feed is one of the primary reasons that vitamin C deficiencies are seen (Fig. 18–39).

The cavy require 0.5 mg/kg body weight dietary ascorbic acid per day because they lack L-gulonolactone oxidase. Guinea pigs *must* be fed species-specific food within 90 days of milling. Fruit and vegetable supplementation is discouraged because of the possibility of disturbing the normal gut bacterial flora.

To sex a guinea pig, the handler must observe the urethral orifice and anus. The male has no break in the ridge between the openings, whereas the female has a shallow U-shaped break.

One boar will service up to 10 sows beginning at 8 weeks of age. The sow becomes sexually mature around 5 to 6 weeks of age.

Gestation length is on the average 63 to 68 days, with litter size ranging from one to six precocious offspring.

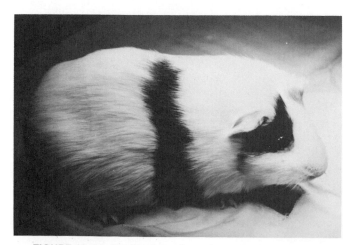

FIGURE 18–35. The English guinea pig, a common house pet.

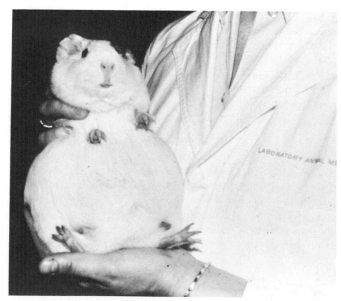

FIGURE 18–37. Proper restraint technique for a guinea pig.

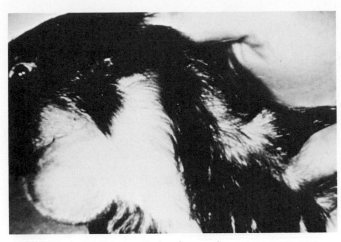

FIGURE 18–38. Submandibular abscess (lumps) in a guinea pig.

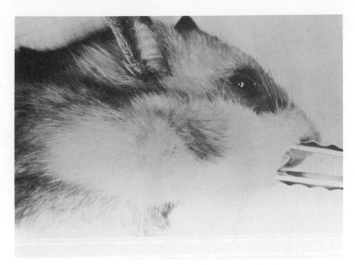

FIGURE 18–40. Hamster cheek pouches extend to the scapula.

Hamster

The golden hamster is a native of Syria and comes in many different color varieties. Check pouches that extend along the head and neck to the proximal dorsum of the back serve as a food transportation device (Fig. 18–40). Along the caudal lateral abdominal region lie the flank glands. A dark brown patch of skin on each side delineates these sebaceous glands that are used to mark territory and in mating rituals.

Hamsters have a tendency to bite and are good at chewing through cage material. To accommodate the animal's physical nature, an exercise wheel should be placed in the cage.

Female hamsters often attack newly introduced males and females. Hamsters live, on the average, 18 to 24 months, with a gestation length of 16 days and offspring averaging five that wean in 20 to 25 days. If disturbed, the female may cannibalize her litter or hide them in her cheek pouches. When the young are hidden in the cheek pouches, they may suffocate. Hamsters can be picked up by the nape skin at the base of the neck or by cupping the hands under the hind limbs.

There are a number of commercially available hamster habitats. An aquarium with a mesh top may be used to house a hamster, with hardwood shavings being the choice substrate. Aromatic shavings such as cedar or pine may cause ocular and respiratory irritation. Sipper bottles are perfect for water dispensing, and nonchewable bowls should be used for food containers or the food should be placed on the floor. All food and water access should be made available to the young.

Males have a greater anogenital distance than females. Hamsters may be mated monogamously or in a harem situation. Females with young should not be disturbed to prevent cannibalism and abandonment of the litter.

Wet tail is used as a general term to describe diarrhea in the hamster. Bacterial infections, cestodiasis and antibiotic administration may also cause diarrhea in these rodents.

Zoonotic Diseases. Lymphocytic choriomeningitis, salmonellosis and hymenolepid tapeworm infections are diseases that may be transferred from hamsters to man. Proper hygiene should be practiced after one has handled these animals.

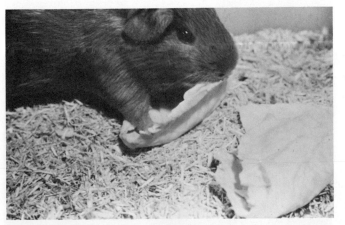

FIGURE 18–39. Vitamin C dietary supplementation is critical for maintaining excellent health.

Gerbil

The Mongolian gerbil is a popular pet native to Mongolia and Northeastern China. It is an active burrowing animal adapted to desert environments. Gerbils have a midventral pad consisting of sebaceous glands used in territorial marking.

The gerbil has a life-span of 3.5 years, with a gestation length of 25 days without lactation and 24 to 48 days with lactation. The litter sizes average five that wean in approximately 25 days (Fig. 18–41). Certain gerbil lines are prone to epileptiform seizure activity. Gerbils are friendly rodents that may be housed in hamster units (Fig. 18–42). These animals are good in escape methods; therefore, the cage should be designed to prevent chewing.

The gerbil's diet may be similar to that of the hamster, and water can be supplied in a sipper bottle. Sexing is accomplished by measuring the urogenital distance. The male has a much longer distance than the female. Males aid in the care of the young.

Gerbils commonly present with a nasal dermatitis caused by

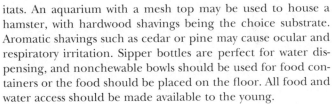

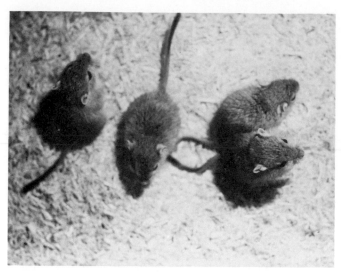

FIGURE 18–41. Young gerbils.

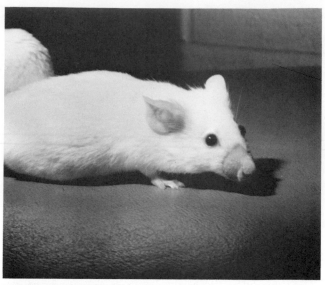

FIGURE 18–43. Trauma (cage mate inflicted hair loss) on a mouse. This is commonly referred to as barbering.

a bacterial infection initiated by their burrowing activity. Topical antibiotic treatment is recommended for resolution of this infection.

Tyzzer's disease may be diagnosed in gerbils and is caused by *Bacillus piliformis.* Dietary change and colibacillosis also cause diarrhea in these animals.

Mouse

Mice are small rodents that are commonly used in the research setting, but make excellent small pets. They are territorial animals and quickly develop a hierarchy when placed in groups (Fig. 18–43). These small animals require small amounts of food and water, but are escape-prone and may develop an unpleasant odor.

Mice should be handled by grabbing the tail with one hand and the back of the neck with the other. Do not use excessive force when grabbing the tail because the skin may be damaged.

Housing should be similar to that of gerbils and hamsters.

Hardwood shavings or chips are recommended instead of the aromatic softwood chips (cedar and pine) because of potential liver damage and epithelial damage.

Housing should be cleaned regularly to prevent odor and health problems. Pelleted rodent feed and fresh water in sipper bottles should be supplied free choice.

Male mice have a greater urogenital distance than females. Female mice become sexually mature at 50 days of age and are best bred in the harem scheme, with one male combined with two to six females.

Rat

Rats are clean and unassuming and can be trained to be good pets. These animals may live up to 3 years or longer and become sexually mature at $1\frac{1}{2}$ to 2 months of age.

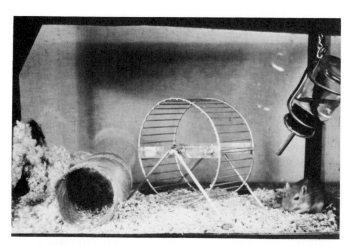

FIGURE 18–42. Typical small rodent cage containing gerbils.

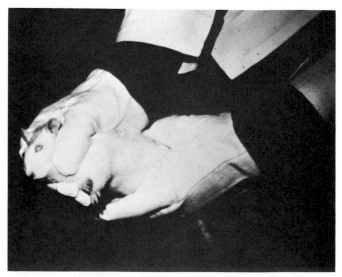

FIGURE 18–44. Proper restraint of a rat.

Restraint is best performed by grabbing the base of the tail and grabbing the animal behind the forelimbs (Fig. 18–44). Rats seldom bite, but caution must be used in a stressful situation.

Commercial rodent cages can be obtained for proper housing. Substrate should be similar to that of other rodents.

Males have a longer anogenital distance than females. The gestation length is 22 days, and nesting material should be provided prior to birth.

Although zoonotic diseases are rare in domestic rats, these animals can carry many diseases transmissible to man. These diseases include rat bite fever, *Yersinia pestis*, leptospirosis, *Streptococcus* sp., cestodiasis and Korean hemorrhagic fever.

Reference

Wise JK and Yang JJ: Veterinary service market for companion animals. JAVMA 201:990–992, 1992.

Recommended Reading

Campbell TW: Avian Hematology and Cytology. Ames, IA, Iowa State University Press, 1988.

Fox JG: Biology and Diseases of the Ferret. Philadelphia, Lea & Febiger, 1988.

Frey FL: Biomedical and Surgical Aspects of Captive Reptile Husbandry. Vols. I and II. Malabar, FL, Krieger Publishing Co., 1991.

Fudge AM (editor): Seminars in Avian and Exotic Pet Medicine. Philadelphia, WB Saunders Co. (Published Quarterly)

Harkness JE and Wagner JE: The Biology and Medicine of Rabbits and Rodents. Philadelphia, PA, Lea & Febiger, 1989.

Harrison G and Harrison L: Clinical Avian Medicine and Surgery. Philadelphia, WB Saunders Co., 1986.

Holmes DD: Clinical Laboratory Animal Medicine. Ames, IA, Iowa State University Press, 1984.

Jacobson ER and Kollias GV Jr. (eds): Exotic Animals: Contemporary Issues in Small Animal Practice. New York, Churchill Livingstone, 1988.

Journal of the Association of Avian Veterinarians. Association of Avian Veterinarians, Lake Worth, FL. (Published Quarterly)

Journal of Small Exotic Animal Medicine. Valley Village, CA, Gray Publishing. (Published Quarterly)

Journal of Zoo and Wildlife Medicine. American Association of Zoo Veterinarians, Lawrence, KS. (Published Monthly)

Mattison C. The Care of Reptiles and Amphibians in Captivity. New York, Sterling Publishing Co., Inc., US Distributors, 1990.

McCelland J: A Color Atlas of Avian Anatomy. Philadelphia, WB Saunders Co., 1991.

Orosz SE, Ensley PK and Haynes CJ: Avian Surgical Anatomy of Thoracic and Pelvic Limbs. Philadelphia, WB Saunders Co., 1992.

Rosskoph W and Woerpel R (editors): Small Animal Practice: Pet Avian Medicine. Vet Clin North Am 21:6, 1991.

19

Veterinary Oncology

MAURA G. O'BRIEN, KRISTA DICKINSON
and STEPHEN J. WITHROW

The treatment of cancer in pet animals has become an important field in veterinary medicine. As the quality of pet care has improved over recent years, dogs and cats are living extended lives, and there has been an associated rise in the prevalence of cancer in these animals. Clients have become increasingly aware of the health care needs of their pets and often seek veterinary care for preventative medicine or in the early stages of the disease. It is no longer acceptable practice to disregard seemingly benign lumps and bumps and hope they are not cancer. The four most dangerous words in veterinary oncology are, "Let's just watch it."

In response to the needs of an educated and dedicated clientele that seek improved health care for their pet, training programs have become established in the discipline of oncology. Trained veterinarians are providing expertise in university referral centers as well as private practice. Significant advances have been achieved by studying tumor behavior and response to treatment in spontaneously occurring tumors in animals. The contributions to both human and animal health that can be made in cancer therapy in animals are countless and can be rewarding to the veterinarians and technicians participating in these clinical research programs.

The recognition of the importance of the human animal bond has also become apparent in veterinary medicine. The emotional aspect of treating cancer in animals cannot be ignored. Many clients have had past experience with cancer, either in themselves or in family members or friends. Such experience makes these clients sensitized to the cancer affecting their pet. The veterinarian and technicians treating the cancer patient must be compassionate and recognize the emotional needs of the client as well as provide quality medical care to the animal.

As part of the veterinary health care team, the veterinary technician's role in providing appropriate case management, quality patient care and client support is vital. Knowledge of the basic principles of oncology will help the technician to understand the diagnostic and therapeutic approach to cancer therapy and to become an active participant in the treatment of the cancer patient.

ONCOLOGY

Oncology is the study of cancer. In general, cancer is defined as an uncontrolled growth of cells on or within the body. This growth can cause clinical signs due to the (1) destruction of local tissue, (2) pain, inflammation, infection or impairment of function of an organ secondary to the cancer, or (3) paraneoplastic syndromes associated with the cancer. Paraneoplastic syndromes are conditions that occur distant to the tumor itself, usually as a result of the various substances produced by the tumor (Table 19–1). Cancer is therefore not a single disease, but a collection of hundreds of diseases that can affect

Table 19–1
EXAMPLES OF PARANEOPLASTIC SYNDROMES AND ASSOCIATED TUMORS

Hypoglycemia
  Hepatocellular carcinoma
  Hepatoma
  Islet cell carcinoma
  Lymphoma
  Hemangiosarcoma
  Leiomyosarcoma
  Oral melanoma
Hypercalcemia
  Lymphoma
  Anal sac apocrine gland
    adenocarcinoma
  Parathyroid tumors
  Thymoma
  Mammary adenocarcinoma
  Multiple myeloma
Disseminated intravascular
  coagulopathy
  Hemangiosarcoma
  Thyroid carcinoma
  Others
Cancer cachexia
  Multiple tumors

Leukopenia
  Lymphoma
  Multiple myeloma
Anemia
  Multiple tumors
Hyperproteinemia
  Multiple myeloma
  Lymphoma
Thrombocytopenia
  Lymphoma
  Hemangiosarcoma
  Fibrosarcoma
  Mammary adenocarcinoma
  Nasal carcinoma
Leukocytosis
  Lymphoma
  Multiple tumors
Gastric ulcers
  Mast cell tumors

Adapted from Ogilvie GK: Paraneoplastic syndromes. *In* Withrow SJ and MacEwen EG (editors): Clinical Veterinary Oncology. Philadelphia, JB Lippincott, 1989, p 30.

---

ferent prognosis. It is also important to realize that the incidence and behavior of cancer in dogs versus cats is often quite different.

Additional methods to further classify tumors and to help in predicting the behavior of a tumor and the prognosis include the tumor's *grade* and *stage*. Established grading systems categorize tumors of the same histopathological type according to shared histological features. The cells in the tumor of one grade may have well-defined cellular architecture (well-differentiated), with few mitotic figures in the nuclei (slow cell division), and exhibit minimal invasion of surrounding normal tissues. The cells in a similar tumor with a different grade may have poorly defined cell architecture (undifferentiated), exhibit numerous mitotic figures (rapid cell division) and appear to invade normal tissues. Unfortunately, most of these systems have been adapted from human pathology and do not always accurately represent the behavior of similar tumors in animals.

Tumors are staged according to their physical characteristics and the extent of tumor present. The World Health Organization's staging system is known as the TNM system and categorizes tumors according to the presence of tumor at the primary site (T), whether there is involvement of regional lymph nodes (N) and whether tumor is present as metastases at distant sites (M). Further divisions, represented as numbers following the T, N, or M, describe the size and extent of the tumor and evidence of any clinical signs of illness (such as "a" means healthy, "b" means sick).

---

all organ systems and tissues as well as various species and breeds. Other terms that have been commonly used to describe cancer include *tumor, neoplasm* and *growth*.

Tumors can be either *benign* or *malignant*. Benign tumors are characterized by an unchecked growth of cells that do not destroy local tissues but can impair function by their presence. An example of this would be a dog with a large lipoma in the axilla, hindering its ability to use the front leg. Malignant tumors are characterized by an uncontrolled growth of abnormal cells that cause local tissue destruction and also have the potential for metastasis. *Metastasis* is the spread of cancer cells from the primary tumor to distant locations such as lung or liver. The exact mechanism of metastasis is not fully understood and varies between tumor types. Basically the metastatic process involves viable cancer cells leaving the primary tumor, entering the lymphatic and/or blood vessels, traveling to distant tissues and then becoming re-established and capable of growing in the tissue of the distant location.

Tumors can be categorized according to the tissue of origin and their histological features (Table 19–2). Carcinomas arise from any epithelial tissue, including skin, mucous membranes, and organs such as liver, kidney, prostate, and so forth. Carcinomas generally spread through the lymphatic system. Sarcomas arise from the mesenchymal tissues (such as blood, cartilage and bone) and generally spread by the circulatory system. A prefix on the tissue type indicates the specific tissue of origin. For example, osteosarcoma would be a sarcoma originating from bone. The suffix of a tumor generally indicates a benign or malignant condition, for example, fibroma (benign) versus fibrosarcoma (malignant). There are exceptions to this rule such as *melanoma, insulinoma* and *thymoma*, which are all malignant tumors. More than 100 histological types of cancer exist, and each may require special treatment and carry a dif-

---

Table 19–2
CLASSIFICATION OF TUMORS IN ANIMALS

Tissue Type	Benign	Malignant
Connective tissue		(Sarcomas)
Bone	Osteoma	Osteosarcoma
Cartilage	Chondroma	Chondrosarcoma
Fibrous tissue	Fibroma	Fibrosarcoma
Fat	Lipoma	Liposarcoma
Myxomatous tissue	Myxoma	Myxosarcoma
Muscle	Leiomyoma	Leiomyosarcoma
	Rhabdomyoma	Rhabdomyosarcoma
Vascular tissue	Lymphangioma	Lymphangiosarcoma
Hemolymphatic cells		Lymphomas
		Mast cell sarcomas
		Multiple myeloma
Epithelial tissue		(Carcinomas)
Skin		Squamous cell carcinoma
Glands	Adenomas	Adenocarcinoma
Sebaceous		
Sweat		
Ceruminous		
Epithelial lining tissue	Adenomas	Adenocarcinomas
Nasal		
Gastrointestinal		
Biliary tract		
Urinary tract		
Undifferentiated	—	Carcinomas and sarcomas
Mixed tissue types	Mammary gland adenomas	Mammary gland adenocarcinomas
		Mesenchymoma

Adapted from Dubielzig RR: Cancer pathology. *In* Withrow SJ and MacEwen EG (editors). Clinical Veterinary Oncology. Philadelphia, JB Lippincott, 1989, p 19.

The exact cause of cancer is not fully understood. Carcinogenesis is the process by which normal cells become transformed into neoplastic cells. The development of cancer is thought to be a multifactorial event. In general, two events must take place before cells transform: *initiation* and *promotion*. During the first event, initiation, it is thought that the cell is exposed to some agent that irreversibly alters the DNA (deoxyribonucleic acid). The promoting factors then appear to enhance replication of the transformed cell. Under appropriate conditions, a single transformed malignant cell may multiply and become an invasive cancer. Carcinogenic influences may include genetic, hormonal, congenital, viral, nutritional, immunological, traumatic, implantation, irradiation or chemical factors. Unfortunately, determination of a simple cause and effect relationship between a carcinogen and tumor development and prevention of that relationship is rare. Cancer causation and subsequent prevention therefore remains a complicated issue.

The search for all the answers in cancer cause and therapy continues with the hope that each new development will bring oncologists closer to understanding tumor behavior, possible prevention and options for treatment.

DIAGNOSTIC APPROACH IN THE CANCER PATIENT

Through early diagnosis and appropriate treatment of cancer, the prospects for cure and/or tumor control are greatly improved. A consistent diagnostic approach and biopsy are essential for establishing the correct diagnosis.

History, Physical Examination, and Minimum Data Base

The first step is taking an accurate history from the client and performing a complete physical examination. There is no diagnostic test that can equal the valuable information obtained from a complete history and physical examination. Knowledge of the signalment (age, breed and sex) of an animal can help in the diagnosis of some tumors and may also help in determining a prognosis. Some types of tumors are known to occur more frequently in certain species or breeds, in either sex, at different ages and at different anatomical sites. Most companion animals that develop cancer are 6 to 15 years old. It is important to remember that the age of the animal should not be a deterrent to aggressive treatment. The physiological age, determined by evaluation of cardiovascular, renal and hepatic function, is more important for predicting risks associated with therapy than is the chronological age of an animal.

The history should include the owner's conception of the primary problem, the clinical signs, the duration of signs, any treatments given and response to treatments. Other concurrent or past medical problems should also be elucidated.

The physical examination should be thorough (see Chapter 2). All organ systems should be examined, not only to assess the primary problem but also to detect concurrent disease. Regional lymph nodes should be palpated for enlargement, especially those close to the cancer. Evidence of tumor extension beyond the primary site into lymph nodes or distant sites will aid in staging the extent of tumor. Any lumps or bumps detected on the body should be measured and their location recorded in the medical record.

A minimum data base generally consists of a complete blood count (CBC), serum chemistry diagnostic profile (profile), urinalysis (UA), and thoracic radiographs. All blood samples should be obtained through venipuncture of the jugular veins if possible. Peripheral veins should be spared in the event that repeated catheterization for anesthesia or chemotherapy administration is indicated.

The CBC is useful in assessing for the presence of any abnormal parameters in the red blood cells and white blood cells, as well as platelets. The biochemical profile will reveal abnormal values in electrolytes, liver enzymes, creatinine, blood urea nitrogen (BUN) and proteins. The UA helps to assess renal function and should be obtained by cystocentesis in order to evaluate the urine sediment for abnormalities that may otherwise be obscured by debris washed out of the urethra in a voided sample. The specific gravity of the urine should also be determined before the animal receives any fluid therapy, since parenteral administration of fluids can lower the specific gravity. Additional diagnostic tests are available to further assess organ function if indicated by abnormalities detected by the minimum data base.

Radiography

Radiology plays an important role in the diagnosis and staging of cancer (see Chapter 7, Diagnostic Imaging). The lungs are a common site for development of metastases from certain malignant tumors. To accurately evaluate all lung fields for metastatic nodules, radiographs should be obtained when the animal is in right lateral *and* left lateral recumbency, as well as in a ventrodorsal position. Views in two planes are mandatory for all radiographic examinations in order to localize the lesion. The use of the additional lateral view improves examination of both lung fields by allowing the "up" lung to be expanded and filled with air, thereby enhancing the radiographic appearance of any nodule that may be present. Additional radiographs of the abdomen or other regions may be required if indicated by findings on the physical examination in order to determine the full extent of the disease.

Ultrasound can be used as a non-invasive method to examine the architecture of specific organs or masses found in the thoracic cavity or abdomen. Computerized tomography (CT scans), magnetic resonance imaging (MRI) and nuclear medicine are additional non-invasive diagnostic tools that are available at many universities and some private veterinary hospitals. Each provides methodology to assess inaccessible areas of the body or silent lesions and to help in staging the extent of the cancer and formulating treatment plans.

Cytology

Cytology is the study of individual cell morphology for the purpose of a diagnosis (see Chapter 4, Clinical Pathology). It is an effective screening tool and can help to differentiate neoplasia from inflammation or infection. Results of the cytological examination may then indicate the need for a biopsy, in order to obtain more tissue to determine a diagnosis. Every lump or bump that is identified should be assessed by either cytological or histopathological examination and not assumed to be benign because of its gross appearance. Collection of populations of cells can be obtained for microscopic examination, with minimal effort, from tissue masses, lymph nodes, bone marrow or fluid in cysts or body cavities.

Adherence to the proper techniques used for obtaining and preparing these samples is important for accurate results. Failure to obtain sufficient cells or distortion of their architecture by poor processing will make diagnosis impossible. Tumors that are easily diagnosed by cytological examination are generally composed of cells that exfoliate, or shed easily, and can be processed onto glass slides with minimal distortion to their architecture (such as mast cell tumors, lymphoma and histiocytomas).

Samples can easily be obtained by fine-needle aspirates of accessible soft tissue masses or fluid-filled spaces; by impression smears of small biopsy samples or ulcerated lesions; or by needle biopsy of bone marrow. These procedures can be performed quickly with minimal discomfort to the patient. Usually it is not necessary to anesthetize or sedate the patient.

Fine-Needle Aspiration

Samples for cytological evaluation of cutaneous tissue masses and lymph nodes are obtained by fine-needle aspiration (FNA). Improvements in ultrasound and in fluoroscopically guided instrumentation have also allowed FNA to be used safely within body cavities. For external masses, a 6- or 12-cc syringe, 22- to 25-gauge needle, and clean glass slides, preferably with a frosted edge to indelibly label the slide, are needed to perform the procedure.

The lesion is swabbed with alcohol and stabilized between the clinician's fingers, and the needle is inserted into its center. The needle may be inserted without the syringe attached and several core samples obtained by redirecting the needle several times (Fig. 19–1). Small portions of the needle contents are then squirted onto clean glass slides.

Slides should be labeled with a permanent marker on the frosted edge of the slide prior to staining. Identification of the slides should include the client's name and identification number and location of the mass that was aspirated. The slides are then air-dried and fixed with appropriate stain. The most common stains available include Wright's stain, new methylene blue, and Romanovsky's stains such as Diff-Quick (American Scientific Products, McGraw Park, IL). Slides can be evaluated in your practice and/or sent to a qualified cytologist for evaluation. Remember that the results of cytology will be useful only if proper technique for sample preparation has been followed and clinical and historical information is complete and made available to the cytologist.

Bone Marrow Aspirate

Evaluation of the cellular elements in the bone marrow is sometimes indicated when abnormalities exist in the erythrocytic, leukocytic or thrombocytic cell lines in the peripheral blood. The bone marrow is also examined to determine the stage of certain tumors such as lymphoma, multiple myeloma and mast cell tumors. The most common technique used to obtain a sample from the bone marrow is aspiration biopsy

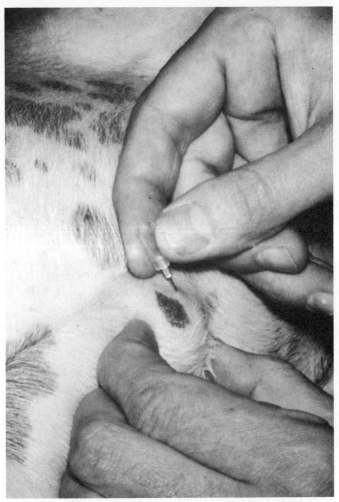

FIGURE 19–1. Fine-needle aspiration of a cutaneous mass. A 22-gauge needle is inserted into the center of a mass. The needle is redirected several times to obtain an adequate cellular sample. A syringe is then attached to the hub of the needle, and the contents are expelled onto clean glass slides.

using 16- or 18- gauge bone marrow needle (see Chapter 4, Clinical Pathology). If this method fails to produce enough cells, a core sample can be obtained by means of a Jamshidi bone marrow biopsy needle (American Pharmaseal Co., Valencia, CA).

The optimal sites for biopsy of the bone marrow are the proximal humerus, the iliac crest and the trochanteric fossa of the proximal femur. Most animals tolerate this procedure after infiltration of the overlying skin with a small amount of local anesthetic; other animals might require sedation.

Histopathology

Determining the histopathological diagnosis is one of the most important steps in the overall diagnostic procedure. The results of a biopsy will determine the method of treatment and the prognosis and will often influence the owner's decision to treat. It is crucial that every mass that is removed be submitted for histopathological examination, regardless of its gross appearance.

A benefit of histopathology over cytology is that the pathologist is presented with more tissue that is not likely to be distorted by procurement and processing techniques. Individual tumors can exhibit cellular heterogeneity and consist of areas of necrosis, fibrosis and inflammation as well as neoplastic cells. Because of this variable cellularity, entire masses or multiple representative sections of large tumors should be submitted for evaluation. All tissue samples are examined to determine cell type, histological grade and the surgical margins.

Common methods used to biopsy tissue include (1) needle core biopsy, (2) incisional biopsy and (3) excisional biopsy.

Needle Core Biopsy

Specialized needles provide a method to obtain multiple core samples of tissues through small, 1- to 2-mm skin incisions. The Tru-Cut needle (Travenol Laboratories, Deerfield, IL) is most commonly used for biopsy of cutaneous or subcutaneous masses. In addition, adaptations of this type of needle can be used for ultrasonically or fluoroscopically guided biopsy of tissues within body cavities. These needles obtain a 1- to 1.5-cm-long sliver of tissue approximately the same diameter as that of the lead in a pencil. The biopsy site is clipped and prepared for minor surgery. The mass is stabilized between the clinician's fingers, and a small incision (1 to 2 mm) is made in the skin. Local anesthetic infiltrated into the incision site renders sedation or anesthesia unnecessary in most cases. The needle is introduced and the sample is obtained (Fig. 19–2). The tissue is gently scraped off the needle blade and placed in 10 percent buffered neutral formalin. Impression smears of this tissue can also be made by gently rolling the sample out onto clean glass slides.

Samples of bone lesions can also be obtained by a closed, needle core biopsy in a similar manner. The animal is placed under general anesthesia for this procedure. Trephine bone biopsy instruments or Jamshidi bone marrow biopsy needle (American Pharmaseal Co., Valencia, CA) can be used for bone biopsy procedures. These instruments retrieve multiple core samples of the bone. Possible complications include pathological fracture of an already weakened bone after biopsy. In order to minimize this risk, the smaller-gauge Jamshidi needle is preferred, and only one cortex of the bone is penetrated. It is possible to obtain multiple samples from the one cortical access site. The preparation of the biopsy site is as for any sterile minor surgery. In order to locate the lesion within the bone, one should have knowledge of normal anatomical landmarks, so as to avoid accidental penetration of nearby joints or major nerves and vessels. In addition, two radiographic views of the bone containing the lesion should be available.

Incisional Biopsy

Incisional biopsy consists of making a small skin incision and removing a wedge of tissue. It is useful for obtaining more tissue than by needle core biopsy, especially when the cancer cells are intermixed with abundant necrotic or inflammatory tissue. It is important to limit the size of the incision and to predetermine the placement of the incision, as in needle core biopsy.

Contamination of the biopsy tract with tumor cells is a potential complication with needle core biopsy and incisional

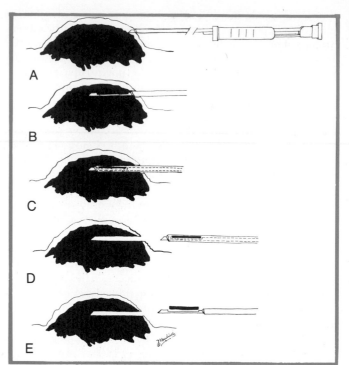

FIGURE 19–2. Mechanism of action of Tru-Cut biopsy needle used for typical nodular biopsy. A, With the instrument closed, the outer capsule is penetrated. A small skin incision is made with a No. 11 blade to allow insertion of the instrument. B, The outer cannula is fixed in place, and the inner cannula with specimen notch is thrust into the tumor. The tissue to be excised then protrudes into the notch. C, The inner cannula is now fixed, while the outer cannula is moved forward to cut off the biopsy specimen. D, The entire instrument is removed, with the tissue sample contained within. E, The inner cannula is pushed forward to expose the tissue in the specimen notch.

biopsy. The biopsy should be obtained through a small incision, with minimal disruption of the surrounding tissue, and the incision should be along the same line as the surgical incision in order that the biopsy tract can be removed with the tumor. It would be best if the surgeon who will perform the definitive surgery also performs the biopsy or is available for consultation.

Excisional Biopsy

Excisional biopsy involves the complete removal of the mass for biopsy. Depending on the results of the histopathological examination, this method of biopsy may be all that is required for diagnosis and treatment. A second surgery or adjuvant therapy may be indicated if the tissue margins are not free of tumor.

Biopsy Preparation

Once the biopsy is obtained, it should be handled gently so as not to distort the cellular architecture. Evaluation of the surgical margins is extremely important for determining the success of the removal of the tumor. The edges or surfaces of the resected tissue that need to be carefully evaluated for presence of tumor should be marked so that the pathologist can identify those sites. The use of India ink to "paint" selected margins has been shown to be extremely helpful in marking

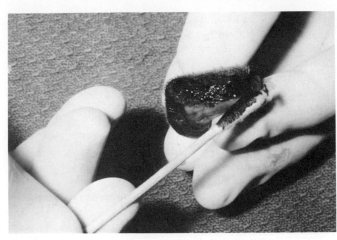

FIGURE 19–3. The cut edge of a resected mass is painted with India ink to mark the surgical margin. The ink is allowed to dry (1 to 2 minutes) before the mass is placed in 10 percent neutral buffered formalin.

surgical margins (Rochat et al., 1992) (Fig. 19–3). Ink will not distort the tissue and can be used to mark the entire margin. The ink will be present as a peripheral black line when the tissue is examined under the microscope. If tumor cells are in contact with this ink-labeled margin, then tumor cells probably remain within the animal, indicating the need for further surgery or alternative treatment.

The tissue should then be placed in 10 percent buffered neutral formalin solution in order to be fixed. The ratio of formalin to tissue for initial fixation should be approximately 10:1. The tissue should be no thicker than 1 cm to allow penetration of the formalin. If it is thicker, it can be cut as is a loaf of bread to allow the formalin to penetrate, but one edge should be left intact so that the pathologist understands the original orientation of the mass (Fig. 19–4). Once the sample has been sufficiently fixed, it can be transferred to plastic bags (two, at least) or commercial mailers with less formalin (1:1 ratio) for transportation to the laboratory.

A detailed information sheet should accompany the sample. Information that should be recorded includes the clinic and veterinarian's name, the owner's name, pet's name, identification number, signalment, site of biopsy, and a brief but detailed clinical history including pertinent treatments and the suspected diagnosis. Any margins that need to be evaluated should be recorded as well. For some tumors, such as mast cell tumors, a histological grade may also be requested to help predict the tumor behavior.

The pathologist is responsible for identifying the tumor type and providing information regarding completeness of surgical margins and histological grade. However, the pathologist is limited by the quality of the sample submitted and the amount of information provided. It is ultimately the responsibility of the attending clinician to assess whether the pathologist's diagnosis appropriately reflects the clinical presentation of the patient.

THERAPEUTIC OPTIONS

Once a diagnosis is made, the method of treatment is planned. The clinician, technician and client should discuss the diagnosis and treatment options in terms of prognosis, benefits and complications associated with each treatment, and cost. The clinician should talk in terms that are understood by the client. Informational handouts are helpful to explain commonly performed procedures (such as amputation, mastectomies, care and monitoring of incisions and bandages). Handouts can also be used to explain the nature, method of action, timing of administration and expected side effects of common chemotherapy drugs.

In oncology, the treatment options generally include surgery, chemotherapy and/or radiation therapy. The use of a single or multimodality protocol is determined for each case.

Surgery

Traditionally, surgery has been the treatment of choice for most types of cancer. It is the best method for removing solitary masses, but its benefits are limited by wide resections that can damage important normal structures or by the extension of tumor to distant sites (metastasis). In such instances, combining surgery with other modalities (adjuvant therapy) or using other modalities in place of surgery is necessary. The oncological surgeon must understand all the potential options for therapy in order to provide the best care.

Surgical resection of malignant cancer requires an aggressive approach. For the surgery to be successful, the tumor must be removed completely with a minimum of cosmetic and functional loss to the patient. An attempt is made to avoid entering the tumor and exposing the surgical field to tumor cells. Tumor cells released in this manner may implant in the wound and result in local recurrence. Instead, the resection should occur in the normal tissues surrounding the mass. Extensive surgical resections and prolonged surgery times in animals that may be debilitated from the cancer or concurrent disease require careful perioperative planning and monitoring to avoid complications.

It is the responsibility of the clinician and technician to make sure the patient has had a complete presurgical work-up and that the surgical team is aware of any conditions that may complicate anesthesia, surgery or recovery. The anesthetic protocol must be tailored to the needs of the individual patient. It is best to perform major surgeries early in the day in order for the animal to receive adequate monitoring in the recovery

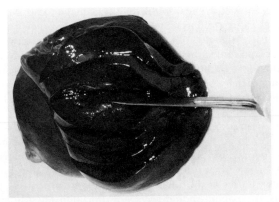

FIGURE 19–4. A large mass is sliced (loafed) into 1-cm sections. A 1-cm-thick base connecting all the slices is left to help orient the pathologist.

period. The preparation for surgery should include clipping wide areas for extensive resections, thorough surgical scrubs and perhaps the use of perioperative antibiotics if prolonged surgery or potential contamination during surgery is anticipated. The benefits of intravenous fluids and regional analgesics (such as epidural anesthesia, local anesthesia in regional nerves) and the parenteral use of analgesic agents provide for an improved recovery in most patients (see Chapter 29, Pain Management).

Another type of surgery used in treating cancer is cryosurgery. This involves the use of a cold source (usually liquid nitrogen) to freeze superficial cancers usually less than 2 cm in diameter. The tissue then undergoes a period of sloughing before healing. Discoloration or loss of hair may be permanent. This technique is useful for small, superficial lesions, such as eyelid, skin and anal masses. A disadvantage of cryosurgery is that the completeness of tumor removal cannot be determined because there is no tissue to submit for margin evaluation.

The goal of surgery may be curative or palliative. Palliative surgery is offered when the tumor is resected in order to improve the animal's quality of life, despite metastasis or poor long-term prognosis. An example would be a dog that presents with an ulcerated or painful mass (such as mammary gland tumor, osteosarcoma) that has metastasized, but the metastatic lesions are not causing clinical signs. Removal of the mass improves the dog's quality of life until the metastatic disease progresses.

Chemotherapy

Chemotherapy means the treatment of disease by chemical agents. Most people associate chemotherapy with cancer therapy, but in reality all drug therapy (even antibiotics) constitutes chemotherapy.

The drugs for cancer therapy are categorized into groups based on their mechanism of action. The majority of these drugs are by nature cytotoxic, and the target is generally the DNA or the protective cellular membrane of the cancer cell. Drugs that disrupt DNA will often target cells that exhibit rapid cell turnover (as in neoplastic cells). Unfortunately, these drugs can also be harmful to normal cells with high cell turnover, such as the cells within the gastrointestinal tract, the bone marrow, and hair follicles.

The dose and timing of administration of each agent are predetermined to achieve maximum cancer cell destruction while at the same time minimizing the damage to normal cells. Dosages can be different for individual species (such as dog versus cat). Dosages are based on the surface area of the body (meter squared) rather than on kilograms or pounds to avoid overdosage or underdosage. Neutropenia is often the dose-limiting toxicity, and the interval between doses is determined by the response time the bone marrow requires to replenish the leukocyte population.

Administration of drugs for cancer therapy requires strict attention to proper dosing, drug handling and technique. These agents are potential carcinogens to both humans and animals, and when using them, one should wear surgical-quality latex gloves at all times. Prior to administration of these agents, the patient should receive a thorough physical examination.

In addition, a CBC and platelet count should be obtained to make sure the patient has adequate cell counts before administration of agents that are known to suppress bone marrow (such as doxorubicin, cyclophosphamide, mitoxantrone). If the agent to be administered is known to be toxic to other systems (e.g., the nephrotoxicity of cisplatin), tests specific to those systems should be performed (BUN, creatinine, UA). The patient should be weighed and the weight converted from pounds or kilograms to meter squared area (M^2). The appropriate dose is then determined. *Remember to **always** double check the body weight conversion and all dose calculations.*

If intravenous administration of chemotherapy is required, a sterile catheter should be placed in a normal peripheral vein, and the patency of that catheter should be carefully checked prior to actually injecting the agent. Two commonly used agents that are known to be extremely irritating to tissues (vesicant) if they are extravasated from a vein are doxorubicin and vincristine. If an accidental extravasation occurs, one should stop administration and draw back on the syringe to retrieve any drug in the catheter. The use of intralesional steroids or saline to dilute the agent in the tissues is controversial. The patient should be closely monitored for signs of continued damage and potential necrosis of tissue.

Once the drug has been administered, all materials that contacted the agent (intravenous [IV] catheters, syringes, connectors and gloves) should be disposed of in proper chemotherapeutic waste bags with warning labels. Specific details on the handling and disposal of these agents can be obtained from the manufacturer. In addition, veterinary oncology textbooks and articles are available that describe indications, administration techniques, dosages and expected toxicities for individual agents (see Recommended Reading).

After each treatment, the patient should be monitored for signs of toxicities. Clients should be given detailed handouts describing known toxicities for each agent. If any abnormalities are detected by the hospital staff or the client, the animal should be re-evaluated. If these drugs are administered properly and the client is educated as to the risks, the toxicities can be minimized and the patient can maintain a good quality of life during therapy. The incidence of serious toxicities for most commonly used drugs or protocols should not occur in more than 5 percent of the cases treated.

Radiation Therapy

Ionizing radiation can also be used for cancer therapy. Radiation causes cell death by disrupting the DNA of the cell or destroying important biological molecules required by the cell. Cell death occurs as a result of the failure of injured cells to repair themselves and/or the inability of subsequent cell generations to divide. Currently, more than 30 radiation therapy facilities are available in the United States to treat animals with cancer.

Radiation therapy can be used as a single therapy or in combination with surgery, chemotherapy and hyperthermia. Routine protocols consist of giving multiple doses (fractions) daily on a Monday, Wednesday and Friday schedule or a Monday through Friday schedule for approximately 15 fractions. Because radiation targets DNA, like chemotherapy, it is most effective in controlling cells with rapid cell turnover. Subsequently, the side effects from radiation therapy are seen in normal tissues with high cell turnover and located in the irradiated field.

The radiation effects observed are divided into acute and long-term effects. Acute effects are seen during the end stages of actual therapy and, although they may require additional nursing care, are temporary. Late effects develop months to years after treatment and usually involve permanent changes such as necrosis or fibrosis of normal tissues.

Acute effects observed with irradiation of oral or nasal tumors results in mucositis of the oral cavity. Irradiation of skin will induce a desquamative dermatitis or loss of the superficial layers of the epidermis. Both conditions will resolve in 2 to 3 weeks with attention to local hygiene and use of analgesics if needed. The use of oil-based topical creams should be avoided, and self-trauma such as licking should be prevented. Hair loss or change in color may be permanent. The owner must be warned of these effects along with the potential benefits of radiation therapy prior to treatment.

EUTHANASIA

Unfortunately, cancer therapy does not always result in a cure. In some cases the best the client and clinician can hope for is a long disease-free interval and a good quality of life. Euthanasia is an important component of pet cancer management. The choice of euthanasia for a pet may be the option chosen by the client at the time the cancer is diagnosed or after therapy has been instituted. In either situation, it is a difficult decision to be made and one that the client should be comfortable with and decide upon after careful consideration of all available treatment options.

The veterinarian and technician must be available to provide all the medical information as well as the emotional support and compassion the client and patient deserve. Many times this support comes from the technical staff. Clients often feel inhibited when talking to the clinician, but can sometimes talk more freely with a nurse or receptionist. Technicians need to be aware of the important role they play in veterinary medicine, not only in providing the treatment for the patient but also in supporting the needs of the client. Good communication and compassion are as important as the treatment in cancer therapy and inherent to its success (see Chapter 25).

Reference

Rochat MC, Mann FA, Pace LW, et al.: Identification of surgical biopsy borders by use of India ink. J Am Vet Med Assoc 201:873–878, 1992.

Recommended Reading

Couto GC (editor): Clinical management of the cancer patient. Vet Clin North Am, Vol 20(4), 1990.
Theilen GH and Madewell BR: Veterinary Cancer Medicine. 2nd ed. Philadelphia, Lea & Febiger, 1987.
Withrow SJ and MacEwen EG: Clinical Veterinary Oncology. Philadelphia, JB Lippincott Co., 1989.

Organizations for Cancer Treatment

Veterinary Cancer Society
c/o Dr. Richard E. Weller
Developmental Toxicology Section
Batelle, Pacific Northwest Labs
P7-52, PO Box 999
Richland, WA 99352
(This organization encourages veterinary technicians to become members.)

American Cancer Society
1825 Connecticut Avenue NW
Suite 315
Washington, DC 20009

rate, blood pressure, bronchial airway tone, body temperature, carbohydrate and fatty acid metabolism and appetite. Although norepinephrine is the primary transmitter substance, epinephrine is also present and is released from the adrenal gland when an animal is stressed through physical, psychological or other stimulatory means.

Since the norepinephrine molecule can be modified extensively and still possess some type of stimulatory properties, numerous agents (more than 30) are commercially available. Manufacturers seek a molecule that accents a certain desired response and eliminates or reduces all the other adrenergic effects.

Epinephrine finds several therapeutic applications in veterinary medicine, though the actual frequency of use is limited. Clinical applications include use for (1) allergic reactions—often lifesaving in the face of shock; (2) bronchospasm—provides rapid relief; (3) cardiac effects—sometimes used in specific heart disorders; (4) local hemostasis—may be used in dilute solutions (1:100,000 to 1:20,000) to control surgical bleeding in highly vascular tissue; and (5) prolonging the effects of the local anesthetics, though there may be undesirable systemic effects from the epinephrine if it is overused.

Norepinephrine that possesses only alpha effects has limited therapeutic value, being used to treat only certain hypotensive shock conditions.

Isoproterenol, which has few alpha effects but has powerful beta effects, is useful as a bronchodilator in respiratory disorders and as a cardiac stimulant in certain heart conditions.

Epinephrine and norepinephrine are not available in oral forms because both are destroyed by stomach acid. In addition, both drugs are relatively short-acting when given by injection. Isoproterenol is available in many preparations for humans that are designed for inhalation use or as sublingual tablets for use under the tongue. Since these forms are not applicable to veterinary use, only the short-acting injectable form has application here.

One synthetic catecholamine that is gaining increased popularity in the treatment of heart disorders involving depressed contractility is dobutamine. In therapeutic doses, the drug has little effect on $beta_2$ or alpha-adrenergic receptors and directly stimulates the $beta_1$ receptors, resulting in cardiac stimulation with perhaps only a slight decrease in peripheral resistance.

Epinephrine and phenylephrine hydrochloride are also commercially available as ophthalmic preparations. They cause the pupil to dilate, but unlike atropine, they directly stimulate those muscles of the eye that are controlled by the sympathetic nerves. This mydriatic effect is useful in selective cases of glaucoma as well as in facilitating ophthalmic examinations.

Sympatholytics

Many chemicals interfere with the function of the sympathetic nervous system. Some of these agents act by interfering with the synthesis, storage and release of the neurotransmitter. Others interfere with the receptors' ability to interact effectively with the transmitter substances. Some blocking agents are specific in their action, for example, prazosin hydrochloride is specific in blocking the alpha receptors. Other agents (i.e., the phenothiazine tranquilizers [e.g., acepromazine]) are more general in their action, blocking alpha and $beta_1$ receptors.

The alpha-adrenergic blocking agents cause vasodilation and are used mainly in humans for lowering the blood pressure or improving blood flow in certain vascular diseases. An older, popular drug, phenoxybenzamine hydrochloride, which is used to dilate blood vessels and lower blood pressure is being replaced by newer drugs, such as prazosin. (There are other hypotensive drugs, such as hydralazine hydrochloride, that act directly on the vascular smooth muscle to cause relaxation.) Phentolamine, an expensive, injectable alpha blocker, is used to diagnose adrenal gland tumors. It is also used during surgery in patients with abnormally high blood pressure.

Beta-adrenergic blocking agents find their therapeutic usefulness as antihypertensive agents and for the treatment of certain heart arrhythmias. Propranolol, an early and popular agent in the human field, is gaining popularity in veterinary medicine.

TRANQUILIZERS (ATARACTICS)

Tranquilizers are drugs that act on the central nervous system to produce a calmness of mind or detached serenity without loss of consciousness or marked depression. Their use in veterinary medicine is to modify the behavior of the animal in order to make it more manageable or less responsive to external stimulation.

Phenothiazines

Phenothiazine was originally used in veterinary medicine as an anthelmintic. Derivatives of phenothiazine, such as acepromazine, promazine, chlorpromazine and so on, have since been developed to improve tranquilizing properties. Most of these derivatives have antihypertensive properties and a varying degree of antihistamine activity. In addition, some are useful antiemetics or anti–motion sickness medicants.

The phenothiazine tranquilizers have found usefulness as preanesthetics by "taking the edge off the animal" and enhancing or prolonging effects of certain anesthetics. Some side effects to be aware of when administering the phenothiazines include a fall in blood pressure, paralysis of the retractor penis muscle in horses and the lowering of the seizure threshold in dogs.

Other Tranquilizers

Of the numerous tranquilizers available for human use, few have found significant use in veterinary medicine. Diazepam is used in animals but more for anticonvulsant effects than for tranquilizing properties. Innovar Vet (Pitman-Moore) contains droperidol as the tranquilizer in the narcotic mixture.

Xylazine and Detomidine (Alpha$_2$-Agonists)

Although xylazine and detomidine in the strictest sense may not be classified as tranquilizers, their sedative and analgesic properties are useful for chemical restraint, especially in the horse. Detomidine is approved for use only in the horse and finds little application in other species. It appears to differ slightly from xylazine by producing greater analgesia and sedation. Although dose-dependent, detomidine's duration of action is longer than that of xylazine.

Both xylazine and detomidine are commonly used in combination with other sedatives, tranquilizers and anesthetic agents. However, the effects of these drugs in combination is greatly potentiated and must be used with caution. Common side effects seen in the horse include muscle tremors, heart block, bradycardia, respiratory changes, sweating and penile prolapse.

Xylazine is used widely in cattle, even though it is not currently approved by the Food and Drug Administration (FDA) for use in food-producing animals. The popularity in ruminants results from its excellent anesthetic properties. Ruminants are sensitive to xylazine, requiring approximately one-tenth the dose (based on body weight) as horses. Adverse effects in cattle also include ruminal atony, intestinal stasis, salivation, diarrhea, bloating and regurgitation with aspiration pneumonia.

Although xylazine is approved for managing hyperexcitable behavior in the cat and dog, it is not widely used in these species. Vomiting is a common side effect seen in the cat, and xylazine is frequently employed as an emetic when this effect is desired (i.e., emptying stomach prior to surgery).

ANTICONVULSANTS

Of the several different causes of seizures (convulsions) in dogs, only about two thirds can be controlled by the various anticonvulsant drugs. Diazepam is perhaps the most popular injectable drug for use during seizures or in other emergency situations. However, diazepam is relatively short-acting ($\frac{1}{2}$ hour to $2\frac{1}{2}$ hours). Phenobarbital sodium is also available for injection when a longer effect (4 to 6 hours) is required.

Oral phenobarbital, which is inexpensive and effective, is employed to treat epilepsy (status epilepticus) and seizures caused by acute encephalitis or meningitis in dogs. For some cases that are uncontrolled by phenobarbital, oral administration of potassium bromide has been found effective. (Note: Potassium bromide is not commercially available for drug use. However, authorization may be obtained from the Food and Drug Administration to compound preparations for treatment of these refractory cases.)

ANALGESICS, ANTIPYRETICS AND ANTI-INFLAMMATORY AGENTS

Analgesics are those agents that alleviate pain. Although local as well as general anesthetics inhibit the sensory perception of pain, analgesics are generally considered to increase the threshold of pain in the pain perception areas of the brain. Antiprostaglandins (e.g., aspirin, flunixin) inhibit the biosynthesis of these natural pain-producing substances and are also considered analgesics.

Opioid Analgesics

The naturally occurring narcotics (e.g., morphine, codeine) as well as synthetic narcotics (e.g., oxymorphone, meperidine) are the most potent analgesics. Although these addictive agents are used for severe postsurgical or post-trauma pain in dogs and horses, their more common use is as an anesthetic or a preanesthetic agent.

The pharmacological effects differ somewhat among the various narcotics, but most will produce the following:

1. Central nervous system depression in the dog, the monkey and humans
2. Central nervous system stimulation (excitement) in the cat and horse
3. Cough sedation in dogs and humans
4. Respiratory depression (panting initially may be seen)
5. Increased tone of intestinal smooth muscle, causing constipation.

Effects are reversed by antagonists, such as naloxone.

Unfortunately, the action of narcotic analgesics is fairly short in the dog and the horse (2 to 4 hours). Gut stasis in the horse is also a concern when considering the use of the opiate analgesics. The potential for central nervous system stimulation in the cat and the horse also discourages use of narcotics. Since the opiate analgesics have questionable efficacy in ruminants, their use in veterinary medicine is limited.

Butorphanol, a morphine congener, has shown promise in dogs as a longer-acting (4 to 8 hours) analgesic. Butorphanol is used in horses as an effective analgesic, though its stimulatory effects must be suppressed by the concurrent use of depressant drugs such as xylazine. Butorphanol is also approved by the FDA as an antitussive in dogs.

Opioid Antagonists

The opioid antagonists reverse the pharmacological effects of the narcotics. Naloxone, discovered in 1960, appears to be the only true antagonist, since it possesses no other pharmacological effect.

Although narcotic antagonists are used commonly in human addicts to reverse overdoses of self-administered narcotics, their principal use in veterinary medicine is to reverse the sedative and quieting effects of analgesics employed for temporary restraint. Dogs receiving narcotic sedation for minor procedures (e.g., hip dysplasia radiographs or suture removal) are easily "reversed" using naloxone. The animal is alert almost immediately. Although the length of action of naloxone is shorter than most narcotics, generally the effects of the unmetabolized analgesic are inadequate to cause the animal to return to its sedated state.

Corticosteroids

Corticosteroids are extremely active compounds that have numerous pharmacological effects on all organ systems. Although they are extremely valuable in the treatment of certain conditions, there is also significant risk when one considers the potential adverse effects.

Since corticosteroids are naturally occurring body substances (i.e., cortisol from the adrenal gland), one indication for the use of steroids would be for replacement therapy to correct a deficiency. Such a deficiency is relatively rare. Most steroids used in veterinary medicine are given for their anti-inflammatory effect. Although the mechanism for the anti-inflammatory

chlorinated hydrocarbons, they should all be treated with caution and used as advised on the container label. Some diluted aqueous suspensions and powders may be applied directly to livestock. Signs of toxicity include vomiting, weakness and other central nervous system effects, such as tremors, incoordination, convulsions, coma and respiratory failure. Young, debilitated or lean animals are more susceptible to the toxic effects. There is no specific antidote for chlorinated hydrocarbon toxicity. The animal should be removed from further exposure and given supportive treatment, such as barbiturates, to control seizures if necessary.

Organophosphates

Although organophosphates is the same class of drugs that was mentioned previously for treatment of intestinal parasites, these agents (ronnel, coumaphos, trichlorfon, fenthion, malathion) are selected or formulated specifically for the treatment of external parasites. As with chlorinated hydrocarbons, a number of preparations exist, such as sprays, dips, foggers, agents to pour on the animal and pest strips. These compounds have good insect-killing ability, but residual effects are related to the vehicle used to apply the agent. Although applied topically, absorption through the skin may occur in amounts adequate to produce signs of toxicity. Signs and treatment of toxicity are the same as those mentioned previously under the section on Internal Parasitism Treatment. People applying these agents should avoid getting them in their eyes or on their skin. Prolonged breathing of spray mists should also be avoided.

Pyrethrins

Pyrethrum flowers (chrysanthemums) have been used as insecticides for centuries, the first powdered form being introduced into the United States in 1855. Before the advent of DDT, importation of pyrethrins reached 18 million pounds per year. Use did drop dramatically with the development of chlorinated hydrocarbons and organophosphates, but recently pyrethrins have again gained popularity. Since they are reported to be nontoxic to mammals as well as having little effect on the environment, our society welcomes their use. Apparently, some toxicity has occurred in cats, however.

Pyrethrins are marketed in numerous formulations for convenient use. Most have chemicals, such as piperonyl butoxide, added to potentiate their killing power. Also, microencapsulation has significantly increased the residual activity of these compounds that were known initially for their quick "knockdown" effect.

Permethrin is a synthetic pyrethroid, its formulation and use being similar to those of natural pyrethrins. However, little can be found in the literature to compare the potency, toxicity, environmental impact, and so on between the natural and synthetic agents.

ANTI-INFECTIVE AGENTS

Antibiotics

Initially, antibiotics (antimicrobials) were defined as substances produced by microorganisms, which in low concentra-

tions destroy or inhibit growth of other species of microorganisms. Today many of these substances may be produced totally or in part by chemical synthesis. Because antibiotics can potentially cure life-threatening infections, they are one of the most popular and useful groups of drugs in veterinary medicine.

It is important not only to know the characteristics and uses of the various antibiotics but also, even more importantly, to have a proper understanding of the principles of antibiotic therapy (chemotherapy). It is beyond the scope of this chapter to present a thorough discussion of chemotherapy; however, some basic principles will be discussed.

Not all microorganisms are harmful or disease-producing (pathogenic). Many bacteria found in the gastrointestinal tract, skin, mucous membranes, and so on are helpful to their host because they compete with pathogens, keeping them in a static state and preventing progression to a disease state.

Each antibiotic is effective against specific groups of microorganisms. Some antibiotics are bactericidal (destroy bacteria), others are bacteriostatic (inhibit growth of bacteria) and some may be both, depending upon the concentration of the antibiotic (Table 20–3). The various species of bacteria that are affected by the antibiotic are known as the antibiotic's spectrum. Broad-spectrum antibiotics are those that are effective against a wide range of microorganisms.

In order for an antibiotic to be effective, it must be able to reach the site of infection in a concentration that is great enough to exert its effect on the microorganism. In addition, the antibiotic concentration must be maintained or reached frequently enough over a period of time to completely destroy all the bacteria or to provide time for the body's natural defense mechanisms to destroy the pathogenic bacteria. Bacteriostatic antibiotics must rely totally on the body's defense response for eradication of the pathogen, whereas bactericidal antibiotics can destroy the pathogens directly.

The length of antibiotic therapy may vary considerably, depending on such factors as the site of infection, the microorganism and the duration of infection. Usually when antibiotics are prescribed, the treatment is for a minimum of 5 days. Although patients may improve with inadequate therapy, it is an unwise practice. Microorganisms exposed to subtherapeutic antibiotic levels may develop resistance to the particular antibiotic. Thus, the antibiotic will be ineffective, even when given at high levels. Not only can bacteria develop resistance to several antibiotics, but they can also pass resistance on to other species of bacteria. Multiple antibiotic-resistant bacteria are a serious problem if they become established in a hospital or clinic, since they can be treated only with the most potent and expensive antibiotics.

The choice of antibiotic is obviously critical to successful therapy. The microorganism must be sensitive to the antibiotic

Table 20–3 ANTIBACTERIAL ACTION AT USUAL SERUM CONCENTRATIONS	
Bacteriostatic	**Bactericidal**
Chloramphenicol	Penicillin
Tetracyclines	Aminoglycosides
Erythromycin	Cephalosporins
Sulfonamides	Trimethoprim-sulfa combinations
Lincomycin	Quinolones

chosen. A sample from the site of infection (blood, urine, tissue) should be collected for culture and antibiotic sensitivity testing to determine the causative organism and the effective antibiotics (see Chapter 6). However, this is not always economically feasible, and so a potentially effective antibiotic frequently is chosen. Administered antibiotics that are not effective may actually worsen the disease by destroying nonpathogenic bacteria that are actively competing with the pathogen. Even when antibiotics are effective against the suspected pathogen, destruction of the nonharmful bacterial flora may allow a second pathogen to manifest itself.

Ideally, it is desirable to choose an antibiotic that is effective only against the identified pathogen. However, even the narrow-spectrum antibiotics are effective against a number of types of bacteria, both pathogenic and nonpathogenic. Therefore, one can only choose antibiotics that are most likely to be effective against the pathogen and are least likely to disturb normal, nonpathogenic bacteria. Indiscriminant use of wide-spectrum antibiotics eventually leads to resistant strains, ineffective antibiotics and expensive, perplexing therapeutic problems.

Penicillins

The discovery of penicillin in 1929 and its subsequent clinical use in 1940 represent perhaps one of the most significant advances in all of medical history. Being the first antibiotic used, it dramatically changed the outcome of many life-threatening infections. Since its discovery, the basic penicillin molecule (Fig. 20–3) has been continuously manipulated and changed to produce a number of improved penicillins having unique characteristics.

Penicillin G (benzylpenicillin), the first clinically used penicillin, is still extensively used in large animals today in its procaine salt form. Procaine penicillin G is poorly soluble and is thus released slowly from its site of injection, providing adequate penicillin levels to allow once daily dosing, though twice daily is usually recommended. When given orally, penicillin G is effective; however, high doses must be administered, since only approximately one fourth of it is absorbed from the gastrointestinal tract. Most of the antibiotic given orally is destroyed by stomach acid, so it should *not* be given directly after feeding, when stomach acid is greatest.

Penicillin acts by blocking bacterial cell wall synthesis in the final stages of replication. Without a cell wall, the bacteria swell and cannot function properly, and some *lysis* (rupturing) may occur. New infections in their high log growth phase are therefore most susceptible to penicillin. Penicillin has no direct effect on mammalian cells, since they do not have cell walls.

One method of classification of bacteria is to determine their tendency to absorb a dye (gentian violet) into their cell wall. Those absorbing stain are referred to as gram-positive and those that do not are referred to as gram-negative (Table 20–4). Penicillin G is effective against most of the gram-positive microorganisms, including many of the streptococcal and staphylococcal species. However, some staphylococcal species have the ability to produce penicillinase, an enzyme that hydrolyzes the lactam ring, rendering penicillin inactive. With high doses, penicillin G is effective against a few gram-negative species.

One alteration of the penicillin molecule was to make it more resistant to hydrolysis by stomach acid. Another improvement was to prepare penicillins that are resistant to the action of penicillinase. (Note: Clavamox [SmithKline Beecham] is a combination product containing amoxicillin and a specific beta-lactamase inhibitor, potassium clavulanate.) Table 20–5 provides some comparisons among various penicillins that are commercially available. Further side chain alterations of the molecule brought forth penicillins that are effective against a wide variety of microorganisms. Some of the penicillins recently released for human use have a broad spectrum of activity and are some of our most important potent antibiotics for use against many gram-negative organisms that may be resistant to most other antibiotics. These penicillins are expensive and should be held in reserve and used when other agents are ineffective.

In general, the penicillins are safe. Allergic reactions, such as skin rashes, fever, urticaria, salivation, cutaneous edema and other hypersensitivities, may occur and lead to justifiable concern.

Aminoglycosides

Aminoglycosides (streptomycin, neomycin, kanamycin, amikacin, gentamicin) have a fairly broad spectrum but are chosen primarily for their activity against gram-negative organisms. None of these agents is absorbed adequately when administered orally, but they may be used orally for intestinal tract infections or "sterilization" of the gastrointestinal tract prior to surgery. Aminoglycosides exert their action by interfering with bacteria protein synthesis. Although toxicity may vary among agents, all are potentially ototoxic as well as nephrotoxic (renal toxicity). Neuromuscular blockage is also an adverse effect that is manifested by apnea and progressive paralysis of skeletal muscle. When giving aminoglycosides to animals

Table 20–4 COMMON ANIMAL PATHOGENS	
Gram-Positive Organisms	**Gram-Negative Organisms**
Streptococcus species	*Escherichia coli*
Staphylococcus species	*Proteus* species
Clostridium perfringens	*Pseudomonas* species
Corynebacterium species	*Klebsiella* species
	Salmonella species
	Brucella
	Vibrio
	Pasteurella species

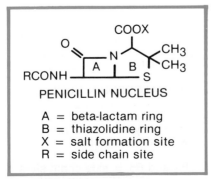

FIGURE 20–3. Penicillin nucleus.

Sulfonamides

Numerous sulfonamides (sulfamethazine, sulfadiazine, sulfadimethoxine) have been formulated, and many have been used clinically since their initial clinical use in 1932. Although their value and usage have declined with the discovery of many of the antibiotics, a few sulfonamides still remain useful for certain conditions. These agents are relatively inexpensive, making them attractive for use in large animals or for herd or flock treatment. The sulfonamides find their usefulness particularly in the treatment of various infections of the respiratory system and the urinary tract, bacterial diarrhea, foot rot and coccidial infections. Unfortunately, bacterial resistance to the sulfonamides limits their effectiveness. A toxicity seen with the original sulfonamides was crystalluria, a condition whereby the sulfa drug formed insoluble crystals in the urine, causing renal damage. Since the solubility of one sulfonamide is independent of other sulfonamides, the formulation of triple sulfa was developed to avert crystalluria. More soluble sulfonamides are now also available, further reducing concern. However, it is important that animals receiving sulfonamides have adequate water available.

The intravenous preparations of sulfonamides have a high (basic) pH and are therefore damaging to tissue when inadvertently given perivascularly. In addition, the intravenous preparations should be given slowly to avoid acute toxicity demonstrated by central nervous system effects, such as salivation, vomiting, diarrhea, weakness, ataxia and convulsions.

Trimethoprim-Sulfonamide Combinations

A popular, effective antibacterial that is being used in veterinary medicine today is a combination product of one part trimethoprim and five parts sulfadiazine or sulfamethoxazole. Ormetoprim with sulfadimethoxine is a comparable combination with similar use and actions. These combinations block two essential sequential steps in the bacteria's replication process, resulting in a synergistic antibacterial action. The combinations are effective against a wide range of organisms, but not *Pseudomonas*. Some resistant strains are seen but are relatively rare.

Undesirable side effects seen with these combinations are infrequent. Although vomiting may occur, one seldom observes diarrhea. Animals that are deficient in folic acid may be prone to develop blood disorders as has been reported in humans.

Nitrofurans

The nitrofurans (nitrofurazone, nitrofurantoin, furazolidone) have been replaced, to a great extent, by newer, more effective, safer antibacterials. Although these synthetic agents have a fairly broad spectrum of activity, they are not effective against *Pseudomonas*.

Although nitrofurazone and furazolidone are not absorbed from the gastrointestinal tract, they were once widely used orally in food animals to treat intestinal bacterial disorders. Except for topical application, their use in food animals is now strictly forbidden by the FDA because of their potential carcinogenicity.

Nitrofurantoin is absorbed well enough to still find some use in small animals for treating urinary tract infections. Nausea and vomiting, common adverse effects, can be reduced by administering nitrofurantoin with food or using the macrocrystal human preparations.

Antifungal Agents

There are numerous agents on the market to treat fungal infections of the skin (dermatomycosis). Griseofulvin is an antibiotic given orally. It has no antibacterial activity, but it inhibits the growth of various skin fungi. It is expensive, so it is not unusual to use other topical agents initially unless the infection is widespread. Common topical agents found in creams, lotions, sprays and other forms include miconazole, tolnaftate, undecylenic acid, iodine compounds, nystatin, various dyes and phenolic compounds.

Treating systemic fungal infections (e.g., cryptococcosis, blastomycosis, histoplasmosis) is usually expensive, requiring lengthy treatment with limited success. Amphotericin B, an antibiotic used for various fungal infections, is toxic, causing kidney and liver damage, central nervous system abnormalities, and so on. Nystatin, another antibiotic, is relatively nontoxic but has a narrow spectrum of effect. Ketoconazole, an expensive antifungal agent, has proved effective against a variety of fungal infections.

HORMONES AND SYNTHETIC SUBSTITUTES

Hormones are substances that are produced and secreted by glands and are carried by the blood, producing an effect on a target organ. There are a number of hormones secreted by several different glands. Our discussion will be limited only to the most clinically significant.

Thyroid Preparations

The thyroid gland is controlled primarily by the amount of thyroid-stimulating hormone (TSH) that is released from the pituitary gland. When stimulated, the thyroid gland releases thyroid hormones consisting primarily of *thyroxine*. Since the thyroid hormones affect the metabolism of carbohydrates, protein and fats, thyroid-deficient (hypothyroid) animals show signs of lethargy, reduced alertness, increased body weight, poor haircoat and other related signs. Inadequate iodine in the diet can result in inadequate production of thyroid hormones. Thyroid hormone deficiencies can be treated with desiccated thyroid, since it is effective orally. Sodium levothyroxine (Synthroid, Flint Labs and Soloxine, Daniels Pharmaceuticals) is perhaps the most popular agent for treating hypothyroidism. Sodium liothyronine (Cytobin, SmithKline Beecham), the other active component of desiccated thyroid, is also commercially available and sometimes used.

Insulin

Insulin is normally produced and released by islet cells of the pancreas. One of its most important functions is to enhance the absorption of glucose into most cells of the body. Animals with inadequate insulin will have abnormally high blood glucose levels (hyperglycemia) and other associated metabolic disorders. Insulin injection (regular Iletin) is a solution of dissolved insulin crystals used for its immediate action and short duration. There are other insulin preparations available that are intermediate- (approximately 24 hours) to long-acting (approximately 36 hours). Isophane insulin suspension (NPH), an intermediate-acting insulin, tends to be the most widely used in small animal medicine. Overdoses of insulin produce hypoglycemia, which if severe may lead to coma and death. Treatment consists of administering dextrose intravenously.

Oxytocin

Oxytocin is a hormone released at the end of pregnancy to stimulate uterine contractions during parturition and induce milk letdown. The synthetically produced oxytocin is therefore beneficial during delayed parturition or for aiding milk letdown.

Prostaglandins

Although prostaglandins (PGs) were discovered in 1935, it has only been in the past two decades that these substances have been extensively studied and developed. PGs are found in many mammalian tissues and have been shown to have a wide variety of effects on a number of body systems, including the central nervous, cardiovascular, urinary, gastrointestinal and reproductive systems. The PGs commercially available, such as dinoprost, prostalene, cloprostenol and fluprostenol, are employed for their effects on the reproductive system.

In cattle, the PGs can be used to regulate the heat cycle so that breeding and consequent calving times for a herd can be planned. The PGs are also approved by the FDA to abort feedlot heifers. For certain conditions in mares, PGs can effectively restore the normal heat cycle so that the animals can be bred.

Since these agents are abortifacients, they should not be handled by pregnant women. Bronchospasms are another potent adverse effect in animals and humans caused by accidental spillage. Consequently, the PGs should not be handled by asthmatics or used on animals with respiratory diseases.

GASTROINTESTINAL DRUGS

Antiemetics

Although certain species, such as horses, rabbits and rodents, are unable to vomit, protracted vomiting may become a problem in dogs, cats and other species.

The vomiting reflex may be stimulated through at least four different pathways. For example, chemical substances in the blood (bacterial toxins or certain drugs) may mediate vomiting via the chemoreceptor trigger zone (CTZ) pathway (medulla of brain). Vomiting arising from movement of the head (motion sickness) is transmitted through another pathway (cortex of the brain). In selecting an antiemetic agent, it is desirable to know the underlying cause of vomiting and the pathway involved, since some antiemetic drugs are specific in their site of action. Since vomiting may be a symptom of an underlying disease, initial attention should be directed to the treatment of the primary disease.

Although independent of their antihistaminic activity, a few of the antihistamines (dimenhydrinate, cyclizine, meclizine) and scopolamine are effective in preventing vomiting induced by motion sickness. The principal side effect of the antihistamines is drowsiness, which may not be undesirable in pets that are traveling.

A number of the phenothiazine tranquilizers (chlorpromazine, prochlorperazine, triflupromazine) are classified as broad-spectrum antiemetics, controlling vomiting by blocking the CTZ at low doses and the emetic center (found in the medulla of the brain) at higher doses. Although these agents have the potential of producing a number of adverse effects, the risk of toxicity is low because of the low dose and short duration of therapy. Some potent broad-spectrum, human antiemetics are finding use in veterinary medicine. Included would be haloperidol and metoclopramide.

Metoclopramide is a unique pharmacological agent that deserves additional comment. Besides its potent antiemetic property, especially for vomiting induced by drugs (e.g., cancer chemotherapy), metoclopramide is also a peristaltic stimulant, increasing gut motility. Thus, it has been employed for gastric stasis in a number of species, including horses and cattle. Also, in order to facilitate radiological examinations of stomach or small intestine, metoclopramide may be used to stimulate gastric emptying and intestinal transit of barium in cases where delayed emptying interferes. Reflux esophagitis in dogs and cats has also been treated with metoclopramide.

Emetics

Agents to induce vomiting are used clinically as a rapid means of eliminating certain poisons or to remove food from the stomach prior to induction of general anesthesia. A once common emetic used in veterinary medicine is apomorphine. Although still commercially available, it is extremely expensive and difficult to obtain. Apomorphine stimulates the CTZ and may be administered orally, intramuscularly, intravenously or via the conjunctival sac of the eye. Since apomorphine depresses the emetic center, repeated dosing is not recommended when the initial dose is ineffective. Apomorphine should *not* be given to cats because it produces extreme excitement. However, xylazine, a sedative analgesic, can be used as an emetic in cats because of the routine vomiting it produces in this species.

Ipecac, once used commonly in cats and occasionally in dogs, has the disadvantage of having to be administered via a stomach tube because of taste. In addition, its effects may be somewhat sporadic, some toxic effects, including death, may be induced in cats. Ipecac syrup does remain a popular, convenient emetic for children for the removal of accidentally ingested noncorrosive poisons.

Antidiarrheal Agents

Diarrhea, like vomiting, may only be a symptom of an underlying problem. Ideally, it is best to identify the specific problem and correct it. Current trends are not to slow the gut but to allow it to remain active in removing any toxins or irritants present. Most small animals with diarrhea recover regardless of therapy. However, persistent diarrhea not only may be offensive to pet owners, but also may require supportive treatment, such as electrolyte and fluid replacement. Anticholinergics, such as the various belladonna alkaloids (atropine, homatropine and scopolamine), have historically been used for treating diarrhea. Although *peristalsis* (propulsive contractions) is reduced with these agents, resistance to flow created by rhythmic contractions is also reduced, thus resulting in a minimal antidiarrheal effect. Because anticholinergics are not without hazards (increased heart rate, dryness of mouth, even diarrhea from gut paralysis), their value is questionable. (As a note of caution, atropine should never be used in horses except as an antidote to life-threatening organophosphate poisoning.)

Opiate drugs, including opium tincture, morphine, codeine and similar derivatives, such as diphenoxylate, are unique in that they increase rhythmic segmentation contractions, which resist intestinal flow and decrease peristalsis. In addition, the opiates increase the tone of the various sphincters and valves in the gastrointestinal tract, which further delays movement of the contents. The commercial product of diphenoxylate (Lomotil, Searle), which is only available with a small amount of atropine, is effective in treating diarrhea in dogs.

An over-the-counter combination suspension of kaolin and pectin is widely used in human medicine. Kaolin is thought to act as an adsorbent, binding toxins and bacteria, as well as a protectant by its coating of the gastrointestinal tract. Pectin may also have some adsorbent and protectant properties. Because of the poor palatability and the volume required per dose, the mixture is difficult to administer to animals. Even though tablets are available, the number of tablets required to be effective makes treating large dogs expensive and cumbersome.

Cathartics (Laxatives)

There are relatively few clinical reasons to use cathartics in veterinary medicine. Occasionally, an older animal may suffer constipation, but usually alteration of the diet will correct the problem. Another indication might be for the treatment of hairballs in cats. Following bowel or anal surgery, stool softeners may reduce stress at the surgery site until healing takes place. Cathartics as well as enemas may also be used prior to gastrointestinal tract radiographic examinations, proctoscopy or elective surgery. One of the most legitimate uses of cathartics is in treating food animals and horses suffering from overingestion of concentrated carbohydrates such as grain. There are a few other unique circumstances in which the use of cathartics is appropriate; however, one is discouraged from overuse because it leads to dependence.

Cathartics increase the motility of the bowel by directly stimulating the smooth muscle or indirectly activating receptors through increased bulk. The irritant laxatives, which directly increase bowel motility, include (1) emodin, found in cascara sagrada, aloe and senna; (2) sodium ricinoleate, a digestive end-product of castor oil; and (3) danthron, a synthetic compound. Bulk-producing cathartics include (1) undigestible materials, such as psyllium seed (Metamucil, Searle), methylcellulose or mineral oil and white petrolatum, which not only increase bulk but also lubricate and soften fecal mass; (2) saline cathartics, such as magnesium sulfate, sodium sulfate, magnesium oxide and phosphate salts, which draw water into the bowel; and (3) stool softeners, such as docusate sodium (DSS, formerly named dioctyl sodium sulfosuccinate) and dioctyl calcium sulfosuccinate (Surfak, Hoechst), which are surface active agents, like soap, that increase bulk through water retention, and they also lubricate and soften the fecal mass.

The cathartics as a group are relatively safe for short-term use, though some may be harsh, causing cramping and diarrhea. Chronic use of the petrolatum-type cathartics may, however, lead to deficiencies in fat-soluble vitamins because of absorption interference.

Ulcer Management Drugs

Gastric ulceration and subsequent blood loss appear to be related to acid damage commonly associated with high doses of corticosteroids or nonsteroidal anti-inflammatory drugs (NSAIDs) as well as to certain medical disorders. Several methods are currently available for treatment and prevention.

Antacids were used initially, but required round-the-clock administration every 2 to 3 hours to truly be effective. A major advance in human medicine for ulcer management was the introduction of cimetidine, a histamine H_2-receptor antagonist. Although these agents are not approved for veterinary use, cimetidine, ranitidine, and others are being employed to block the acid-producing effects of histamine on the gastric parietal cells.

Sucralfate in an acid environment forms an ulcer-adherent complex providing a protective, Band-aid like barrier for the damaged mucosa. Sucralfate also inhibits pepsin activity.

Omeprazole is a new agent that acts directly on the parietal cell, blocking acid secretion. Misoprostol not only blocks gastric acid secretion but also appears to enhance natural gastromucosal defense mechanisms.

INVENTORY CONTROL

To maintain an active working inventory requires both planning and continuous monitoring. Failure to keep abreast of usage and needs results in shortage, inefficient utilization of time, increased costs and added stress. Therefore, the time invested to sustain appropriate levels of stock is beneficial to the overall practice operation.

Veterinary technicians who demonstrate an active inventory concern may find themselves acquiring an increasing role in inventory control and maintenance. Assuming this additional responsibility not only increases one's value in the practice but also adds to job satisfaction.

Ideally, the quantities of each item stocked should be as small as possible without running out between reasonable ordering periods. Since shortages of certain items are worse than having extra, most practices lean toward a higher inventory than actually required. Inventory turnover (the total cost of goods sold annually divided by the average inventory level) should be at least four to six times per year. With the assistance of a computer monitoring daily usage and keeping helpful records, this turnover can usually be increased.

Inventory Maintenance

The primary disadvantage of having a large inventory is the expense of having working capital tied up in drugs and supplies. However, there are other factors, such as the difficulty in switching to better or less expensive products until the current supply is exhausted. In addition, there is greater potential for outdating, breakage, spoilage and obsolescence. Some states have inventory taxes that provide added incentive for keeping working stock to a minimum.

Occasionally, there is some justification for increasing one's purchase of certain products. The "savings" claimed through many of the "deals" offered by vendors should be approached with caution. Unless one can predict accurately the usage of certain products, quantity buying is difficult to justify. In order to participate in most marketing promotions a significant financial commitment is usually required. Before entering into these agreements, one should truly determine whether the products offered are desirable and will be used within a reasonable period and whether the "savings" really merit the capital commitment.

Processing small individual orders is costly because the time commitment required to process the order is not much different than that of a larger order having several items. One is justified in increasing quantities on these small orders, especially if the items are inexpensive, in order to reduce ordering frequency and cost of acquisition.

A factor that will affect one's inventory turnover will be the availability of replacement goods. With some items one may be able to predict monthly usage accurately and maintain a few weeks' supply. Unfortunately, the usage of most items cannot be readily anticipated, which results in larger inventory requirements, especially if the replacement stock cannot be readily obtained.

Procurement

Veterinary Suppliers

One may purchase supplies through veterinary wholesale suppliers (distributors) or directly from manufacturers. Distributors may specialize in one class of item, such as surgical supplies or bulk pharmaceuticals, but many offer a complete line of veterinary products, ranging from buckets to gas machines. In dealing with wholesalers, one has the advantage of reducing the number of small orders that would be required in purchasing from several individual outlets. A few manufacturers, however, only sell their products directly to veterinarians rather than through distributors. A fairly complete reference of veterinary pharmaceutical companies and their product lines is found in Veterinary Pharmaceuticals and Biologicals (Veterinary Medicine Publishing Co., 1992) or the Compendium of Veterinary Products (North American Compendiums Inc., 1993).

Veterinary Clinics

For immediate crisis needs, it is nice to enjoy a good relationship with another clinic in the area. A borrowing relationship is encouraged rather than a buying one. If someone borrows, you know they are going to order the item and return it. If they are buying it from you, you may end up being their supplier, especially for expensive short-dated items.

Pharmacies and Drug Wholesalers

Utilizing the services of a retail pharmacy is nearly essential to practice quality veterinary medicine. Retail pharmacies may not stock many injectable products, but they can help with most ophthalmics, with topical preparations and with some oral products. The veterinarian will have need for various products for humans that may not be obtainable through routine veterinary suppliers. In some locations, one may find drug wholesalers for humans that deal with the small, individual practitioner directly. Most, however, do not welcome these small accounts and deal only with hospitals and pharmacies. Therefore, the practitioner must make arrangements with pharmacists to obtain human products for clinic or client use. Most pharmacists will welcome this opportunity to serve the veterinarian. It is hoped that the days of direct competition between professions are limited.

Hospitals and Hospital Suppliers

Local hospitals may be a valuable resource for the veterinary clinic. However, recent federal law restricts hospitals with special buying privileges from selling to anyone outside their institution. As a result, veterinarians and their clients cannot easily obtain some of the more potent, expensive and rarely used medical supplies, except in an emergency. Human hospital contacts should be made to determine which supplies and drugs are available locally. The hospital's library and clinical laboratory may also provide some welcome assistance at times.

Some practices may have local human hospital suppliers available, which stock items such as syringes, needles, cotton balls and tongue depressors. Although one may not purchase routinely from the local supplier, at times of shortages do not overlook them as an immediate supply source.

Other Sources of Supplies

Major chemical suppliers not only will stock chemicals (ammonium chloride, magnesium sulfate, sodium bicarbonate and so on) but also will have glassware, balances, disposable beakers, brushes and carboys, as well as many other labor- and time-saving devices that would be useful in a veterinary clinic. Most of these suppliers are located in metropolitan areas and have addresses and telephone numbers listed in the telephone directory.

Numerous mail order suppliers exist, providing not only pharmaceuticals but also a wide variety of veterinary products and equipment. Quality of products and service may vary greatly between these outlets. Of major concern is the company's return policy for handling inferior or unacceptable items.

Professional journals and, more commonly, trade magazines advertise a wide variety of veterinary products. Most likely a telephone number and/or address is provided so that one may obtain additional product and ordering information.

Feed stores and lay veterinary drug outlets can be used for an occasional urgently needed item. One may at times also want to take advantage of certain specials offered through these suppliers.

ORGANIZING THE PHARMACY

Whether planning a major hospital complex or rearranging a small portion of one, a comprehensive list should be prepared of all activities conducted within the area as well as the activities interacting with other areas or outside agencies. Activities related to the pharmacy include storage (refrigeration, security), ordering, receiving, clean-up, dispensing, withdrawal and administration of medication, compounding and manufacturing, product information, and so on. In one's design, the location for each activity needs to be determined and each activity coordinated with other areas when required. Although most areas will be multifunctional, such as office space being used for ordering, references, correspondence or storage of reports, some activities may be unique and have their own special requirements.

A detailed list of activities pertaining specifically to the pharmacy inventory would include:

1. Ordering, which requires a telephone, desk, file and calculator
2. Receiving, which should be near an outside door and have temporary counter or floor space
3. Returns, which is an area for holding broken items, outdated items and so forth
4. Storage, which includes working inventory, back-up inventory, refrigeration and secure storage for volatile or hazardous bulk materials
5. Pricing, which involves the price book, mark-up tables, records and so on

In addition, one would have to consider the movement of items to areas of use or dispensing. The monitoring of the inventory level of all items for usage and reorder would also need consideration.

Arrangement of Inventory

Working inventory should be placed on shelves in an organized fashion. One method is to arrange items by dosage form. Categories would include:

1. Oral solids (tablets and capsules)
2. Oral liquids
3. Oral miscellaneous (boluses, powders, pastes)
4. External liquids
5. External miscellaneous (sprays, powders, ointments, creams)
6. Ophthalmics (ointments, suspensions, solutions)
7. Otics
8. Small-volume injectables
9. Large-volume injectables
10. Mastitis preparations
11. Miscellaneous (e.g., chemicals for compounding)

Each section should be further arranged, perhaps by generic name or brand name or by the more common name used by individuals in the practice. One may wish to make exceptions for items that are popular, but they should be limited.

A different type of arrangement would be to group items by their most common therapeutic use. Classification would be similar to that in the discussion of drugs found in the first portion of this chapter.

1. Anesthetics
2. Tranquilizers

3. Anticonvulsants
4. Analgesics
5. Anti-inflammatory drugs
6. Cardiovascular drugs
7. Fluids and electrolytes
8. Diuretics
9. Parasiticides
10. Antibiotics
11. Other antibacterials
12. Antineoplastics
13. Hormones and related substances
14. Gastrointestinal drugs
15. Vitamins

The grouping could be further subdivided into more specific uses, such as gastrointestinal drugs into antiemetics, emetics, antidiarrheals, and so on, and then placed on the shelf according to name. However, some classes may only have two or three items. Another disadvantage is poor use of shelf space. Unless a number of exceptions are made, gallon jugs may end up next to ampules.

Another arrangement is to group items by company or vendor. This method may be acceptable for back-up stock because it is helpful when preparing orders. However, in an active inventory, there is again poor use of shelf space. Perhaps the greatest disadvantage is trying to recall the last supplier for rarely used items. Purchasing generic items from multiple vendors would probably lead to multiple locations of the same item and duplicate stock.

Pharmacy organization is desirable and has advantages, primarily by assisting each individual in locating items. However, the best method of organizing stock is probably a combination of the various arrangements above. Each practice should design its own method. In addition to the methods listed, placing selected items in areas where they are frequently used should also be considered.

DRUG LAWS

Federal Laws

Although the Food, Drug and Cosmetic Act of 1938 has been amended numerous times, it is still the basic federal law governing drugs in the United States. This law assures the public that drugs have been prepared through approved manufacturing standards and are safe as well as effective for the claims made. The Durham-Humphrey Amendment (1951) restricted the availability of certain drugs to prescriptions through licensed practitioners. Such drugs bear the legend "Caution: Federal law restricts this drug to use by or on the order of licensed veterinarian" or "Caution: Federal law prohibits dispensing without prescription." This class of drugs, which is referred to as *prescription drugs* or *legend drugs,* is that class deemed unsafe for lay medication. *Nonprescription* or *over-the-counter* drugs may be sold directly to clients but must bear extensive labeling, which includes warnings as well as instructions for proper use.

State Laws

Most state pharmacy laws are primarily concerned with the distribution of drugs within the state. These laws specify who is authorized to prescribe and dispense legend drugs, the licensing of outlets, records required and certain processing standards.

Since state laws are unique to each state, it is the responsibility of those practicing veterinary medicine to know the laws that apply to them. Most states have regulations governing dispensing practitioners, though these regulations are directed primarily toward physicians. Two important concerns that veterinary clinics should address regarding dispensing of drugs are proper labeling and proper dispensing records.

Labeling requirements vary between states but may include (1) name, address and telephone number of the clinic, (2) name of client, (3) species or name of pet, (4) date, (5) prescribing veterinarian, (6) adequate directions for proper use of medication, (7) name of medication (optional) and (8) prescription transaction number (optional). Auxiliary labels may also be required to caution or inform the client. Examples would include "shake well," "keep refrigerated," "do not use after (date)," "poison," "external use only," "for veterinary use only."

The ultimate responsibility for any medication dispensed through a veterinary practice is with the authorizing veterinarian. In some states, the technician may be allowed to assist the veterinarian by typing labels, counting or pouring, attaching labels and pricing. However, *technicians should not refill or issue medications without the veterinarian's approval.* For most medications, this would be in violation of federal law.

Readily retrievable dispensing records may be required by some states in order to safeguard the public's health. Accidental ingestion of prescription drugs by small children is not uncommon. Proper records can provide attending physicians with the name and the amount of medication dispensed so that proper treatment may be initiated.

The federal Poison Prevention Packaging Act passed in 1970 requires pharmacists and physicians to dispense medications intended for oral human use in childproof containers. Although this act does not apply directly to veterinary drugs, childproof container usage is considered "state of the art."

Veterinary clinics failing to employ such a safeguard would be highly vulnerable to legal action in a case of accidental poisoning.

Controlled Substances

The Controlled Substances Act of 1970 was passed to combat drug abuse by defining certain legal and illegal acts regarding substances of high abuse potential. It furthermore established and authorized the Drug Enforcement Administration (DEA) to enforce this law. The law is designed to provide an approved means for proper manufacture, distribution, dispensing and use of controlled substances through licensing of legitimate handlers of these drugs. This "closed" system has been effective in reducing widespread diversion of these drugs into the illicit market. Controlled substances are classified into five categories (schedules) according to their use or abuse potential (Table 20–6).

All veterinarians using these drugs in the course of their practice are required to have a DEA license number. Those who engage in administering or dispensing controlled substances in schedules II, III, IV and V are required to keep records of such transactions for 2 years. Receiving records or reports of controlled substances received must also be kept for 2 years. In addition, practitioners having controlled substances in their possession are required to take an initial inventory, followed by an inventory every 2 years, of all controlled substances. Records for *schedule II substances* must be kept separate from all other records, whereas records for substances in schedules III, IV and V must only be "readily retrievable."

It is best that those persons responsible for handling controlled substances be familiar not only with federal laws governing them but also with state laws, which may be more strict. Agencies such as the State Board of Pharmacy or the local DEA office are quite helpful in answering questions concerning compliance.

The law states that, "A practitioner who has controlled substances stored in his office or clinic must keep these drugs in a securely locked, substantially constructed cabinet or safe." A secure area is usually interpreted as a double-locked container that cannot be picked up and moved. Examples would be a locked metal box stored inside a floor safe or an attached

			Table 20–6		
		SCHEDULE OF CONTROLLED SUBSTANCES			
Schedule	**Abuse Potential**	**Dispensing Limits**	**Distribution Restrictions**	**Schedule Examples**	**Comments**
I	High	Research use only	DEA form 222 required	LSD, heroin	No accepted medical use
II	High	Requires written prescription, no refills	DEA form 222 required	Oxymorphone, sodium pentobarbital injection	Abuse may lead to severe dependence
III	Less than I and II	Oral or written, refills up to five times within 6 mo	DEA registration number	Hycodan, Tylenol with codeine, anabolic steroids	Abuse may lead to moderate dependence
IV	Low	Oral or written, refills up to five times within 6 mo	DEA registration number	Diazepam, phenobarbital	Abuse may lead to limited dependence
V	Low	No DEA limits	DEA registration number	Lomotil, Robitussin AC	Lowest potential for abuse

locked wall cabinet. The responsibility for access to controlled substances should be restricted to only one or two people in the clinic practice. Practitioners experiencing theft or significant loss of controlled substances must report such loss to the DEA Regional Office and the local police department when the loss is discovered.

The state of Colorado developed and published an excellent, comprehensive set of guidelines for the proper handling of controlled substances in a veterinary practice. These guidelines were "de-regionalized" and included in the Appendix of *Veterinary Drug Handbook 1992*. Some of the material incorporated into the guidelines was obtained from a government publication entitled the *Physician's Manual, An Information Outline on the Controlled Substances Act of 1970*. This government manual may be obtained free by request from the following:

U.S. Department of Justice
Drug Enforcement Administration
1465 "I" Street, N.W.
Washington, D.C. 20537

References

Plumb DC: Veterinary Drug Handbook. White Bear Lake, MN, PharmaVet Publishing, 1992.
Spinelli JS and Enos LR: Drugs in Veterinary Practice. Minneapolis, Alpha Editions, Div. of Burgess Publishing Co., 1978.

Recommended Reading

Booth NH and McDonald LE: Veterinary Pharmacology and Therapeutics. 6th ed. Ames, IA, Iowa State University Press, 1988.
Compendium of Veterinary Products. Port Huron, MI, North American Compendium, Inc., 1993.
Gilman AG, Rall TW, Nies AS and Taylor P: The Pharmacological Basis of Therapeutics. 8th ed. New York, Pergamon Press, 1990.
Kirk RW and Bonagura JD: Current Veterinary Therapy XI: Small Animal Practice. Philadelphia, WB Saunders Co., 1992.
Upson DW: Upson's Handbook of Clinical Veterinary Pharmacology. 3rd ed. Manhattan, KS, Dan Upson Enterprises, 1988.
USPDI: Drug Information for the Health Care Provider. 12th ed. Rockville, MD, USPC, 1992.
Veterinary Pharmaceuticals and Biologicals 1992–1993, 8th Ed. Lenexa, KS, Veterinary Medicine Publishing Co., 1993.

21

Clinical Nutrition

STEPHEN W. CRANE and SHEILA R. GROSDIDIER

The professionalism and knowledge displayed by the veterinary technician strongly complements the veterinarian's provision of nutritional information to clients. Information most commonly sought is what to feed and how to feed. Education of the owner prior to a patient's discharge is important at transitional feeding periods, that is, when foods are being changed. Nutritional assessment and specialized feeding for anorectic and hospitalized patients represent another major role for the technician.

Additionally, nearly every veterinary practice dispenses dietary animal foods, and many provide well-animal pet foods. The technician will be seen as a source of authoritative advice and a complement to the veterinarian's recommendations.

This chapter defines nutrients and their use, distinguishes nutrients from ingredients, and suggests nutrient intake levels for pets, horses and livestock. Determination of food dosage for pet animals, true feeding costs (cents per calorie) and quality assessment guidelines for livestock forage and prepared animal foods are also discussed. A summary of companion animal clinical nutrition familiarizes the reader with dietary therapy. Basic assisted feeding techniques for hospitalized animals are also described.

OVERVIEW OF NUTRITIONAL OBJECTIVES AND PRINCIPLES

Nutritional goals differ sharply between agricultural and companion animals. As in human nutrition, the goal of feed-ing pets is to maximize length and quality of life by reducing food intake risk factors that work against wellness (Morris et al., 1987). The other aspect of well-pet nutrition is to elect nutrient intake patterns consistent with current physiological need. Feeding an adult dog for maintenance, instead of as a puppy, is one example.

In production animal agriculture, feed conversion efficiency and least-cost ration formulation are important aspects of nutritional management. Production animals require perfect targeting of nutritional objectives to meet growth and lactation requirements because the cost of animal feed is a major percentage of production costs. Veterinary technicians working in dairy and beef herd health areas often participate in detailed nutritional analysis. Nutrition in the poultry, swine and aquacultural finishing industries is usually managed by nutritionists rather than veterinarians.

ENERGY-PRODUCING NUTRIENTS

A nutrient is any substance ingested to support life and may be classified as an energy-producing nutrient or a non–energy-producing nutrient. Energy-producing nutrients are sugars, amino acids, and fatty acids. While nutritionally different, each nutrient class possesses a common availability and structure of hydrocarbon, making them suitable as metabolic "fuels." Digestion, assimilation and metabolism of nutrients produce the chemical energy for the "fire of life." The energy released from metabolism of food fuels deposits in chemical bonds that are held in a ready-to-use form in storage molecules (adenosine triphosphate, ATP). The storage molecules are the source of energy for cell maintenance, reproduction, repair, heat production, muscle contraction and the synthesis of new tissue.

Carbohydrates: Sugars, Starches and Fibers

"Carbohydrate" is a general biochemical classification that includes sugars, starches and fibers. Sugars are numerous and include mono- and disaccharides and more complicated sugar molecules. Multiple sugars can bond and link to form complex sugar polymers. Polymerized sugars are the starches and fibers. The starch or fiber type depends on sugar species and type of polymer linkages. Glucose (a monosaccharide blood sugar) and lactose (a disaccharide milk sugar) are two important animal sugars. Glycogen is an animal-specific starch and can quickly depolymerize to release its glucose content. Glycogen storage in the body is limited.

In the plant kingdom, starches and fibers are numerous and diverse. Feed grain starches are an energy source of fundamental importance to animals. Cellulose and other fiber are structural elements of grass, plants and wood. Mammals lack fiber-degrading enzyme systems, so fiber is not digestible by the monogastric mammal. However, fiber is digestible by bacteria and protozoan microbes in the rumen and cecum of herbivorous animals. Short-chain fatty acids result from fiber digestion and these are transformable to glucose. Fiber thus serves as a major energy source for grazing animals. Debates over the environmental impacts and costs of cattle grazing and feedlot finishing sometimes ignore the creation of high-quality animal-sourced protein from inedible plant tissues. In monogastrics, fiber reduces digestibility and effective caloric density yet maintains dry matter bulk. This effect finds applications in reducing caloric density for weight control foods. Some metabolic and gastrointestinal (GI) tract transit disorders also respond to fiber therapy (Blaxter et al., 1990; Dimski, 1992).

Lipids, Fatty Acids, Fats and Oils

Fatty acids are building block components of vegetable and animal fats. The type and distribution of constituent fatty acids determine the physical, nutritional and biological characteristics of the fat or oil. Lipids have one to three molecules of fatty acids, are highly digestible and have twice the caloric density of a similar quantity of carbohydrate or protein. Fat imparts significant food flavor that often improves its acceptability and palatability. Fat also facilitates digestion and assimilation of fat-soluble vitamins (A, D, E and K). The technician will see literature referring to types of fatty acids. The length of the carbon chain "backbone" identifies a fatty acid as "long-chain," "medium-chain" or "short-chain." Short-chain fatty acids (1 to 8 carbon atoms in length) from rumen fluids and gases are important sources of energy, but their distribution ratio can be unbalanced by rapidly changed roughage:concentrate ratios in feeds. Long-chain fatty acids (12 to 20 + carbon units) are the most common components of dietary fats and oils.

The degree of hydrogen saturation (numbers of hydrogen per carbon) is variable, and "saturated," "unsaturated" or "polyunsaturated" denote hydrogen content. A high quantity of unsaturated or polyunsaturated fatty acid distribution usually yields the oil form of a lipid at room temperature. More saturated fatty acid content produces fats with a higher melting point. Positioning of double-bond carbon to carbon linkages within the fatty acid leads to further subclassifications. "Omega 6" and "omega 3" fatty acids designate some of these positioning features. The ratio of "omega 6" to "omega 3" distribution has different biological effects in several body systems and has increasingly important therapeutic applications in clinical nutrition (Bauer et al., 1989; Campbell, 1992).

Amino Acids and Protein

Amino acids are the building blocks for plant and animal protein. Gastric and intestinal digestion subdivides protein into progressively smaller peptide units. The digested protein yields the amino acids that are assimilated into a common amino acid pool. The amino acids are then available for protein synthesis. The turnover and depletion of the pool determine the current amino acid requirement. Growth and lactation increase requirements more than maintenance and exertional work or exercise.

Amino Acids as Energy Sources

Amino acids can serve as energy nutrients as well as synthesis units for new protein. Any amino acid intake beyond requirements of the circulating pool is metabolized into energy. This is because there is no way to "store" extra amino acids from excess dietary protein as new viscera or muscle. Conversion of extra amino acids into energy is a several-step process. Removal of the amino (nitrogen-containing) group from the hydrocarbon skeleton of the amino acid is the first step. The conversion of the hydrocarbon skeleton into ATP, CO_2 and water is the second step. The nitrogen content must be eliminated as the third step. In addition to being "expensive energy," the metabolism of excess amino acids increases liver and kidney processing and excretory requirements for the urea and organic acid waste by-products.

Essential Amino Acids

All 22 amino acids are necessary for synthesis of new protein. As the body synthesizes 12 amino acids, an "essential" amino acid is one requiring supply from oral intake or ruminal synthesis (Table 21–1). The quantity and distribution of essential amino acids in a protein are important features determining a protein's biological quality. All proteins are not of equal worth, and an "ideal" protein contains the exact essential amino acid distribution profile to meet a specific requirement (Schaeffer et al., 1989; Van Horn, 1991). When profiles are not "ideal" (the case in practical diets), a higher biological quality of protein better fulfills amino acid requirements with more efficiency and lower total nitrogen content than a low-quality protein. A "limiting" amino acid is one cause of a decreased protein quality. When an otherwise high biological value protein has a missing essential amino acid and, therefore, a more limited quality, the full potential of the biological value of the protein is restored when the limiting acid is added. This is one reason why mixed animal and plant protein sources are often complementary to each other in food formulation.

Table 21–1
ESSENTIAL AMINO ACIDS
Arginine
Histidine
Isoleucine
Leucine
Lysine
Methionine
Phenylalanine
Threonine
Tryptophan
Valine
Taurine*
Glycine†

*Cats only
†Poultry only

Amino Acids as Emergency Fuels

Amino acids can produce energy during starvation or other negative energy balance situations. As starch and fatty acid stores are depleted, amino acids mobilize from skeletal muscle and visceral proteins to provide glucose for energy. Gluconeogenesis (chemical breakdown of protein for glucose) is a valuable survival mechanism but "wastes" vital circulating and structural proteins. Loss of muscle mass and strength is a common clinical observation during anorexia and illness/injury, and muscle atrophy is a fundamental signal to the technician that protein is supplying energy.

Protein Requirements

Clients often inquire about the "best" protein intake for animals. Crude protein quantity (on the label) is the usual concern, and clients assume that "more is better." However, a "high protein number" is not always the defining criterion for food quality. Chemical analysis for crude protein measures only total nitrogen content. The essential to nonessential amino acid profile, protein digestibility, and amino acid bioavailability are neither measured nor stated. Lower quantities of a higher biological quality protein usually represent a higher-quality food and a more appropriate nutritional objective.

In cats, gluconeogenic amino acids are a major source of energy, and cats are specifically adapted to high protein intake (Morris and Rogers, 1989). Herbivores evolved eating seasonal grasses and plants and have rumen or cecal microbes capable of synthesizing a portion of the amino acid requirement (Simons and Hand, 1993). Therefore, herbivores have lower amino acid requirements. Supplying a nonprotein nitrogen source (urea) to ruminants also assists the microbes in their synthetic activity.

NON–ENERGY-PRODUCING NUTRIENTS

Oxygen and Water

Oxygen is a "nutrient" because it permits the "burn" of the energy substrate. If oxygen is the most limiting of all nutrients, water is the most important of the orally ingested nutrients.

Water quality issues matter greatly to animals. In production animal agriculture, the provision of an accessible and potable water supply is a fundamental, and perhaps limiting, husbandry resource (Carson, 1993). Dehydration from heavy sweat and prolonged work can be compensated for in animals by periodically watering them while they are working if that is possible. Frozen water can result in dehydration of animals, and a functioning stock tank heater or ice-breaking is needed for livestock under conditions of prolonged freezing weather. Dehydration is a common and frequently major clinical problem in sick patients unwilling or unable to eat and drink.

Minerals

"Macro" and "micro" describe two mineral intake levels. Calcium, phosphorus, magnesium, sodium, potassium, chlorine and sulfur are dietary macro minerals. Macro minerals are constituents of bone and structural proteins, and they participate as cofactors and catalysts in many biochemical reactions. When minerals circulate as ionized cation or anion electrolytes, they participate in osmotic fluid balance, nerve conduction, muscle contraction, blood clotting, blood pH buffering and numerous other physiological processes.

Requirements for the macro minerals are expressed as parts per hundred (percent). Deficiency of macro mineral intake produces serious clinical effects, but these are uncommon with proper feeding of appropriate foods. Deficiency most frequently follows anorexia, starvation or poor-quality food. Excess macro mineral intake results from supplementation or poorer-quality foods high in mineral-containing ingredients such as meat and bone meal. Owner supplementation leads to excess when a food is already adequate in macro minerals. The technician most commonly encounters this situation among well-intentioned, but uninformed, purebred animal hobbyists. When adequate calcium and vitamin D in foal or puppy foods are supplemented for "support" of rapid skeletal growth, a resulting hypercalcemia may actually inhibit normal bone growth and cartilage maturation.

Micro Minerals

Important micro or "trace" minerals are iron, zinc, manganese, copper, iodine and selenium. Dietary requirements for these minerals are in parts per million (mg/kg) instead of the percent levels for macro minerals. Hemoglobin, thyroxin, and many enzymes and cofactors contain micro mineral constituents. Trace mineral deficiency and intoxication syndromes are potentially important in all species. Iron-deficient intake and chronic blood loss leads to depleted iron stores. Trace mineral deficiency can also result from bioavailability reductions from a competitive inhibition of assimilation. High calcium and/or phytate content may reduce bioavailability of zinc, copper and other minerals, and zinc-responsive dermatoses are seen in hogs and dogs fed inferior, high-mineral foods.

Selenium deficiency and intoxication states are important in herbivore livestock. Deficient selenium intake contributes to a specific muscle disease (white muscle disease). Selenium intoxication occurs when grazing animals consume selenium-accumulating plants. There is a diverse geographical distribution of both low- and high-selenium soils. The technician should consult the agricultural extension service for local soil characteristics and learn to identify selenium-accumulating forages and weeds (James, 1993; Lewis, 1982).

Vitamins

"Vitamin" (from "vital amine") describes essential dietary cofactors that participate in many biochemical reactions. Vitamins have both common and chemical names. Vitamins are classified as fat-soluble (A, D, E and K) or water-soluble (all B and C), based on water solubility and route of excretion. Vitamins are not energy nutrients, and intake in excess of requirements does not improve performance. However, vitamins are often ascribed mystical performance enhancement values, and the "more-is-better" philosophy is frequently encountered. In the world of performance athletes, where vitamin megatherapy is routinely encountered, abusive oversupplementation levels of fat-soluble vitamins may lead to hypervitaminosis syndromes.

"Nutrients" Versus "Ingredients"

The terms nutrient, ingredient, formula and nutrient profile are easily confused and sometimes used interchangeably. *Nutrients* are fundamental energy and metabolic substrates and cofactors such as lysine, glucose or zinc. *Ingredients* are the materials used to manufacture a finished feed. The *formula* selects and apportions ingredients. The *nutrient profile* describes the resulting quantitative distribution of the individual nutrients within the finished formula. These definitions are important in client education efforts when nutrient profile becomes confused with ingredients. In particular, some pet food advertising focuses on the presence of a particular ingredient as a brand point of difference. However, at the absorptive surface of the small intestinal mucosa, the ingredient of origin for a nutrient is immaterial.

Additives and Preservatives

"Additives" are non-energy, non-nutrient components added to protect nutrient stability or enhance acceptability. Clients sometimes question additives and preservatives from the standpoint of necessity and food safety. The technician will need an opinion on the subject of natural versus synthetic additives in particular.

Colors, flavors, palatability enhancement digests, emulsifying agents, stabilizers, thickeners and dough conditioners are examples of additives. Preservation of the nutrient profile is an important need achieved by both physical and chemical means. Dehydration is an important form of food preservation as seen in dried meats, dry pet food and dry hay. Drying can protect nutrients for months. Canned pet foods use heat sterilization, an anaerobic environment, and a physical vacuum as a preservative and antioxidant system. Chemical preservatives are additives that retard oxidation, discoloration or spoilage.

Organic acids or inorganic salts, such as common table salt, have preservative effect through their antimicrobic activity (salted meats). Humectants are a preservative additive that binds water to inhibit mold and fungal growth. Chemicals that inhibit oxygen's destruction of vulnerable bonds are antioxidants. These agents primarily protect fatty acids and fat-soluble vitamins from rancid oxidation and loss of potency. Over the

food's shelf life, a significant percentage of an antioxidant is "consumed" doing its job. One may question the need for additives such as colors. However, the additives generally protect product quality and have good safety records based on years of application in animal agriculture and in pets (Mumma et al., 1986).

ESTIMATING ANIMALS' ENERGY REQUIREMENTS

Energy requirement estimates are used to calculate feeding quantity. There are several predictive equations for energy requirements based on the animal's species and size (Table 21–2). Maintenance energy requirements are simply the calories needed to maintain neutral weight for the animal's current activity and environment. This number is a range affected by several activity and environmental factors (Fig. 21–1). Work, lactation and growth further modify energy requirements, and such multiples over maintenance are sometimes called production energy requirements.

Predictive equations are useful, but judging the body composition and condition is the key issue for energy balance assessment. The guideline for maintenance energy requirements is simply "To feel but not see the ribs." Production commensurate with genetic potential assesses adequacy of production energy intake.

COMPANION ANIMAL NUTRITION

Feeding Dogs

Dogs are highly social pack animals and cooperative team hunters. Wild-type feeding is both hierarchical and competitive with intrapack feeding order maintained by the alpha dominant animal. Food intake in wild canids is distinctly omnivorous, although pet food advertising emphasizes the carnivorous aspects of intake ("meatier is better"). Wild dogs eat intestines and intestinal contents of herbivorous prey, as well as organs and flesh. Many domesticated dogs will eat vegeta-

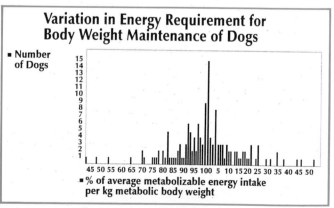

FIGURE 21–1. Different energy intake may be required to maintain stable body weight in the same breed of dog kept under the same kennel conditions. Different activity level and resting metabolic rate help to explain easy versus hard "keepers."

Table 21-2
CALCULATION OF ENERGY REQUIREMENTS AND FOOD DOSAGE

Calculation Steps:
1. Estimate maintenance energy requirement (MER)
   MER (Kcal/day)
   Dog = 2 (30 Wt kg + 70)
   Cat = 1.5 (30 Wt kg + 70)
   For animals greater than 2 kg and less than 45 kg
2. Factor MER, as follows:

Activity	
Inactive pet = 0.6 to 0.8 × MER	1 hr light work = 1.1 × MER
1 day light work = 1.5 × MER	1 day heavy work = 2 to 4 × MER

Growth	
Weaning to 3 mo = 2 × MER	Giant breed puppies
3 to 6 mo = 1.6 × MER	3 to 9 mo = 1.6 × MER
6 to 12 mo = 1.2 × MER	9 to 24 mo = 1.2 × MER

   Reproduction
   Gestation: 1st 6 wk = MER; last 3 wk = 1.3 × MER
   Lactation. (≈3 wk) − [1 + (0.25 × # in litter)] × MER
3. Select specific food and determine energy density

Dog food (generic, private label and popular)	
Dry	350 Kcal/cup
Soft-moist	275 Kcal/cup
Canned	500 Kcal/15 oz can
Cat food (generic, private label and popular)	
Dry	300 Kcal/cup
Soft-moist	250 Kcal/cup
Canned	400 Kcal/15 oz can
	180 Kcal/6.5 oz can

4. Divide energy requirement by energy density of food, to obtain food
   dosage in cups or cans

bles, grains and pastas, meat, processed foods, various dairy products and even fruit. Dental and digestive anatomy and nutritional biochemistry further document the dog as omnivorous, and it is fair to say domesticated dogs can adapt well to a varied dietary intake (Morris and Rogers, 1989). However, when domesticated dogs eat grass and/or feces, owners complain that the pet is not behaving as a carnivore. While such ingestive behavior is natural, behavior modification (cayenne pepper sauce on the feces) may reduce the objectionable activity.

Canine Pediatric Nutrition

Puppies usually nurse soon after birth. Postsurgical nursing of the canine who has undergone cesarean section specifically notes colostrum production by the dam and intake by puppies prior to discharge from the hospital. Colostrum provides fluid for vital postpartum circulatory expansion and maternal immunity factors (globulin antibodies) for absorption by the intestine. Most puppies are healthy and are capable and active in nursing. Most mothers are lactating well and attentive to the litter. Therefore, no assistance is needed from the technician or owner. The possible exception is in extremely small, toy-breed puppies for whom frequent, assisted hand-feeding for several weeks after birth may be needed to preclude hypothermia and hypoglycemia. When there is concern about lactation, a quick indicator for quality and quantity, in addition to examining the milk itself, is to weigh the puppies. A normal growth rate for puppies is 2 to 4 g/day/kg of anticipated adult weight. Weight gain below this rate accompanied by restless hungry acting puppies is a sign of feeding distress.

Raising Orphan Puppies

Neonatal puppies unable to nurse require a canine milk replacer formula. Canine milk is higher in protein and lower in lactose than bovine milk, so water, not cow's milk, should be used to mix formula. The orphan formula dose is initially 15 percent of the puppy's body weight per day divided into several doses. Food dose adequacy is usually announced by the puppy's becoming content and going to sleep after feeding. Assisted feeding of neonates is by feeding syringe and a flexible, rubber feeding tube (Fig. 21-2A). If there is adequate nursing vigor, one may substitute a pet nurser system (Fig. 21-2B). At litter discharge from the hospital, the technician should pre-test flow rate from all nipples dispensed and give explicit instructions for sanitation and formula mixing. When the puppy reaches 2 to 3 weeks of age, the food dose approximates 25 percent of the body weight divided into 4 to 6 daily feedings.

Weaning Puppies

Peak lactation occurs at 4 weeks, and weaning concludes at 6 to 8 weeks. Begin introducing puppies to semisolid gruel made from 2 parts of water to 1 part of a high-quality, dry, canine growth/lactation pet food. Three weeks of age is a suitable time to introduce a semisolid gruel except for toy breeds and weak animals. Mash the mixture with a fork, and place the gruel in a shallow pan. Gruel ingestion inevitably follows a play period and begins acclimating the puppies to intake of particulate solids. At 5 weeks of age, puppies are reducing their intake of mother's milk and consuming significant amounts of gruel. The ratio of water can be reduced as the puppies approach total weaning onto dry or moist foods.

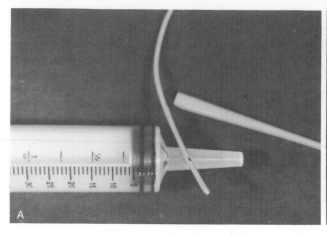
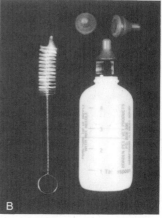

FIGURE 21–2. A, Orphan puppies and kittens are raised on species-specific milk replacer. Tube gavage with flexible feeding tube and a "catheter tip" syringe is an easy and safe technique in neonatal puppies and kittens. B, Pet nursers are used in neonates with adequate sucking vigor. Always test flow and temperature of formula in advance and sanitize equipment between uses.

Feeding Growing Dogs

Absolute and relative nutritional requirements change rapidly during a puppy's growth. Rate of growth, as well as final adult size, is obviously and dramatically different between various dog breeds. Most growing puppies eat four to five times daily during the post-weaning period, but meal frequency declines as gastrointestinal capacity increases. The quantity of food can be determined in several ways, and Table 21–2 demonstrates some model calculations for establishing a food dose. Slide rule calculators and computer programs are also useful in volume-restricted feeding situations.

Growth/lactation foods are recommended for puppies until they reach 90 percent of their skeletal maturity. The methods of feeding puppies require specific consideration. The ad-lib feeding method clearly causes excess nutrient intake in many puppies. When the puppy overconsumes energy and calcium, developmental bone disease may surface (Kallfelz, 1989B). This is especially evident in the rapidly growing members of the large and giant breeds. Unfortunately, some growth type pet foods contain excessive calcium even at appropriate levels of dry matter intake (Kallfelz, 1989A, 1989B). Energy overconsumption, by itself, was studied in two groups of Labrador Retriever puppies (Kealy et al., 1992). One group ate ad-lib, and the second group was limited to 75 percent of the ad-lib quantity. Serial pelvic radiography for two years showed significant reductions in hip laxity in the meal-limited group.

"Roly-poly" puppies also risk current and future obesity. The technician should emphasize the risk of juvenile overfeeding as a part of the client education program. This is especially true when the animal is a member (or cross breed) of obesity-prone breeds (Table 21–3).

Feeding Adult Dogs

A primary objective in feeding the adult dog is finding energy requirements and food doses that maintain neutral energy balance (Fig. 21–3). In adult dogs, ad-lib feeding is less labor-intensive for animal colony and kennels. Late detection of anorexia and timid animals not having adequate intake are potential problems with this method. When dogs are individually penned or can eat from self-feeders, these problems are eliminated.

Individual meal feeding is best whenever possible (Fig. 21–4). In the time-restricted method, feed from one to three times daily with an ad-lib consumption for 10 to 15 minutes. If the dog consistently leaves a little food in its dish and also maintains an ideal body condition, the conclusion must be that animal is self-regulating its food intake at its energy requirement. Time-restricted feeding works well for many dogs and their owners. However, some dogs ravenously overeat during the allotted time. In those dogs that overeat, try volume-restricted meal feeding by serving a calculated food dose. To determine the daily volume, divide the energy requirement by the food's caloric density. Then feed one half to one third of the daily volumes two to three times per day. An average caloric density guideline for pet foods is listed in Table 21–2. Other aids for food dose calculations are suggested feeding amounts on labels, food dose calculators, and technical information from manufacturers.

It should also be recommended that table scraps be eliminated or used in moderation (10 percent or less). Fat trimmings quickly unbalance a base diet and lead to "finicky" behavior and predisposition to obesity. Avoid feeding animal bones, as sharp fragments may wedge between teeth or lacerate the esophagus. Nylon bones and chew toys are safe substitutes for natural bones. Table 21–4 lists guidelines for assessing pet foods used in life-stage feeding. Maintenance pet food is recommended for the average house pet.

Feeding Adult Dogs with Increased Energy Needs

Increased energy is important in working dogs and stressed animals. Supply extra energy by using pet foods of increased caloric density and digestibility. This permits dry matter intake and gastric fill to remain at familiar, non-excessive levels. In-

Table 21–3 BREED EFFECTS ON OBESITY	
Obese Prone	**Non–Obese Prone**
Labrador Retriever	Yorkshire Terrier
Cairn Terrier	Whippet
Cocker Spaniel	Doberman
Shetland Sheepdog	Boxer
Dachshund	Greyhound
Basset Hound	Sealyham Terrier
Beagle	Staffordshire Bull Terrier

Modified from Edney ATB and Smith PM: Study of obesity in visiting veterinary practices in the United Kingdom. Vet Rec 118:391–396, 1986.

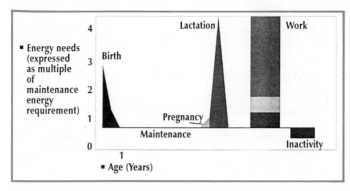

FIGURE 21–3. An important monitoring and counseling role for the technician is to periodically assess the pet's energy balance. Except for a few short periods, the majority of the life cycle is spent in adult "maintenance."

creasing the quantity and/or frequency of a regular food is a secondary option.

The technician can provide a high-quality client service by reminding hunting dog owners to aerobically condition animals before extensive field work. Training for 3 weeks prior to work conditions the muscles and cardiovascular system, and induces enzyme changes in the muscle that allow more efficient use of fatty acids as muscle fuel. The aerobic use of fatty acids spares the rate of consumption of muscle glycogen and can increase the interval to exhaustion.

When aerobic conditioning begins, convert the dog(s) to the more calorie-dense food and suggest feeding the majority of daily calories after completion of training to help prevent hunting dog hypoglycemia. Unfortunately, the more obvious feeding recommendation would seem to be the reverse—feeding prior to work. However, insulin release follows glucose assimilation following the meal's digestion, allowing a high rate of glucose transfer into the cells. If the animal simultaneously begins hard work, the combination of the two glucose-consuming activities may precipitate hypoglycemia. If animals show consistent signs of hunting dog hypoglycemia, even after conditioning, they may be fed 10 to 15 percent of the daily calorie dose as a light feeding at 2-hour intervals during work. Clients should also be reminded of the importance of adequate water.

Feeding During Pregnancy and Lactation

Early and mid-term pregnancy is a nutritional "non-event," but requirements increase modestly during the last one third of gestation. Recommend a growth/lactation formula to meet the increased requirements. Lactation markedly increases energy, protein, and mineral requirements. After whelping, the bitch returns to her regular body weight and eats to service increased needs (Fig. 21–5A). Expect food intake to rise rapidly by 50 percent the first week and by 200 to 400 percent by the fourth week of lactation. This level of demand is equivalent to those of heavily pulling sled dogs, and the loss of fat and even muscle is common during lactation. This potential underfeeding situation can be helped by allowing ad-lib intake of a high-quality growth/lactation pet food. Supplements are *not* needed for normal animals when high-quality pet foods are used.

Weaning the Litter

Food intake should be terminated for 24 hours to help the bitch slow and stop her milk production. The food intake can

be resumed using maintenance foods at one third of the customary maintenance level. On the second day, use two thirds feeding and full intake on day three. When lactation quickly dries from acute calorie deprivation, the bitch will more readily reject the puppies' attempts to continue to nurse.

Obesity-Prone Animals

Definition and Causes of Obesity

The malnutrition of obesity is at epidemic proportions. Canine obesity estimates are 30 percent, with feline obesity as

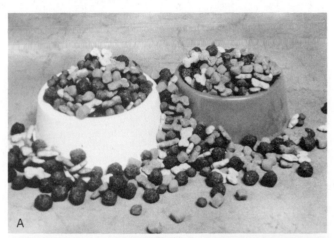

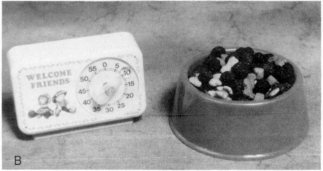

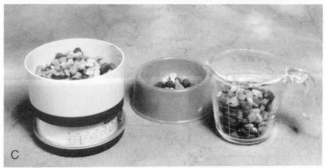

FIGURE 21–4. A, Free choice (ad-lib) feeding is frequently unsuitable for adult maintenance because of pets' overconsumption. This method is indicated during lactation or heavy work or in animals that prefer to "graze" over the day and are not prone to be obese. Ad-lib feeding is most suited to dry pet food. B, Time-restricted meal feeding offers free choice consumption limited to 10 to 15 minutes. The owner helps the pet to self-regulate food intake by removing uneaten food after that interval. This method does not work for highly voracious animals. C, Volume-restricted meal feeding controls calorie intake in self-engorging animals. The owner must control calorie intake by scheduling and measuring meals.

Table 21–4
NUTRIENT GUIDELINES FOR LIFE-STAGE PET FOODS*

Life Stage	Food Characteristics	Comments
Cat Kittens 8 weeks–1 year Gestation/lactation	Metabolizable energy 4.5 Kcal/g dry matter Digestibility ≥80% Protein 35%–49% Fat 17%–30% Fiber ≤5% Calcium/phosphorus ratio 1.0–1.8 to 0.8–1.6 Magnesium ≤20 mg/100 Kcal	Transition the queen to a growth diet at 3 weeks of gestation. Ad-lib feeding is acceptable to kittens and queens.
Adult cat	Metabolizable energy >3.75 Kcal/g dry matter Digestibility >78%† Protein 26%–45% Fat 9%–25% Magnesium <20 mg/100 Kcal	Maintain optimum weight. Meal feed to help prevent obesity.
Obese-prone cat	Metabolizable energy <3.50–3.75 Kcal/g dry matter Digestibility >75% Fiber 7%–12% Protein 35%–45% Fat 8%–17% Magnesium <20 mg/100 Kcal	Feed multiple meals (3–4) daily. Fiber provides satiety and decreased caloric density.
Dog Puppies Gestation/lactation	Metabolizable energy >3.9 Kcal/g of diet Digestibility >80% Protein 27%–30% Fiber <4% Calcium/phosphorus ratio 1.0–1.8 to 0.8–1.6	Avoid excessive weight during pregnancy. "Puppies" are "adults" at 90% skeletal maturity (9 months for miniature breeds and 16–24 months for giant breeds).
Adult dog	Metabolizable energy >3.5 Kcal/g of diet Digestibility >75% Protein 15%–25% Fat 7%–17% Fiber ≤5%	Food and feeding consistency encouraged.
Obese-prone dog	Metabolizable energy <3.5 Kcal/g of diet Digestibility ≥80% Protein 15%–25% Fat 6%–10% Fiber 7%–15%	Free feeding can contribute to obesity.
Increased activity or stressed dog	Metabolizable energy >4.2 Kcal/g of diet Digestibility >82% Protein 25%–32% Fat 23%–27% Fiber < 4%	
Geriatric dog	Metabolizable energy = 3.75 Kcal/g of diet Digestibility >80% Protein 14%–21% Fat 10%–12% Fiber >4% Control sodium	The average dog is considered geriatric after 7 years. Giant and large breeds are geriatric at 5 years of age.

*Information presented is expressed on a dry weight basis. These general guidelines may require adjustment to meet an individual's needs.
†% digestibility = (stool dry weight + food dry weight) × 100.

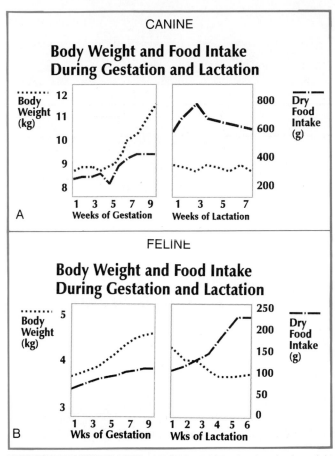

CANINE

Body Weight and Food Intake During Gestation and Lactation

FIGURE 21–5. Different patterns of pre- and postpartum body weight and food intake are observed between the bitch (A) and the queen (B). (See text for explanation.)

Fifth, multi-animal households or other group feeding situations may provoke competitive eating. The control measures are volume-restricted feeding and separation of the competitive animals by time and/or place of feeding. Most owners can "engineer" these circumstances with a little thought and coaching.

Sixth, surgical neutering of males and females deregulates satiety and increases the desire to feed. One may suggest less calorically dense foods concurrent with post-neuter suture removal. This seems especially prudent in obesity-prone breeds of dogs (Edney and Smith, 1986).

Diagnosis and Treatment of Obesity

One can assess the quantity of the patient's fat by examining the subcutaneous deposits visually and by palpation over the ribs, groin and tail head. This method substitutes for objective methods of measuring body composition. Radiographs of the abdomen and thorax will also reveal fat accumulations. Weighing only indirectly measures body composition. Using ideal weight tables for purebred animals is useful (Hand et al., 1989). Obesity is best prevented but can be treated by caloric restriction and exercise. Specific treatment requires teamwork among the owner, the veterinarian and the technician.

The equation of energy consumed versus energy expended is accurate, but weight control is rarely as easy as it sounds and long-term weight reduction fails more often than it succeeds (MacEwen, 1992). As success is precious, some practices focus most strongly on identifying those clients most able or most likely to be educated and motivated. In monitoring any treatment program, the veterinary technician is of fundamental importance as educator and cheerleader. Part of the dietary management program is building awareness of extraneous contributions of calories such as treats, including both human snack foods (Table 21–5) and commercial pet treats (Table 21–6). By following consistent feeding guidelines, one can control calorie intake in dogs and cats (Table 21–7).

Feeding the Geriatric Animal

The definition of "geriatric," as it pertains to the dog, is not precise because of breed variability in the natural life span and because "miles as well as years" influence the "wear-and-tear" of physiological aging. As a generality, toy- and small-sized breeds are "geriatric" at 7 years, medium-sized dogs at 6 years, and large and giant breeds as early as 5 years of age.

Loss of reserve capacity of organ function (eyes to bones) is universal with the normal aging change. Chronic progressive renal disease, due to aging changes alone, is of high incidence in dogs and cats (Markham and Hodgkins, 1989). There is no proven cause for or prophylactic strategy against the scourge of renal aging. However, the progressive loss of renal reserve ultimately reduces the animal's capability to excrete phosphorus, urea and other waste by-products of protein metabolism. Controlling excesses of intake during the geriatric period does no harm even in the absence of clinical signs of renal failure. Therefore, the recommendation to restrict excessive protein, phosphorus and sodium seems medically prudent.

In renal failure the veterinarian will prescribe specific intake restrictions of protein, phosphorus, and sodium and, perhaps, other measures to control hyperphosphatemia (Polzin et al.,

high as 40 percent (MacEwen, 1992; Sloth, 1992). Obesity is a body composition with a ratio of too much fat to lean tissue. ("Overweight" is not always an accurate measurement for "overfat.") There are several known causes for obesity, and as a confidant of the owner, the technician is vital in the crusade to prevent and treat this epidemic.

One cause for obesity-prone animals is overfeeding when young. A positive calorie balance during juvenile growth induces increased numbers of fat cells (hyperplasia) (Hand et al., 1989). Once formed, these fat cells are present for life and have minimal volumes of triglyceride content below which they cannot shrink (Crane, 1991). Therefore, a lifelong predisposition for excess weight develops. Needless adipocyte hyperplasia is prevented by using meal feeding for puppies, kittens and foals. A second cause of obesity is genetic predisposition. Several lines of evidence establish genetic inheritance as influential on the resting metabolic rate (Crane, 1991). This means "easy keepers" with less food intake required.

Third, a declining lean body mass and declining activity level are part of the normal aging process. Decreases in energy requirements may be considered in a geriatric feeding program (Markham and Hodgkins, 1989).

Fourth, animals may overeat just because they like the high palatability of the food. Volume-restricted meal feeding and control of the intake of treats will be needed when this situation is identified. Using a less palatable food is also a measure for control of intake.

Table 21–5
NUTRIENT CHARACTERISTICS OF HUMAN SNACK FOODS*

Food	Svg Size	Kcal/svg	Kcal/g	Protein (g)	Fat (g)	Na†
Cow's milk (3.5%)	1 c = 244 g	150	0.6	8	8	122/81
Whole egg (boiled)	1 egg = 50 g	79	1.6	6.1	5.6	69/87
Ice cream (van., 10% fat)	1 c = 133 g	266	2.0	4.8	14.3	116/43
American cheese	1 oz	93	3.3	5.6	7	337/362
Cottage cheese (low fat, 2%)	1 c = 226 g	203	0.9	31	4.4	918/452
Jell-O	1 c = 280 g	162	0.6	3.2	0	108/67
Hot dog (beef)	8/lb = 57 g	180	3.2	6.9	16.3	585/325
Bologna (beef)	1 slice = 23 g	72	3.1	2.8	6.6	226/313
Big Mac	1 sand = 200 g	570	2.9	24.6	35	979/172
Peanut butter (smooth)	2 tbsp = 32 g	188	5.9	9	5.4	234/124
Popcorn (w/butter)	3 c = 37 g	192	5.2	2.8	11.5	273/142
Corn chips	1 oz	153	5.5	1.7	8.8	218/142
Potato chips	1 oz	148	5.3	1.8	10.1	133/90
Pretzels	1 oz	110	3.9	3.0	1.2	543/493

*Metabolizable energy for humans. All values from Pennington JAT: Food Values of Portions Commonly Used. 15th ed. New York, Harper & Row, 1989.
†Sodium content per serving/sodium content per 100 Kcal.

Table 21–6
NUTRIENT CONTENT OF COMMERCIAL TREATS

Nutrient Content of Commercial Dog Treats

Treat Name	MFG	WT/ Piece (g)	Cost ($/LB)	Water	Protein	Fat	Na	Ca	P	CA:P	Mg	Ash	NFE†	Fiber	Kcal/G†	Kcal/ Treat†
Liver Snaps	Alpo	3.5	1.57	9.1	25.1	4.8	0.57	0.11	0.37	0.3:1	0.14	3.5	63.8	2.8	3.2	11
Stew Biscuit	Alpo	8.5	1.46	9.5	28.3	12.2	0.31	1.1	0.82	1.34:1	0.2	6.5	49.2	3.9	3.4	29
Recipe Dog Treats	Champion Valley Farms	1.6	1.36	9.9	18.9	11	2.3	0.07	0.33	0.2:1	0.1	2.3	64.4	2.8	3.5	6
Jerky Strips (Beef)	Alpo	8.1	6.88	21.4	43.6	25.6	1.03	1.53	0.97	1.6:1	0.18	10.4	16.5	3.8	3.4	28
100% Natural Treats	Ken-L-R Chix BACN	7.6 5.7	1.18	7.8	18.6	8.5	0.52	0.07	1.08	0.06:1	0.16	3.5	67.4	3.3	1.6	12
Milk Bones (small dog)	Nabisco	5.7	1.46	9.2	24.8	7.7	0.42	1.2	0.88	1.4:1	0.14	6.4	57.7	3.3	3.2	18
Beggin' Strips	Purina	11.5	6.50	19.9	25.1	7.2	1.2	1.01	0.8	1.3:1	0.1	6.9	56.4	4.4	2.8	32
Hearty Chews	Purina	Pkg = 50 g Pcs. 1.9	22	2.3	33.7	11.3	2.08	2.07	1.69	1.2:1	0.13	16.4	32.1	6.5	2.5	5
Short Ribz	Purina	4.5	1.50	8.6	23.1	12	0.37	1.1	0.68	1.6:1	0.13	5.8	50.3	8.0	3.3	15
Cheese Dawgs (Beef)	Purina	7.7	3.26	26.8	29.9	16.3	0.42	1.04	0.57	1.8:1	0.08	6.0	42.3	5.5	3.6	28
BONZ	Purina	19.9	1.08	8.1	14.9	9.4	0.29	1.2	0.76	1.6:1	0.11	5.66	65.7	4.4	3.3	66
Snausages (Beef)	Ken-L-R	5.4	2.78	32	33.8	13.6	1.13	1.47	1.03	1.4:1	0.15	12.3	38.1	2.2	2.5	14
Meaty Bone (Beef)	Star Kist	9.5	1.59	9.6	15.6	10.7	.80	0.09	0.33	0.3:1	0.12	4.0	64.7	5.0	3.4	32
Jerky Treats	Star Kist	6.7	6.37	24.5	51.9	30.5	3.4	0.43	1.1	0.4:1	0.07	10.5	3.3	4.0	3.5	23

Nutrient Content of Commercial Cat Treats

Treat Name	MFG	WT/ Piece (g)	Cost ($/LB)	Water	Protein	Fat	Na	Ca	P	CA:P	Mg	Ash	NFE†	Fiber	Kcal/G†	Kcal/ Treat†
Bonkers (Liver)	Martha White Foods	1.8	2.60	29.6	40.5	20.9	0.99	1.7	1.6	1.1:1	0.09	21	9.4	27.8	1.4	3
Whisker Lickins	Purina	.7	6.47	11.7	33.9	17.6	1.03	1.36	1.13	1.2:1	0.12	33	7.7	35.8	5.1	3
Puss 'N Boots Pounce	Quaker Oats	1.3	3.68	34.2	38.3	19.9	0.3	1.06	0.7	1.5:1	0.06	23	7.0	32.5	2.3	3
9 Lives Finicky Bits	Star Kist	.8	4.64	34.1	36.4	17.3	0.52	1.82	1.46	1.3:1	0.17	68	10.3	30.8	4.6	3

*By analysis
†By calculation

Table 21–7
FEEDING DOGS AND CATS

Do	Don't
Feed for ideal weight.	Allow excess calories. Obesity increases disease predisposition.
Feel but not see the ribs.	
Meal feed for control of calorie intake.	Ad-lib feed obese-prone dogs.
Provide fresh clean water.	Provide stagnant or frozen water.
Provide a consistent food and ritualize the time and place of feeding.	Rotate flavors or brands on a frequent basis.
Use life-stage feeding concept.	Use growth/lactation diets for adult maintenance.
Select treats with nutrient profile and caloric density considerations	Supplement a good diet.

1989). Cats have elevated potassium requirements during renal insufficiency and renal failure, and managing and monitoring all such patients is a considerable challenge (Fettman, 1989). Many animals with renal insufficiency and failure will be in their geriatric period of life.

Calorie control may begin or be continued in older animals. On the other hand, other older animals may have inadequate calories due to systemic illness, dental or oral pain, failing sight and smell, or progression of "finicky" tastes or fixed food addictions. Blanket feeding recommendations based solely on age are unwise without consideration of the individual. Pet foods specifically intended for "seniors" emphasize moderate energy density with good palatability and reductions of some excess nutrients, as found in all-purpose pet foods.

Feeding Cats

Cats are not "small dogs" and are physically, physiologically and behaviorally adapted as solo-hunting, carnivorous predators. Use of amino acids as important energy sources translates into twice the protein requirement of the more omnivorous dog. The percentage of total dietary calories originating from an ideal protein source (biological value of 100 percent) is 8 percent in adult cats but 4 percent in adult dogs. Other feline specific requirements include taurine as an eleventh essential amino acid (McDonald et al., 1984). Provision of animal origin types and/or sources of vitamin A, niacin, pyridoxine and arachidonic acid (a fatty acid) are other feline-specific requirements. Feeding dog food to cats for convenience or economy is ill advised. If the technician encounters this dietary history, the veterinarian should be alerted for educational intervention.

Feeding Kittens and Adult Cats

One must confirm adequate colostrum intake for all kittens. Like puppies, the orphan kitten can be raised by tube gavage or nurser administration of queen's milk replacer. Kittens are weaned later than puppies—generally at 7 to 9 weeks. Growth-sustaining kitten foods are then meal-fed twice to three time daily until the kitten is 10 months of age.

As adults, feral cats have "nibbling" eating patterns as they hunt mice and other small animals most of the night and part of the day. Nibbling minimizes the effect of the postprandial alkaline tide—a physiological event alkalinizing the urine following meal feeding. This may help to protect against urinary crystalluria, but twice daily meal feeding is practical and works well for indoor cats.

A consistent feeding product and schedule should be recommended during adult maintenance. Decreased finickiness results from this approach, but flavor rotation is a perspective of some owners in response to the large number of cat food flavors present on supermarket shelves. Flavor rotation is unnecessary for variety and a transient "newness" factor increases food intake when the new flavor is introduced. The result is the owner's perception of doing the cat a "favor" (expressed as increased intake). However, weight homeostasis may be upset by the flavor rotation approach. Adult feline maintenance pet food is recommended, and vegetarian-type diets are specifically discouraged for cats.

Commercial feline treats are usually clones of dry cat food (see Table 21–6). As such, they are appropriate for treating when given in moderation and dietary restriction is not needed. Some cat owners prefer "natural" treats such as raw or cooked poultry necks, oxtails, or liver. While little harm results from such treats in moderation, finicky behavior and nutritional imbalance are potential hazards. Liver contains an inverted Ca:P ratio (1:17), and potentially toxic levels of vitamin A (hypervitaminosis A) can occur with long-term use (Goldman, 1992).

Feeding Cats in Gestation and Lactation

There are significant differences in food intake between the bitch and the queen during the initial stages of lactation (Fig. 21–5B). The queen apparently will forgo postpartum hunting to attend her kittens. As a solitary hunter, she hunts less and uses the body fat stored during gestation to support her lactation. The practical significance is that clients may question low food consumption in their new mother cat. Such clients are advised that the queen will eat heavily, as expected, by the third week of lactation.

Feline Lower Urinary Tract Disease (FLUTD)

Domestic cats evolved from desert-adapted ancestors. Urine specific gravity greater than 1.070 indicates excellent ability to concentrate dissolved urinary solutes as a water conservation mechanism. High solute concentration may favor formation of urinary crystals (crystalluria). Specific minerals dissolve into solution or precipitate as solids at specific urine pH levels. Controlling urine pH to reduce crystalluria requires a knowledge of the mineral to be inhibited. This is because struvite and oxalate, the two most common stones, form most readily in alkaline and acidic urine respectively.

It is an oversimplification to state that controlling urine solutes of magnesium or pH always controls FLUTD. This is because the FLUTD syndrome is multifactorial, and all causative agents or combinations of contributory factors are presently unknown. However, maintaining a physiological urine acidity (pH 6.2 to 6.4) and controlling magnesium intake to non-excessive levels are prudent risk control measures for struvite crystalluria.

the "as is" basis. This often means water-containing ingredients list high in the ingredient ordering when a dry ingredient actually predominates on a dry matter basis.

Nutritional Adequacy Statement

The nutritional adequacy statement may be as simple as "totally nutritious" or "complete and balanced" or the statement may be more elaborate. The technician should interpret the method used to determine the nutritional adequacy statement. The statement "meets or exceeds NRC guidelines" (or similar wording) indicates only a laboratory analysis for a minimal chemical content. Such testing is not an animal feeding performance trial and says nothing about adequacy, bioavailability or excesses.

The "AAFCO Protocol Feeding Test" statement, however, indicates that a representative product was used in animal feeding tests and performed at a defined level. Thus, the consumer knows that living animals have been test-fed, and the technician should recommend products with the AAFCO rather than the NRC statement when there is a choice. A nutritional adequacy statement is not needed on treats or dietary management foods intended to be used within the context of a professional diagnosis and relationship.

The Percentage Rules

The designator and modifying wording on pet food labels contains considerable information regarding content of the named ingredient in a product. According to AAFCO rules, when a label statement identifies only one ingredient, at least 70 percent of the total product will consist of that named ingredient (e.g., beef). When modifying words accompany the named ingredient, the amount of the named ingredient that must be present declines to 10 percent (chicken *dinner*, fish *entree*, liver *stew* and so forth). When a named ingredient is modified by the word "with" (e.g., with beef), the total portion of the named ingredient declines to 3 percent. When the term "flavor" is used (e.g., cheese flavor), the named flavor must only be "detectable" by the animal. The designator "food" ("dog food") means that there are no rules regarding minimal content of ingredients. Indirectly, the technician may gather further quality information about a product through understanding these nuances of pet food labeling.

Technician's Role

Actually, the technician is in a position to assess pet food and livestock food quality by far better means than reading even the most informative of labels. That method is the direct assessment of an animal's performance. Feeding performance in daily use defines the real "gold standard" of quality assessment.

Feeding Costs for Dog and Cat Foods

There are substantial variations in actual daily feeding costs (see Table 21–8). When cost comparisons are calculated, a pet food perceived as "expensive" may actually be cheaper on the per calorie and actual feeding cost basis. Unfortunately, unit price comparison rather than feeding cost information influences the purchasing decision.

COMPANION ANIMAL CLINICAL NUTRITION

"Thy food is thy remedy"

HIPPOCRATES

Clinical nutrition is a medical subspecialty having the objective of modifying the cause, progression or end-stage effects of illness by applying specific nutrient profiles. The application of prophylactic or therapeutic dietary management is the expression of this objective. Purpose-specific dietary management has a long history of efficacy in large, small and exotic animal species. However, the use of altered nutrient profiles should be justified by professional diagnosis, judgment and monitoring.

Numerous nutrient profiles support various prophylactic and therapeutic applications in small animal patients. Examples are as follows: high protein/low carbohydrate; high protein/fat/micronutrient; low protein/high nonprotein calorie; low fiber/high digestibility; fiber enhanced; low sodium; very low sodium; low mineral; low fat/high fiber/low calorie; low copper; and restricted/novel protein sources. Specific effects on urine acidification or alkalization and restriction of urinary solutes such as magnesium are attained from specific formulations. Meat-free, soy-free, lactose-free, corn- and wheat gluten–free, and additive-free nutrient profiles are available in various commercially available products. Nutrient control objectives are fulfilled with either hospital-formulated/owner-cooked feedings or commercially prepared formulas. Table 21–9 summarizes objectives and nutrient profile for selected applications.

Feeding Hospitalized Small Animal Patients

Medical-surgical malnutrition is a major clinical problem for patients unable or unwilling to eat. To complicate the food deficit, hypermetabolic energy requirements often follow significant illness or injury (Chandler et al., 1992). A state of "accelerated starvation" and lean tissue catabolism follows protein-calorie malnutrition (Crowe, 1986A). Decreased immune function, delayed wound healing (rate and strength), loss of muscle and visceral mass, delayed general recovery and increased mortality all result from protein calorie malnutrition (Crane, 1989). The veterinary technician is a critical interface in daily cage-side nutritional management. A "wait-until-ready-to-eat" passivity is not beneficial, and no patient has yet been starved into wellness (Armstrong, 1992; Armstrong et al., 1990; Bright and Burrows, 1988; Chandler et al., 1992; Crowe, 1986B; Labato, 1992). Even when the patient is overweight, an acute hospitalization is not the setting for weight reduction.

Patient Selection for Assisted Feeding

The technician frequently uses *subjective global assessment* (SGA) to determine nutritional status. SGA considers the dietary history, the body's condition and the current morbidity

Table 21–9
SUMMARY OF SMALL ANIMAL CLINICAL NUTRITION[1]

Disease	Objectives	Considerations	Product[2]	Comments
Allergy, food				
Dog	Reduce antigen ingestion.	Novel protein source Reduce total protein. Simplify food. Distilled H_2O	Prescription Diet Canine d/d Prescription Diet Feline d/d	6 week trial period Avoid antigen intake in treats.
Cat		Same as dog except: Control Mg^{++} intake. Provide taurine. Control urine pH.		
Anemia	Support RBC production.	↑ Iron, cobalt and copper ↑ B-complex vitamins ↑ Protein	Prescription Diet Canine p/d Feline p/d	

Anorexia	Prevent protein/calorie
	  malnutrition.
	Stimulate appetite.
		Establish fluid/electrolyte
		  balance.
		Acid base balance
		↑ Protein and fat
		↑ Micronutrients
			Prescription Diet
			Feline/Canine a/d
			Canine p/d
			Feline p/d
				Cat foods are suitable dog
				  foods in acute care.

Ascites	Reduce fluid retention.	Restriction of sodium
		Maintain hydration
			Prescription Diet
			Canine h/d, k/d
			Feline h/d, k/d
				h/d = marked Na^+
				  restriction
				k/d = moderate Na^+
				  restriction

Bone loss and fracture
  healing
	Correct deficiency of energy
	  and protein.
		↑ Protein
		↑ Energy
		Avoid supplementation.
			Prescription Diet
			Canine p/d
			Feline p/d
				Dietary calcium excess does
				  not increase rate of
				  fracture healing.

Colitis	Normalize GI motility. Rebalance microflora. Provide local healing factors.	Small meals—3–6 times day Control dietary antigens. Vary levels of dietary fiber.	Prescription Diet Canine w/d, i/d, d/d Feline w/d, d/d	
Constipation	Normalize GI motility. Maintain stool water. Maintain stool bulk.	>10% fiber	Prescription Diet Canine w/d Feline w/d	No table scraps or bones Increase exercise. Cats—Keep litter box clean.
Copper storage disease	Restrict copper intake.	<1.2 mg copper/100g dry diet	Prescription Diet Canine u/d	No table scraps or treats

Debilitation	Replete tissue, plasma and
	  nutrients.
		↑ Protein
		↑ Fat
		↑ Macro and micro
		  nutrients
			Prescription Diet
			Canine/feline a/d
				Assist feed if needed.

Diabetes mellitus	Even rate of glucose
	  absorption.
	Consistent caloric intake.
		>10% fiber
		↓ Soluble carbohydrates
			Prescription Diet
			Canine w/d
			Feline w/d
				Weigh animal frequently and
				  note in medical record.

Acute diarrhea	Normalize gastrointestinal
	  tract, motility and
	  secretion.
		Withhold food 1–2 days.
		Feed small amounts 3–6
		  times day.
		↓ Fiber
		↓ Sugar
		↑ Digestibility
			Prescription Diet
			Canine i/d
			Feline c/d
				Electrolyte disturbances and
				  dehydration are common.

Eclampsia	Provide calcium/phosphorus
	  in correct quantity and
	  ratio prepartum.
		High digestibility of diet
		Balanced minerals/vitamins
			Prescription Diet
			Canine p/d
			Feline p/d
				Avoid supplementation.

Flatulence	Decrease aerophagia.
	Avoid food fermentation.
		Avoid milk or milk products.
		Feed small meals 3–6 times
		  day.
		↑ Caloric density
			Prescription Diet
			Canine i/d
			Feline c/d
				Feed in a flat open dish.
				Avoid vitamin
				  supplementation. Separate
				  competitive eaters.

Gastric dilatation/bloat
  (postoperative)
	Prevent gastric distention.	Avoid exercise before and
		  after feeding
		↑ Digestibility of diet
		Small frequent feedings
			Prescription Diet
			Canine i/d
				Diet form or type is *NOT*
				  related to risk of
				  occurrence or recurrence.

Heart failure				

Dogs	Control sodium retention.	Dogs:
		↓ Sodium intake
		Maintain energy and protein
		  intake.
		↑ B-complex vitamins
			Prescription Diet
			Canine h/d
				Prescription Diet k/d has
				  moderate salt restrictions.

Cats		Cats: ↓ Sodium intake ↑ Taurine Control Mg^{++} levels.	Prescription Diet Feline h/d	Avoid high-sodium treats and water (see Table 21–5).
Hyperlipidemia	Control fat intake.	↑ Fiber intake ↓ Fat intake Limit sugars.	Prescription Diet Canine w/d Feline w/d	Common in Schnauzers. Consider fat in treats, scraps and supplements.
Hyperthyroidism		↑ Energy intake ↑ Vitamins and minerals ↑ Protein	Prescription Diet Feline/canine a/d	
Cats	Support increased energy need.			
Liver disease (fat tolerant)	Reduce protein metabolism. Maintain liver glycogen. Prevent ammonia toxicity.	↑ Digestible energy Protein restriction High biologic value proteins Control sodium intake.	Prescription Diet Canine k/d Feline k/d	May feed small meals (4–6 times day).

Table continued on following page

Table 21–9
SUMMARY OF SMALL ANIMAL CLINICAL NUTRITION[1] *Continued*

Disease	Objectives	Considerations	Product[2]	Comments
Lymphangiectasia	Decrease dietary fat.	↓ Intake of long-chain triglycerides Control protein levels. Consider medium-chain triglycerides.	Prescription Diet Canine w/d or r/d	Medium-chain triglyceride oils and powder can increase caloric density.
Obesity	Maintain intake of all nutrients except energy.	↓ Energy digestibility Replace digestible calories with indigestible fiber. Increase bulk to control hunger.	Prescription Diet Canine r/d Feline r/d	Requires professional advice and teamwork. Obesity is better prevented than treated.
Vomiting	Minimize gastric secretion. Gastrointestinal rest.	↑ Digestibility ↑ Caloric density	Prescription Diet Canine i/d	Frequent, small meals
Acute pancreatitis (recovery phase)	Control pancreas secretions.	↓ Fat ↑ Digestibility Feed small meals 3–6 times daily.	Prescription Diet Canine i/d Feline w/d	Frequent, small meals
Pancreatic exocrine insufficiency	Reduce requirements for digestive enzymes.	↓ Fiber ↓ Fat Highly digestible carbohydrates. ↑ Caloric density.	Prescription Diet Canine i/d	Pancreatic enzymes complement highly digestible food.
Regurgitation	Decrease gastric acid secretion. Maintain caloric intake.	Low bulk. Slurry of ½ food and ½ water for 72 hours	Prescription Diet Canine i/d Feline c/d	Elevate the food bowl. Try different food texture.
Renal failure Dogs	Reduce signs of uremia.	Dogs: ↓ Protein (↑ biologic value of protein) ↑ Non-protein calories ↓ Phosphorus and sodium Increase B-Complex vitamins.	Prescription Diet Canine k/d Prescription Diet Feline k/d	Small meals several (4–6) times a day Conversion to a protein-restricted diet may take 7 to 10 days.
Cats		Cats: ↓ Protein ↑ Biologic value of protein ↓ Phosphorus, calcium and sodium (control Mg^{++})		
Canine urolithiasis (struvite) *Treatment*	↑ Urine volume ↓ Urine pH Restrict Mg^{++}, NH$^+$, PO$_4$.	*Treatment:* ↓ Protein ↓ PO$_4$, Mg^{++} ↑ Sodium ↓ Urine pH (5.9–6.1)	Prescription Diet Canine s/d	Evaluate and treat urinary tract infection. Average duration of stone dissolution is 36 days. Follow via radiography.
Canine urolithiasis (struvite) *Prevention*	Maintain physiologic level of urinary solutes and urine pH.	*Prevention:* Control protein excess. ↓ Calcium, phosphorus, magnesium ↓ Sodium mildly ↓ Urine pH 6.2–6.4	Prescription Diet Canine c/d	Monitor urine sediment for crystalluria and infection.
Canine urolithiasis (ammonium urate) *Prevention*		*Treatment:* ↓ Protein ↑ Nonprotein calories ↓ Nucleic acids ↓ Calcium, phosphorus, magnesium, sodium Urine pH (6.7–7.0)	Prescription Diet Canine u/d	Drugs plus diet may be successful treatment. Monitor urinary crystalluria. Prevention may require long-term drug treatment.
Canine urolithiasis (calcium oxalate and cystine) *Prevention*	↓ Urinary concentration of calcium oxalate or cystine	↓ Protein ↑ Nonprotein calories ↓ Calcium, phosphorus, sodium magnesium ↑ Urine pH (6.7–7.0)	Prescription Diet Canine u/d	*Treatment* by surgical removal. *Prevention* by dietary management ± drugs.
Feline urolithiasis (struvite) *Treatment*	↑ Urine volume ↓ Urine pH (5.9–6.1) Restrict Mg^{++}, Ca^{++}, PO$_4$.	*Treatment:* ↑ Caloric density ↓ Phosphorus and calcium Magnesium >20 mg/100 Kcal ↑ Sodium Urine pH (6.2–6.4)	Prescription Diet Feline s/d	Average dissolution is 35 days after negative radiographs. Recurrence is high if prevention is not implemented.
Feline urolithiasis (struvite) *Prevention*	Maintain physiologic levels of urinary solutes and urine pH.	*Prevention:* Magnesium >20 mg/100 Kcal (0.1% DMB) ↓ Phosphorus ↑ Caloric density Urine pH (6.2–6.4)	Prescription Diet Feline c/d	In obesity use calorie-restricted diets that maintain urine pH 6.2–6.4. (Prescription Diet w/d is suggested.)
Feline urolithiasis (calcium oxalate) *Prevention*	↑ Urine volume ↓ Urinary Ca^{++}, oxalate ↑ Urine pH	↓ Protein ↑ Nonprotein calories ↓ Phosphorus, calcium, sodium Magnesium <20 mg/100 Kcal	Prescription Diet Feline k/d	Monitor urinary crystalluria.

[1]Nutrients expressed on a dry weight basis.
[2]Prescription Diet is a registered trademark of Hills Pet Nutrition, Inc., Topeka, KS. Other North American brands of dietary management food are: Cadillac, CNM (Pro Visions); Hi Tor; Neura; Protocol; VMD (MediCal); and Waltham.

index of the illness or injury. Body scoring is by physical examination, with 0 = cachexia and 5 = obese. Albumin, globulin and other "markers" for malnutrition decline with energy deprivation and protein-calorie malnutrition. However, these objective indicators change too slowly to be functional prognosticators, and use of SGA permits the same clinical conclusion of "nutrient depletion and negative nitrogen balance" earlier (Armstrong, 1992; Labato, 1992). The most important outlook for the hospital is an awareness of the critical "need to feed" and the need to do so early. These steps reduce catabolism and improve responses to virtually all other therapy.

Indications for nutritional support include recent weight loss of more than 10 percent, absent or poor food intake for more than 2 days, presentation of acute illness or injury with a high trauma index, acute muscle wasting and heavy GI or urinary system losses of protein or electrolytes. The technician assesses daily needs and progress in conversation with the veterinarian and by the daily patient progress notes. The trauma index, the patient's desire and ability to eat, and response to therapy can all rapidly change.

Enteral Versus Parenteral Feeding

Total parenteral nutrition (TPN) is a complete intravenous nutrition technique whose objective is complete bypass of the seriously impaired GI tract. Parenteral nutrition technique is the controlled infusion of special feeding fluids of concentrated dextrose and amino acids. Special fat emulsions and micronutrient modules may also be added. Even during TPN, partial enteral intake supports the enterocyte cells of the small intestinal mucosa (Allen and Hand, 1992). Maintaining enterocyte function is important to reduce TPN complications of bowel atrophy and bacterial translocation across the intestine into the circulation (bacteremia).

Enteral feeding is more physiological, safer and cheaper than parenteral nutrition. Therefore, feeding by mouth or tube is used if the GI tract can absorb nutrients (Abood and Buffington, 1991; Armstrong, 1992). Contraindications to enteral nutritional feeding are the need for complete GI secretory rest and a high risk of aspirating vomitus.

Methods of Assisted Enteral Feeding

Coax feeding, appetite stimulation with drugs, forced oral feeding and various tube administration techniques are four separate enteral feeding methods. At the "easiest" level, place a warmed pet food directly into the patient's mouth. This may tempt some animals back to normal oral intake as may an owner's hand-feeding of a favorite food. As olfaction is more important than taste for short-term acceptance, the animal's nares should be cleaned of debris and exudate as needed.

Assist oral feeding with finger, spoon, tongue blade or feeding-tipped dose syringe. These techniques employ more persistence than "coaxing" and intend to deliver substantial quantities of oral nutriment. It is important to appreciate patient stress involved with this feeding method and to monitor food swallowed versus that rejected. Then, multiply the volume swallowed by the caloric density to measure caloric support. For example, Prescription Diet Canine/Feline a/d (Hill's, Inc.) has a caloric density of 1.2 Kcal/ml and provides 120 Kcal per 100 ml.

Pharmaceutical stimulation of feeding is effective in about 50 percent of patients to "jump-start" or maintain appetite in a partially anorectic patient. The benzodiazepine tranquilizers appear most effective, and many veterinarians are familiar with these methods. However, glucocorticoid, anabolic steroid and B vitamins are not of proven benefit in "breaking" anorexia.

Feeding tubes should be used only after assisted enteral feeding techniques have failed. Veterinarians usually place the largest possible feeding tube as far proximal as possible in the GI tract (Armstrong et al., 1990; Crowe, 1986B). Orogastric tubes are reserved for short-term use, although some animals permit repeated tubing. Orogastric tubes have the advantages of quick placement and can rapidly deliver large quantities of blenderized pet food. Disadvantages are that restraint needs and patient stress may be substantial.

Transnasal tubes (nasogastric or nasoesophageal) are well tolerated by both dogs and cats. There is some choice of materials for tube comfort, but any of the tubes may be used with an acceptable complication rate (Abood and Buffington, 1992A). A transnasal tube is placed under general anesthesia or by analgesia from anesthetic nose drops. A "pig-nose" maneuver of lifting the soft portion of the nose upward better exposes the ventral nasal meatus. This method makes transnasal tube placement an easy and routine procedure (Abood and Buffington, 1991; Abood and Buffington, 1992B). The major disadvantage of transnasal tubes is their size restriction of less than 10 French (Fr) in dogs and less than 6 Fr in cats. This limits feeds to a nonparticulate liquid or a highly homogenized pet food.

Large-bore pharyngostomy tubes require surgical installation under general anesthesia. Although popular, these tubes may have several potential complications including esophageal irritation, gastric reflux and interference with laryngeal mechanics. Close monitoring is maintained for saliva aspiration, difficulty in swallowing or breathing, gagging and attempts to vomit or paw out the tube. Suspicions of any complication should be reported to the veterinarian earlier rather than later.

Esophagostomy tubes combine advantages of nasoesophageal and pharyngostomy placements (Crowe, 1986B). A 12- to 16-Fr tube extends from the lateral neck into the proximal esophagus with the tip resting in the caudal esophagus. Esophagostomy permits use of slurried diets, and these are well tolerated for intermediate term feeding needs.

The gastrostomy tube is a powerful method of both short- and long-term feeding. As a major advantage, gastrostomy tubes are large-bore (12 to 20 Fr) and may be reliably used for weeks or months (Fig. 21–8A). Placement is usually left-sided into the gastric fundus, but right-sided pyloric placements are equally effective. Gastrostomy tubes are surgically placed during midline celiotomy or by a left flank approach to the stomach. Percutaneous placement techniques using endoscopic and non-endoscopic techniques are described, and both will require technical assistance (Bright and Burrows, 1988; Fulton and Dennis, 1992).

The technician must carefully monitor all feeding tubes for mechanical blockage or kinking. This is a critical monitoring obligation for small-bore tubes. Water is flushed through the tube to clear debris after each feeding. Capping the tube prevents air from entering the catheterized viscus between uses. It is preferable for the same person to feed, as this may allow quicker notation of flow and resistance changes in the tube.

It is also important to monitor GI tolerance during the refeeding of the animal. The objectives of repletion feeding may

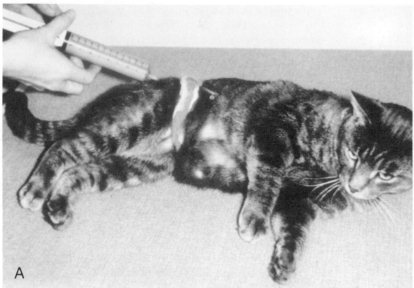

FIGURE 21–8. A, Feeding for convalescence, repletion and recovery should extend past hospital discharge. This cat is anorectic and has received blended pet food by tube gastrostomy for 5 months. Most owners can be coached in food preparation for tube feeding techniques. B, Feeding of ill and injured animals helps to curtail accelerated catabolism and negative clinical outcomes. Assisted alimentation is a fundamental aspect of nursing, and food dose calculators allow convenient determination of injury energy requirement (IER) recommendations for a particular food.

be at odds with the patient's best interests when serious vomiting and diarrhea follow feeding.

Steps in Enteral Alimentation Calculations and Food Selection

1. Calculate resting energy requirement (RER) as:

   A. $RER = 70 \, (BW \text{ in } kg)^{0.75}$

   or

   B. $RER = 30 \, (BW \text{ in } kg) + 70$

2. Factor the RER to obtain illness/infection/injury energy requirement (IER). (Multiply RER × Trauma Index.) An IER of 1.25 to 1.5 times RER is commonly used for many critical care applications (Armstrong, 1992; Chandler et al., 1992; Crowe, 1986A) (see Table 21–10 and Fig. 21–8B).

3. Consider the distribution of fuel sources among protein, carbohydrate and fat. Dogs receiving more than 16 percent of energy from protein (protein calories) and cats receiving more than 24 percent protein calories recovered well when human liquid enteral products were enterally supplied (cats were supplemented with casein-based protein sources) (Abood and Buffington, 1992A). However, these protein levels are considered minimal, and higher levels may be prudent (Donoghue, 1989).

4. Consider physical form and other nutritional characteristics prior to final selection of feeding products. Note that oral calorie paste supplements are extremely deficient in protein and that meat baby foods are neither complete nor balanced. Five percent dextrose does not provide adequate calorie concentrations and is devoid of protein. Table 21–11 summarizes the nutrient profile of selected foods and enteral products used in small animal patients.

5. Establish the food dose, administration rate and feeding schedule. A conservative rate of patient re-feeding is needed after prolonged anorexia or GI disease. Controlling the size and frequency of the per feeding dose by giving small frequent feedings can be a critical factor in improving patient tolerance. Calorie and volume intake at IER levels may require a 3 day transition period.

FEEDING PET BIRDS

Avian nutrient needs are diverse and the technician may variously accommodate insectivorous, frugivorous (fruit-eating), nectivorous, carnivorous, seed eating and omnivorous species of birds. The origins and ecological niche of common pet birds vary greatly. For example, the common budgerigar is a desert-adapted bird, while many parrots are acclimated to rain-forest environments. When one considers the range of canaries, finches, parakeets, cockateels, lovebirds, conures, macaws, and various parrots and cockatoos, a dangerous generalization would be that they all "eat seeds." Unfortunately, the knowledge of nutrient requirements and wild-type feeding behaviors is incomplete for some species.

The history for the pet bird should include the amount of free flight (if any), water intake, and the brand and type of avian pet food provided. If birds eat from the owner's kitchen, note the general distribution of food types. Question the use of treats, supplements, fresh foods, cuttle bone and grit. Some seed mixes are supplemented with protein, vitamins and minerals and are labeled as "fortified." If owners do not know whether seeds are fortified, one should request the label.

Table 21–10
ENTERAL FEEDING WORKSHEET

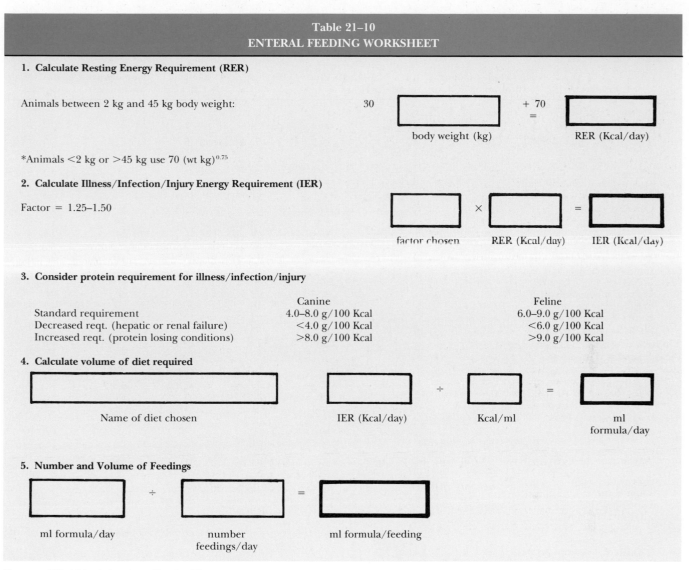

1. Calculate Resting Energy Requirement (RER)

Animals between 2 kg and 45 kg body weight:

30 [　body weight (kg)　] + 70 = [　RER (Kcal/day)　]

*Animals <2 kg or >45 kg use 70 (wt kg)$^{0.75}$

2. Calculate Illness/Infection/Injury Energy Requirement (IER)

Factor = 1.25–1.50

[　factor chosen　] × [　RER (Kcal/day)　] = [　IER (Kcal/day)　]

3. Consider protein requirement for illness/infection/injury

	Canine	Feline
Standard requirement	4.0–8.0 g/100 Kcal	6.0–9.0 g/100 Kcal
Decreased reqt. (hepatic or renal failure)	<4.0 g/100 Kcal	<6.0 g/100 Kcal
Increased reqt. (protein losing conditions)	>8.0 g/100 Kcal	>9.0 g/100 Kcal

4. Calculate volume of diet required

[　Name of diet chosen　] [　IER (Kcal/day)　] ÷ [　Kcal/ml　] = [　ml formula/day　]

5. Number and Volume of Feedings

[　ml formula/day　] ÷ [　number feedings/day　] = [　ml formula/feeding　]

Courtesy of Mark Morris Associates, Topeka, KS.

Quantity of food consumption is often difficult to judge. This is true both in smaller passerines, which may go several days between seed cup refreshment, and in large psittacines, which frequently waste a sizable fraction of the food supplied. Food preferences and addictions are important to note, but many owners are unaware of an addiction until making an attempt to change the food. As with any other animal, direct observation of anorexia and body condition is important to physical diagnosis.

An increasing percentage of companion birds are being hand-raised in captivity. Breeder hatching and hand-feeding of baby birds increases socialization to humans and their value as pets. Hand-feeding baby birds permits the growing and weaning foods to be adjusted to intake requirements. At "weaning," complete and balanced avian pet foods should be selected as the basis of feeding (Fig. 21–9A, B). Some avicultural hobbyists and veterinarians recommend that mixed, fresh foods also be provided for nutritional diversity.

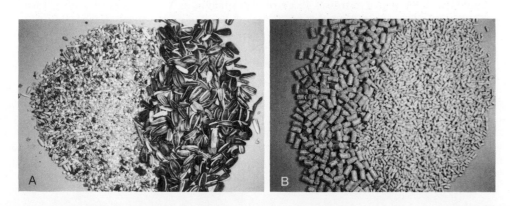

FIGURE 21–9. A, Seeds are an important part of many avian diets. However, high-oil seeds and nuts, such as sunflower seeds and peanuts, may cause addictions and nutritional imbalance. Oil seeds are deficient in protein relative to calorie content and have deficiency of calcium and micro nutrients. B, Complete and balanced avian foods are available as fortified seed mixtures and extruded and pelleted foods.

Table 21–11
COMPOSITION OF SOME ENTERAL FORMULAS

Product	Caloric Content (Kcal/ml or Kcal/g)	Protein Content (g/100 Kcal)	% Prot. Cal.	Fat Content % Fat Cal.	Carbohydrate Content % CHO Cal.	Osmolarity (mOsm/kg)	Cost Cents/Kcal
Veterinary							
Feline p/d*	0.9	9.3	37	56	7		0.2
Feline k/d†	0.9	4.4	21	67	13		0.2
Feline c/d†	0.6	8.9	33	52	15		0.2
Canine k/d†	0.6	3.1	13	49	39		0.2
Canine u/d†	0.7	1.9	8	48	45		0.2
Canine i/d†	0.6	5.9	24	31	45		0.2
Canine & Feline a/d	1.2	8.9	36	51	13		0.4
CliniCare Canine powder	0.9	6.0	24	64	12		2.5
CliniCare Canine liquid	0.9	5.5	25	59	16	340	3.5
RenalCare Canine liquid	0.8	2.8	14	66	20	260	3.7
CliniCare Feline powder	0.8	9.1	36	53	11	340	2.6
CliniCare Feline liquid	0.8	8.6	36	84	16	368	4.2
RenalCare Feline liquid	0.8	5.6	25	60	15	260	4.0
Triage Canine powder	5.3	5.5	22	67	11		0.8
Triage Feline powder	4.4	8.5	34	46	20		0.9
Nutri-Cal paste	4.6	0.3	1	62	37		1.2
Sheba Turkey cat food	1.2	10.2	41	57	2		0.6
Dyne liquid	5.2	0.7	3	74	23		1.3
Human Polymeric							
Jevity	1.1	4.2	18	30	52	310	
Pulmocare	1.5	4.3	17	55	28	490	
Osmolite HN	1.1	4.4	17	30	53	310	
Sustacal	1.0	6.8	24	21	55	530	
Ensure HN	1.1	6.0	23	40	38	470	
Baby food, turkey	1.0	14.6	58	42	0		1.0
Human Monomeric							
Peptamen	1.0	4.4	16	33	51	260	
Supplements							
Promod (protein)	4.0	23.6		0	0		
Casec (protein)	4.0	30.7	0	100	0		
MCT oil (medium-chain triglyceride)	47.7	0	0	100	0		
Vegetable oil (long-chain triglyceride)	9.4				0		

*Blenderized 1/2 can (224 g) + 3/4 cup (170 ml) water
†Blenderized 1/2 can (224 g) + 1 1/4 cups (284 ml) water

Nutritional Disease of Pet Birds

Malnutrition of pet birds is common and potentially tragic. Obesity is common in pet birds, but not so common as in mammalian pets. Lack of exercise (no flying) and high fractions of oil seeds are usually incriminated. Sunflower, safflower, other oil seeds and peanuts are lipid-rich and have a low protein content for their energy content. Seeds also lack vitamin A, and epithelial distress is a sign of hypovitaminosis A (Fig. 21–10). The exceptional palatability of oil seeds commonly leads to addictions. Changing from seeds to complete foods may seem to be easy, though it might be difficult. Fresh foods and/or specific transitional feeding products may be the "bridge" to complete avian diets. Protein, vitamin and mineral fortified mixtures may be given as an alternative.

Hypo- and hypervitaminosis D, hypovitaminosis E, calcium deficiency, and unbalanced Ca:P ratios are other common malnutritions. When a nutritional disease is clinically evident with physical signs it is considered advanced. Specific drug and dietary therapy will be urgently needed. Vitamin A and other nutrients are more reliably given parenterally than by medicated water or food. Some patients benefit from enteral feeding by crop gavage. Place the feeding tube between the beak commissures (not beak tip), past the pharynx and into the esophagus or crop. Palpate the tube in the crop to ascertain that the trachea has not been entered. Gentle technique and practice are necessary to ensure proper tube feeding (Fig. 21–11A).

Enteral feeding solutions for avian critical care will vary by species. For generally debilitated psittacines, use slurries of baby bird growth formula. These may be specifically supplemented according to the diagnosis. Raptorial species do well on a meat and organ tissue–based mammalian repletion formula such as Prescription Diet Canine/Feline a/d (Hill's, Inc.). Any formula should be freshly prepared, carefully strained and warmed to a temperature not to exceed normal body temperature. Overheating foods may cause thermal burns to the esophagus or crop (Fig. 21–11B). Suggested gavage volumes in milliliters per feeding are as follows: budgerigars, 1 to 2; lovebirds, 2 to 3; cockateels, 3 to 6; conures, 4 to 12; parrots, 15 to 35; cockatoos, 20 to 40; macaws, 35 to 60. All equipment for feeding sick birds should be sanitized or sterilized between uses.

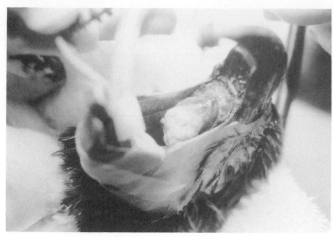

FIGURE 21–10. An abscess of a parrot's hard palate secondary to hypovitaminosis A. The vitamin A deficiency resulted from an exclusive intake of sunflower seeds. (Courtesy of Dr. Jeffrey Jenkins.)

PRODUCTION ANIMAL NUTRITION

Equine Nutrients

Nutrients of concern for horses are water, energy, protein, calcium, phosphorus and vitamin A. While all animals require access to good-quality water on an ad-lib basis, this is especially true for an animal capable of copious sweating (Carson, 1993; Lewis, 1982). Hot, exhausted horses should rest and perhaps consume some hay while cooling. A waiting period of 30 minutes should occur before allowing water after heavy exercise.

Horses evolved eating grass and other range forages. Not surprisingly, grass and hays serve well as a foundation for feeding all horses. *Good-quality* grass or legume hay, free-choice water, calcium and phosphorus as needed and trace mineralized salt are the only foods needed by the adult horse at maintenance.

The role of grain and protein meal "concentrates" is to complement forages during periods of higher than maintenance nutrient demand. Unfortunately, some horse feeding programs overlook quality forages and focus on elaborate programs of concentrate supplementation. The technician attending performance horses will also encounter a wide variety of owner- and trainer-selected supplements. These are diverse and may well match the current nutritional fad. Time-proven horse feeding programs emphasize simplicity and quality forage foods.

Equine food dose calculations are based on the horse's weight, and an amount of feed per 100 pounds of horse is a simple and frequently used method. Therefore, a horse weight tape is a simple and inexpensive tool worth having and using. For example, a 6-year-old, 1000-pound light-breed gelding is at rest in a backyard paddock. The animal receives only 1 hour per week of light work. This horse is considered to be at "maintenance"—an activity requiring 1.5 percent of the horse's body weight (BW) per day as dry matter. This means that 15 pounds of a good quality hay will suffice in addition to salt and water. If a 6-inch hay "flake" weighs 5 pounds, then feeding three per day (one in the AM and two in the PM) can be suggested as a food dose. Table 21–12 summarizes different dry matter intake levels for various activity and physiological states. As in small animals, equine overfeeding is a problem,

and a routine portion of all horse evaluations is body condition assessment (Fig. 21–12).

Some hays or hay/grain combinations need calcium and phosphorus supplementation. Most commonly, a source of phosphorus is added when a good legume hay is the sole source of nutrition. One best determines mineral supplement needs from a feed analysis or by consulting tables listing the mineral content of the type of hay being fed. The absolute quantity of total dietary calcium and phosphorus is more important than the calcium/phosphorus ratio. If macro mineral supplementation is needed; calcium, phosphorus, or combination calcium/phosphorus supplements are found as dicalcium phosphate, calcium carbonate, monosodium phosphate, and Purina 12:12 (Purina Mills). These powdered mineral supplements are often mixed with loose rock salt and provided free choice.

The micro minerals zinc, manganese, iron, copper, cobalt and sometimes iodine are contained in "trace mineralized" salt blocks. These are provided ad-lib in a location protected from rain.

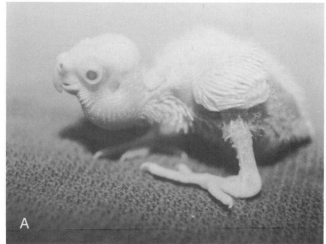

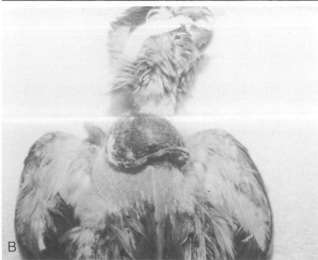

FIGURE 21–11. A, Hand-feeding baby birds formula by cannula or tube must be gentle. Esophagus perforation resulted from heavy technique. (Courtesy of Dr. Jeffrey Jenkins.) B, A full-thickness crop burn resulted from overheated formula. Temperature of formula should never exceed 40°C (104°F), and microwave heating is hazardous because irregular warming may result in "hot spots." (Courtesy of Dr. Jeffrey Jenkins.)

Table 21–12
NUTRIENT SUPPLY FOR HORSES*

Age	Energy	Protein	Vitamins and Minerals	Comments
Nursing foals	Supplement mare's milk if foal is very thin.	>16%	Calcium >0.85%	At 2–3 months of age begin 1 lb concentrate mixture/months of age/day.
			Phosphorus >0.5%	Adequate calcium, phosphorus, trace minerals in grain mix.
			Copper >25 mg/kg	If creep feeding, mix 50:50 chopped hay to grain.
			Vit. A 50 IU/kg BW	Wean at 4 months.
Weaning	Adequate to feel but not see the ribs.	15%	Calcium 0.7%	Dry matter intake = 3% of body weight.
			Phosphorus 0.4%	Free choice good roughage and trace mineral salt.
			Vit. A 50 IU/kg BW	1 lb concentrate mix/month of age/day 7–9 lb max.
Yearling	Adequate to feel but not see the ribs.	13%	Calcium 0.5%	Dry matter intake = 2.5% body weight.
			Phosphorus 0.3%	Free choice good roughage, trace mineral salt.
			Vit. A 50 IU/kg BW	1 lb concentrate mix/month of age/day 7–9 lb max.
				Feed as mature horse at 90% of mature weight.
Adult *Maintenance*	Adequate to feel but not see the ribs.	8.5%	Calcium 0.3% Phosphorus 0.2% Vit. A 50 IU/kg BW	Dry matter = 1.5% body weight. 1½ to 1¾ lb roughage/100 lb body weight. Free choice trace mineral salt.
Adult *Working*				
Light (pleasure ride)	Add .5–1.5 lb of grain/hour of activity/day.	8.5%	Calcium 0.3% Phosphorus 0.2%	Amortize grain supplement over the week.
Moderate (ranch work, roping, cutting, jumping, barrel racing)	Add 2–3 lb of grain/hour of activity/day.	8.5–10%	Vit. A 50 IU/kg BW	
Heavy (race training, polo)	Add 4 or more lb of grain/hour of activity/day.	8.5–10%	Calcium 0.3% Phosphorus 0.2% Vitamin A 50 IU/kg body weight	Dry matter = 1.75% body weight.
Adult Reproduction *Mares*	Feed at maintenance until late pregnancy.	8.5%–10%		
Late pregnancy	Needs 20% more energy.	11%	Calcium 0.5% Phosphorus 0.35% Vitamin A 50 IU/kg body weight	Feed 1½ to 1¾ lbs grass hays/100 lbs body weight with addition of ½ to ¾ lb grain or concentrate mix/100 lbs body weight. Free choice trace mineral salt–mineral calcium/phosphorus mix.
Last 3 weeks pregnancy	Needs 30% more energy.		Needs 100% more calcium and phosphorus Vitamin A 60 IU/kg body weight	1¾ to 2 lb legume hay/100 lb body weight. Free choice trace mineral salt–mineral calcium/phosphorus mix.
Lactation	Allow 75% energy increase at peak lactation.	14%	Calcium 0.5%	Dry matter = 1.75%–2.0% BW Free choice grass hay.
			Phosphorus 0.35% Vitamin A 60 IU/kg body weight	Add 1½–2 lb/100 lb BW of concentrate. Add calcium/phosphorus mix, and trace mineralized salt. At weaning: Stop concentrate; return to maintenance forage.
Stallions	Feed for maintenance.			

*Free choice, potable water should be available at all times.

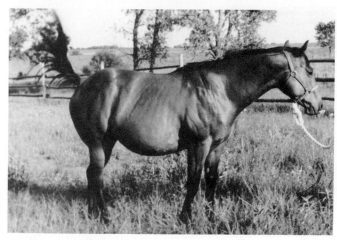

FIGURE 21–12. The last third of gestation elevates nutrient requirements for the mare. However, these elevations are modest, and the mare is not "eating for two." This animal shows good prepartum body condition because she was not overfed.

Routine horse feeding problems include overgrazed pastures, ingestion of sand and weeds, underfeeding due to poor-quality forage, too much grain, too fine a grind in pelleted feeds, various nutrient imbalances and toxic supplementation. Unfortunately, horses are not routinely or easily weighed in the typical setting, and changes in condition may be insidious. Accidental engorgement of grain may precipitate colic or founder with morbid or even tragic results (Table 21–13).

Feeding Sick Horses

Hospitalized horses develop the same protein-calorie deficits, hypermetabolic stress and catabolic wasting states as small animals. These have identical negative clinical effects, and early interventional feeding is vital in equine critical care. Major gastrointestinal tract (colic) surgery is especially challenging in the perioperative period. The animal needs a feed rich in protein, calories and micronutrients, but has reduced gastrointestinal motility (Ralston and Naylor, 1991). The veterinarian will focus closely on when GI motility returns. Homogenized, moistened, alfalfa pellet mashes are high-protein, high-energy and non-irritating repletion formulas. These may be given as slurries through nasogastric tubes and are often enriched with nutriment modules. Liquid enteral formulas based on mare's milk replacer and commercial equine critical care formulas are available and well tolerated. These formulas should be given in small frequent feedings via indwelling nasogastric tubes.

Feeding Ruminants

Ruminant nutrition varies from simple to complex. A beef cow does well on good range forage and a watering hole, while the heavily producing dairy cow requires 45 gallons of water, a 16 percent dietary protein concentration and very heavy energy intake. It appears that some metabolic disturbances in dairy cows follow exceptional energy requirements. Milk fever, grass tetany, rumen acidosis and left displacement of the abomasum have significant incidence and specific control measures (Allen and Sansom, 1993; Oetzel, 1988).

Llamas, goats and sheep may subsist on ranges unsuitable for cattle, but also may be intensively reared for wool, work, reproduction, meat or milk (Bretzlaff, 1993; Bulgin, 1993; Hutcheson, 1993; Kimberling and Marsh, 1993).

Young ruminants may have particular problems with cold stress, and high perinatal calf or lamb mortality is economically devastating. The health team perspective is that nutrition for thermogenesis and shivering must complement the provision of windbreaks and shelter (Cole, 1993; Olson, DP, 1993).

Livestock ranchers are sensitive to availability and quality of

Table 21–13 FEEDING PROBLEMS IN HORSES			
Disease	**Clinical Signs**	**Causes/Prevention**	**Comments**
"Colic"	1. Restlessness 2. Rolling 3. Intermittent flank kicking 4. Sweating 5. Rapid pulse 6. Altered GI movement	*Causes:* 1. Overload of grain 2. Toxic plants 3. Chronic parasite infestation 4. Foreign materials (sand) *Prevention:* 1. Avoid rapid feed/water changes 2. Internal parasite control program	1. May be life-threatening 2. Wide variety of severity
Laminitis (founder)	1. Anorexia 2. Severe hoof pain 3. Reluctance to walk	*Causes:* 1. Drinking cold water when overheated 2. Grain overload 3. Metritis	
"Milk fever" (hypocalcemic parturient paresis)	1. Sweating 2. Tremors 3. Incoordination	*Causes:* 1. Lactation and stress 2. Lush pasture *Prevention:* 1. Keep mare off lush pasture 8–10 days after foaling	Most common in draft breed horses

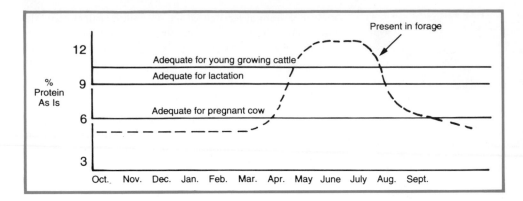

FIGURE 21–13. In the ruminant animal, rumen microbes create amino acids from nonprotein nitrogen sources and have a variety of nitrogen recycling systems. These abilities permit reduced protein intake when quality or quantity of forage is in decline. The highest percentage of protein present in forage occurs in May through August. Protein content is highest during the period of late gestation, lactation and weaning.

feed and water. Pastures become marginal or deficient in nutrient value during seasonal decline or drought, but grazing animals have several adaptive mechanisms (Figs. 21–13 and 21–14). However, pasture analysis, as the basis for customized supplemental rations, is an important concept and should be considered (Kothmann, 1993).

A summary of more common ruminant nutritional disorders is listed in Table 21–14. Table 21–15 describes generalized nutrient intake levels for various classes of farm ruminants. When nonprotein nitrogen sources partially fulfill crude protein requirements, the nonprotein nitrogen levels are limited to preclude palatability and metabolic problems (Simons and Hand, 1993; Van Horn, 1991).

Swine, Poultry and Fish

Swine, poultry and aquacultural nutrition is highly specialized in the intensive "agribusiness" rearing format. Long-term animal health usually is not involved in the planning for the nutritional care of these animals, as the nutritional objective is maximal growth rate. As a growing hog consumes 4 to 6 pounds of feed per 100 pounds of body weight per day, least-cost ration formulation programs are indispensable in controlling production costs (Table 21–16). In non-intensive hog operations, the management level may be lower and the technician may see dehydration (heat stress or under watering), protein/energy undersupply, and lysine, B vitamin, zinc and iron deficiency (Table 21–17) (Conner, 1993; Thaler and

Weaver, 1993). Nonconfinement hog operations may turn the pigs into pasture or fields to "hog down" crops. When pigs self-harvest, there is less labor and lower feeding costs, but a slower rate of growth than in the intensive confinement rearing mode.

Assessing Livestock Forages and Grains

The veterinary technician can assist the veterinarian as an extra set of eyes and ears around the horse and livestock feedbunk. Confirming access to good water and the quality pastures and hays are important starting points.

A feedbunk "rule" for horses is not to exceed a 50:50 ratio of concentrate to roughage. Oats and corn are the two most common feeds, and noting their relative energy content is important (Fig. 21–15A). Various horse grains, mixed concentrate supplements, and several totally complete extruded or pelleted horse feeds will be encountered on horse calls (Fig. 21–15B, C). If horses consume only complete extruded or pelleted feeds, an issue may be an adequate roughage intake. The sudden onset of fence chewing when only a complete pelleted food is used suggests the need for at least some long-stem or coarse chopped hay.

Forage quality varies greatly by soil quality, species of grass, season of year, rainfall, overgrazing, pasture rotation, weed control and the presence of toxic weeds (Burrows and Case, 1993; James, 1993). The quality of silage and haylage depends on ensiling conditions as well as the quality of the original

Text continued on page 477

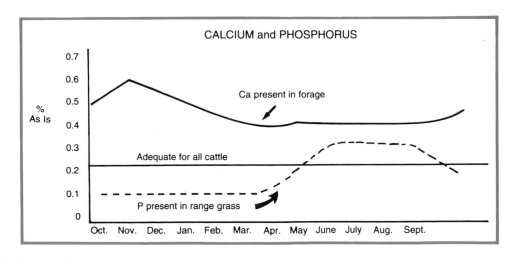

FIGURE 21–14. Nutrient quality in forage is influenced by soil quality, species of plant, and the plant's growth stage. Animals are able to store the macro minerals calcium and phosphorus in skeletal reservoirs during period of intake adequacy.

	Table 21–14 FEEDING PROBLEMS IN RUMINANTS*		
Disease	**Clinical Signs**	**Causes/Prevention**	**Comments**
Bloat	1. Gas or froth 2. Respiratory distress 3. Distention of the left side 4. Salivation, cyanosis	*Causes:* 1. Overeating 2. Fine ground feeds 3. Bacterial overgrowth 4. Certain pasture types *Prevention:* 1. Pasture <50% legumes 2. Avoid heavy grain intake 3. Gradually increase grain or alfalfa	All ruminants, but particularly cattle.
Grass tetany (hypomagnesemia)	1. Disorientation 2. Paddling 3. Convulsions	*Causes:* Heavy intake of lush pasture *Prevention:* 1. Mineral blocks 2. Magnesium	Most common in adult beef cows and ewes. Calves may have inadequate absorption of magnesium.
Left displaced abomasum	1. Intermittent anorexia 2. Decreased stool output 3. Left flank fullness	*Causes:* 1. Heavy feeding of grain 2. Parturition 3. Ketosis 4. Toxemia 5. Metritis *Prevention:* High grain and low fiber are risk factors	
Milk fever (parturient paresis)	1. Unsteadiness 2. Anorexia 3. Subnormal temperature 4. Dull expression 5. Paralysis	*Causes:* Heavy lactation *Prevention:* Acidifying diet during late pregnancy	Most often in dairy cows 5 to 9 years old within 3 days of parturition. May occur in dairy goats.
Urinary calculi	1. Urinary straining 2. Hematuria 3. Kicking at abdomen 4. Secondary rectal prolapse 5. Rupture of bladder or urethra	*Causes:* 1. ↓Fresh water supply 2. ↑Mineral excretion 3. Genetic predisposition *Prevention:* Fresh water and balanced mineral intake	Feeder cattle and wethers are predisposed. Most often in the winter months.

*Data from Caple IW and West DM: Ruminant hypomagnesemic tetanies. *In* Howard JL (editor): Current Veterinary Therapy: Food Animal Practice 3. Philadelphia, WB Saunders Co., 1993, pp 318–321.

Table 21–15
NUTRIENT SUPPLY FOR LIVESTOCK*

Species	Protein	Energy	Minerals and Vitamins	Comments
Cattle *Beef* Growing-finishing Steer/heifers Calves and yearlings	Crude protein, 14%–15% (weanling), 12%–13% (up to 900 lb), 9%–11% (finishing); protein is affected by environment, growth rate and age.	200–750 lb/body weight = 2.6–7 lb TDN 750–1100 lb body weight = 7–8.5 lb TDN	Calcium/phosphorus ratio 1.5:1 Readily available salt and trace minerals Vitamin A 20–40,000 IU Vitamin D 275 IU	Muscle tissue growth rapidly diminishes after 900–1000 lb of weight. See references for cold and heat stress in beef cattle.
Beef breeding herd	Crude protein, (dry, pregnant cows) 5.9%–7.0% Crude protein (lactating cows) 9.2%–10.9%	TDN = 7.7–8.8 lb/day (52% digestibility) or TDN = 10.7–13.7 lb/day (55% digestibility)	Calcium/phosphorus ratio 1:1 Readily available salt and trace minerals Vitamin A 35–40,000 IU Vitamin D 275 IU	1. Dry cows intake = 1.5% of body weight. 2. Average cows = 1.75% of body weight. 3. Poor condition cows = 2.25% of body weight.
Dairy† Lactation	Crude protein, 13.9%–18% (dependent on milk production)	TDN 8.8–18.7 lb/day (70% digestibility)	Calcium/phosphorus ratio 1.3:1 Vitamin A 28,000 IU Vitamin D 500 IU Salt and trace minerals	Lactating cows will drink 15–45 gallons/day.
Dry cows		TDN 8.8–18.7 lb/day (70% digestibility) *Dry cows:* First 5–7 days 10–15 lb poor quality hay TDN 1% of total body weight (55% digestibility) 2–5 lb grain/day	Salt and trace minerals Calcium/phosphorus ratio 1:1 Vitamin A 28,000 IU Vitamin D 500 IU	Energy and protein intake influences milk production.
Calves	Crude protein, 18%	Milk replacer at least 10% fat Calf starter: 4–5 lb grain/day	Calcium/phosphorus ratio 4.1 to 3.2 Young heifers 3.4 to 2.6 Salt and trace minerals Vitamin A 1600 IU Vitamin D 250 IU	
Replacement stock	Crude protein, 8.6%–10%	*Yearling heifers:* TDN = 3.9–4.8 lb/day 2-year-old heifers: 4.6–5.8 lb/day	Calcium/phosphorus ratio 1.3:1 Salt and trace minerals Vitamin A 25,000 IU Vitamin D 500 IU	
Sheep/Goat Ewes/nannies: Maintenance/early gestation (first 15 weeks)	Crude protein, 10%–12% (ewes)	Total energy intake 1.2–1.5 lb/day (first 15 weeks)	Calcium/phosphorus ratio 1.1:1 Vitamin A 1275–2040 IU Vitamin D 278–444 IU	Do not exceed 1 ppm selenium. Learn regional soil Se++ content.
	Crude protein, 10%–13% (nannies)	Total energy intake 3.0–3.7 lb/day	Calcium/phosphorus ratio 1.3:1 Vitamin A 4250–6800 IU Vitamin D 278–444 IU	Loose salt available to flock.
Late gestation (last 6 weeks)	Crude protein, 12%–16%	Total energy intake 3.3–4.3 lb/day	Calcium/phosphorus ratio 1.4:1 Vitamin A 4250–6800 IU Vitamin D 278–444 IU	Use trace mineral blocks.
Lactation	Crude protein, 10%–13%	Total energy intake 1.7–3.1 lb/day	Calcium/phosphorus ratio 1.5:1 Vitamin A 1700–5100 IU Vitamin D 222–666 IU	Readily available fresh water.
Replacement stock Lambs/kids (early weaned)	Crude protein 10%–13%	Total energy intake .97–2.25 lb/day	Calcium/phosphorus ratio 1.5:1 Vitamin A 850–2550 IU Vitamin D 67–200 IU	Confirm dietary sulfur content if finishing with nonprotein nitrogen sources.
Finishing lambs/kids	Crude protein 10%–13%	Total energy intake 1.8–2.9 lb/day	Calcium/phosphorus ratio 1.6:1 Vitamin A 765–1400 IU Vitamin D 166–305 IU	
Orphans	Milk protein >25%	Milk replacer: Fat >30%	Calcium/phosphorus ratio 1.5:1 Vitamin A 850 IU Vitamin D 67 IU	Average intake on twice daily feeding is ½ to ¾ lb dry milk replacer dry or 2–4 pints liquid milk. Wean at 25–30 lb.

*Nutritional requirements vary with breed, age, activity and environment. Use these figures as a guide only. Feed to maintain optimum weight.
†Dairy cattle vary greatly.

Table 21–16
NUTRIENT SUPPLY FOR SWINE

Swine Species	Protein	Energy	Minerals and Vitamins	Comments
Weaning to market	Crude protein, 13%–20%	1473–1489 Kcal ME/lb* diet	Calcium 0.75% Phosphorus 0.60% Salt 0.1% Vitamin A 591–1000 IU Vitamin D 68–100 IU	Free feeding is common. Restricted feeding improves feed efficiency.
Bred gilts and sows	Crude protein, 12%	1481 Kcal ME/lb diet	Calcium 0.75% Phosphorus 0.60%	Bred gilts and sows are fed similarly to market animals during early gestation.
Breeding boars			Salt 0.15% Vitamin A 1818 IU Vitamin D 91 IU	
Lactation Gilts and sows	Crude protein, 13%	1481 Kcal ME/lb diet	Calcium 0.75% Phosphorus 0.60% Salt 0.20% Vitamin A 909 IU Vitamin D 91 IU	

*Kcal ME refers to number of calories of metabolizable energy per pound of ration consumed.

Table 21–17
NUTRITIONAL DISORDERS OF SWINE

Disease	Clinical Signs	Cause/Prevention	Comments
Iron deficiency anemia	Weakness, poor growth, anorexia	*Cause:* Poor placental transfer, rapid growth rate, low concentration of iron in milk *Prevention:* Fortify iron in latter part of gestation for gilts and sows	This is common, and there is some genetic predisposition.
Lysine deficiency	Reduced growth rate Reduced milk production	*Cause:* Incomplete diets *Prevention:* Use complete and balanced rations	Lysine is the first limiting amino acid in home-made corn-soy rations.
Nutritional secondary hyperparathyroidism	Twisted snouts Lameness	*Cause:* Unbalanced rations too high in phosphorus *Prevention:* Avoid excess wheat bran	

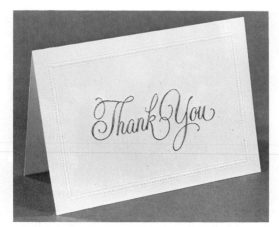

FIGURE 22–18. Example of thank-you card.

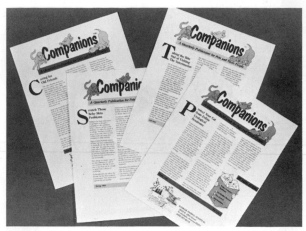

Figure 22–19. Commercially prepared newsletter. (Courtesy of Hill's Pet Nutrition, Inc., Topeka, KS.)

client deal with the loss and also allows the client to understand the "I care" attitude of the practice.

Newsletters. Charles, Charles and Associates have reported use of newsletters is related to increased number of clinic visits of dog owners (Troutman 1988). The utilization of newsletters will increase client activity through improved understanding and education about veterinary services. Educational goals for newsletters should be to inform animal owners of signs of illness, to make seasonal animal health care recommendations (i.e., heat stroke in summer), to review health care programs and to introduce key staff members. Many clients do not understand how to tell whether an animal is ill or in serious condition. This lack of knowledge is especially true for cat and horse owners.

The horse is difficult for the average client to evaluate when experiencing abdominal pain from colic. Unless the owner is familiar with the specific signs of abdominal pain, the animal's condition may become critical before attention is sought. It is also difficult to tell when a cat is ill. Normally cats sleep a lot, cover their feces and urine and tend to be loners. It becomes difficult to really know when they are ill unless the owner has a little knowledge.

Newsletters will allow the client to be exposed to specific pieces of information that will help the owner to know when to call a veterinarian for help. Total health care plans can also be explained to allow the owner to be aware of full-service health care that extends beyond vaccinations. The newsletter should help market the benefits of healthy animals.

Newsletters can be sent to specific segments of clients in the practice computer base. However, they can also be provided through a hand-generated list or passed out to each client as they enter the practice. Most veterinarians do not have the experience or time to compose a complete newsletter three or four times per year. Careful thought should be given to purchasing a professionally edited newsletter service. Several services are available from which to choose, with direct mailing from the publisher to the client as an option (Fig. 22–19).

Each newsletter should be personalized by the practice to allow the reader easy access to the practice's location and phone number. Another advantage newsletters have in overall marketing is the ability to reach the nonuser. If the client receiving the newsletter passes it on to a nonclient friend, the nonclient has an opportunity to be exposed to various veterinary services.

Specialty Services. Practices can expand services or add new services to increase their market share. In a small animal practice, market expansion might be in the areas of birds and exotic service, bereavement counseling, prepurchase evaluation of pets to determine suitability for family, nutritional counseling (i.e., puppy, adult, senior), dental care (i.e., endodontics, periodontics, orthodontics), geriatric care, cremation service, emergency care and intensive care unit. Since most small animal clinics cater to dogs, many cat owners do not feel welcome or comfortable in an environment of dog pictures on the walls and barking dogs in the reception area. Practices that want to increase feline clients might be well rewarded by considering the needs of cats and cat owners when remodeling. Having a separate reception area for cats and keeping cats in a separate ward should be a starting point. Our own attitudes about feline care may be the primary reason for serving only 70 percent of the cat owners with professional veterinary care (Wise, 1992).

Sales Point Displays. When displays are being considered as an internal marketing technique, several important points must be contemplated if they are to be maximally successful. First, the practice must define the clients' needs. The specific products must be carefully selected and priced. An appropriate location(s) must be established in the clinic or hospital that may be monitored at *all* times by the technical staff (Fig. 22–20). The products must be attractively arranged and kept neat and clean. Prices must be clearly marked on all products.

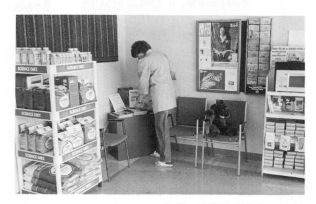

FIGURE 22–20. Professional display in reception area being monitored by a staff member.

The most important difference between a hospital or clinic display and a retail store display is the *professional* advice that goes along with each item sold. Professional counseling is not available at the feed store, grocery store, department store or mail order outlets. The technical staff will play a key role in product information for the client.

Professional displays may be limited product lines confined to an examination room, a specific area of the reception room or a special room adjacent to the reception room.

Animal Care Talks. Veterinary technicians and veterinarians can both become involved in providing veterinary medical care talks to grade school and high school students as well as to clients. These presentations can provide information on routine animal health care, first aid activities, signs to look for when an animal is ill and general information of educational requirements of veterinarians and technicians. These presentations can help to change the established "norms" about animal care.

When a presentation has become polished, service clubs in the community make excellent audiences. Talks to service clubs are helpful to the individual practice and the profession. A slide presentation that features both veterinarian and technician in their "team" roles is effective.

The veterinary technician could present information on care of the new puppy or kitten, information on exotic pets and birds, first aid, feeding the pet, whelping and queening, hip dysplasia, parasite control, pet obedience training and pet selection. Client education programs should be given on a regular basis and offered at convenient times. Attendees should be provided with handout material to take home for future reference.

When the education program is held at the practice, a complete tour of the facilities should be planned. Clients are interested in seeing hospital equipment and understanding more about hospital care. A hospital open house is an excellent image builder to clients. Having a "behind the scenes" tour is something most clients have not had an opportunity to experience. Children are especially impressed with "show and tell" demonstrations.

By providing client education opportunities, the client becomes more bonded to the practice. When veterinary problems arise, the client is more apt to contact the practice who has provided the inside look and veterinary medical information.

External Marketing

Most external marketing activities are aimed at expanding current client activity and identifying new nonclient activity. External marketing can be carried out by an individual practice, group practice, organized veterinary medicine and commercial companies.

Some types of external marketing are currently being utilized in many practices. The use of newsletters (direct mail to nonclients), telephone yellow page listings, building signs, client education nights, community service activities and utilization of the American Veterinary Medical Association's National Pet Week materials all expand the image of the practice to clients and nonclients. When a practice wants to penetrate into the nonclient base, one must make use of advertising.

Professional Advertising. Professional advertising includes hospital signs, telephone book listings, practice newsletters, vaccination reminders, professional business cards, and so forth. However, the focus on advertising in this discussion will center on the more "hard core" forms of advertising: yellow pages of the telephone book, newspapers, magazines, radio, direct mail and television.

Attitudes concerning advertising differ between the professional and the consumer. A great majority of professionals (physicians, dentists, attorneys, veterinarians) themselves are against advertising for a variety of reasons: unprofessional, unethical and lowers status, credibility and sense of dignity. Just as professionals feel strongly negative toward advertising, consumers feel strongly positive. Consumers generally feel advertising by a professional would not compromise that professional's credibility, status, image, or dignity. In fact, most consumers believe advertising by professionals would help them make a more intelligent choice (McCurnin and Thompson, 1986).

Telephone Yellow Pages. Veterinarians have been strongly encouraged by yellow page sales staff to market their practice through increasingly larger telephone advertisements. Many major metropolitan area telephone books now carry a variety of one-quarter, half and full page advertisements for individual veterinary practices. Investing in a larger and larger telephone advertisement is not the long-term solution to market expansion. Unfortunately, some practitioners have not considered other forms of practice marketing. When most practitioners in a specific area are using quarter- or half-page telephone advertising, the consumer impact is the same as when practitioners are all using one-line listings. The only difference is the increased costs of the larger listings that must eventually be passed on to the client.

When developing a new practice, a larger telephone listing is effective, but using an ever-increasing sized listing does not replace a multi-approach marketing plan. If a particular practice area is in need of greater client exposure, the individual practitioner's cost can be reduced by group advertising. As an example, the local Veterinary Medical Association could sponsor a "practitioner locating service" by using a full yellow page listing grouping practitioners by location within the area. These location guides are helpful to the consumer and represent a savings to the practitioners, yet provide a full page of veterinary advertising.

When a yellow page advertisement is deemed appropriate for external marketing purposes, several guidelines should be followed. First, the advertisement should not be larger than one-quarter page. Advertisements larger than one-quarter page are perceived as being more unprofessional by the consumer. Second, the advertisement should be set in one color (preferably black). The use of multiple color (such as red and green) is again perceived by the consumer as being less professional.

Newspapers. Newspaper advertising, like telephone yellow page advertising, is useful for initial impact when opening or expanding a practice. Many professionals will have a newspaper listing when opening a new practice, when relocating an existing practice or when adding new associates to an existing practice. The continual use of newspaper advertising by veterinarians has been largely prohibited by cost.

In large multilocation practices, newspaper advertising might be used effectively if professionally prepared. However, the cost-benefit ratio would need careful monitoring.

Probably the best form of newspaper advertising for veterinarians is the "animal care information" format. Weekly animal care information columns are a public service, and newspapers are always seeking educational material. "Pet columns" have become popular reading as the public begins to acknowledge and understand the human-animal bond. To address the need for weekly newspaper columns, several private column services have sprung up that will provide the practitioner with 52 professionally written stories on animal care each year. This service can be purchased by individual veterinarians or through associations.

In the larger metropolitan areas, newspapers can become restrictive as to the stories they print. If a veterinarian (or association) is unsuccessful in obtaining agreement for publication of a regular column, one should explore the neighborhood papers in the area. These "weekly" local neighborhood papers are usually well read and circulated and are always open to new material.

Radio and Television. Two of the most powerful advertising mediums are radio and television. Both are expensive and are generally out of financial consideration of most veterinarians. Consumers are being exposed to increasing numbers of commercials for services provided by attorneys, dentists, opticians, physicians and chiropractors as professional competition increases.

A few large, multilocation veterinary group practices advertise services on television. If a large practice is considering radio and/or television media, an advertising consultant should be retained and the cost-benefit ratio closely evaluated.

Veterinary associations can obtain air time essentially free by participating in talk shows. The subject of animals, animal care and animal behavior is a fascinating subject to most listening and viewing audiences. A number of the larger radio and television markets have regularly scheduled talk shows (some hosted by veterinarians) that have a question and answer format devoted to animal care. The talk show format is an excellent opportunity for those associations that have articulate and knowledgeable veterinarians and technicians to sell veterinary medicine for the profession as a whole.

The bottom line for all individual practices and most smaller group practices is advertising is too expensive to be carried out on a regular basis. The only medium that has consistently been used to attract nonclients is the telephone yellow pages. Other forms of advertising (i.e., television, newspaper, magazines, radio) must be supported by organized veterinary medicine and commercial companies. Increased interest in promoting veterinarians and veterinary practice has come from commercial companies upon the realization that individual practice expansion results in commercial expansion.

Community Activities. Veterinary practices that are engaged in community activities have a much wider client contact base. Veterinarians and technicians can both become involved in community service through Girl Scouts, Boy Scouts, school board, humane society, breed club, country club, Rotary, Lions and church activities. Potential client contacts are made in the course of "being involved."

One should not join a community activity only to make client contacts. Practice is too time-consuming for both veterinarian and technician to become involved in too many activities or activities that are not personally rewarding. However, these activities are an important marketing tool in addition to being necessary for the community.

Equipment and Building Maintenance

The largest capital investments of a veterinary hospital practice are the building, land and equipment. Clients continue to evaluate the level of animal care by the appearance of the building and grounds. Maintenance of building and grounds through painting and repair of the interior and exterior of the building along with meticulous care of the lawn, shrubs, trees and flowers translates into a caring feeling to the client.

General maintenance within the building is an ongoing responsibility. Floors, flat surfaces, walls, cages, runs and stalls must be kept sparkling clean and odor-free. To reach this goal, *everyone* in the practice must assume some of the responsibility. No one should hunt for someone else to clean up a fresh urine or fecal deposit; it is quicker and easier to clean it up by yourself!

Equipment maintenance and cleaning should be an ongoing activity as well. Each major piece of equipment should be assigned to a specific member of the hospital team. Certain items should have a specific recorded maintenance schedule to ensure proper servicing (e.g., anesthetic machines, x-ray tank solutions, autoclave, microscope, clinical pathology laboratory instruments, computer terminals, central vacuum system). Other items need to be cleaned or serviced, or both, after each use, such as electric clippers, surgical instruments, endoscopes, otoscope, ophthalmoscope, Bard-Parker instrument tray and gas levels of oxygen and nitrous oxide.

If each equipment item has an assigned responsible maintenance person, all equipment will last longer and will always be ready when needed. Nonmedical equipment, such as typewriters, calculators, air conditioning and heating units, lawn mowers and hospital vehicles, must also be assigned to those responsible for their use.

In conclusion, practices that will flourish in the twenty-first century will be those that integrate well-trained technicians with responsible client communication, deliver high-quality medicine and surgery, maintain good client-patient and personnel-business management, practice in attractive facilities aided by a good location and practice preventative maintenance on the facility, equipment and grounds. These flourishing practices will be exciting and rewarding for clients, patients and staff.

References

McCurnin DM: Marketing your practice and the profession. *In* McCurnin DM (editor): Veterinary Practice Management. Philadelphia, JB Lippincott Co., 1988, pp 113–137.

McCurnin DM and Thompson A: Professional advertising, JAVMA:188(12):1387–1389, 1986.

Schwarz JH: Personnel management. *In* McCurnin DM (editor): Veterinary Practice Management. Philadelphia, JB Lippincott Co., 1988, pp 41–67.

Troutman CW: The Veterinary Services Market. Overland Park, KS Charles, Charles and Associates, 1988.

Wise JK: The Veterinary Service Market for Companion Animals 1992. Schaumburg, IL. AVMA, 1992.

23

Basic Necropsy Procedures

DOO-YOUN CHO and TERRY R. SPRAKER

INTRODUCTION

Necropsy (Greek = viewing death) is the postmortem examination of a dead animal. The word autopsy (Greek = viewing self) should not be used in veterinary medicine because of its reference to humans. The necropsy is an important part of the veterinary medical practice for many reasons, the major reasons being (1) to determine the cause of death of the animal; (2) to determine the nature and course of the disease and/or pathological process; and (3) to assess the accuracy of the clinical diagnosis and the effectiveness or success of the treatment. Necropsy may also need to be performed for medicolegal reasons. In these situations, however, it may be better to submit the animal to a qualified veterinary pathologist. This is important, especially if a particular case were to be challenged in court.

Since the postmortem examination involves dissection of the body and organs and recognition of pathological changes in the tissues, systematic dissection techniques and a knowledge of anatomy are required. During necropsy, proper tissue samples are collected and submitted to the appropriate laboratories for further evaluation.

Knowledge gained through necropsy will aid and enhance the quality of the practice of veterinary medicine in the future.

PERFORMING THE NECROPSY

Records

The necropsy record is commonly overlooked or poorly completed by veterinarians. The most common excuse is "not

enough time." If one is going to take time to do a necropsy, one should "take time" to write down the findings. The necropsy record is important for future reference, especially in medicolegal problems. Pathology or necropsy records should contain at least five items: (1) signalment, (2) anamnesis (history), (3) gross necropsy findings, (4) tentative diagnosis and (5) tissues submitted to the laboratory.

The signalment should contain the owner's name, address and phone number and the animal's species, age, sex and name. The signalment should also include the animal's clinical case number, date of death, postmortem interval (hours since death), date of necropsy and necropsy number.

The anamnesis should contain a brief medical history, including clinical signs, duration of illness and treatments. If the veterinarian is referring the animal to a pathologist and has a special diagnostic request (e.g., removing the spinal cord), this request may be stated in the anamnesis.

The next portion of the necropsy report should contain a brief gross description *(not interpretation)* of organs and lesions. The gross description should contain comments on size, shape, color, consistency, texture and odor of all organs and a detailed description of all lesions. The last statement of the gross description should list the organs or tissues that were clinically suspected to be involved but are found to have no gross abnormalities.

Following the gross description, a tentative diagnosis is made. The interpretation and discussion of lesions and the cause of death of the animal are stated here. The interpretation of lesions should *not* be included in the description of the gross findings.

Finally, a short note should be added if tissues are submitted to a laboratory for microbiology, toxicology, parasitology or histopathology studies. If tissues are being sent to the laboratory, one copy of the necropsy report with a cover letter explaining specific requests should be mailed with the tissues. Another copy of the necropsy report should be placed with the medical record of that particular animal. (Additional information concerning the medical record can be found in Chapter 3.)

Fixatives

If the veterinarian requests histopathological studies on tissues from the case, the tissues must be properly preserved. *Fixatives* are chemicals that preserve the natural architecture of tissues by causing alteration of proteins, lipids and carbohydrates and thus prevent *autolysis* (self-destruction). For histopathological studies to be of value, tissues must be taken as soon as possible after death and must be properly fixed. If an animal has been dead for longer than 24 hours or has been exposed to the sun for several hours, autolysis of the tissues will prevent meaningful histopathological studies. The size of tissue to be fixed in the fixative is also important. Tissues should not be more than 0.5 cm in thickness. The only exception is when fixing brain (which should be hemisected and placed in formalin), eye and lung tissue.

The most practical fixative for the practicing veterinarian is 10 percent neutral buffered formalin (formalin can be used for all tissues). Formalin is actually a 3.7 percent formaldehyde solution and is acidic. The solution has to be buffered to a pH of 7, or it will cause acid digestion of tissues. Formalin can be easily made and, in tightly closed containers, has a shelf life of a minimum of 6 to 8 months. All solid tissues should be 0.5 cm or less in thickness when placed in the formalin. The total volume of formalin to solid tissues should be approximately 10:1. The 10:1 ratio will allow proper fixation of tissues. If too much tissue is placed in the formalin, the tissues will tie up all of the fixative leaving some of the tissue unfixed. This unfixed tissue will then undergo autolysis.

Other fixatives of which the veterinary technician should be aware are *Zenker's* and *Bouin's fixatives*. Zenker's is an excellent fixative for eyes, but to benefit from this rapid fixative the eyes should be placed in it within 10 to 15 minutes after death; otherwise formalin is as effective. Bouin's is the preferred fixative for reproductive organ tissues. Neither Zenker's nor Bouin's is recommended for use in private practice because of the involved fixation procedures and cumbersome disposal requirements of the chemicals involved. All fixatives must be clearly labeled, and the proper precautions must be taken to avoid a direct contact with these chemicals. See Table 23–1 for formulation of the fixatives.

Equipment

The equipment used for necropsies includes three major categories: (1) protective clothing, (2) instruments and tools and (3) fixatives. Protective clothing should be worn during every necropsy and includes coveralls or aprons, rubber gloves and boots. Some infectious diseases are transmissible from animals to humans (zoonotic diseases). When one is performing a necropsy on animals suspected of a zoonotic disease, includ-

Table 23–1 FORMULATION FOR FORMALIN, ZENKER'S AND BOUIN'S SOLUTIONS	
Buffered Neutral Formalin Solution	
37%–40% formalin	100.0 ml
Distilled water	900.0 ml
Sodium phosphate monobasic	4.0 gm
Sodium phosphate dibasic (anhydrous)	6.5 gm
Zenker's Solution*	
Distilled water	1000.0 ml
Mercuric chloride	50.0 gm
Potassium dichromate	25.0 gm
Sodium sulfate	10.0 gm
Bouin's Solution	
Picric acid, saturated aqueous solution	750.0 ml
37%–40% formalin	250.0 ml
Glacial acetic acid	50.0 ml

*Add 5 ml of glacial acetic acid to 95 ml of Zenker's solution before use. The solution does not keep well after the addition of the acetic acid.

ing birds (especially psittacines), a mask should be worn in addition to the routine protective clothing and gloves.

The instruments needed to do a necropsy for both large and small animals include knives, scalpels, scissors, forceps and saws of various sizes and shapes (Fig. 23–1). Knives should be kept sharp. Dull knives tend to tear and compress tissue and cause compression artifacts on histopathological study. The prosector also has to apply more pressure for cutting, and one is more apt to cut oneself when using a dull knife. Cleavers or saws can be used for removing the brain or spinal cord. Pruning shears intended for cutting branches from trees are useful for cutting ribs of large and small animals. Necropsies should be done in areas that are easily cleaned and disinfected and *not* in surgery or treatment rooms.

A covered instrument tray filled with disinfectant, containing scissors, forceps and scalpels, should be kept near the necropsy table for collection of sterile samples for microbiology (see Chapter 6). Properly labeled fixatives and collection bottles should also be available for tissue samples.

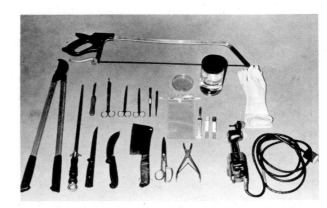

FIGURE 23–1. Instruments commonly used during a necropsy include saws, knives, scalpels, scissors, forceps, formalin and gloves.

General Procedure

An important point to remember about a necropsy is that autolysis begins immediately after the animal dies. Therefore, necropsy should be done immediately following death of the animal. If it cannot be done immediately, the carcass should be refrigerated. The carcass should not be frozen if a meaningful histopathological evaluation is desired. Freezing disrupts cells by crystallization and melting of intracellular water. In general, the longer you wait to do a necropsy following the death of an animal, the less information the necropsy will provide. Before the necropsy is started, the signalment and anamnesis should be reviewed.

There are various techniques for doing a necropsy. The veterinary technician should develop a standard technique that allows examination of all organs and meets the requirements of the veterinarian. The prosector should have a knowledge of anatomy, including normal size, shape, color, consistency, texture and odor of all major organs. At first, the veterinary technician should follow a step-by-step outline of a necropsy. As the technician gains experience, some alteration in the basic outline may become necessary in order to check for specific lesions.

Necropsy Technique for the Bovine

The animal that most commonly undergoes necropsy by veterinarians is the bovine. The reason is the "herd health approach" to bovine medicine. If a farmer has several sick calves, several morbid calves will often be presented for necropsy so that a definite etiological diagnosis can be determined. Following necropsy, the veterinarian will usually be able to provide information on prevention of the disease and specific treatments for the other sick calves.

Position

Most ruminants (cattle, goats, sheep) are positioned with the left side down, since the rumen is on the left side, and if the animal is examined from the right side, the internal organs are more easily visualized. Before the animal is opened, a complete examination of all external surfaces should be completed with special attention to eyes, ears, nose, feet, anus and hocks. For example, a calf with staining of the hocks and tail region with feces suggests scours. This would provide additional insight into the problem and may suggest tissues that need to be taken for histopathological and microbiological studies prior to opening the carcass. Following the external examination, the skin is incised from the chin along the ventral midline encircling the external genitalia (and mammary glands in adult females) to the anus. The skin is reflected on the right side, including right forelimbs and hindlimbs (Fig. 23–2). Reflection of the limbs may be accomplished by raising the leg and cutting the axillary muscles of the forelimb and by cutting the muscles, joint capsule and round ligament of the coxofemoral (hip) joint of the hindlimb. As the legs are reflected, the brachial plexus of the foreleg and the sciatic nerves of the hindlimb should be examined. Alternatively, when necropsies are performed on large cattle, the limbs may be reflected first before the skin is reflected. The exposed right side of the animal should be examined. Muscles and external lymph nodes should be checked. If the animal is an adult female, the

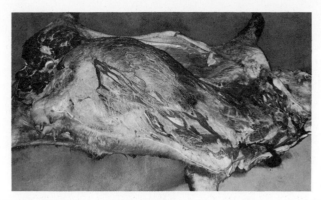

FIGURE 23–2. The skin, forelimb and hindlimb have been reflected in this bovine.

mammary glands, including the mammary lymph nodes, should be removed from the carcass and examined.

Exposure of Abdominal and Thoracic Cavities

The abdominal cavity is opened by making an incision through the abdominal wall, starting behind the ribs down to the sternum then posteriorly along the ventral aspects of the vertebrae (dorsal flank region) down to the pelvic rim. This creates a large abdominal wall flap. This flap is reflected downward. Opening the carcass in this manner allows replacement of the viscera back into the carcass and reattachment of the abdominal wall flap to the vertebrae. This technique will allow easier removal of the carcass from the rancher's pasture.

Once the viscera are exposed (Fig. 23–3), they should be examined for size, position, adhesions, and so on. The prosector should run his or her hand between the reticulum and the diaphragm in adult cattle to check for adhesions (hardware disease). Next, the diaphragm should be punctured with a knife, and the prosector should listen for the inflow of air into the thoracic cavity. An animal with pneumonia or *pneumothorax* (air in the thoracic cavity) will have a reduced amount of negative pressure within the thoracic cavity. This will result in reduced sounds of inflowing air. Next, the entire right side of the diaphragm should be removed along its costal arch to allow observation of the thoracic cavity. Now, using the pruning shears, the dorsal aspects of the ribs are cut, and the costochondral junctions are cut with the knife, allowing the rib cage to be removed (Fig. 23–4).

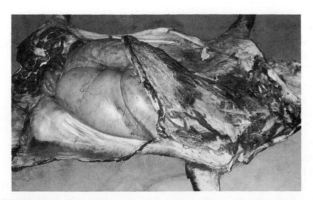

FIGURE 23–3. Skin reflected, abdominal flap removed and viscera exposed in a ruminant.

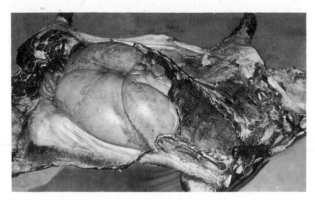

FIGURE 23–4. Skin reflected and abdominal flap and rib cage removed to expose viscera, lungs and heart in a bovine.

The thoracic and abdominal cavities are now exposed, and all organs are inspected in situ for displacement, size, shape and color. If organs are noted to be abnormal and cultures are desired, now is the best time to take the samples before tissues are handled and further contaminated. For example, if a pneumonic lung is observed, the culture should be taken before removal from the thoracic cavity. All microbiological specimens should be taken with sterile instruments and placed in sterile containers (see Chapter 6).

Removal of Primary Organs

The viscera are now removed from the abdominal cavity. First, take four pieces of string and double ligate the terminal rectum and proximal duodenum. After transecting the rectum and duodenum between the double ligatures, begin to pull out the small intestine. Remove the mesentery and cut the attachments to the liver. Next, remove the liver and set it aside. Remove the rumen by pulling it ventrally and cutting its dorsal attachments. Another double ligature is placed around the esophagus as it enters the rumen, thus preventing spillage of rumen contents into the thoracic cavity when transected. The spleen will be attached to the dorsal left side of the rumen and will be removed with the rumen. The urinary and reproductive systems and adrenal glands remain in the abdominal cavity. These systems are removed en masse and are set aside for further examination. The pluck (includes tongue, thyroid glands, trachea, lungs, thymus and heart) is removed en masse and set aside. This is done by incising the medial side of both mandibles close to the bone; this will free the tongue. Next, pull the tongue downward to the hyoid bones, cutting through the large prominent keratoepihyoid joints of the hyoid bones. The teeth and hard and soft palate should now be examined. Continue to pull the tongue and trachea posteriorly and cut the tissue between the aorta and the ventral aspects of the vertebrae. Continue the cut between the mediastinum and pericardial sac to the sternum, transecting the aorta, vena cava and esophagus at the level of the diaphragm.

Head

The head is removed by extending the head and transecting the ventral neck muscles down to the level of the atlanto-occipital joint. If cerebral spinal fluid is needed, insert a needle attached to a syringe into the subdural space of the spinal cord and collect the sample. Oftentimes 10 to 12 ml of clear cere-

brospinal fluid may be obtained in this way. Next, cut the ventral ligaments of the atlanto-occipital joint, transect the spinal cord and cut the dorsal ligaments of the joint and the dorsal neck muscles. The oral cavity and teeth should be examined at this time. Place the head aside.

Musculoskeletal System

The muscles of the hindlegs and the forelegs should be incised several times and carefully evaluated for muscular lesions. At this time, the prescapular lymph nodes (just anterior to the midscapular region), the prefemoral lymph nodes (just anterior and dorsal to the stifle joints) and the popliteal lymph nodes (under the ventral aspects of the semitendinous and semimembranous muscles and adjacent to the sciatic nerve and femoral artery) should be checked. Stifle and hock joints should be opened in both hindlimbs and at least the carpal joints of the forelimbs should be opened. If joint lesions are found, all joints should be opened. If a culture is needed of joint fluid, open the joint by first cutting the skin over the joint with a clean knife (Fig. 23–5), then use a sterile scalpel to cut the joint capsule. Open the joint and swab the inside, being careful not to touch the cut edges of the joint capsule (Fig. 23–6).

The internal organs are now examined carefully. The order in which they are examined is a matter of personal preference. For the sake of organization, the techniques used to examine organ systems will be described in the following order: head; lungs, trachea and thyroid glands; thymus and heart; great vessels and esophagus; liver and gallbladder; spleen; kidneys, adrenal glands and bladder; genital organs, small and large intestines; pancreas and mesenteric lymph nodes and forestomachs.

Eyes

The head should be taken to a chopping block and the skin over the cranium and around the eyes should be removed,

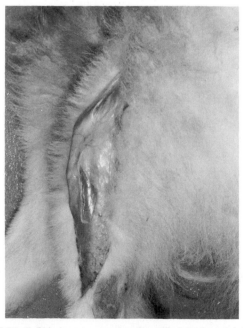

FIGURE 23–5. Skin is cut, exposing the stifle joint for a joint culture.

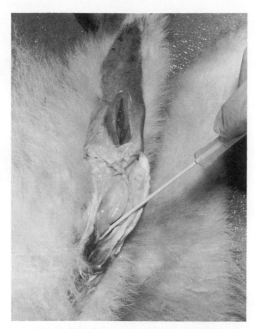

FIGURE 23-6. Stifle joint is opened and a culture is taken.

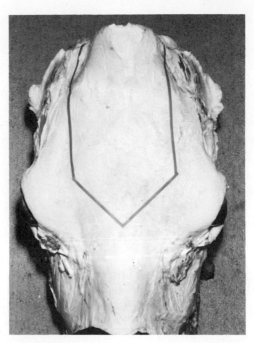

FIGURE 23-7. Skin reflected from the skull of a bovine. Note the line indicating the location of the skull cut.

leaving the skin around the nose. The skin is left around the nose to enable the prosector to hold the head with more stability. The eyes are removed by grasping the skin that is left around the eyes or the conjunctiva with a pair of forceps, then cutting the loose tissue around the eye with a sharp pair of scissors. The ocular muscles, vessels and optic nerve are cut, and the entire eyeball is removed. For best fixation remove all of the loose tissue and muscles from the eyeball. If there are lesions in the eyes or if the animal was known to be blind, the eyes should be removed first. If the animal died by euthanasia, the eyes should be removed within 3 to 5 minutes after euthanasia and placed in Zenker's solution. If the postmortem interval is beyond 20 to 30 minutes, the eyes can be fixed in formalin. If the animal has cataracts, the best fixative is formalin, regardless of the postmortem interval.

Brain

The brain is removed by cutting away all of the major muscle masses covering the lateral aspect of the cranium (Fig. 23–7). Using a cleaver or saw, two parallel cuts are made, starting at the upper lateral edge of the foramen magnum and progressing anterior to the cranial aspects of the eye sockets. The anterior portions of this cut should be connected. As these two parallel cuts are connected, the frontal sinuses will be entered. These structures should be inspected before cutting the bony covering of the brain. After the bony cap is removed (sometimes prying the bony cap with a screwdriver or the tip of the cleaver is helpful), the dura should be cut. Sometimes (especially in young animals), one has to cut the dura as the bony cap is being removed (Fig. 23–8). Make sure that you cut the tentorium cerebelli (the thick portion of dura between the cerebrum and the cerebellum) before removing the brain. If the tentorium cerebelli is not cut, the brain cannot be removed intact and will be divided between the cerebrum and the cerebellum. Now that the dura and tentorium cerebelli have been incised and removed, grasp the head by the nose and hold it upright. Tap the head lightly on the chopping

block to loosen the brain. If brain cultures are desired, they should be taken before removal from the skull. Cultures should include the subdural space, especially around the optic chiasma. Tilt the head backward to allow the brain to roll out of the cranial vault. The optic and remaining cranial nerves must be severed to allow removal of the brain from the skull. Care must be taken not to let the brain drop on the table or on the floor. If histopathological studies are to be done, the brain should be hemisected by cutting along the longitudinal fissure and placing both halves in 3 to 4 liters of formalin. If the brain is not to be fixed, the brain should be transected in 0.5-cm slices and inspected grossly for lesions. The pituitary gland, gasserian ganglion (fifth cranial nerve) and cerebral retes should be removed and placed in formalin. These struc-

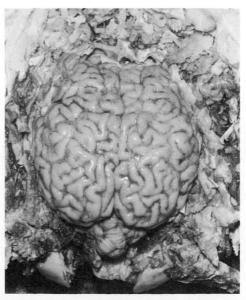

FIGURE 23-8. Bony cap of the skull and dura removed from a bovine to expose the brain.

tures are removed by making a cut posterior to the optic chiasma lateral to the left and right gasserian ganglion and posterior to the pituitary gland. With a pair of forceps, grasp the dura covering the gasserian ganglion and pull upward, using a scalpel to cut the tissue away from the nerve and the anterior aspect of the fifth cranial nerve as it enters the foramen on both sides. Then peel out the square of tissue that contains the pituitary gland in the center surrounded by the cerebral retes and the gasserian ganglion.

Pluck

The pluck (tongue, esophagus, trachea, thyroid glands, parathyroid glands, thymus, heart, great vessels and lungs) is examined next (Fig. 23–9). First, locate the thymus gland. In young animals, the thymus should be large and located anterior to the heart under the left apical lobe of the lungs. In ruminants (cattle, goats and sheep), a large portion of the thymus is located on the ventral aspect of the trachea and can extend to the thyroid glands. The tongue is incised at 1-cm intervals and is inspected. The thyroid and parathyroid glands located just posterior to the larynx should be checked. The esophagus is opened and inspected from the oral cavity to the rumen. The trachea is opened along its dorsal aspects down to the bifurcation. The lungs and pleura are inspected. The lungs are examined by palpation. The lungs should be light pink, soft and spongy, and the pleura should be shiny and smooth. Red, rubbery lungs usually are edematous and congested. Firm, dark red lungs are usually pneumonic. In bovines, the pleura covering the dorsal aspects of the diaphragmatic lobes is normally thick and opaque. Remove both lungs from the heart and dissect out the aorta. Using scissors, open the trachea, main stem bronchi and the smaller air passages of the lung (Fig. 23–10). Locate the thick-walled artery and, using scissors, open this vessel and check for emboli. Locate the large, thin-walled pulmonary veins and cut along these vessels checking for thrombi. If histopathological studies are desired on the lungs, use a pair of forceps to grasp a small portion of lung tissue and, using a sharp scalpel, remove a small wedge of lung parenchyma. Do not squeeze lung tissue to be examined histopathologically, since this causes extensive artifacts.

Heart

If you are right-handed, hold the heart in the left hand so that the right ventricle is on your left. The fat encircling the

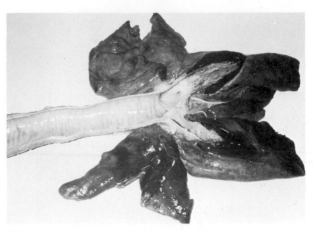

FIGURE 23–10. Lungs with trachea and main stem bronchi opened for inspection.

coronary vessels should be checked. An animal that has had a chronic disease or has been in a malnourished condition will have serous atrophy of fat around the coronary vessels instead of white opaque fat. The heart is opened in the same sequence as the flow of blood. The right atrium is opened and inspected. The atrioventricular valves are checked. The right ventricle is opened by starting in the opened right atrium (Fig. 23–11), cutting along the interventricular septum to the tip of the ventricle, then upward and into the pulmonary artery outflow tract (Fig. 23–12). The atrioventricular valves can be more closely inspected now. One should look into the pulmonary artery to check for stenosis (narrowing of the lumen) or other lesions before cutting through it. Now cut through the semilunar valves and up the pulmonary artery. The left atrium is now opened, and the left atrioventricular valves are inspected. The left ventricle is opened by making a straight incision from the atrioventricular valve down to the tip of the heart. The aorta is opened by inserting scissors under the medial cusp of the left atrioventricular valve (Fig. 23–13). As you are opening the aorta, turn the scissors slightly to the right or clockwise; this is done to avoid cutting through the orifice of the ductus arteriosus. The semilunar valves of the aorta should be examined. The atrial septum should be checked for an open foramen ovale, and the ventricular septum should be checked for septal defects. Among the more common heart defects in cattle are

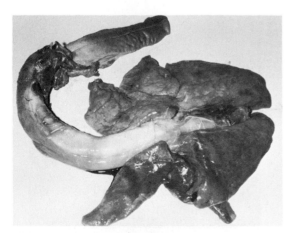

FIGURE 23–9. The pluck includes the tongue, esophagus, trachea, thyroid glands, thymus, heart and lungs.

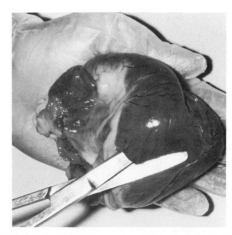

FIGURE 23–11. The right atria and ventricle are opened first during examination of the heart.

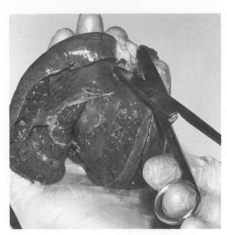

FIGURE 23–12. Following opening of the right ventricle, the pulmonary artery is opened.

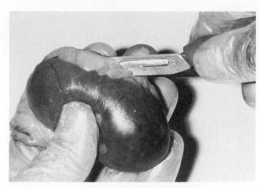

FIGURE 23–14. The kidney is incised longitudinally down to the renal pelvis.

high ventricular septal defects. Check the orifices of the left and right coronary arteries (just under the semilunar valves of the aorta). Now make multiple cuts in the myocardium, checking for small foci of degeneration or necrosis. If no lesions are found in the heart, and a section is desired for histopathological study, a small section of the left papillary myocardium is the best place to sample.

Liver and Gallbladder

The liver is examined by first inspecting the capsule and external surfaces. The gallbladder is opened, and its mucosal surface is examined. Remember, an animal that has not eaten for several days prior to death will have a distended gallbladder filled with a thick green bile. In order to check for a swollen liver, make one deep cut into the parenchyma and wait 10 to 15 seconds, then try to appose the tissue back together. If the liver is swollen, the cut edges below the capsule will bulge, and the cut edges will not match, whereas if cellular swelling is not present, the cut edges will match. The texture of the liver is evaluated by making two deep cuts into the liver parenchyma approximately 0.5 cm in thickness. Using the thumb and forefinger, squeeze the tissue between your fingers. A liver from an animal with chronic heart failure (as with high mountain disease) will be firm. However, the texture of a liver from a cow with ketosis (fatty liver) will be soft and greasy. The portal

and hepatic veins should be opened and checked for thrombosis. Next, with the liver lying flat on a table, make multiple incisions into the parenchyma approximately 1 cm in thickness. This opens the organ, thus exposing internal lesions. If histopathological studies are desired, a small wedge of liver tissue, including the capsule, should be placed in formalin.

Spleen

The spleen should be examined next. The technique for inspecting the spleen is similar to that for inspecting the liver—that is, multiple cuts are made throughout the organ, thus exposing the internal parenchyma. A small wedge of spleen should be taken for histopathological study.

Adrenal Glands

The adrenal glands should still be attached to the anterior pole of the kidneys. The size and shape of the adrenal glands should be noted, and multiple incisions should be made through both organs. Hemorrhagic adrenal glands are often found in calves that have died of acute endotoxemia and scours. Animals that have undergone extensive chronic stress usually have bilateral enlargement of the adrenal glands.

Kidneys

Examine the external surface of both kidneys. Open the kidney longitudinally (Fig. 23–14), extending the incision to the level of the renal pelvis (Fig. 23–15). Inspect the paren-

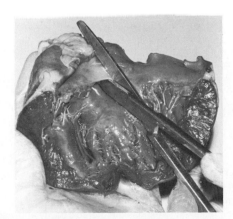

FIGURE 23–13. The aorta is opened by inserting scissors under the medial cusp of the left atrioventricular valves and cutting upward.

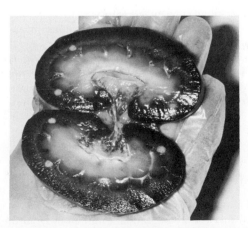

FIGURE 23–15. A kidney opened and ready for inspection.

chyma. In order to check for swelling, fold the kidney back together. The cut surfaces should match. If the cut surfaces do not match but bulge instead, this indicates that the organ is swollen. A small wedge of kidney including capsule, cortex, medulla and pelvis should be taken for histopathological study. Next, the capsule is peeled from both kidneys, and the organ is sectioned in multiple areas. The parenchyma can then be examined thoroughly. With a small pair of scissors, open both ureters. Open the urinary bladder and examine the mucosal surface. Extend the incision through the trigone of the bladder down through the urethra.

Reproductive Tract

In the male, both testicles should be opened and multiple incisions made in both organs so that the inner parenchyma can be examined. The penis and prepuce should be examined and the urethra opened to the glans penis. In females, the vagina and uterus should be opened. Both ovaries should be incised multiple times to inspect the inner parenchyma. The vulva should be checked for lesions also.

Digestive System

The only system remaining is the digestive tract. When the intestinal tract was removed from the abdominal cavity, it was removed in two parts. One part contained the small intestine and large intestine, and the other portion contained the rumen, reticulum, omasum and abomasum. The small and large intestinal tracts are usually examined first. The intestine is removed from its mesenteric attachment and is laid out on the floor. While this is being done, the mesenteric lymph nodes are examined. Next, the intestine should be opened. This is best done by opening the intestine with a pair of enterotome scissors (scissors made for opening the intestine) over a garbage can. As the prosector opens the intestine, lesions such as ulcers, parasites, necrosis of Peyer's patches and so on should be noted.

The rumen should be opened, and the inner surface and the contents examined. The reticulum and omasum should be opened and examined. The abomasum should be opened along its greater curvature. The mucosae should be checked carefully for lesions, such as ulcers and parasites.

Spinal Cord

The spinal cord is the most commonly overlooked system because of the difficulty in removing it. The easiest method to remove the spinal cord on a bovine is to first remove all of the muscles on the right side of the spinal column from the neck to the pelvis. Next, using a large cleaver, cut away the lateral aspects of the cervical, thoracic and lumbar vertebrae. Be careful as you near the spinal cord so that the cord is not crushed with the cleaver. The entire cord can be exposed with the use of the cleaver. Using a pair of forceps, grasp the dura over the anterior aspect of the spinal cord and pull upward. Use a scalpel or pair of scissors, or both, to cut the left spinal cord nerves and gently pull the spinal cord upward.

Necropsy Technique for the Equine

The basic technique for doing a necropsy on a horse is similar to that for a cow. Only the variations from the bovine

will be covered in this section. The prosector should refer back to necropsy technique for the bovine for a more detailed description of the examination of individual organs. If the horse is undergoing necropsy for insurance purposes, photographs of the entire horse should be taken for proof of identification. The inner lips and ears should be checked for tattoos. In gross necropsy reports of such cases, all identifying marks, such as white socks on specific feet, stars and tattoo numbers, should be included.

Horses should be placed with their right side down (just the opposite of cattle). This allows the best exposure of the spleen, stomach and large colon. The external parts (especially all orifices) should be examined first. If sections of skin are needed, they should be collected. The animal is opened, as is the cow, by making an incision from the chin to the anus and reflecting the skin. Both left limbs are abducted by transecting the muscular attachments of the forelimb and coxofemoral joint of the hindlimb. The abdominal wall and rib cage are opened (Fig. 23–16). The best time to examine proper locations of internal organs and displacement colics or torsions is immediately following exposure of the internal organs. Any specific cultures that are needed for microbiological procedures should be taken at this time to help prevent contamination.

It is usually easier to remove the abdominal organs first, then the thoracic organs. After opening the abdominal cavity and exposing the abdominal viscera, check the intestines for torsions or displacements. Discoloration of the wall and disorganization of the arrangement of organs are usually the first clue of displacement. Sometimes, the large bowel is so filled with gas that the organs immediately bulge out of the abdominal cavity. When this happens, several small holes should be punctured in the wall of the large colon to deflate the distended bowel. Following visual inspection for the location of organs within the abdominal cavity, the bowel and mesenteric attachments should be palpated in search of twists or torsions.

Next, the abdominal organs should be removed in a systematic fashion. First, grasp the pelvic flexure on the left side located just anterior to the pelvic inlet. Pull the pelvic flexure outward, thus removing the entire large colon. Place the large colon at right angles to the body. This allows a good view of this organ. Vessels of the large colon can be examined now. The spleen is removed and examined. The left adrenal gland

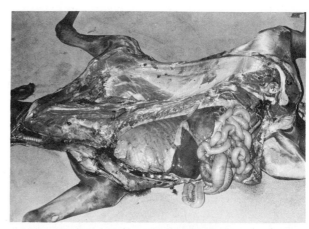

FIGURE 23–16. Skin reflected, abdominal wall and rib cage removed and left limbs reflected to expose the thoracic cavity and viscera of an equine.

and kidneys are now removed and examined. The abdominal aorta is exposed and should be opened in its entirety. One should also dissect the anterior celiac and mesenteric arteries to check for verminous arteritis resulting from *Strongylus vulgaris.*

Next, the terminal rectum should be located, doubly ligated and transected. Remove the small colon by spearing this organ from its mesenteric attachment. The small colon should be followed to the right dorsal colon. Another double ligature should be placed around the small colon just posterior to the large dorsal colon. The small colon should now be removed from the abdominal cavity and placed aside for further examination. The ileum should be located just as it enters into the cecum. The ileum has a much thicker wall than the remaining small intestine. The ileum is then double ligated and cut. The large colon is now free and can be removed from the abdominal cavity and laid on the floor for further examination. The small intestine is now traced proximally to the duodenum and stripped from its mesenteric attachments and is placed on the floor. The duodenum is double ligated, transected and removed from the abdominal cavity. Next, double ligate the esophagus, transect it and remove the stomach. The right adrenal gland and kidney are removed and examined. The liver can be removed and examined. The urinary bladder and genital organs are removed and examined.

Removal of the pluck is more difficult in the horse because of the long, narrow mandible. Removal of the tongue and pharynx is facilitated by separating the left and right mandible by cutting the mandibular symphysis with a cleaver or saw. The teeth and the hard and soft palates are examined. The tongue/pharynx/trachea are then pulled caudally, and the heart and lungs are removed as in the bovine. The thyroid glands should be checked at this time. It is difficult to remove the heart with the intact pericardial sac. Thus, if excessive pericardial fluids or specific lesions within the pericardial sac are noted, the prosector should open the pericardial sac while the heart is still in the thoracic cavity. Otherwise, when the heart is pulled out with the lungs, the pericardial sac will tear, and the fluid within the sac will be lost.

The inner surfaces of the thoracic and abdominal cavities can now be examined for puncture wounds, such as bullet holes.

Large incisions should be made in all major muscle masses in order to search for lesions deep in muscles. Keep in mind that intramuscular injections (especially antibiotics) can cause massive areas of necrosis. All joints should be opened and examined. Removal of the head and brain is similar to their removal in the cow. Since the pituitary gland is much larger than in the cow and most of the organ is not covered by dura, it is slightly more difficult to remove the pituitary gland and gasserian ganglion. However, it can be removed with the same technique described for cattle, but additional care should be taken.

The animal's individual organs—that is, heart, lungs, brain, liver, kidney, endocrine glands, and lymphohemopoietic and reproductive organs—are evaluated as described for cattle. The only major difference is the examination of the digestive system. The stomach should be opened above its greater curvature. Common lesions in the stomach are small ulcers due to stomach bots *(Gasterophilus)* and small abscesses just below the margo plicatus caused by *Habronema* spp. The small intestine, the small colon, the large colon and the cecum should be

opened and their mucosal surfaces examined. It is common to see multiple, small 1- to 3-mm lymphoid nodules within the mucosa of the large bowel in horses with moderate to heavy parasite loads.

Necropsy Technique for Small Animals

Most of the necropsy procedures for small animals are similar to the procedure for the bovine, except for positioning and the initial removal of organs. The necropsy technique used on the dog will be described; moreover, this same technique can be used for other monogastrics, such as cats, ferrets, pigs and rodents.

The initial step is to examine the skin thoroughly on both sides and especially around the head, neck, ears, paws and perineum, checking for lesions such as lacerations or swelling (abscesses or tumors). The mouth and teeth should be examined next. If ocular lesions are suspected, the eyes should be removed first. If the animal died by euthanasia, the eyes should be fixed in Zenker's solution. If the dog has cataracts, the fixative of choice is formalin, regardless of whether the dog died by euthanasia.

Position and Initial Exposure

The animal is now placed on its back, and an incision is made through the axillary region and muscular attachments of the scapula bilaterally. Another incision is made in each groin area through the muscles of the hindlimbs, transecting the coxofemoral joint capsule and round ligament of each hip. All four legs should now be lying flat on the table, thus stabilizing the carcass. An incision is then made from chin to anus (Fig. 23–17). The skin is reflected on both sides of the animal nearly to the back (Fig. 23–18). Another technique commonly used on small animals is to first make the incision from chin to anus (Fig. 23–19) and then reflect the skin, cut the muscular attachments to the scapula and disarticulate the hip joints, in that sequence (Fig. 23–20). Peripheral lymph nodes should now be examined, especially the prefemoral, prescapular and popliteal nodes.

The abdominal cavity is opened by starting an incision at the pubis, incising along the lateral abdominal wall and ending in the center of the last rib. When this incision is made on both sides, and this flap of abdominal muscle is reflected cranially, one can visualize the size, shape and location of most of the abdominal organs (Fig. 23–21). A small stab incision is made in the diaphragm on both sides to check for negative pressure. Dogs that have been hit by cars commonly have fractured ribs and pneumothorax. With the pruning shears (or scissors, depending on the size of the animal), the ribs are cut in the

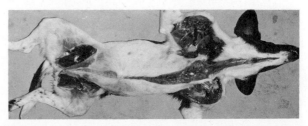

FIGURE 23–17. All four limbs have been cut and laid flat on the table. An incision is made from the chin to the anus of a dog.

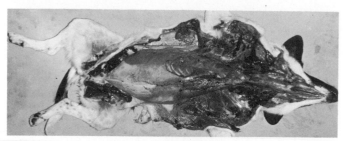

FIGURE 23–18. The skin is now reflected down to the back of the dog, thus exposing the chest and abdominal wall.

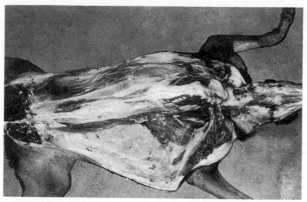

FIGURE 23–20. Skin, including limbs reflected, of a dog. The abdominal and chest wall are thus exposed.

midregion starting with the last rib and progressing to the first rib. The ribs and sternum are removed. The entire abdominal cavity and thoracic cavity are now open (Fig. 23–22). This complete exposure allows close examination of the organs without moving them (checking for displacement, tumors, and so on) and also allows collection of microbiological samples.

Internal Organs

The sequence for removal of internal organs varies with the pathologist and the observation of various lesions during the initial inspection. For the sake of organization, the sequence that follows will be used. Double ligate the terminal rectum if the animal had diarrhea; otherwise transect the rectum without ligation. Hold the rectum with one hand and begin to pull it out of the abdominal cavity. With scissors, cut the mesenteric attachments of the intestine. While removing the intestines from the abdominal cavity, inspect the mesenteric lymph nodes. As the duodenum is approached, the pancreas will be found. Inspect this organ carefully; pancreatitis is a common disease in dogs. Continue to remove the small intestine, including the stomach. Double ligate the esophagus just behind the diaphragm and anterior to the stomach. Cut between the ligatures. The digestive system from the stomach to the anus can be removed and set aside for further examination. The liver and spleen are removed and set aside. The pelvis is cut so that the kidneys, adrenal glands, ureters, bladder and female genital organs can be removed en masse. With males, the genital organs usually remain attached to the carcass.

The pluck (tongue, trachea, thyroid and parathyroid glands, esophagus, lungs and heart) is removed as described for the bovine. As the tongue is removed, tonsils and teeth should be carefully examined. The head is removed as described for the bovine.

All muscles should be examined carefully by making incisions deep into the muscle masses. All joints should be opened and examined. The stifle joints and both anterior cruciate ligaments should be given special attention in the dog (especially in the smaller breeds such as the poodle).

Head

The head is examined in a manner similar to that used for the cow. The skin and muscles covering the skull are removed. This exposes the salivary glands and parotid lymph nodes. These organs should be examined and several deep incisions made in order to check the inner parenchyma for cysts and tumors. The brain is removed by means of a small cleaver or stryker saw. In small dogs, a pair of bone rongeurs may be used to easily remove the brain. The pituitary gland and gasserian ganglion are removed as described for the horse. Remember that the gasserian ganglion is an important tissue to examine histopathologically for rabies. With cases submitted for rabies, the veterinarian should submit either the entire head or one half of the brain frozen and one half of the brain in formalin to a local diagnostic laboratory. The frontal sinuses should be opened and examined, especially in pigs, to check for atrophic rhinitis.

Pluck

The lungs, trachea, esophagus, parathyroid, thyroid and thymus should be examined as described for cattle. In dogs, the parathyroid glands are more prominent and should be checked, especially in older dogs with chronic renal problems.

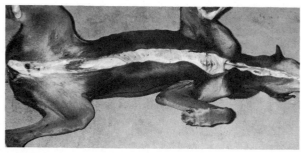

FIGURE 23–19. Dog with primary skin incision from chin to anus.

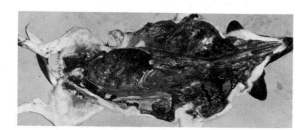

FIGURE 23–21. Skin and limbs reflected and abdominal wall removed to expose the abdominal cavity of a dog.

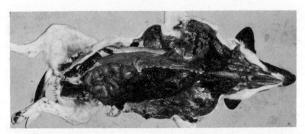

FIGURE 23–22. *Skin and limbs reflected with abdominal and chest wall removed to expose the thoracic and abdominal organs of a dog.*

Heart

The heart, great vessels and valves should be examined. The right and left atrioventricular valves should be carefully checked because of the common problem of degenerative lesions (valvular endocarditis) within the valve leaflets in older dogs. Occasionally, a chorda tendineae cordis is ruptured, and this must be checked before the ventricle is opened. The method to check a ruptured chorda tendineae cordis is to open the atrium only. Then the clotted blood is washed from the ventricle, and the ventricle is filled with water. Using the hands, the ventricle is compressed from the bottom upward. If the chordae tendineae cordis are ruptured, they will flow up and be visualized. This method also helps to evaluate competence of the valves, especially in cases with valvular endocarditis. The heart should now be open as described for cattle. The heart should be incised in 0.5- to 0.75-cm thick pieces to examine the inner myocardium. Occasionally, dogs with diabetes will have atherosclerosis of coronary vessels, which may result in myocardial infarction.

Urogenital and Digestive Tract

The kidney, bladder, urethra, adrenal glands and genital organs should be examined as described for cattle. In male dogs, the prostate gland (posterior to the trigone of the bladder as it enters the pelvic canal) should be carefully checked for neoplasia, hyperplasia or infection. The digestive system is best examined by opening the stomach along its greater curvature, continuing through the pylorus and the intestinal tract along the mesenteric border to the anus. If there is suspicion that the dog has been poisoned, the stomach contents should be saved for analysis. The external surface of the pancreas is examined, then multiple slices are made to inspect the inner parenchyma of the organ.

Cosmetic Necropsy

A procedure that is commonly requested for pet animals is a "cosmetic" necropsy. A cosmetic necropsy should be discouraged, because it precludes a thorough examination, which may result in lesions being missed. A cosmetic necropsy is a postmortem examination done through a small abdominal incision similar to that made for a routine laparotomy. The animal is placed on its back and a 10- to 12.5-cm incision (depending on the size of the animal) is made through the skin and linea alba of the abdominal wall. All of the abdominal organs are removed through this incision. Next, the hand is inserted into the empty abdominal cavity, the diaphragm is cut and the heart and lungs are removed. The organs are now examined as described earlier. The empty abdominal cavity is stuffed with paper to give the dog a "full appearance," and the abdominal incision is sutured.

The brain can be removed during a cosmetic necropsy. Wet the hair of the skull, part the hair and make the skin incision from behind the eyes to the external occipital protuberance. Peel the skin laterally in both directions, separate the muscles of the jaw from the skull and, using a Stryker saw, remove the skull cap. With practice, the intact brain can be removed in this manner. The skull cap is now replaced; sometimes it helps if two small holes are made in the skull cap (one on each side), and an opposite hole is made in the lower portion of the skull. Using a small piece of wire or string, the skull cap can be secured. The skin is sutured, and the hair is flattened. If the eyes have to be removed during a cosmetic necropsy, the eyelids should be sutured using a subcuticular suture pattern so that the suture is not observed.

The spinal cord can be removed during a cosmetic necropsy, but it is difficult and time-consuming. The procedure is similar to that of removing the brain. The dog is placed in ventral recumbency, and the hair over the back is moistened and then parted. An incision is made from the first cervical vertebra distad to the base of the tail. The skin is reflected 5 to 7.5 cm on each side of the incision down the carcass. The muscles of the spinal column are dissected from the bone. Using bone rongeurs or a Stryker saw, the dorsal wall, including the dorsal processes, is removed. The cord with the dorsal root ganglia can be removed. The muscles are put back in place, and the entire incision is sutured.

Necropsy Technique for Birds

Avian medicine (including caged-bird medicine and raptor rehabilitation) in the veterinary profession has greatly increased in the last 10 years. Veterinarians and veterinary technicians should be acquainted with a necropsy technique for birds. Remember that psittacine birds may have psittacosis (an important zoonotic disease of humans), and if this disease is suspected, the bird should not undergo necropsy by the veterinarian but should be mailed or hand-carried to the nearest state health department or state diagnostic laboratory.

The history should be carefully reviewed as with any necropsy. All psittacine birds should be dipped in a bucket of soapy water prior to necropsy. This is done for several reasons: one reason is that it wets the feathers and helps to prevent aerosolization of organisms that have dried on the feathers, especially *Chlamydia* (psittacosis). The external surfaces of the bird are examined with particular attention to the body orifices. The wings and legs are palpated to check for fractures.

Small birds may be placed on cardboard, and pins may be used to hold the wings open. The bird is placed on its back, and a line is made from the lower beak down over the keel to the cloaca by parting the wet feathers. An incision is made through the skin from the beak to the cloaca along this line. The skin is reflected on both sides, and the legs are disarticulated from the coxofemoral joints (Fig. 23–23). This provides good visualization of the pectoral muscles and abdominal wall. One blade of the scissors is inserted through the bird's mouth and into the pharynx. A cut is made down through the cervical esophagus and crop, thus exposing the upper digestive system. The abdominal wall is grasped with a pair of forceps, and a

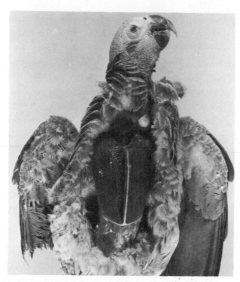

FIGURE 23–23. Skin is reflected from this African gray parrot to expose the chest muscles and abdominal wall.

flap of abdominal wall is removed from the posterior tip of the keel to the cloaca. This exposure opens the abdominal cavity and abdominal air sacs. The sternum and pectoral muscles are removed by cutting through the ribs and coracoid bones with a heavy pair of scissors or poultry shears. As the sternum is removed, the thoracic air sacs, pericardium, heart, lungs, liver, thyroid and parathyroid glands can be easily examined (Fig. 23–24). The heart is removed and examined first. The liver should be removed and examined. The spleen is best found by rotating the ventriculus outward and counterclockwise. The spleen is located at the junction of the proventriculus and the ventriculus. The esophagus is grasped with forceps and is transected anterior to the proventriculus. The esophagus may be removed by pulling posteriorly. This results in removing the entire digestive system from esophagus to cloaca. Incise the skin around the external cloacal opening and set the digestive system en masse to the side. If histopathological study is de-

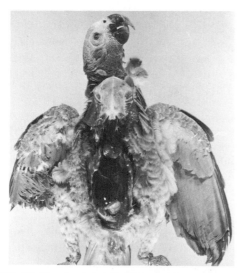

FIGURE 23–24. The chest and abdominal wall have been removed to expose the lungs, heart, air sacs and viscera.

sired on the lungs, kidneys, adrenal glands and gonads of small birds, it is easier to leave these organs attached within the cavity of the bird. Place this mass of tissue in formalin intact. In larger birds, the lung should be removed. The kidneys, adrenal glands and gonads are then removed en masse. The gonads are located on the anterior pole of the kidneys, and the adrenal glands are just under the gonads. Remember that only the left ovary is present in birds. The brain is removed in a manner similar to that described for other animals, except that scissors only are needed to cut through the thin calvarium. The spinal cord is rarely examined in birds because of the difficulty of its removal. The easiest way to examine the spinal cord is to place the whole spinal column in formalin and let the cord fix; then, using bone rongeurs, cut the dorsal wall of the vertebral column and remove the fixed cord. This prevents destruction of the small, soft, unfixed spinal cord. All joints should be opened and slices made in muscle masses (pectoral, leg and thigh muscles) to check for lesions. All internal organs are examined essentially as described for other animals.

COLLECTION OF SPECIMENS DURING A NECROPSY

Proper collection and identification of specimens during necropsy is a must; otherwise false laboratory results may follow. Some of this information has been covered in previous chapters, so only highlights will be discussed here.

Clinical Pathology

Blood deteriorates rapidly following death, especially in large animals. One of the few tests that is somewhat accurate is the use of serum in serological tests for bacterial or viral diseases. This is probably good for the first 4 to 5 hours after death. The best place to obtain serum in an animal that has been dead for several hours is the atrium of the heart or the posterior vena cava. Urine is somewhat stable and can be collected from the bladder with a needle and syringe. If poisoning by ethylene glycol is suspected, urine should be collected from the dog or cat and submitted for analysis. Two common tests done on urine in large animals are ketone bodies (dairy cattle with ketosis) and glucose (lambs with *Clostridium perfringens* type D enterotoxemia). As with diabetes mellitus, a dog that has glucosuria will have a positive glucose test for several hours after death. Remember, however, that bacteria are in the bladder, and they will utilize glucose fairly rapidly.

Body fluids and cerebrospinal fluid are stable 4 to 5 hours following death if the animal is cooled. These fluids can be collected with a needle and syringe and placed in either a clot tube or an EDTA (ethylene diamine tetra-acetic acid) tube. Joint fluids are stable following death, since they usually cool rapidly because of their peripheral location. If one is checking joint fluid for cellular components, the fluid will be representative of the live state for 3 to 4 hours post mortem. However, joint fluid enzymes deteriorate rapidly, and following death they lose their value. Occasionally impression smears are made during a necropsy to diagnose infections or tumors. Impression smears are made by first blotting the tissue so that most superficial blood is removed. Touch impressions on a clean glass slide are then made. (For further discussion of collection and handling of specimens for clinical pathological studies, see Chapter 4.)

Toxicology

Collection of specimens for toxicological analysis is common in both small and large animals. The two most common types of poisoning in small animals are ethylene glycol (car antifreeze) and strychnine. Stomach contents and urine should be collected when ethylene glycol is suspected. Stomach contents only should be collected when strychnine is suspected. If heavy metals are expected (i.e., arsenic, lead or mercury), 20 to 30 g of kidney and liver should be collected. Nitrate toxicity is common in cattle; however, analysis of tissues cannot be used. Thus, if nitrate toxicity is suspected, the animal's feed and water must be analyzed. If nitrate poisoning is suspected in an aborted bovine fetus, ocular fluid (aqueous humor) should be collected in a syringe and then placed in a glass tube and submitted to a laboratory for nitrate levels. Further discussion of various toxins is not within the scope of this book. Consulting a general toxicological textbook is recommended.

Microbiology

The most common samples taken during a necropsy are for microbiological culture. Remember that within 5 to 10 minutes after death (and even before death with many debilitating diseases), motile intestinal bacteria may invade the blood and can seed many organs. Bacterial and viral cultures are best taken just after the carcass is opened to minimize contamination. Viral cultures must be taken within 20 to 30 minutes after death; otherwise the pH change in the tissue inactivates most viruses. A few exceptions do occur, such as contagious ecthyma (sore mouth of sheep) and rabies. Bacterial samples are usually diagnostic for the first 8 to 15 hours after death, depending on how rapidly the animal cooled following death or the specific bacterial organism, or both. When an enteritis is observed and a culture is desired, using sterile instruments, first remove one large mesenteric lymph node and place it in a sterile Whirl-Pak (Fisher Scientific, Englewood, CO). Then, tie off a loop of small intestine (approximately 2.5 cm in length) with string and place it in a sterile Whirl-Pak. If you suspect an infection in a solid organ (e.g., hepatitis or pneumonia), remove a wedge of tissue (approximately 2.5 to 5 cm in thickness) using sterile instruments and place the tissue in a sterile Whirl-Pak. When an infection of the brain is suspected, two types of cultures should be taken. The first is a swab of the subdural space. This swab is taken under the brain just after the skull cap has been removed, and the head is turned over and tapped so that the brain will fall forward before the optic nerve cord and other cranial nerves are cut. The second type of culture is obtained by submission of one half of the entire fresh brain to the laboratory in a sterile Whirl-Pak.

Joints should be opened carefully; otherwise they are easily contaminated. A method to culture joints is to wash the skin with alcohol and make an incision through the skin over the joint with a sterile scalpel (see Fig. 23–5). Then, using another sterile scalpel, incise through the joint capsule and open the joint to its maximum. Do not touch the cut joint capsule, but swab the far end of the joint space (see Fig. 23–6). All swabs should be placed in either aerobic or anaerobic transport media in an effort to preserve the organisms during transport to the laboratory.

When an animal has died of bacteremia (bacteria in the blood stream), three culture sites are important: (1) heart blood, (2) spleen and (3) blood from a lower leg vein. Usually, heart blood is the first to be contaminated by intestinal organisms, followed by the spleen. Many times, even though heart blood and spleen are contaminated, a pure culture of an organism (e.g., Pasteurella) can be isolated from blood of the lower leg. The reasons for this are that the blood in the lower extremities cools rapidly and the lower extremities are farther from motile intestinal flora.

Samples obtained for fungal culture are taken in the same manner as described for bacterial samples.

Samples for virus isolation are obtained in the same manner as described for bacteriological cultures except that they must be taken within 10 to 15 minutes after death. The samples should be cooled and immediately taken to the laboratory. If the samples cannot be taken to the laboratory within 30 minutes, the tissues should be frozen. Most viruses are not stable or do not maintain viability if frozen in a refrigerator freezer; thus these samples should be packed on dry ice and taken to the laboratory as quickly as possible.

Samples for fluorescent antibody tests should be collected with clean scissors and forceps. Small pieces of tissue, approximately 0.5 cm^2, are adequate. For example, if one suspects infectious bovine rhinotracheitis (IBR) in a bovine fetus, several small pieces of liver and lung should be submitted to a laboratory for fluorescent antibody testing for IBR. These samples should be kept cool during transportation to the laboratory. If the transportation time to the laboratory is greater than 24 hours, the tissue should be transported frozen.

A test commonly being used in the laboratory is the electron microscopic scan. This test involves concentrating viral particles from intestinal contents and then identifying viruses with the use of the electron microscope. The technique is especially useful in calves and pigs with scours and with parvovirus enteritis in dogs and cats. A satisfactory sample would be 5 to 10 ml of the lower small intestine contents (in a syringe) for parvovirus in dogs and cats. The sample from pigs and calves is best taken from a mixture of the lower small intestine, rectum and spiral colon, since the viruses seem to be concentrated in these locations, even though virus replication occurs in the upper and middle small intestine. (For further detailed discussion of the collection and handling of specimens for microbiological cultures and tests, see Chapter 6.)

The procedures for collection of specimens for parasitology at the time of necropsy are fairly straightforward. A 4- to 5-g sample of feces from the terminal rectum is best for routine fecal flotation. This will be adequate for cestodes, trematodes, nematodes and Coccidia ova or larvae. If parasites are found intact (e.g., lungworms in cattle, liver flukes in sheep or intestinal nematodes in dogs), the easiest method to preserve these specimens is 10 percent buffered formalin. If the parasites are still alive, it is best to cool them in saline prior to placing them in formalin. (For further detailed discussion of collection and handling of specimens for parasitology, see Chapter 5.)

SHIPMENT OF TISSUE

Microbiological Samples

All microbiological samples should be tightly packed in either transport media or sterile Whirl-Paks. Specimens should be chilled and placed in small styrofoam containers. Two to three ice packs should be included in the container. If transportation time is greater than 24 hours, the samples should be frozen and packed with dry ice (there are a few exceptions; see Chapter 6). Most samples are shipped via mail or bus.

Toxicological and Parasitological Samples

Specimens shipped for most toxicological tests should be frozen and placed in styrofoam containers containing frozen ice packs. Specimens should be double packaged, and tops of the styrofoam containers should be well sealed. Parasitological samples should be kept cool, and parasites should be preserved in formalin. These samples can then be packaged in styrofoam containers and shipped. The two most common means of transporting samples are by bus and the U.S. postal service.

Clinical Pathology Samples

Transportation of clinical pathology specimens to the laboratory should be done as quickly as possible. Several private laboratories have a carrier service to pick up samples and deliver them to the airport, then transport them to the laboratory by air. These laboratories usually have special shipping instructions that should be consulted. Otherwise, clinical pathology samples should be cooled, packaged in a styrofoam container and shipped to the laboratory as soon as possible. Serum should be transported frozen and on dry ice. (For further discussion of collection and handling of specimens for clinical pathological studies, see Chapter 4.)

Histopathology Samples

Samples for histopathological study should be placed in small, well-sealed glass or in plastic containers containing formalin. The tops of the containers should be taped to ensure that shaking or vibrations that occur during transportation do not loosen the lids and allow formalin to leak. If multiple tissues are to be sent via mail or bus, tissues should first be allowed to fix properly in the proper volume of formalin (10:1, formalin to volume of tissue); then the tissues can be placed in a smaller jar filled with formalin and shipped to a diagnostic laboratory. This procedure reduces the weight of the package to be shipped. For example, if an expensive insured stallion has undergone necropsy, the tissues collected may fill two 4-liter jars of formalin (remember the 10:1 formalin to tissue ratio). Formalin weighs approximately 4 kg per 4 liters. This would result in more than 8 kg of substance. The best way to reduce the weight is to allow the tissues to fix for 3 to 4 days, then place all the tissue in a 1-liter jar and cover the tissue with formalin. This will adequately keep the tissues during transportation.

Recommended Reading

Andrews JJ (editor): Necropsy techniques. Vet Clin North Am Food Animal Practice, Vol 2/No 1, 1986.

Strafuss AC: Necropsy. Procedures and Basic Diagnostic Methods for Practicing Veterinarians. Springfield, IL, Charles C Thomas, 1988.

Van Kruiningen HJ: Veterinary autopsy procedure. Vet Clin North Am 1:163–189, 1971.

24

Euthanasia

JOSEPH TABOADA

Old Dog

When the old dog had to die after long years full with love and honor,
When the weight of time grew wearying and she was content to have it finished,
I brought my old dog to our friend.
Old dog lay soft against me, old eyes already closed, waiting.
Our friend's hand was gentle on the weary body, with its ragged fur,
So gentle to find the frail small vein where death could enter.
DIFFICULT,
Old blood runs sluggish, old veins slackly resisting.
So patient, our friend, his knowing hands, all I can see through silent tears.
I watch capable strong hands lightly coaxing, and at last a small red flower
blooms briefly in the crystal before he eases the plunger in.
Old dog only sighs very softly.
The weary heart slows and stops as the joyful spirit leaps free.
We wait a quiet minute, my tears dropping unheeded, into the soft fur.
Our friend withdraws, his gentle hands leaving old dog's cast-off body.
My head bowed over the weathered white mask for a moment before I let her lie
by herself and draw the blanket over her.
I wish the old dog had made it easier for him.
To bring even a kindly death brings sadness.
He asked how many years she had, and I heard more than that in his voice.
I wish I could thank him for keeping zest in her years, for making a good end of
them, for his capable hands, for his gentle word, and caring heart.
I took the old dog home, and laid her as if sleeping, wrapped in her worn
blanket and sheltered deep in the kindly silent earth.

ANONYMOUS

Perhaps no single issue in veterinary medicine conjures up the range of emotion, ethical deliberation and stress occasioned by euthanasia. There is a tremendous diversity of opinion and tolerance among veterinary professionals, both within the United States and abroad. Euthanasia was defined by the 1986 American Veterinary Medical Association (AVMA) Panel on Euthanasia as, "the act of inducing painless death," but "the act" is only one small aspect of the larger issue facing the profession.

The word euthanasia is derived from the Greek root *Eu*, meaning good, and *thanatos*, referring to death. Few in the veterinary profession would argue that when used in the context of relieving suffering, the word runs counter to its Greek roots; however, as the word is currently defined, it also pertains to the killing of unwanted, abandoned, stray or phenotypically undesired animals by the veterinary profession. Euthanasia, therefore, can present veterinary professionals with problems in balancing conflicting interests. It is not always in the common interest of the patient, the client, and the veterinarian that euthanasia is performed. Euthanasia is an emotionally charged issue, with members of the profession varying significantly in their acceptance of the practice and in their views as to its utility. On one hand it might be viewed simply as "convenience killing," whereas on the other it might be viewed as a means of furthering respect and love through the compassionate termination of hopeless suffering. No matter how one looks at it, the animal health professional may be caught in the middle, experiencing doubts, confusion and moral questions over participation in the ending of an animal's life. It is an ethical dilemma that does not have an easy or even an absolutely right or wrong answer. It is an issue that all of us must wrestle with, individually and collectively.

THE DECISION

The decision to perform euthanasia is one of the most difficult decisions that the owner of a companion animal will ever have to face. Some owners may make the decision quickly because of financial constraints or fear of what the illness may eventually cause, while others may never be able to make the decision, preferring to let their pet die naturally. The decision is often made more difficult by the fact that few pet owners have an adequate support group available that understands the bond that develops between an animal and the recipient of its unconditional love.

Most owners who elect to have euthanasia performed make the decision because they perceive that their pet's illness involves some degree of suffering. Suffering is difficult to define, and perceptions of animal suffering differ markedly between individuals and from case to case. The place the pet holds in the owner's family circle, how long the pet has been owned, the relationship between the pet and other loved ones, the financial resources available to the owner, and the disease process afflicting the pet are other factors that most owners take into consideration when trying to make the decision.

The veterinary team (veterinarian, veterinary technician and animal health care providers) can play an important role in the decision-making process. The veterinary staff often serves as a sounding board for the client who is trying to make the decision. We can help with the decision by approaching the subject professionally with compassion and respect. The most important help that the team can give is the providing of information. What the owner can expect from the disease process, what treatments are available, the prognosis with and without treatment, and what costs are involved are all questions that should be answered by the veterinarian. The veterinary technician can play a vital role as a client resource by answering questions about euthanasia. How euthanasia is performed, whether the animal will feel pain, how long the procedure will take and what happens to the body afterward are all areas that a technician may be asked to address.

When interacting with an owner considering euthanasia, the veterinary professional should go to great lengths to lay out all the options available while being careful not to make the decision for the client. Too many veterinary professionals make judgments as to the "value" of an animal (both monetary and personal) that only the owner can make. Questions such as "What would you do if he were your animal?" are difficult to address and are perhaps best answered by urging the client to verbalize what he sees as the pros and cons of each choice. In doing this, it may become obvious that the client has already made the decision and is looking for support or validation. The client may feel guilt, anger, sadness, depression, pain and helplessness during the decision-making process and after euthanasia has been performed (see Chapter 25). The veterinary professional can help by assuring the owner that these feelings are normal, and indeed expected, and by assuring the client that he is not alone in the pain that he is feeling.

Once an informed decision has been made, it should be supported, even if it may not have been the decision that the veterinarian or veterinary staff would have made. Pet owners are sensitive to the actions of hospital personnel, and for this reason it is extremely important that persons interacting with the client or handling the animal in the presence of the owner be supportive, gentle and empathetic.

AS THE END DRAWS NEAR: THE BEGINNING OF THE END

The death of a pet can be a devastating experience that can drastically affect the relationship between client and veterinarian. As many as 40 percent of clients change veterinarians after a pet has died. This number probably approaches 100 percent if euthanasia is handled in a manner that causes the client to perceive a lack of care, concern or respect on the part of the veterinarian or other staff members. On the other hand, much can be done to foster a long-lasting relationship through the professional and compassionate handling of a euthanasia. It is often true that the client who loudly sings the praises of a veterinarian and his staff is not the owner of an animal saved through long hours of hard work and outstanding medical care, but the owner who was treated with compassion, care and concern at and around the time of the loss of a pet.

Preparations for pet loss should begin as soon as it becomes apparent that death is a possibility. The veterinarian will often discuss euthanasia with a client early so that he understands that it is an available option. However, it is important to discuss all of the other medical or surgical options first. Euthanasia should not be presented in such a manner that it is either completely discounted or viewed as the only reasonable course. Remember that the initial reaction of a client receiving bad news is often denial or feelings of numbness or shock. It is important to allow time for this initial reaction to fade and for the entire family to be given time to discuss the various options before allowing the client to make such a difficult and important decision.

While discussing options with the client, the veterinarian may use alternative jargon terms for euthanasia such as *put to sleep, put down, put away, humanely destroy, rock, shoot,* and so forth. Use of such terms is appropriate only when their meaning is understood by all individuals involved. Confusion will result from the use of a term such as *put to sleep* when talking to a companion animal owner who perceives the phrase to refer to anesthesia instead of euthanasia. Children are especially confused by the term "put to sleep" and may be afraid that they might die when going to sleep at night. Whatever term is used to describe the act of euthanasia, it is important that it be fully understood by all parties involved.

Once the decision has been made to have an animal undergo euthanasia, there are many choices that a client must make. When and where should the euthanasia take place? Should they or other family members be present during the euthanasia? What is to happen to the body following euthanasia? Should a necropsy examination be allowed? What special method, if any, will they use to memorialize the pet? It is best to discuss these concerns thoroughly in advance so that everyone understands precisely the wishes of the client.

The client, together with the veterinarian, should decide who will be present during the euthanasia. This is sometimes a difficult decision for both the client and the veterinarian. Some veterinarians do not offer this option to the client in the mistaken view that it will be too difficult for the client to watch. Contrary to this view, many clients will grieve more easily and accept more quickly the loss of their pet if they have had the opportunity to say good-bye in this most personal way (Fig. 24–1). The chance to hold their pet and let it know that it is loved dearly while sharing its last moments is sometimes an important first step in the grief process. However, with the benefits to the client can come problems for the veterinarian and his staff. The veterinary team must realize that having the client present can increase their own stress level associated with euthanasia, and every attempt should be made to understand and minimize its effects (see The Stress of Euthanasia in this chapter).

When the client or family members are to be present, euthanasia should be scheduled for a time of the day when interruptions are unlikely, the waiting room is empty, and the potential for embarrassment by public exposure is minimized. Early mornings, evenings, or during the lunch hour may be suitable. It is best to schedule at least 30 minutes. The most important aspect of the euthanasia to consider is communica-

tion. The unexpected should be avoided at all costs, and prior to the procedure, the client should be given a detailed explanation of exactly what is about to happen to the pet and what he is about to see. Then the client should be talked through each step of the procedure. The euthanasia should proceed at a pace with which the client feels comfortable. Occasionally pets will urinate, defecate, vocalize, twitch, or gasp after they have become unconscious. Although these reflex acts can be minimized, they will still occasionally occur and will have a far less negative effect if they are expected and if the client is told that they are not a reflection of pain or suffering.

Deciding where the euthanasia is to take place can be important. Utilizing a hospital space that is less sterile than the typical stainless steel hospital examination room is preferred. If the examination room is to be used, at least a blanket should be placed over the table and there should be a chair where the client can sit down. Some clients will request that the euthanasia be performed at home or at some special place. Many veterinarians will honor these requests or utilize the services of a house call practice for this need. Sometimes just being outside the "normal" environment of the veterinary facility is a fair and acceptable compromise. A blanket on the floor, the lawn beside the clinic, even the back seat of the family car might serve this purpose. One important consideration for the veterinarian in choosing the place is that many clients will feel uncomfortable coming back into the room where a pet previously underwent euthanasia. Indeed, many clients switch veterinarians because of a lack of sensitivity to this fact by the veterinary staff. To minimize this potential conflict in the future, it is best to choose a space that will not be routinely used for other client-related activities.

Clients who choose not to be present during euthanasia may still wish to see the body of the animal after it is dead. Seeing the animal dead conveys finality and also allows the client the opportunity to say good-bye. Many clients have a difficult time proceeding through the grief process if they have not been given this chance.

Make arrangements in advance concerning how payment for services is to occur. Discuss with the client whether payment is going to be made in advance, at the time of services, or is to be billed later. This can be an uncomfortable subject to broach after euthanasia has occurred.

AT THE END

All of the preparations having been made, the euthanasia should be performed with skill and concern. Each member of the veterinary team should be well trained, know his responsibilities, and be available. The key, as already mentioned, is to expect and plan for the unexpected. Although many methods of euthanasia are deemed acceptable by the AVMA panel on euthanasia, only those that are aesthetically acceptable should be used when the client is going to be present.

If the examination room is to be used, the table should be covered with a cloth or blanket. Some owners will want to bring a favorite blanket for the pet to spend its last few moments on. It is important that they understand that it is possible, indeed likely, that the blanket will be soiled by feces or urine when euthanasia occurs. If the pet is likely to be aggressive, or ex-

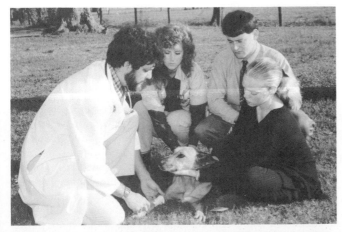

FIGURE 24–1. Being present during the euthanasia of their companion animal helps clients to say good-bye and complete the responsibilities of pet ownership. At times clients will want to have euthanasia performed in a "special place," making the event more personal and meaningful.

tremely apprehensive, tranquilizing it ahead of time should be considered. If the client is to be present, the animal should be taken away briefly so that a peripheral vein can be catheterized for smooth delivery of the euthanasia solution. It is advisable to put the catheter into a vein in a back leg; this will allow the client to hold the animal and pet its head without being in the way of the veterinarian while the injections are being given. Once the catheter has been placed, the client should be given the opportunity to be alone with their pet for a few moments.

Before administering the euthanasia solution, a saline solution should be injected into the catheter to ensure its patency. Next, the patient should be anesthetized with an ultrashort-acting barbiturate. This will decrease the incidence of excitement after the euthanasia solution is injected. Once the animal is anesthetized, the euthanasia solution can be injected. Sodium pentobarbital is the most commonly used euthanasia solution. It is a member of the barbiturate family of drugs that depress the entire central nervous system.* When large doses of this drug are administered, as for euthanasia, unconsciousness occurs first, and then breathing stops owing to depression of the respiratory center. This is followed by cardiac arrest. The pentobarbital dose concentration and the rate of administration determine the speed of action. When the drug is administered intravenously, animals die swiftly and quietly. Although intravenous administration is preferred, the drug is also effective when injected intrahepatically and, to a lesser extent, into the peritoneal cavity. Death following intraperitoneal injection may take as long as 15 minutes, however, because of relatively slow absorption. Pentobarbital for euthanasia is available alone or in combination with other drugs. The concentration of pentobarbital in most euthanasia solutions is approximately 20 percent by weight. The recommended dose is 2 ml for the first 4.5 kg of body weight and 1 ml for each additional 4.5 kg of body weight. Sodium pentobarbital should be administered as rapidly as possible in order to provide the quietest and swiftest form of euthanasia. The veterinary team should be completely familiar with the use of the euthanasia solution chosen and the possible reactions that might be seen.

As the cerebral cortex is affected by general anesthetic, predominant emotions may take over and the animal may show fear behavior, which is usually characterized by struggling and vocalization. Experimental studies indicate that the animal is not conscious of these feelings at the time. People who have undergone the "excitement" phase during general anesthesia do not remember that it took place. Although trained individuals may understand this "excitement phase" from the clinical standpoint, it is difficult for the owner to understand that struggling and vocalization is not due to pain or discomfort. Thus, the owner's perception is that the animal is not experiencing a peaceful death. Clients who choose to be present should be warned that this phase may occur. The use of an ultrashort-acting barbiturate first will minimize the "excitement" phase.

*Note that all barbiturates are strictly controlled by federal regulations, and accurate accounting of the use of these agents is required. The Drug Enforcement Agency (DEA) of the U.S. Department of Justice is responsible for enforcement of laws governing the use of barbiturates. Sodium pentobarbital is a Schedule II controlled substance and can be obtained only by a licensed medical practitioner, such as a physician, dentist, veterinarian or approved institution. In addition to the DEA paperwork involved with procuring barbiturates like sodium pentobarbital, careful handling of the drug is necessary after the drug is on the hospital premises. Thorough record keeping is required by law.

THE END AS A BEGINNING. . . . AFTER THE END

A gentle touch,
barely audible she purrs,
good-bye, oh good-bye,
a final glimpse of life drifting away,
a lifeless stare;
. . . and then, I am alone.

J. TABOADA

Many veterinary professionals are good at the technical aspects of euthanasia but fall short in supplying what the client needs after euthanasia has been performed. The animal's death is often only the beginning of a long and difficult odyssey that the client is about to face. Some clients will feel a great sense of relief immediately following the pet's death, but most will soon feel empty, numb or alone. They may question whether they did the right thing. We can help them by again stressing that the pet's death was painless, assuring them that they did the right thing, and focusing on some of the positive things that the pet brought to their life. At the time of euthanasia it is important that an environment be fostered that says, "It's all right to cry, it's all right to be emotional, it's all right to begin to grieve." Few of us have the gift of being able to say the right thing at the right time, so sometimes consolation can best be offered in a touch or an embrace. A touch on the arm or a simple embrace will often express best what the client needs to hear: "We care and you are not alone."

Many clients, whether present for the euthanasia or not, need assurance that the animal is dead. Clients will feel more assured by the veterinarian who takes the time to listen to the animal's thorax with a stethoscope and shines a pen light into the animal's eyes before pronouncing the patient is dead. For those who choose not to be present, allowing them to view the animal's body can alleviate some of this fear. Before bringing the body to the client it should be made as presentable as possible. It must always be treated with dignity and respect. Clean any blood from the fur, remove any catheters or bandages, place the tongue in the mouth, and close the eyes. Placing a drop of cyanoacrylate glue* in each eye will keep the eyelids closed. If time permits, bathe and brush the animal before laying it on a clean paper, blanket, or towel in a sturdy box. This will help to make the viewing as pleasant an experience as possible. If the animal's body is sealed in a box (commercially made boxes for home burial are available), let the client know how the body is wrapped and whether any signs of trauma or surgery are present. Even the client that assures the veterinarian that he will not open the box before burial or cremation often changes his mind after leaving the office.

Having the client bring someone who will be able to drive him home will help him feel less alone and will also ensure a safe trip. It is nice to call clients after they have arrived home to check on them. Attempts should be made to call all clients who have lost a pet to answer any questions and to show concern. The veterinarian or a staff member may call. The show of concern is always appreciated, helps the client who is having difficulty in dealing with grief and assures the client that a relationship with the clinic fostered in life has not been ended

*Krazy Glue, B. Jadow & Sons, Inc., New York, NY 10010

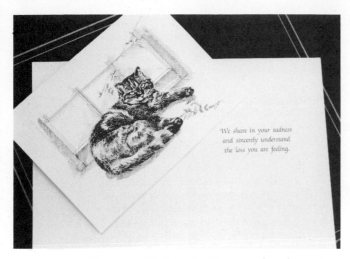

FIGURE 24–2. After a pet has died, condolence cards or letters from veterinary professionals are appropriate symbols of support. Many clients will return to a practice that shows this type of caring gesture when they eventually invest in a new relationship with another pet.

by the death of their pet. Most clients will eventually choose to get another pet. A sympathy card or a handwritten note is usually appreciated. Many beautiful sympathy cards designed for veterinary use are available (Fig. 24–2).

One of the biggest concerns of clients who have just lost a pet is disposition of the body. When possible, all arrangements should be made in advance. The veterinary staff should be prepared with information to assist the client in making these arrangements. Know the laws concerning burial in the practice area. Make available names and phone numbers of places that offer cremation and pet cemetery burial. If the client chooses to have the veterinarian handle the remains, it is best not to lie to the client concerning the disposal of the animal's body.

Memorializing the pet is a step that many clients find comforting. It can be an important part of grieving for many clients. Offering the client a lock of hair and returning collars or leashes may facilitate these wishes. Having a memorial service, planting a special plant in memory of the pet, framing a photograph, keeping a lock of hair, writing a poem or special letter, or offering a memorial scholarship at a veterinary school are actions that clients may use to memorialize their pet (Fig. 24–3).

THE STRESS OF EUTHANASIA

Euthanasia is stressful not only to the client but also to the veterinarian and veterinary staff. Frequent performance of euthanasia is a primary cause of burnout within small animal practice. It is at times even more stressful to the technical staff than it is to the veterinarian because they usually have little control over the situation. Euthanasias that go smoothly as well as "difficult" euthanasias will both create stress. "Difficult" or inherently stressful euthanasias include euthanasia in which technical problems arise, instances in which the animal reacts badly to the injections in the presence of the client, and the euthanasia of one's own pet, healthy animals, young animals and animals for whom one has put a great deal of time and

medical effort into fighting their disease. Euthanasia with the client present usually creates more stress on the veterinary staff than when the procedure is performed in the absence of the owner.

Each individual will have to decide for himself in what type of euthanasia he is able to participate and what his tolerance is for euthanasia. A technician may not be able to work effectively in a practice in which the veterinarian's views on euthanasia are vastly different from his own. Stress can become intense if these differences are not discussed and reconciled. Veterinarians differ markedly in their views on euthanasia. A survey of British veterinarians revealed that 74 percent would perform euthanasia on a healthy animal if the owner requested it. A similar survey in Japan revealed that 63 percent would not. There is room within the veterinary profession for this divergence of views; indeed, the diversity of opinions is one of the profession's strengths.

One of the most important mechanisms of coping with the stress brought on by euthanasia is discussion with colleagues. Having sessions for the hospital staff in which people can openly express their feelings is a good outlet for emotions that, if unexpressed, can cause further stress and lead to burnout. This type of communication allows members of the veterinary team to understand their colleagues' feelings and tolerances for different situations. Members of the team may need to temporarily pass responsibility for euthanasia to their colleagues when they have reached the limit of their tolerance. Other mechanisms of managing stress include taking time off, making time for self, adopting recreational habits, helping clients deal with their grief and finding strength in relationships formed with colleagues that experience the same stresses. Dark humor is often used to relieve stress. Such humor reduces tension by acknowledging death as part of the setting, but also minimizing, for the moment, its tragedy and finality. In animal shelters or practices where large numbers of euthanasias are performed, veterinary staff often cope by shifting moral responsibility for killing animals away from themselves

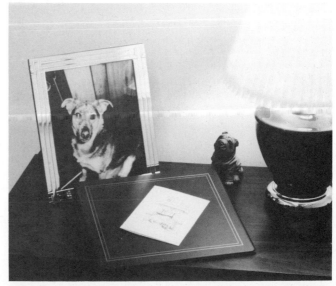

FIGURE 24–3. Memorializing a pet who has died can be an important part of grieving. A framed photo and a scrapbook are two effective ways to memorialize.

to the owners. Care must be taken not to develop an attitude that will be detrimental to the client-veterinarian relationship. (Additional information concerning stress management may be found in Chapter 28.)

EUTHANASIA OF LARGE ANIMALS

Euthanasia of large domestic animals presents specific hazards and problems not encountered in companion small animals. Safety must be a major consideration. The jugular vein should be used for injection whenever possible because this will place the person injecting the euthanasia solution in the safest position. On rare occasions, the jugular veins may be thrombosed from disease, and the cephalic vein must be used. However, this puts the individual under the animal's forequarters and in a dangerous position.

Euthanasia-strength pentobarbital can be administered with a large-gauge needle (16 to 14 gauge). The volume of solution is large, and even with a large-gauge needle, the time it takes to inject the solution is relatively long. The animal may go through the same "excitement" phase as that experienced by small animals, and it may come crashing to the ground upon becoming unconscious. Generally, large-animal euthanasia should be performed in an area with vehicle access to allow removal of the body. In some instances, the client may wish to bury a large animal. It should be remembered that all of the same emotional concerns encountered in small-animal euthanasia pertain to large animals when a bond has formed between the owner the animal.

CONCLUSION

Euthanasia is a skill that, like any other skill, must be well thought out and practiced. The entire veterinary team should be involved in a well-coordinated and professional manner. Euthanasia, if performed poorly, can be a disastrous experience for both the client and the veterinary practice. If performed with practiced care and gentle concern, it can be remembered positively for a long time.

Recommended Readings

Arluke A: Coping with euthanasia: A case study of shelter culture. J Am Vet Med Assoc 198:1176–1180, 1991.

AVMA Council on Research: Council Report: Report of the AVMA panel on euthanasia. J Am Vet Med Assoc 188:253–268, 1986.

Fogle B and Abrahamson D: Pet loss: Attitudes and feelings of practicing veterinarians. Anthrozoos 3:143–150, 1990.

Grier RL and Schaffer CB: Evaluation of intraperitoneal and intrahepatic administration of a euthanasia agent in animal shelter cats. J Am Vet Med Assoc 197:1611–1615, 1990.

Hart LA, Hart BL and Mader B: Humane euthanasia and companion animal death: Caring for the animal, the client, and the veterinarian. J Am Vet Med Assoc 197:1292–1299, 1990.

Kay WJ: Euthanasia. Trends 1(5):52–54, 1985.

Kogure N and Yamazaki K: Attitudes to animal euthanasia in Japan: A brief review of cultural influences. Anthrozoos 3:151–154, 1990.

Peters TG: Commander. JAMA 260:1460, 1988.

Tannenbaum J: Veterinary Ethics. Baltimore, Williams & Wilkins Co. 1989, pp 208–236.

Walshaw SO: Consoling bereaved clients. Compendium of Continuing Education 2(6):414, 1981.

25

Client Bereavement and the Grief Process

JOSEPH TABOADA and SANDRA BRACKENRIDGE

Domestic animals have lived in association with humans for thousands of years. The dog was probably the first animal to be domesticated, a process that probably began at least 15,000 years ago. The domestication of the cat may have begun as early as 7000 BC. Initially these animals were tools used for hunting, hauling and protection, but over time they have assumed a variety of other roles, not the least of which is companionship.

Today, with over 53 million families owning one or more companion animals,* pets are considered part of the "extended family network." Surveys and clinical experience indicate that many people consider their pets to be like children, partners or best friends. Family structures have evolved from traditional nuclear families to single-parent, step-parent, never-married and widowed elderly families. Owing to changing family structure and because more people are living alone, companion animals have taken on larger roles in people's support systems. With these changes have come added expectations of veterinary health care professionals. Members of the veterinary medical profession must realize that they are not treating just dogs, cats, birds, rabbits or horses but important members of their clients' family and an important part of their clients' support system (Fig. 25–1).

THE HUMAN–COMPANION ANIMAL BOND

During the twentieth century, society has evolved at a remarkable rate. As a result of the industrial revolution and

---

*Source: Nielson Marketing Research.

technological advances, modern society is largely urban rather than rural; thus the need for companion animals as hunters and herders has decreased. Millions of Americans restrict themselves and their animals to urban life styles. Animals live indoors in apartments or houses with their owners, increasing familiarity, dependency and bonding.

Society is also more mobile than ever before. It is not unusual for people to change locales and residences several times within a 10-year period. Additionally, the family itself is radically different from the nuclear family of the past. No longer do most Americans live within a short distance of their extended families, and the nuclear family is smaller, consisting of an average of less than two children per family. More than half of American couples divorce, and the single-parent family is becoming common. Since 64 percent of American women work outside the home, many school-age children return home to be greeted not by their mother, but by the family pet. Companion animals provide both parents and children with stability, constancy and security in a twentieth century littered with losses and personal adjustments.

More and more adults live alone, and more and more couples opt to remain childless. Many of these people fill the void with pets who provide a unique outlet for their owners' needs to nurture and to be loved. As health and medical care improves, the number of people in the age group above 60 has increased—nearing 25 percent of the population. Pets fulfill many needs for the elderly, including needs for interaction, exercise, companionship, protection and motivation to remain active and independent.

Recently, special populations have benefited from contact

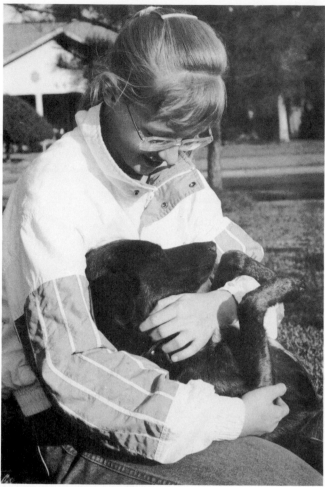

FIGURE 25–1. Pets have become important members of the "extended family network." They provide tactile contact that can be important for young and old alike.

The Attachment Between Animals and Humans

The attachment between animals and people is based on such factors as the frequency of contact, the pleasant emotional states produced during these contacts, and the pleasing behaviors, facial expressions and body postures displayed during interactions. Pets can generate a sense of well-being, of being wanted, needed and unconditionally loved and can provide warm, soft, tactile contact (see Fig. 25–1). They can also help people to feel happy by greeting them in familiar and endearing ways.

Strong attachments can form between owners and any type of animal, but are probably recognized most commonly in veterinary practice with dogs, cats and horses. The degree of attachment varies greatly from the utilitarian attachment between a rancher and his cattle to the parent/child–type bonding that may occur between some people and their dog or cat. Over the past decade the cat has supplanted the dog as the most popular pet in the United States, with more than 55 million being owned.* It has recently been estimated that about 50 percent of these cat owners classify their attachment to their pet as "strong." Of these "strong attachment" owners about half see their cat(s) as reflections of themselves or of their tastes, who are dependent upon them for love, affection and care. The other half of the "strong attachment" owners go so far as to report a reliance on their cat(s) as an emotional crutch, supplying unconditional love and affection, sometimes acting as a substitute for family, friends or children.

As pets are used to meet many of the changing psychosocial needs of modern society, the intensity of attachment has increased. When pet loss occurs, intensity and duration of attachment are determinants of the significance of the loss and intensity of grief that follows. Attachment is more intense when the animal has functioned in many roles for the owner. The owner of an assistance dog may therefore suffer more intense bereavement than the owner of a dog used only for herding or hunting. Owners who have experienced previous significant losses, adjustments or traumas and have been comforted by their pet's presence may also exhibit strong attachment and thus intense bereavement.

Benefits of Attachment

As reminders of both pleasant and traumatic events in people's lives, pets can take on symbolic meaning. If a pet is associated with a particular friend, relative or stage in life, the attachment to the pet can take on added significance. If the pet represents a tangible link to a person or relationship that is now gone owing to death, divorce or other loss, the pet's death may stimulate recurring grief for the lost loved one as well as for the animal itself. Even when the pet is simply another family member, grief can be intense. Grief is also very individual, and each family member may grieve in his own way.

Casey, an 8-year-old male Doberman, is brought into the clinic for lethargy and anorexia. After a work-up he is diagnosed as having Doberman cardiomyopathy. Even with appropriate treatment, the prognosis for a long lifetime is poor.

with animals. As society has realized the special talents of pets, we have found new utilitarian functions for them. Dogs are now used with success to assist the blind, the hearing impaired and the physically challenged. These specially trained animals provide their owners with independence, companionship, social lubrication, protection and love. Both cats and dogs have been used successfully in animal-assisted therapy programs for people with all types of physical and mental disabilities. Animals facilitate interaction with people who may be reluctant to interact, and their presence reduces anxiety, lowers blood pressure and decreases heart rate. Results of some studies indicate that animals may alleviate and/or prevent depression. Survival rates for cardiac patients who are pet owners are higher than for those who do not own pets. In fact, pet ownership is considered an important predictor of survival for patients with coronary artery disease.

In short, the relationships between people and animals have become physically closer, and the role of animals in the daily lives of their owners has become more emotional and less utilitarian as society has changed. Of the over 53 million families owning at least one pet, 87 percent describe their pets as "family members" and cite companionship, love and friendship as the most important derivatives of the relationship.

*1989 AVMA Statistics.

Casey is owned by a 72-year-old widow named Emily who lost her husband to cancer 5 years earlier. During her husband's fight against the disease, Casey was his constant companion. Emily can still vividly remember how Casey, as a young puppy, used to make her husband laugh by chewing on her shoes while always leaving her husband's alone.

Casey was brought to the veterinarian for what was perceived to be a minor problem, but a severe, life-threatening disease was diagnosed. Emily is likely to feel numb initially. The diagnosis is likely to be hard to accept. An important part of Emily's attachment to Casey comes from her relationship with her late husband. Casey represents a tangible link between Emily's life now and the many memories of her life with her husband. Casey's death is not only going to be hard because of the loss of a faithful companion/family member, but it is also going to bring back many of the emotions that were associated with the death of her husband.

PET LOSS AND VETERINARY MEDICINE

Veterinarians and veterinary technicians are daily confronted with complex issues of attachment, loss and grief in the course of their patient's illness and death. The diagnosis of life-threatening or terminal disease can be a difficult time for both the client and the veterinary professional (Fig. 25–2). Considering all the emotional and utilitarian aspects of the human–companion animal relationship in modern society, it is not surprising that the breaking of the bond due to the death of the pet is a significant event in the lives of many pet owners. The loss of the pet for many owners is made even more intense and personal in that the pet is often grieved by no one other than themselves. Daily routines are filled with reminders of activities once performed for or with the pet. The loss of a pet often means that a unique, irreplaceable member of the family is gone.

A person's support system is made up of people (and pets) that interact with one another on a day to day basis, providing support, comfort and social interaction. Support systems are especially important during times of loss. Unfortunately, most people who make up these support systems do not understand the full extent of attachment between a pet owner and their pet. This lack of understanding can present serious problems for the owner facing the odyssey of grief after the death of a pet.

Because of the general lack of social support from standard support systems for clients that have experienced pet loss, and because of the caregiving role veterinarians and veterinary technicians fill, pet owners often turn to veterinary professionals as sources of support, comfort and understanding at and around the time of their pet's death. Veterinary professionals usually have a good understanding of attachment. Additionally, veterinary professionals are often looked upon as an important part of the pet's life.

The tendency for people to turn to the veterinary staff during the period of grieving the death of a pet places veterinary professionals in an awkward position, however. It demands that they have knowledge that is typically outside the boundaries of traditional veterinary medicine and requires that they find a comfort level in talking about death and the grief process. This is why the areas of attachment, animal behavior, human bereavement and grief counseling are becoming more and more relevant to veterinary medicine.

In the sections of the chapter that follow, we will describe the normal grief responses to pet loss and offer veterinary technicians and other veterinary professionals a framework from which they can develop a level of comfort with grief and support of the grieving pet owner. The goal is not to transform veterinary professionals into therapists, but to give them an understanding of grief and the grief process that will be useful in the day to day practice of veterinary client relations. It is best to remember that in most cases, grief responses are normal and healthy, and require little or no intervention beyond validation and compassion.

WHEN THE BOND IS BROKEN

Our society has been described as "death denying" because many people are uncomfortable talking about death. We know little about the experience of death, and we fear the unknown. Yet veterinarians and their staff must frequently discuss death, participate in causing it, witness it and deal with the emotions triggered by these experiences.

Although people in the midst of grief have a need and a right to understand what is happening to them, there are few places they can go to get helpful, supportive information about grief. This is particularly true when the loss they are grieving is that of a beloved pet. Like most of society, veterinarians and veterinary technicians rarely have formal training in this area. Few curricula offer more than a cursory introduction to the concepts of death, grief and bereavement. On-the-job training is almost always inadequate because few veterinary professionals, especially technicians, have the extent of client follow-up needed to see and understand the full spectrum of effects that grief has on owners. Despite this fact, veterinary professionals are still often the people clients instinctively turn to for support.

Making the job more difficult is the fact that grief and bereavement are emotional and often irrational areas of human

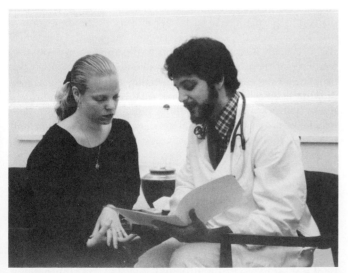

FIGURE 25–2. The diagnosis of a disease can be a difficult time for both clients and veterinary professionals.

interaction. The bereaved may, at times, seem out of control or out of touch with reality. When this happens, those around the griever, including the veterinary professional, may feel uncomfortable; few of us are taught how to support or to deal with people who are irrational or emotional. Compassion is an important sensitivity to draw on when interacting with clients experiencing grief.

Grief is the companion to death. It is the mental anguish experienced by any human being confronted with the loss of an object of attachment. Grief may ensue as an effect of any loss; the loss may be through death, divorce, loss of a job, or even moving or having friends move away. It can be intensely emotional and can affect mind, body and spirit. Also, grief is a major stressor, able to produce any of the symptoms of stress listed in Chapter 28. When confronted with grief, the bereaved individual goes through a grief process. The term *grief process* implies that there is an intended end or result to be produced through grieving. Thus, the grief process is the means of letting go of the object of attachment in order to feel better, reinvest, emotionally grow, and attach again.

The veterinary staff is in a unique position to assist clients going through the process of grief. They, by way of their unique role in the life of the owner and pet, may be the only people who knew the pet and understood the bond that had developed between owner and pet. Additionally, the veterinarian and the owner may have interacted uniquely in choosing the time of the pet's death (as occurs when euthanasia is performed). In order to assist clients during the difficult bereavement period, it is helpful to understand the normal grief process and the manifestations of it as applied to pet loss.

Pet Loss and the Grief Process

The death of a pet is all too often regarded as a trivial loss by society, perhaps owing in part to the mistaken belief that pets can be easily replaced. There are no socially sanctioned rituals like funerals or memorial services to help grieving pet owners gain support once the bonds between them and their companion animals have been broken. Furthermore, people are rarely granted time off from their jobs in order to care for sick animals or to make arrangements for them after their deaths. Society also does not allow adequate time for mourning the death of a pet. Most people feel pressured to be "back to normal" within a few days of their pet's death in order to avoid being labeled as neurotic, hysterical or overly attached. However, crying, taking time away from work, and wanting to memorialize a pet are healthy responses to the death of a pet. They should not be discouraged, nor should they be judged.

One of the most effective ways for veterinary professionals to assist grieving clients is to educate and reassure them that their feelings and behaviors are normal parts of the grief process. Other ways that veterinary professionals can help are listed in Table 25–1.

The Normal Grief Process

As stated earlier, the word process implies movement toward some end or result. In regard to grief, this movement is accomplished by passing through what have been termed stages, phases or tasks. The basic emotional process in pet loss is the same as in human loss. However, veterinary professionals who assist clients are aware of some differences and particulars.

Several models of the grief process can be modified to describe the emotional process that occurs during pet loss. Some important ones are exemplified in Table 25–2. For our purposes, we will use the classic model supplied by Elisabeth Kübler-Ross (1969) and extrapolate for the situations peculiar to pet loss.

Dr. Kübler-Ross was one of the first to work extensively with the dying and their families during the late 1960s. She described the grief process as consisting of five "stages": denial, bargaining, anger, depression, and resolution. She used the stages to describe the passage through grief, but it is helpful to remember that these stages are not a linear odyssey. Although people may travel through the grief process in a straight line, they more often fluctuate between stages, bounce back and forth, and feel the entire gamut of grief within minutes, within days or within months.

Stage 1: Denial

Denial is a normal defense mechanism that buffers a human being from some unbearable news or reality. It is important to recognize the word "normal" here, as many individuals experiencing denial at the time a poor prognosis is given or during bereavement will seem to all observers to be out of touch with reality. The veterinary staff may wonder whether the client has even heard the veterinarian stating the seriousness of an animal's illness. A client in denial may listen attentively to a diagnosis of cancer with a poor prognosis, but ask only if the toenails can be clipped or if their current flea shampoo is correct. A client informed of the death of their pet while it was hospitalized may chatter on about activities for the weekend. A simple form of denial is exemplified by the client who states repeatedly, "It can't be. I don't believe it."

It is tempting when presented with a client experiencing denial to insist that they recognize the seriousness of the situation. Many veterinarians and veterinary technicians worry that the client does not comprehend or has not heard correctly. There is no harm in repeating oneself to a client in denial (Fig. 25–3). In fact, restating diagnoses, prognoses, treatment plans and particulars is advisable. However, clients in denial will only accept the unbearable reality of the situation when they are ready internally; attempts to push them may backfire, resulting in frustration. Usually, a client will begin to ask appropriate questions about the time they arrive home and may phone the veterinary office. Some may even seem to return to reality before your eyes while those toenails are being attended to. The veterinary professional must feel assured that the client has been told the basic information that needs to be given. Remember, however, that it may not have been fully understood; therefore, always leave the door open for further communication.

Although denial reappears later during the grief process, at that time it is usually of little significance to the veterinary staff. Later-stage denial may be manifested as clients reporting during a phone call or visit that they were sure they had seen their pet that morning, or they had absent-mindedly purchased pet food several weeks or months after their pet's death. Denial is reflected by the client's eyes and demeanor, and by incongruous questions. The veterinary staff should not feel respon-

Table 25–1

THE STAGES OF GRIEF: HOW VETERINARY PROFESSIONALS CAN HELP

Denial

What the client needs most is time, support, understanding and permission to grieve.

PRIOR TO DEATH

- Arrange to communicate with the client in person, if possible, where you both can sit down to talk without interruption or distraction. Recognize denial as a normal part of grief.
- Communicate clearly, and reiterate patiently. Phrase statements in words that are concrete and simple for the layperson. Avoid using medical jargon and lapsing into complicated medical explanations.
- Listen actively: Maintain eye contact, use attentive body language, and paraphrase or clarify the client's statements as you respond to him. Give him permission to express his feelings.
- Give the client time to think about and to grasp the reality of information that has been given. Some clients need only a slight pause in the conversation or a few minutes alone. Other clients may need more time to themselves before they comprehend the news of severe illness or actual death.
- Refrain from judging the client as "stupid" or "out of it."
- Remain nonjudgmental and unhurried toward the client, and state that you are available to talk about specifics or about his feelings whenever he's ready.
- NEVER attempt to force the client to "come to his senses" or to move out of denial. He will comprehend at his own pace.

AFTER DEATH

- Encourage the client to view the body, say goodbye.
- Reveal a bit of personal experience (self-disclosure) that relates to the situation. (Self-disclosure allows clients to feel comfortable and not alone in what they are feeling and gives them permission to grieve.)*
- Give permission to grieve.

Bargaining

- Understand that bargaining is an attempt to control or reverse a dire situation. The client feels irrationally compelled to bargain during the grief process and does not mean to doubt the professionals involved.
- When the patient is terminally ill, do not become defensive or threatened when clients ask for other opinions or consider alternative treatments. Giving information and readings, and referral for second opinion will ameliorate bargaining attempts and facilitate commitment to treatment.
- After the death, be sympathetic and educative about the stage of bargaining when clients confide their feelings and bargaining behaviors, such as prayers and dreams (or daydreams) of the pet still alive. Reassure them that the emotional basis for their behaviors and feelings is normal even though it may seem irrational.
- When clients inquire as to when to "replace" their pet, educating them about the role bargaining plays in shopping for a new pet can alleviate future disappointment. State that their dead pet was unique and cannot be replaced, but encourage them to obtain a new pet whenever all members of the family feel ready. Help them to find the type of animal they are looking for while gently steering toward one that is slightly dissimilar to the dead pet. Encourage them to choose a different breed, color or gender, and a brand new name should be chosen.

Anger

- Listen actively and let the client know that you understand.
- Arrange for communication in a private room with no distractions. Sit at eye level, and use attentive body language. Take notes if the client is complaining or criticizing.
- Give the client permission to ventilate his feelings. Listen actively using attentive body language, maintaining eye contact, nodding and responses that paraphrase, clarify and indicate your understanding of the client's feelings. (Example: "I can see that you're very angry . . ." or "You feel that diagnosis could have been made sooner. . . .")
- If the client is directly angry at the veterinarian, technician(s), or clinic staff, take a mental step backward, pause with either a deep breath or by counting to 10.
- DO NOT BECOME DEFENSIVE OR RESPOND IN LIKE MANNER to the client.
- Relieve guilt by assuring the client that he did the right thing.
- Educate the client about the grief process and about the role of anger and guilt. Let him know that as he is able to let go of his anger/guilt, he will move toward resolution of his grief.

Depression

- Encourage depressed clients to talk about their feelings in regard to their pet. Follow up clients whose pets have died with a phone call in a few days and then 2 weeks afterward.
- Listen actively.
- Attend to the client by positioning yourself at eye level, offering tissues and/or a drink of water, and leaning slightly toward him. A nonthreatening yet compassionate touch on the forearm or on the shoulder communicates empathy and understanding.
- Offer a place to sit, a place to be out of the "public eye."
- Tell the client that it is all right, and even good for him, to cry. Listen supportively and actively, and touch the client gently on the shoulder or forearm. Some clients are known well enough to embrace, and this can be helpful as well.
- Validate the feelings of sadness by letting the client know that he is normal.
- Offer to call a family member or friend.
- Be a friend.
- Encourage and suggest means by which clients can memorialize their pet. Making scrapbooks, planting a tree, writing a letter to the pet or writing the pet's life story all are cathartic activities that alleviate depression due to grief.
- If a client expresses continued depression several weeks following the death of his pet, if his support system is poor or if a client expresses a personal wish to die, referral to a compassionate professional counselor is necessary. Although referral may feel awkward, many clients appreciate the technician who states, "Grief due to pet loss is normal, but sometimes there can be no one to talk to, or the grief can be overwhelming. I know of a person who understands what you're going through. Would you like her (his) telephone number, or may I have her (him) call you?" Today, several schools of veterinary medicine employ counselors experienced in pet loss. Many communities have established support groups, and private counselors increasingly view pet loss as significant bereavement.†

Resolution

- Acceptance is achieved once the above four stages have fallen into the background of the client's life. At this point, the bereaved can channel emotional energy into a new relationship. The veterinary professional can help clients reach the resolution stage by offering insight into the grief process through their actions and by offering suggestions of reading material or seminars on the grief process.

*When using self-disclosure, take care not to monopolize the time with your own experiences. A short comment that lets the client know that your own experiences parallel and thus validate their emotions is sufficient.
†For a complete list of referral counselors or for a referral, write the Delta Society (address and phone number is footnoted in the text).

Table 25–2
POPULAR MODELS OF THE GRIEF PROCESS

Kübler-Ross	Worden	Rosenberg	Dersheimer
STAGES	TASKS	STAGES	PHASES
Denial	I. To accept the reality of the loss	Denial	Shock
Bargaining	II. To experience the pain of grief	Anger/guilt	Acute grief
Anger	III. To adjust to an environment in which the deceased is missing	Grief	Straightening up the mess
Depression	IV. To withdraw emotional energy and reinvest it in another relationship	Acceptance	Reinvesting and re-engaging in life
Acceptance			

sibility to "break through" a client's denial. The client will move out of denial, accepting the reality of the situation, when he is ready. The veterinary staff's recognition of the client's denial can prevent impatience and frustration during the veterinary contact.

Soft Paw, a 15-year-old female domestic shorthair cat, is brought into the clinic for vomiting and anorexia that the owner thinks is due to the ingestion of chicken bones. Physical examination reveals Soft Paw to be thin and pale. Further evaluation reveals that Soft Paw is severely anemic due to renal failure. The prognosis is poor.

Soft Paw is owned by a 20-year-old college student named Ashley who found the cat as a kitten. Ashley has owned Soft Paw since she was 5 years old. When told that Soft Paw's problems were not caused by chicken bones but were due to end-stage renal failure Ashley at first did not seem to hear what the doctor had said. A blank stare washed over her face, and for a moment she appeared to be daydreaming. The doctor continued by explaining that there were some treatments that may prolong Soft Paw's life, but they should be considered palliative and not potentially curative. After hearing the doctor's assessment Ashley smiled, picked up her cat and turned to leave. "Thank you for your time today," she said as she turned to leave. "I'll try not to let her get into the chicken bones in the future. Oh, by the way, can you trim Soft Paw's front claws? They are getting kind of long."

Ashley came to the veterinarian's office for what she perceived to be a problem brought on by Soft Paw's dietary indiscretion. Ashley had probably not seen her cat eat chicken bones but was grasping for an explanation for why Soft Paw was vomiting, losing weight and acting lethargic. In all probability, Ashley had been denying that Soft Paw was sick for some time even before making the appointment with the doctor. When the doctor told Ashley the diagnosis her initial reaction appeared to be that of shock. Ashley's shock, seeming not to hear the results of the evaluation, and asking the doctor to perform something seemingly inappropriate like a nail trim is part of denial, the first stage of grief.

When a client like the one presented above is encountered, the veterinary professional must realize that the response is a normal part of the grief process. The conversation up to that point may or may not have been heard, but it certainly has not yet been clearly comprehended. The client will be able to acknowledge the seriousness of the situation only when he or she is ready internally. The veterinary professional should repeat things and not become frustrated or impatient. Clip the nails and call the client at home later for further discussions. At that time the client may be ready to acknowledge the reality of the bad disease, and meaningful discussions concerning treatment options can then occur.

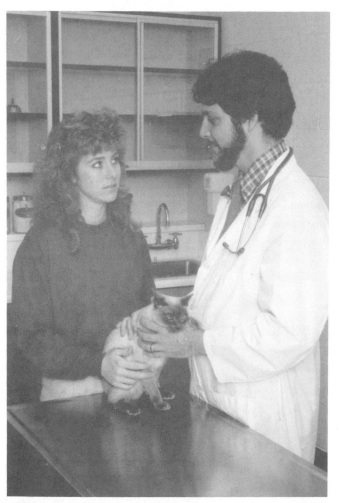

FIGURE 25–3. Even when dealing with attentive clients, veterinary professionals may be required to repeat themselves several times while clients decide on a course of treatment for their pet.

Stage 2: Bargaining

Once the reality of death or impending death is realized, the client may show various impotent attempts to control or to reverse the reality. The client is grappling with the stage of the grief process that Dr. Kübler-Ross called bargaining. During this stage, the client maneuvers personally and privately, possibly praying and negotiating with God for miracles. They might add various herbs and old family remedies to food. Children behave like little angels, hoping to be rewarded with a reversal of bad news. The veterinary staff may be subject to various inquiries by the client at this stage, such as, "Have you ever heard of avocado in the food? I read that it may reverse cancer." It is while bargaining that a pet owner may also request permission to obtain a second (and sometimes third, fourth or fifth) opinion. Bargaining during terminal illness rarely results in harm to the patient, and veterinary staff should reassure themselves of their clients' normality. Be compassionate and when possible answer their questions. Help clients to understand that this stage of grief is normal.

Bargaining after death has occurred may go on without the knowledge of the veterinary professionals involved. Seeking to "replace" the lost animal without grieving at all is a form of bargaining. Many pet owners seek a new pet too soon, and they purchase the same species, the same color, and name them the same or a similar name. Leaving dishes or the dead pet's belongings down for an obviously unusual length of time is another subtle form of bargaining. Through bargaining the client is unconsciously attempting to control or subvert the grief process.

It is important to recognize bargaining as part of the normal grief process. The veterinary professionals who understand the stages of bargaining and denial will avoid frustration in their attempts to provide quality patient care and client service.

> *Three days after the euthanasia of his Doberman "Saber," Ron came into the clinic to pay his bill. After reviewing the bill, he asked to speak to the veterinarian who was busy at the time. Maggie, the technician, led Ron to an examination room and then inquired as to how he had been doing. Ron told her that he had not been sleeping well because of dreams of Saber. He stated that the dreams were pleasant, but he would awaken hoping that Saber's death had been a nightmare. He said, "Sometimes I'll keep my eyes closed for an extra ten seconds and pray that she's come back, somehow, healthy and happy. But of course, it never works." In addition, he said, "I want to see Dr. Roberts today because I can't stop thinking about Saber's treatment. I know Dr. Roberts is the best vet around, and I'm grateful to him for being so kind to me and Saber. But I feel like maybe something more could have been done."*

> *Ron met with Dr. Roberts for only a few minutes. During this time Maggie was asked to bring tissues to the room. As Maggie handed him a tissue, Ron said tearfully, "I looked at the whole record. Even while I was doing it, I realized that no information could bring Saber back to life. For some reason, I had to look anyway. Now, maybe, I can let her go."*

Although Ron understands that Saber died, he feels compelled to try controlling the situation. Childlike and irrational behaviors such as his closing his eyes and wishing or praying that Saber was alive are manifestations of the bargaining stage of grief. Ron's request to view the record might have been viewed by the veterinarian and the technician as challenging or accusatory. Yet Ron was not looking for information which could be damaging, he was hoping again to somehow reverse the illness and death of Saber. Bargaining can be frustrating for veterinary professionals unless they understand and assist the client in working through these irrational attempts to "bring their beloved pet back."

Stage 3: Anger

During the grief process, clients may move in and out of the stage called anger. Clients coping with this stage may exhibit anger in a wide variety of direct or indirect manners. The anger may be specific or nonspecific in the way that it is directed. Anger may also be exhibited in the form of guilt, which can be defined as anger turned inward.

Anger is a particularly difficult emotion to deal with when a client directs it toward the veterinary professional. Whether or not the client is justified in his stated cause for anger, staff members must use tolerance and patience to avoid responding defensively. Bereaved clients may complain that the illness which resulted in death should have been discovered sooner, should have been treated differently or should not have been allowed to happen. They may complain that their pet died while hospitalized owing to neglect or inappropriate treatment rather than to the tumor revealed by necropsy.

Anger may be apparent in the form of guilt. Clients feeling guilt use language with an abundance of "I should've" statements. They often seek the listening ear of the veterinary professional to ask questions pertinent to absolution from guilt. They may ask whether or not the food they fed their pet could have contributed to the illness or death. They often ask whether or not it was the pesticide in their home or in the shampoo that caused a tumor or cardiac arrest. Clients may believe they allowed their pet to be too active or too fat; others may believe they caused the kidney failure in their cat by feeding insufficient diet. These clients can direct anger at themselves, but frequently they cannot find a specific crime that they committed. When possible, the veterinary professional can assist the client by assuaging their guilt. Reassuring the client that, in your opinion, they did everything possible for their pet, that they did only what they thought would benefit their pet and that they made the right decisions for their pet will relieve much of the client's guilt or anger and assist him in moving through the grief process.

The client showing indirect and nonspecific anger is not as threatening to the veterinary professional as those who direct their anger specifically toward the veterinarian or veterinary technician. The client who is feeling this type of anger may be gruff or rude and generally hard to get along with. Stating that he is angry, he may be at a loss to express with whom or what he is angry. This type of anger is common in American society. These clients yell at the cashiers, waitresses and telephone operators; and they drive their cars with aggressiveness and anger. Giving the angry client an opportunity to express his feelings (ventilation) is an effective way for the veterinary professional to help. At times, all that is needed is for the sensitive veterinary professional to explain that, considering the client's loss, anger is a normal feeling. This explanation gives the client permission to grieve effectively.

Indirect and specific anger in a client is most often exhibited by reluctance to pay the bill. Upon receiving an inquiry by telephone, the client implies that nonpayment is due to anger at treatment by the veterinarian or by the technician, the pet was neglected, that the illness was mistreated or that he (the client) was treated insensitively. Bereavement support can alleviate this client's anger. Listen attentively, state your apologies, if any, and follow up with this client. No admission of mistakes need be made, but the client needs to feel significant and understood.

Although all of the types of anger may be exhibited by one client, it is guilt that may be hardest for the client to relinquish. Yet, direct and specific anger, when justified (or perceived to be justified), is difficult to work through, as well. In continuing to feel guilt and anger, the client avoids letting go of the beloved pet, and the grief process is stymied. Once the client

---

Table 25–3

HOW TO HELP CHILDREN WHEN A PET DIES

When children's companion animals die, many parents follow their instincts to protect them from pain and grief. Some parents make decisions regarding the pet without discussing them with their children. Some may even lie to their children about the actual circumstances of the pet's "disappearance," preferring to tell them that a beloved pet ran away or was stolen rather than died. These tactics are not used maliciously by parents. They develop from a desire to spare children feelings of pain and from a belief that they, as parents, are inadequately prepared to discuss loss, death and grief with their children.

Children, however, are tuned into their parents' emotions and, almost without exception, know that *something* is going on in the family. They don't know what that *something* is, but they do know that it upsets mom and dad. Consequently, children may feel anxious, confused, left out and even guilty because, without honest explanations of a family crisis, children often feel that they are somehow responsible for the tension level in the home. At later ages, children may also feel betrayed by the parents they trusted when they discover the "truth" about their childhood pet's "disappearance."

The knowledge, skills and tools for dealing with loss and grief that are developed in childhood are the same ones used in adolescence and adulthood. It is of utmost importance, then, that children be given honest support and information about loss and death so their grief-coping strategies will be healthy, rather than unhealthy, ones.

How Technicians Can Help

Parents will often turn to veterinary professionals for assistance in telling their children about the death of a pet. Having books available for them to read and having information yourself to share can help ease an otherwise traumatic situation. Here are some suggestions:

● Always encourage parents to be honest with their children throughout a companion animal's illness, treatment and death. Never agree to participate in a lie that the parents may want to tell their children in order to protect them. In the long run, lies create more problems for everyone involved and can be more damaging to children than the pet's death itself.

● Children under the age of 8 do not really understand that death is final. They may believe that a dead pet can return or that they will need food in their grave with them. Young children are also egocentric and believe quite strictly in the law of cause and effect. Thus, they may develop the idea that they did something to cause the pet's death. Therefore, they must be reassured repeatedly that the pet died because it had a disease or an accident or was very old.

● Straightforward explanations and concrete words like dead and died should be used, then, when talking to children about death. Young children don't understand euphemisms and can become upset when they hear terms like "put to sleep." Since they go to sleep every night, and don't want to die like their pet did, attempts at "softening the blow" can actually make the situation more difficult and frightening for children.

● Children need to be held, reassured and allowed to ask questions. Open communication about death is the desired atmosphere for keeping death anxiety manageable. Pets' names should be used in conversation whenever possible and memories of them should be shared by the whole family. Older children should be included in the euthanasia process, the memorial ceremonies and the goodbye rituals to whatever extent they wish to be and should be encouraged to demonstrate their sensitivity and compassion.

● It is always helpful to contact children's teachers, care providers, relatives and other significant adults so they can help acknowledge the loss and grief process. Adults may observe children playing "funeral" or overhear them talking to friends about a pet's death. While these activities may seem alarming and even morbid to adults, they are normal, healthy responses for children. Children deal with issues through play and experimentation. Unless they are in physical danger, their activities do not, in most cases, require interference.

● For more information about helping children deal with pet loss, consult the following books:

Balk DE: Children and the death of a pet. Manhattan, KS, Cooperative Extension Service, Kansas State University, 1990.

Jewett CL: Helping Children Cope with Separation and Loss. Boston, Harvard Common Press, 1982.

Nieburg HA, and Fischer A: Pet Loss: A Thoughtful Guide for Adults and Children. New York, Harper and Row, 1982.

Quackenbush J and Graveline D: When Your Pet Dies: How to Cope with Your Feelings. New York, Simon and Schuster, 1985.

Shirl-Potter JW and Koss GJ: Death of a Pet; Answers to Questions for Children and Animal Lovers of All Ages. Stanford, Guideline Publications, 1991.

Stein S: About Dying: An Open Family Book for Adults and Children. New York, Walker and Co., 1974.

Viorst J: The Tenth Good Thing about Barney. New York, Atheneum, 1972.

Reprinted with additional readings from Lagoni L and Hetts S: Bereavement *In* McCurnin DM (ed): Clinical Textbook for Veterinary Technicians. 2nd ed. Philadelphia, WB Saunders Co., 1990.

Table 25–4
BOOKS ABOUT PET LOSS FOR ADULTS

Anderson M: Coping with Sorrow on the Loss of Your Pet. Los Angeles, Peregrine Press, 1987.

Church JA: Joy in a Woolly Coat. Tiburon, CA, HJ Kramer, Inc., 1987.

Kay WJ, Nieburg HA, Kukscher AH, Ross MG, and Fudin CE (editors): Pet Loss and Human Bereavement. Ames, Iowa State University Press, 1984.

Kay WJ, Cohen SP, Nieburg HA (editors): Euthanasia of the Companion Animal: The Impact on Pet Owners, Veterinarians, and Society. Baltimore, The Charles Press, 1988.

Nieburg HA and Fischer A: Pet Loss: A Thoughtful Guide for Adults and Children. New York, Harper and Row, 1982.

Quackenbush J and Graveline D: When Your Pet Dies: How to Cope with Your Feelings. New York, Simon and Schuster, 1985.

Reprinted from Lagoni L and Hetts S: Bereavement. *In* McCurnin DM (editor): Clinical Textbook for Veterinary Technicians. 2nd ed. Philadelphia, WB Saunders Co., 1990.

special to remember Missy. After a short pause the youngest sister says that they would like to plant a tree in remembrance of Missy. They have even picked a special place in front of the clinic where Missy spent her last few days. A week later a small tree is planted on the clinic lawn during a short ceremony in which Missy is remembered. The two sisters, their mother, the veterinarian and the veterinary technician attend. Afterwards the veterinary technician cries with the sisters. All three feel the sadness of the loss but can smile in shared memories.

Two months after Missy's death, the girls show up at the clinic with proud smiles on their faces and a new puppy in their arms. Archie is a beautiful little Schnauzer puppy that they adopted from the local humane society. "He is a ball of fire," laughs the older sister. "You should have seen what Archie did to his favorite stuffed doll yesterday!" Both the veterinarian and the veterinary technician smile.

The girls are doing well. They have grieved for their lost pet—a process made easier by the compassion and concern shown by the veterinary staff. In being present during the euthanasia they had a very special opportunity to say goodbye, and by memorializing Missy with a ceremony and by planting a tree the girls were not only able to remember Missy in a special way, but they were able to share it with people at the veterinary office who had become part of Missy's (and therefore their) extended family. Through the process of grieving, the girls, and indeed the veterinary staff in this instance, have experienced a degree of personal growth. The resolution is symbolized by the channeling of emotional energy into a new relationship with Archie. Missy is not forgotten!

Recommended Reading

Beadle M: The Cat: History, Biology, and Behavior. New York, Simon and Schuster, 1977.

Beaver BV: Feline Behavior: A Guide for Veterinarians. Philadelphia, WB Saunders Co., 1992.

Bowen M: Family psychotherapy with a schizophrenic in the hospital and in private practice. *In* Borzormenyi-Nagy I and Framo JL (editors): Intensive Family Therapy. New York, Harper and Row, 1965.

Bowlby J: Attachment and Loss. 2nd ed. London, Hogarth Press, 1982.

Brackenridge SS and Elkins AD: Euthanasia and patient death: Stressors in veterinary practice. Vet Pract Staff 4:1, 8–10, 1992.

Cain AO: A study of pets in the family system. *In* Katcher AH and Beck AM (editors): New Perspectives on Our Lives with Companion Animals. Philadelphia, University of Pennsylvania Press, 1983.

Cohen SP and Fudin CE (editors): Animal Illness and Human Emotions. Prob Vet Med 3(1):1–121, 1991.

Cusack O: Pets and Mental Health. New York, Haworth Press, 1988.

Dershimer RA: Counseling the Bereaved. New York, Pergamon Press, 1990.

Fogle B and Abrahamson D: Pet loss: A survey of the attitudes and feelings of practicing veterinarians. Anthrozoos 3:143–150, 1990.

Frey WH: Crying: The Mystery of Tears. Minneapolis, Winston Press, Inc., 1985.

Haig RA: The Anatomy of Grief: Biopsychosocial and Therapeutic Perspectives. Springfield, IL, Charles C Thomas, 1990.

Harris JM: Nonconventional human/companion animal bonds. *In* Kay WJ, Nieburg HA Kukscher AH (editors): Pet Loss and Human Bereavement. Ames, IA, Iowa State University Press, 1984, pp 31–36.

Katcher A: Interactions between people and their pets: form and function. *In* Fogle B (editor): Interrelations Between People and Pets. Chicago, IL, Charles C Thomas, 1981.

Kübler-Ross E: On Death and Dying. New York, Macmillan Publishing Co., 1969.

Lagoni L and Hetts S: Bereavement. *In* McCurnin DM (editor): Clinical Textbook for Veterinary Technicians. 2nd ed. Philadelphia, WB Saunders Co., 1990.

Messent PR: Social facilitation of contact with other people by pet dogs. *In* Katcher AH and Beck AM (editors): New Perspectives on Our Lives with Companion Animals. Philadelphia, University of Pennsylvania Press, 1983.

Rosenberg MA: Clinical aspects of grief associated with loss of a pet: A veterinarian's view. *In* Kay WJ, Neiburg HA, Kukscher AH (editors): Pet Loss and Human Bereavement. Ames, IA, Iowa State University Press, 1984, pp 119–125.

Salmon PW and Salmon IM: Who owns who? Psychological research into the human-pet bond in Australia. *In* Katcher AH and Beck AM (editors): New Perspectives on Our Lives with Companion Animals. Philadelphia, University of Pennsylvania Press, 1983.

Smith SL: Interactions between pet dog and family members: An ethological study. *In* Katcher AH and Beck AM (editors): New Perspectives on Our Lives with Companion Animals Philadelphia, University of Pennsylvania Press, 1983.

Veevers JE: The social meanings of pets: Alternative roles for companion animals. *In* Sussman MB (editor): Pets and the family. Marriage and Family Review 8(3/4):11–30, 1985.

Voith VL: Attachment of people to companion animals. Vet Clin North Am Small Anim Pract 15:289–296, 1985.

Walshaw SO: Role of the animal health technician in consoling bereaved clients. *In* Kay WJ, Nieburg HA, Kukscher AH (editors): Pet Loss and Human Bereavement. Ames, IA, Iowa State University Press, 1984, pp 126–134.

Wilbur RH: Pets, pet ownership, and animal control: Social and psychological attitudes. Proceedings of the National Conference on Dog and Cat Control. Chicago, American Veterinary Medicine Association, 1976.

Worden JW: Bereavement. Semin Oncol 12(4):472–475, 1985.

Worden JW: Grief Counseling and Grief Therapy: A Handbook for the Mental Health Practitioner. 2nd ed. New York, Springer Publishing Company, 1991.

26

Animal Behavior

SUZANNE HETTS

"My cat has started urinating outside her litterbox! How can I make her stop?"

"My dog is tearing things up and going to the bathroom in the house when I'm at work. Do you have any advice?"

Technicians and veterinarians are asked questions like these almost every day in clinical practice. Often, the answers to these questions are based on personal experience, or on information provided from others. Technicians may not have had the opportunity to obtain scientific and practical information about animal behavior that is based on learning and behavior theories. The goal of this chapter is to introduce the field of animal behavior, provide basic principles that can be applied to animal behavior problems, and help to provide guidance for more informed referrals to behavior specialists when needed.

HISTORY OF THE DISCIPLINE OF ANIMAL BEHAVIOR

Classical Ethology

Animal behavior is a specialized field of study. A few of the best-known classical animal behaviorists are Charles Darwin, Niko Tinbergen and Konrad Lorenz. Classical animal behaviorists, or ethologists, observed and described behavior with four important questions in mind: (1) *causation*—what is the immediate (short-term) reason or cause for the behavior, (2)

ontogeny—how does a particular behavior develop or change throughout the life span of the animal, (3) *evolution*—how does behavior change as species evolve and are subjected to natural (or artificial) selection and (4) *function*—what role does the behavior play in the adaptation of the animal to its environment? *Classical ethology* focused on describing behavior in an animal's natural habitat, comparing similar behaviors in closely related species, and did not look favorably on the sole study of domestic animals.

Animal Psychology

Classical animal psychologists studied animal learning and attempted to elucidate general laws of behavior by studying laboratory species (such as rats and pigeons) under controlled experimental conditions. Important early animal psychologists include E.L. Thorndike, B.F. Skinner and Ivan Pavlov.

Contemporary Animal Behavior

The *contemporary* science and study of animal behavior reflects the input from many different disciplines and a blurring of the distinctions between classical ethologists and animal psychologists. Ethologists have moved away from strictly descriptive studies and have become more sophisticated in their use of the experimental method, statistical analyses, experimental controls and theoretical models. Animal psychologists have become more aware of the narrow focus and possible distortions resulting from studying only the behavior of laboratory species solely in the laboratory. The field of contemporary animal behavior has benefited from the contributions of many disciplines, including zoology, entomology, physical anthropology, behavioral ecology, physiology, social psychology, comparative psychology, ethology, wildlife biology, animal science and veterinary medicine.

APPLIED ANIMAL BEHAVIOR

Applied animal behavior is the application of the body of knowledge about behavior to practical problems and situations. Animal behavior has applications for wildlife management, management of zoo animals, food animal production and management, and issues related to the welfare of laboratory animals. The resolution of behavior problems in companion animals, often called animal behavior counseling, is the type of applied animal behavior that is the focus of this chapter.

Animal Behavior Counseling

Animal behavior therapy or counseling can be defined as the process of working with the owner to assist the owner in modifying those behaviors displayed by an animal that present a problem for the owner. First of all, it is important to note that it is the owner who becomes the agent of change for the animal's behavior. Second, it is the owner who defines the problem. A dog who jumps on people may be a problem for one owner but not for another. The majority of behavior problems in companion animals represent *normal* behavior for the animal but *unacceptable* behavior for the owner. Owners usually judge behaviors to be unacceptable if they occur in excess or in inappropriate contexts or locations. For example, it is normal for both cats and dogs to establish surface and location preferences for elimination. This normal behavior becomes a problem if the preferences include the Persian rug in the dining room.

Animal behavior counseling involves determining the cause of the behavior problem, recommending techniques for resolving the problem and follow-up of the progress toward resolution. Analyzing the cause of the problem is accomplished with a detailed behavioral history and, ideally, observations of the animal and its environment. A sample of a possible format for obtaining a behavioral history is shown in Table 26–1. Techniques for resolving the problem are clearly explained to the owner. A written summary of the recommendations is provided, and if necessary, techniques are demonstrated by working directly with the animal.

A behavior counseling session may last 30 minutes to 2 hours or more, depending on the nature of the problem. The counseling session can take place in the client's home, in the veterinary clinic or, in some cases, by telephone. Advantages and disadvantages associated with each alternative are summarized in Table 26–2.

Follow-up visits or telephone calls are done at intervals appropriate to the problem and may range from 1 day to several

Table 26–1
FORMAT FOR A BEHAVIORAL HISTORY

(1) Signalment
Species, breed, age, gender, spayed, neutered, or intact
(2) Early History
When, where, why obtained
Behavior of sire/dam (if known)
Behavior in the litter
House-training procedures
Socialization experiences
(3) Current Environment
Time—inside/outside
Feeding—schedules/routines
Other animals/family structure
Description of "typical day"
(4) Training
Methods
Who trained
Commands to which animal responds
Methods used for punishment/discipline
(5) Presenting Problem
Owner's description
When, how it began
When, where it occurs
Developmental course
Eliciting, inhibiting stimuli
Frequency of occurrence
Owner's reaction, attempts at resolution
(6) Additional Information
Other problem behaviors
Pertinent medical history

weeks. Animal behavior counseling requires time, energy, commitment and effort from both the behaviorist and the owner. Behavior problems cannot be solved in "25 words or less," and animal behavior counselors provide a *professional* service for which a fee is charged; they do not give "tips" or "advice."

Qualifications of Applied Animal Behaviorists

The field of animal behavior counseling has grown significantly in the past 10 years. Some aspects of this growth have been notably positive, resulting in increases in the number of applied animal behaviorists, an increase in the amount of research being conducted and an increase in public awareness of the field. Unfortunately, there has also been an increase in the number of people (primarily dog trainers) calling themselves "animal behaviorists" who have no training in animal behavior. Professional ethics should dictate against this practice. This has unfortunately led to confusion for pet owners when they seek assistance for behavior problems. Animal trainers and animal behaviorists often approach behavior problem resolution differently. Most pet owners do not have sufficient knowledge to be able to determine which approach is best. Thus, it is important that the veterinary technician know what an animal behaviorist is, how a behaviorist is trained, how to evaluate behaviorists closest to the practice location and how to refer a client to a behaviorist.

In February 1991, professional certification for animal be-

product and service. Therefore, look for longevity and number of installations.

A vital element to look for is support for both hardware and software. This is a feature that is not given enough attention but is of extreme importance. Most companies concern themselves primarily with software and provide the hardware as a service to the customer. What kind of software support do they provide and during what hours of the day do they provide support? The vendor should know its program inside and out; there are often features or shortcuts that are not documented in the instructions. Even those of us who think we know what we are doing with computers have to rely heavily on software support because the systems are proprietary. Without easily reached, competent support, the system will *never* survive. A monthly support fee will usually provide telephone support and upgrades when new programs are developed. The number of upgrades and the regularity with which upgrades are issued is another indicator of the stability of the program and the company. A progressive company will consistently be improving its product.

Probably the last feature to evaluate is hardware. There is an idiom in the computer world that states that one should always select the software first; there will always be a computer to make it run. Networking and multi-user, multitasking computers have changed greatly since the early 1970s. Computer hardware has become so inexpensive and powerful that it is much less a concern than before. The prices of powerful computers have come down drastically in the last few years and there are wide selections of computers and operating systems that actually work!

Most vendors offer a package system of software and hardware, and in general, it is worth buying the package. Most practice personnel do not have enough knowledge or time to buy and install their own computers and networks. Prices at the local computer store may look slightly better than those of the software vendor, but the local person is probably not knowledgeable about the particular practice management software package to be of real support. The software vendor has tried and developed the software on a particular type of computer on which he or she knows it will work. The vendor probably will not provide hardware support, and possibly not even software support, if you do not comply with their hardware specifications.

The larger software companies usually provide an on-site demonstration by a trained representative; this is highly desirable. This is the time to get a good overview of the software. It also is the time to ask questions. "Can the computer do . . . ?" "How does the computer do . . . ?" It is a good time to let the staff use the system and see how easily it will do the everyday functions. Smaller companies may not have the resources to send a representative but will allow on-site evaluation of the system for some period of time. Evaluation of systems at meetings is an alternative, but usually things are too hectic to be able to really sit down and do a good evaluation.

It is during the demonstration or the evaluation period that a decision should be made regarding what portions of the program are needed. Most programs are built in modules that can be added to the basic system. A small-animal boarding and grooming package would be of no use to an equine practice. An equine trainer list would be of no use to a small-animal practice. This is a good way to hold down prices by buying just what the practice can use.

The Decision to Buy—What Happens Next?

After the decision to buy is made, what happens next? Depending on the agreement with the vendor, your delivered computer system will be set up either by you or by the vendor. If a single-user computer system has been purchased and the software is already loaded into the computer, setup will be minimal. It is usually worth the extra expense to have the vendor set up a networked system. Network operating systems are complex and require trained personnel for installation and management. Extensive network maintenance is far beyond the capabilities of most practices.

After installation is complete, the next step is training on the actual system. Most of the large vendors provide on-site training for some period of time, usually 2 to 5 days. During the training period, a reduced appointment schedule is recommended as it becomes too hectic to handle a normal business load and learn the computer system. This is the time when all staff members need to be deeply involved in the new system.

No matter how easy the program is to use and no matter how intelligent the staff, the initial stages of computerization are traumatic. It is amazing, though, how soon things return to "normal." Most programs are well organized and intuitive so that everyday functions become second nature in a matter of days.

A major area of trauma will be working with two systems for a period of time, using both the computer system and the old paper record system. If the practice is new and client records are not extensive, it is better to completely switch to the new computer system and not to use the old paper system. Transferring data from the old paper system to the computer system is extremely time-consuming and labor-intensive.

Recommended Reading

Acerson KL: PC Magazine Guide to WordPerfect for Windows. Emeryville, CA, Ziff-Davis Press, 1992.

Baer J et al.: Windows 3.1 Complete, Abacus, Grand Rapids, MI, 1992.

Danuloff C and McClelland D: Encyclopedia Macintosh. San Francisco, Cybex, 1990.

Laurisch D: Novell NetWare Lite—Step by Step. Grand Rapids, MI, Abacus, 1992.

Trends, American Animal Hospital Association, June/July 1991, pp 15–17, 26–39.

Venit S: Using PageMaker 4.0 for Windows. Carmel, IN, Que Corp., 1991.

Veterinary Forum. St. Simons Island, GA, Forum Publications, Inc., September, 1992, pp 78–103.

Rosen KH, Rosinski RR and Farber JM: UNIX—System V Release 4, An Introduction. Berkeley, CA, Osborne McGraw-Hill, 1990.

Glossary

ASCII—American Standard Code for Information Interchange. A standard format for representing characters. This format is used in text files and is useful when files are shared between programs.

AUTOEXEC.BAT file—A file containing DOS commands written in ASCII text form which is automatically executed when the computer is turned on or booted.

Batch file—An executable file with DOS commands written in ASCII text, which is used for automating frequently used commands.

BIOS—Basic Input/Output System. This is part of the read only memory (ROM) of the central processing unit (CPU), which is installed in the form of a chip and which controls how the CPU interacts with the screen, keyboard, printer and other peripheral devices.

Bit—Unit of data in binary form; the smallest storage unit for data in a computer.

Byte—A fixed number of bits that represents a character. The most common byte size is eight bits.

CPU—Central Processing Unit. That part of a computer or computer system responsible for the actual computations.

CRT—Cathode Ray Tube. This is the electronic tube making up the visual display of the terminal or the computer.

Database—A collection of interrelated data stored together with a minimum of redundancy to serve multiple applications.

DOS—Disk Operating System. This is software that controls movement of information in a computer and allows the central processing unit to use peripheral devices, such as printers, diskette drives and fixed disk drives.

Driver—A set of commands that are used to run a peripheral device, such as a printer.

EGA—Enhanced Graphics Adapter. This acronym refers to the ability of a computer to display graphic images in color.

E Mail—Electronic Mail. An electronic method of communication between network users.

Extended memory—The random access memory (RAM) of a computer in excess of 1 megabyte.

Expanded memory—The random access memory (RAM) of a computer in excess of 640 kilobytes and less than 1 megabyte.

Facsimile—A device for transmission of graphic files from one location to another. The graphic image is converted to digital signals by the sending device, and the receiving device converts the digital signals to a graphic image. Facsimile machines act as remote copying machines.

File—A collection of one or more records.

Fixed disk—A high-volume magnetic storage device that is usually built into the computer.

Floppy disk—Small, portable, magnetic storage devices for storage of computer programs and data.

Font—A specific typeface, including its point size and weight.

Graphics display—A cathode ray tube or monitor that is capable of displaying graphical images.

Hardware—A digital or analog device that is capable of detecting, transmitting or processing electronic signals.

LAN—Local Area Network. An electronic network permitting communication between the central processing units (CPU) and/or CPU's and peripheral devices, such as terminals, printers and plotters.

Language—A computer language is a particular format in which programs are written, e.g., BASIC, Fortran, Cobol and MUMPS.

MB—Megabyte. One million bytes; refers to amount of memory available or used. To be more specific, it is 1024 kilobytes or 1,048,576 bytes.

Modem—A device that accepts a digital signal and converts it into an analog signal and accepts an analog signal and converts it to a digital signal.

Operating system—Software that enables the computer to run the application software programs.

Optical scanner—A device that converts printed text and/or graphic images to digital files.

Printer, daisywheel—An impact printer that functions by a device striking a wheel containing the alphabet and the numbers 1 to 10.

Printer, dot matrix—An impact printer that functions by pins striking the inked ribbon to form the letters, numbers and graphical forms. Dot matrix printers have from 9 to 32 pins. The more pins in the print head, the better the quality of print.

Printer, ink jet—A relatively inexpensive, letter-quality printer which operates by fluid ink being forced through nozzles and transferred to the paper by resistive heaters.

Printer, laser—A printer that produces high-resolution images utilizing the same process as photocopy machines.

RAM—Random Access Memory. Memory that is used to store application programs and data while the program is in use. All data in RAM will be lost when the computer is turned off.

ROM—Read Only Memory. That part of a computer memory that contains prewritten instructions. These instructions cannot be erased or rewritten by application programs.

Software—Written instructions that enable the computer to conduct desired functions. The software includes the operating system, application programs, utility programs and other types of programs.

Tape drive—A high-speed storage device that reads from and records data on magnetic tape. This type storage device is often used for archiving or "backing up" programs and data.

Terminal—An input/output device with a visual display and keyboard that is utilized to send and receive data from the central processing unit. Terminals are referred to as "dumb" terminals because they are incapable of processing information.

VGA—Video Graphics Adapter. A board installed in a computer which allows one to view graphical images in color.

WAN—Wide Area Network. This is usually a network linking two to several LAN's.

Windows—An operating system with a graphical interface that allows two applications to be active at the same time and the transfer of information between applications.

WYSIWYG—What You See Is What You Get. This acronym refers to programs that print exactly what is seen on the display screen.

thermoregulation, viral infections, parasitism, and developmental and heritable defects of the immune system.

Blood stream invasion is usually by the more common bacteria such as *Staphylococcus, Escherichia, Klebsiella, Enterobacter, Streptococcus, Enterococcus, Pseudomonas, Clostridium, Bacteroides, Fusobacterium,* and *Salmonella* spp., and of these, gram-negative bacilli most often occur. Sources from which gram-negative bacilli enter the blood stream include gastrointestinal tract and peritoneal infection, respiratory tract infection, skin and wound infection, and urinary tract infection.

Signs of Neonatal Illness

The clinical manifestations of neonatal illness do not always allow specific identification of the causative condition. Furthermore, many puppies and kittens have unusual or a wide variety of clinical presentations, which may not be immediately recognized as being associated with a specific illness. Death can occur so suddenly that noticeable signs are virtually absent. More typically, however, puppies and kittens will cry a lot, show signs of restlessness, weakness, hypothermia, diarrhea, altered respiration, hematuria, failure to thrive, and cyanosis, and in advanced stages may slough parts of their extremities.

The diagnosis of a neonatal illness is usually based on the case history and physical findings. Ideally, a complete blood count, plasma chemistry profile, urinalysis, urine and/or blood culture, and culture of suspected sources of infection are obtained. When dealing with neonatal sepsis, it is imperative to conduct a thorough search for the primary source of infection and collect appropriate bacterial culture samples before initiating antimicrobial therapy.

The hemograms of septicemic puppies and kittens are usually characterized by a normochromic normocytic anemia. Thrombocytopenia and mild to moderate neutrophilia with a left shift may be present. Another laboratory finding that is consistent with, but by no means specific for, neonatal sepsis is hypoglycemia. The remaining laboratory values from the plasma chemistry profile and urinalysis may reflect a specific organ failure.

Management of Neonatal Illness

Early, prompt care for the ill puppy or kitten is required for satisfactory results. Because many neonatal diseases may cause sudden death, puppies and kittens suspected of having a severe illness should be treated immediately. In most instances, rewarming, fluid replacement and antimicrobial therapy are started empirically. Severely ill puppies and kittens may also require glucose therapy if hypoglycemia is present (Table 30–2).

Meaningful advances in treating bacterial infections have been made in recent years, particularly in the development of antimicrobial agents. Many of these antimicrobial agents have either an increased spectrum of activity or a diminished toxicity relative to previously available antimicrobial agents. However, specific pharmacokinetic data for many of the antimicrobial agents have not been obtained in adults or in puppies and kittens, and therefore the veterinary use of these antimicrobial agents remains somewhat empirical.

Unfortunately, clinical information necessary for appropriate dosing of antimicrobial agents in septicemic puppies and kittens is not always available. Drug distribution, especially in puppies and kittens younger than 5 weeks of age, differs from that of adults because of differences in body composition, such as lower total body fat, higher percentage of total body water, lower concentrations of albumin and poorly developed blood-brain barrier. Because of these differences, modifications of

---

Table 30–2
MANAGEMENT OF A SEVERELY ILL PUPPY AND KITTEN

I. External warming procedure
   A. Use circulating hot water blanket and hot water bottle
   B. Take at least 20 to 30 minutes for gradual warming of the patient
   C. Turn the patient every hour
   D. Record rectal temperature every hour
II. Parenteral fluid therapy
   A. Use multiple electrolyte solution supplemented with 5 percent dextrose solution
   B. Supplement the fluids with potassium chloride solution if plasma potassium concentration is less than 2.5 mM/liter
   C. Administer warm fluids slowly by intravenous or intraosseous route
III. Glucose replacement therapy
   A. Administer 5 percent dextrose solution intravenously or intraosseously, to effect
   B. Administer 1 to 2 ml/kg of a 10 to 25 percent dextrose solution to the patient that is profoundly depressed or having seizures
   C. Maintain plasma glucose concentration at 80 to 200 mg/dl for euglycemia
IV. Antimicrobial therapy
   A. Collect bacterial culture samples (whole blood, urine, exudate, feces) before initiation of antimicrobial therapy
      1. For blood culture, collect one ml of whole blood aseptically and inoculate blood directly into enriched tryptic or trypticase soy broth, dilute the whole blood 1:5 to 1:10 in enriched broth, and examine broth for bacterial growth 6 to 18 hours later
      2. For urine culture, collect urine by cystocentesis and culture it by standard methods
      3. For exudate and fecal cultures, collect and culture by standard methods
   B. Empirical treatment with antimicrobial agent(s) begins immediately after collection of appropriate bacterial culture samples
   C. Adjust the dosage and dosing interval of antimicrobial agent(s) selected
   D. Administer the antimicrobial agent by intravenous or intraosseous route
V. Provide oxygen and nutritional therapy
   A. Administer oxygen by mask or intranasal catheter to counteract tissue hypoxemia
   B. Encourage food intake once patient is normothermic and adequately hydrated
VI. Monitor the effectiveness of medical management
   A. Observe for improvement in the patient's general demeanor
   B. Regularly assess the cardiopulmonary status (it is extremely easy to overhydrate the severely ill puppy or kitten, and so attentive monitoring of breathing pattern is helpful for early recognition of overhydration)
   C. Weigh the patient three to four times a day to record weight gain
   D. Observe for moistness of mucous membranes and clearness of urine in assessing for adequate hydration (healthy puppies and kittens have clear, colorless urine when normally hydrated—any color to the urine usually indicates dehydration)

dosing amounts for adults, as much as 30 to 50 percent reduction of the adult dose, or changes in dosing frequency may be necessary when antimicrobial agents are administered to septicemic puppies and kittens.

Furthermore, fluid replacement therapy and antimicrobial agents should be administered intravenously or intraosseously in severely ill puppies and kittens, as systemic absorption following oral, subcutaneous or intramuscular administration may not be reliable. Most drugs ingested by the lactating bitch or queen appear in her milk; the amount generally is 1 to 2 percent of the mother's dose. Therefore, severely ill puppies or kittens should never be treated by only treating the lactating mother. The beta-lactam antimicrobial agents are considered to be the first choice in the treatment of septicemic puppies and kittens. The beta-lactam antimicrobial agents include the penicillins, cephalosporins, and the combination of beta-lactam antimicrobials and beta-lactamase inhibitors.

FOAL

The critically ill foal is perhaps the most intensively managed of all veterinary patients. With the advent of specialized centers for the treatment of foals, great advances have been made in understanding the physiology and disease states of the equine neonate. With these advances, the overall survival rate for foals entering intensive care is improving, and foals of younger gestational age are surviving. The most critical factor influencing a foal's survival is, undoubtedly, diligent nursing care. Successful foal management requires a team approach, and competent veterinary technical support has become the foundation of the team. The skills required of equine neonatal technicians are extensive. This chapter provides only an overview of these skills, and individuals with aspirations in this area should consult other textbooks that focus on equine and human neonatal care. Additional clinical training can be obtained in most university teaching hospitals that have a foal neonatal care unit.

The High-Risk Foal

The term "high-risk foal" refers to the foal that is not necessarily ill but is at high risk of becoming ill. Sick foals generally appear normal for the first 24 hours of life and then quickly decompensate. Because survival depends on early recognition of disease, during the period of vague clinical signs, foals at high risk of becoming ill are assumed to be abnormal and are treated accordingly. During the initial examination, physical, historical and laboratory factors that may classify the foal as high-risk are identified.

Assessment of the foal should attempt to identify factors relative to the dam that increase the foal's risk of being diseased. Foals from mares that have had prior foaling difficulties, including abortion, stillbirth or twinning, are considered to be at high risk. If the mare experienced poor nutrition, vaginal discharge, illness, prolonged transport or abdominal surgery during gestation, the foal is at high risk of being diseased. Retained, inflamed or infected fetal membranes, induced or prolonged labor, and dystocia all increase the risk of disease in the foal. The mare's udder should be inspected for the presence and quality of colostrum. Good colostrum should be

sticky and have a specific gravity of 1.060 on colostrometer reading. A full, tight udder is presumptive evidence that the foal is not nursing adequately and is not normal.

The classic early signs of disease in the foal are lethargy, depressed suck reflex, depressed appetite, increased recumbency and sleeping, and decreased affinity for the mare. Historical factors relative to the foal that increase its chance of being "high-risk" include in utero meconium passage (evidenced by staining of white hair and hooves), the presence of twins, abnormal birth behavior (see physical examination), abnormal physical findings, failure of passive transfer, and prolonged or shortened gestational length.

The equine gestation length may range from 315 to 365 days, the average being 341 days. Prematurity refers to foals that are born prior to 320 days of gestational age. Physical signs of prematurity include low birth weight, weakness, delayed standing post partum, soft pliant lips and ears, flexor tendon laxity, prominent forehead, soft silky haircoat and incomplete ossification of the carpal and tarsal bones. Any of these physical abnormalities will categorize the foal as high-risk. The terms prematurity, dysmaturity and immaturity are often used incorrectly. Dysmature foals are of a gestational age greater than 320 days with physical signs of prematurity. Immaturity is a blanket term encompassing all foals with physical signs of prematurity regardless of gestational age. Because the foal's haircoat matures from the head to the rump, the hindquarters should be closely examined for the presence of silky hair. It is noteworthy that miniature horse foals normally have a prominent forehead. Technicians working with foals should remember that external signs of immaturity correlate with immaturity of other body systems and greater susceptibility to disease and injury. For example, foals with soft silky haircoat are likely to have incomplete skeletal ossification, which can result in crushing injury to the carpal and tarsal bones by simple weight bearing. Individuals involved with foal care should be aware of the fragile nature of the equine neonate and take appropriate precautions.

Physical Examination

Recognizing high-risk foals requires familiarity with normal peripartum history and behavior. After birth, the normal equine neonate will exhibit a suck reflex in 20 minutes, stand within 1 to 2 hours and nurse within 2 to 3 hours. Foals should urinate within 10 hours of birth and pass meconium, the dark first feces, by 24 hours of age. The mare should pass her placenta within 4 to 6 hours of delivering the foal.

The physical examination of the foal begins at a distance. The awake foal should be alert and easily aroused by stimuli in its environment. The respiratory rate is 20 to 40 at birth, increasing to 60 to 80 within 1 hour. The respiratory rhythm is regular in the awake state but may be irregular while the foal is sleeping. The degree of inspiratory and expiratory effort should be noted. Foals should develop a strong bond with their mare by 1.5 hours of age. Foals generally sleep by 3 hours after birth and after each feeding. Foals nurse an average of 7 times per day. Head bobbing while searching for the udder is normal. Within 24 hours of birth the normal foal should be strong, alert and capable of running.

As the examination continues, the foal's body systems should be thoroughly evaluated. Because the foal has its own list of

Table 30-3 DISEASES OF FOALS	
Infectious:	Septicemia/bacteremia, pneumonia, meningitis, omphalophlebitis, nephritis, septic arthritis, osteomyelitis, septic peritonitis
Gastrointestinal:	Meconium impaction, gastric and duodenal ulceration, enteritis, peritonitis, intussusception, intraluminal obstruction, volvulus, cleft palate, prognathism, brachygnathism, atresia coli, atresia recti, atresia ani
Respiratory:	Respiratory distress complex, pneumonia, meconium aspiration, persistent pulmonary hypertension
Cardiovascular:	Ventricular septal defect
Musculoskeletal:	Flexural deformities, angular limb deformities, incomplete skeletal ossification, osteochondrosis, physitis, rib fracture
Urogenital:	Patent urachus, rupture of the ureter, bladder, urethra or urachus, umbilical hernia, scrotal hernia
Immunologic:	Failure of passive transfer, combined immunodeficiency
Hematologic:	Neonatal isoerythrolysis, anemia
Neurologic:	Neonatal maladjustment syndrome, brain and spinal hemorrhage, epilepsy
Ocular:	Corneal ulcer, entropion, ectropion
Miscellaneous:	Hypoxemia, hypoglycemia, hypothermia

common diseases (Table 30-3), special attention should be directed toward their early identification. The heart rate is 40 to 80 bpm within five minutes after birth, increasing to 130 bpm from 6 to 60 minutes, and stabilizing at 90 to 100. The heart rate will increase to 130 or higher upon exertion (as when standing). Normal rectal temperature ranges from 37.2 to 38.9°C (99 to 102°F). The integument should be inspected for decubital ulcers, urine and fecal scalding.

Evaluating cardiovascular stability begins by palpating the extremity for temperature and for the quality, regularity and rate of the arterial pulses. The arterial pulse is easily identified at the facial artery, which courses beneath the ramus of the mandible; the brachial artery, located at the medial aspect of the elbow; and the great metatarsal artery, which is palpable on the lateral aspect of the third metatarsal bone (Fig. 30-1). This latter vessel is ideal for the collection of arterial samples for blood gas analysis. The foal should not have pulse deficits, jugular distention or a jugular pulse. Cardiac auscultation generally reveals a grade II to grade VI machinery or holosystolic murmur at the left heart base, which abates by 72 hours post partum. Rarely, the murmur may continue for 30 to 60 days. This murmur is suspected to be associated with closing of the ductus arteriosus. Rate and rhythm of the heart should also be assessed. The capillary refill time should be less than 2 seconds. Mucous membranes of the mouth, eyes, nares, vulva and urethra should be pink and moist. Cyanotic, jaundiced or injected membranes are abnormal. All membranes should be closely inspected for ulceration or petechiae. It should be noted that membrane color is not an adequate assessment of oxygenation in the foal. Adequate oxygenation can only be assessed by means of arterial blood gas analysis.

A complete auscultation of the lung fields should be per-

formed. The respiratory tract is a major route for exposure to organisms causing septicemia. The boundaries of the equine lung begin at the seventeenth intercostal space at the level of the tuber coxae and slope in an arc to an area just above the olecranon. Careful auscultation of these areas and the trachea should be performed in a quiet room. As allowed by the foal's temperament and status, a rebreathing bag may help to identify abnormal areas. The benefits of this procedure should be carefully weighed against the potential stress on the foal.

A foal's lung sounds are normally harsh, making evaluation subjective. An elevated respiratory rate, which exacerbates harsh lung sounds, can occur with many systemic diseases in the absence of lung disease. The slightest wheeze or crackle should be taken seriously. Note that auscultation is extremely insensitive for the detection of lung disease in the foal. The chest should be carefully examined for possible rib fractures. Because pneumonia and other lung diseases can be ruled out only by radiographic examination of the thorax, all high-risk foals should have thoracic radiographs performed on admission.

In examining the gastrointestinal system, the passage of meconium should be assured, as meconium impaction is the primary cause of neonatal colic. Foals should have fecal matter on the thermometer. If none is present, the possibility of a nonpatent gastrointestinal system (atresia ani, atresia coli) in a foal that exhibits abdominal pain or straining to defecate should be considered. Diarrhea is a significant finding because the gastrointestinal system is a second major route for exposure to bacterial organisms causing septicemia. Borborygmi should be detectable by auscultation. Abdominal distention or "pings" noted on auscultation are abnormal findings. The mouth is examined for cleft palate and abnormal dentition. Foals with clefts in the soft palate often require endoscopic examination to identify the abnormality.

The musculoskeletal evaluation focuses predominantly on the joints and growth plates. All joints are placed through their full range of motion in order to identify contracted tendons. The foal is encouraged to stand and move to identify flexor tendon laxity (walking on heels or fetlocks), lameness and angular limb deformities. Each joint and physis must be carefully palpated to detect swelling, heat or pain. Careful palpation of these areas can detect infection prior to the onset of lameness, improving response to treatment. Any lameness in the foal should be assumed to be infectious until proved oth-

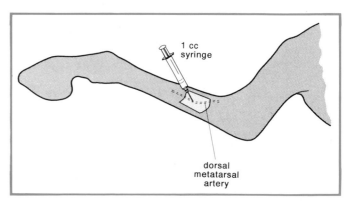

FIGURE 30-1. Location of dorsal metatarsal artery for collection of arterial blood samples in the foal.

erwise and is an emergency situation. It is a misconception that mares step on their foals.

The urogenital system is another area for intense examination. For many years the significance of the umbilicus as a major route of infection has been recognized. The umbilical stump, palpable outside the abdomen, consists of remnants of the urachus (which connected to the bladder in utero), one umbilical vein and two umbilical arteries. Within the abdomen the umbilical vein courses forward to the liver, and the umbilical arteries travel caudally entering the wall of the bladder. The umbilicus is closely inspected for infection, increased size and moistness, which suggests patency. Because the predominance of the umbilical structures are within the abdomen, thorough examination requires ultrasonic imaging. The umbilical, inguinal and scrotal areas are palpated for hernias and distention. Abdominal distention or pitting edema of the perineal or inguinal areas may indicate impatency of the urinary tract. Because of its liquid diet, the normal foal passes dilute urine frequently.

The neurological system of the foal is relatively unique compared to that of the adult horse. When the foal stands for the first time, it assumes a base-wide stance and, as it tries to ambulate, takes exaggerated steps. Exaggerated response to visual, auditory and tactile stimuli and exaggerated jerky movements are normal. The recumbent foal will normally have hyperreflexive spinal reflexes even as severe as myoclonus (rhythmic muscle contraction) when one is eliciting the patellar reflex. The normal foal also exhibits a crossed extensor reflex (extension of a limb in response to squeezing the opposite limb) for as long as 4 weeks. When restrained, the standing foal initially struggles, then falls limp into the arms of the person restraining it, as if sleeping. Loosening the restraint causes the foal to support its weight once again.

During the neurological examination, the eyes must not be neglected. Foals do not have a menace reflex for 2 weeks after birth. When excited, the pupillary light reflex of the foal may be slow. The presence of entropion or ectropion should be noted as such conditions and associated corneal ulceration are common. The eyes are carefully examined for corneal abrasion and ulcers, uveitis, hyphema (blood in the anterior chamber), hypopyon (purulent exudate in the anterior chamber) and congenital cataracts. Detection of hyphema and hypopyon requires diligent examination of the dependent portion of the anterior chamber. The sclera should be checked for hemorrhage and injected blood vessels, which can be the result of trauma during birth or sepsis.

Laboratory Examination

The hematological values and serum chemistry values of the foal differ somewhat from those of the adult horse (Table 30–4). The ranges provided are from the laboratory of the University of Florida College of Veterinary Medicine. Because of interlaboratory variations in technique and equipment, reference ranges should be established at each laboratory. The packed cell volume (PCV) of the normal foal is greater than that of the adult during the first 24 hours of life and falls into the low normal range of the adult from two weeks to one year of age. Total red blood cell count (RBC) for the foal remains above that of the adult from birth through 1 year of age. Band neutrophils are uncommon in the normal foal and greater than 100 to 150 cells/μl should be considered abnormal. Plasma protein concentrations of the foal are expected to be much lower than those of the adult prior to absorption of colostral immunoglobulins, but as noted, the normal range of

Table 30–4
SELECTED LABORATORY VALUES OF THE EQUINE NEONATE

Age	PCV (%)	RBC ($\times 10^6/\mu$l)	Plasma Protein (g/dl)
Pre-suckle	40–52	9.3–12.9	4.5–5.9
≤12 hours	37–49	9.0–12.0	5.1–7.6
1 day	32–46	8.2–11.0	5.2–8.0
1 day – 1 month	28–46	7.2–11.6	5.1–7.9
Adult	31–47	5.9–9.9	6.2–8.0

	Serum Protein (g/dl)	ALP (IU/liter)	GGT (IU/liter)	SDH (IU/liter)
Pre-suckle				
<12 hours	4.0–7.9	152–2835	13–39	0.2–4.8
1 day	4.3–8.1	861–2671	18–43	0.6–4.6
1 day – 1 month	4.4–7.76	137–1462	8–169	0.6–8.4
Adult	5.5–7.9	64–214	5–28	0.5–3.0

	Glucose (mg/dl)	Creatinine (mg/dl)	BUN (mg/dl)
Pre-suckle			
<12 hours	108–190	1.7–4.2	12–27
1 day	121–233	0.4–4.3	9–40
1 day – 1 month	101–221	0.4–2.1	2–29
Adult	57–96	0.9–2.0	12–24

Data from Koterba AM, Drummond WH and Kosch PC: Equine Clinical Neonatology. Philadelphia, Lea & Febiger, 1990; and University of Florida, College of Veterinary Medicine.

Table 31–2
CANINE VACCINES*

Vaccine	Manufacturer	Type‡	CDV	CAV	CPI	PV	LEP	BR	RB	CV	MV	BO
Adenomune-7	Fermenta Animal Health	A/I	X	X	X	X	X					
Adenomune-5-L	Fermenta Animal Health	A/I	X	X	X	X						
Adenomune-7-L	Fermenta Animal Health	A/I	X	X	X	X	X					
Annumune	Fort Dodge Laboratories	I								X		
Bronchicine	Fermenta Animal Health	I						X				
Companion	Haver/Diamond Scientific	I	X	X	X	X	X					
CoughGuard-B	SmithKline Beecham Animal Health	I						X				
CoughGuard-BP	SmithKline Beecham Animal Health	A/I			X			X				
CPV/LP	A.M. BioTechniques	A				X						
Cytorab	Coopers Animal Health	I								X		
DuaMax	A.M. BioTechniques	A/I				X				X		
Duramune Cv-K	Fort Dodge Laboratories	I								X		
Duramune DA$_2$P + Pv	Fort Dodge Laboratories	A/I	X	X	X	X						
Duramune DA$_2$LP + Pv	Fort Dodge Laboratories	A/I	X	X	X	X	X					
Duramune DA$_2$PP + CvK	Fort Dodge Laboratories	A/I	X	X	X	X				X		
Duramune DA$_2$PP + CvK/LCI	Fort Dodge Laboratories	A/I	X	X	X	X	X			X		
Duramune KF-11	Fort Dodge Laboratories	A				X						
Duramune-Pv	Fort Dodge Laboratories	A				X						
Duramune PC	Fort Dodge Laboratories	A/I				X				X		
Dura-Rab 1	Fermenta Animal Health, ImmunoVet, Vedco	I							X			
Dura-Rab 3	Fermenta Animal Health, ImmunoVet, Vedco	I							X			
D-Vac-7	Bio-Centic Laboratories	A/I	X	X	X	X	X					
Endurall-K	SmithKline Beecham Animal Health	I								X		
Endurall-P	SmithKline Beecham Animal Health	I								X		
Epirab	Coopers Animal Health	I								X		
Firstdose CPV	SmithKline Beecham Animal Health	A				X						
Firstdose CV	SmithKline Beecham Animal Health	I								X		
Firstdose CPV/CV	SmithKline Beecham Animal Health	A/I				X				X		
Fromm D	Solvay Animal Health	A	X									
Galaxy DA$_2$L	Solvay Animal Health	A/I	X	X			X					
Galaxy DA$_2$PL	Solvay Animal Health	A/I	X	X	X		X					
Galaxy 6 MHP	Solvay Animal Health	A	X	X	X	X						
Galaxy 6 MHP-L	Solvay Animal Health	A/I	X	X	X	X	X					
Galaxy 6 MP-L	Solvay Animal Health	A/I	X	X	X	X	X					
Imrab	Rhone Merieux	I							X			
Imrab-I	Rhone Merieux	I							X			
Intra-Trac-II	Schering-Plough Animal Health	A			X			X				
LymeVax	Fort Dodge Laboratories	I										X
Naramune-2	Bio-Ceutic Laboratories	A			X			X				
Parvocine	Fermenta Animal Health	I				X						
Parvocine-MLV	Fermenta Animal Health	A				X						
Parvoid 2	Solvay Animal Health	A				X						
Performer-One	Agri Laboratories	I				X						
Performer-Seven-K	Agri Laboratories	A/I	X	X	X	X	X					
Performer-Seven-L	Agri Laboratories	A/I	X	X	X	X	X					
Quantum	Rhone Merieux	A				X						
Quantum 4	Rhone Merieux	A	X	X	X	X						
Quantum 6	Rhone Merieux	A/I	X	X	X	X	X					
Quantum Parvovirus	Rhone Merieux	A				X						
Rabcine-3	SmithKline Beecham Animal Health	I							X			
Rabguard-TC	SmithKline Beecham Animal Health	I							X			
Rabvac 1	Solvay Animal Health	I							X			
Rabvac 3	Solvay Animal Health	I							X			
Sentrypar	SmithKline Beecham Animal Health	A				X						
Sentrypar DHP	SmithKline Beecham Animal Health	A	X	X	X	X						
Sentrypar DHP/L	SmithKline Beecham Animal Health	A/I	X	X	X	X	X					
Sentryvac DHP	SmithKline Beecham Animal Health	A	X	X	X							
Sentryvac DHP/L	SmithKline Beecham Animal Health	A/I	X	X	X		X					
Solo-Jec-7	Anchor	A/I	X	X	X	X	X					
Tissuvax 5	Rhone Merieux	A/I	X	X	X		X					
Tissuvax 6	Rhone Merieux	A/I	X	X	X		X					
Trimune	Fort Dodge Laboratories	I							X			
Trirab	Coopers Animal Health	I							X			
UnaMax	A.M. BioTechniques	I								X		

Table 31–2
CANINE VACCINES* *Continued*

Vaccine	Manufacturer	Type‡	Vaccine Components†									
			CDV	CAV	CPI	PV	Lep	Br	Rb	CV	MV	Bo
Vanguard 5	SmithKline Beecham Animal Health	A	X	X	X	X						
Vanguard 5/CV	SmithKline Beecham Animal Health	A/I	X	X	X	X				X		
Vanguard 5/CV-L	SmithKline Beecham Animal Health	A/I	X	X	X	X	X			X		
Vanguard 5/L	SmithKline Beecham Animal Health	A/I	X	X	X	X	X					
Vanguard CPV	SmithKline Beecham Animal Health	I				X						
Vanguard DA₂MP	SmithKline Beecham Animal Health	A	X	X	X						X	
Vanguard DA₂P	SmithKline Beecham Animal Health	A	X	X	X							
Vanguard DA₂PL	SmithKline Beecham Animal Health	A/I	X	X	X		X					
Vanguard 5/B	SmithKline Beecham Animal Health	A/I	X	X	X	X		X				
Vanguard D-M	SmithKline Beecham Animal Health	A	X								X	
Vanguard DMP	SmithKline Beecham Animal Health	A	X		X						X	
Votar	Coopers Animal Health	I					X					

*Compiled with the assistance of Compendium of Veterinary Products. 1st ed. Port Huron, MI, North American Compendiums Inc., 1991, and Compendium of Animal Rabies Control, 1992. J Am Vet Med Assoc 200(2):145, 1992.
†CDV = canine distemper virus; CAV = canine adenovirus (infectious canine hepatitis); CPI = canine parainfluenza virus; CPV = canine parvovirus-2; Lep = leptospirosis (usually *L. canicola* and *L. icterohaemorrhagiae*); Br = *Bordetella bronchiseptica* (kennel cough); Rb = rabies; CV = canine coronavirus; MV = measles virus; Bo = *Borrelia burgdorferi* (Lyme disease).
‡A = attenuated (modified live virus or MLV); I = inactivated (killed); A/I = combinations of attenuated and inactivated.

that the puppy is receiving adequate nutrition (nutritional information is found in Chapter 21).

Physical inspection begins by checking the head and oral cavity for evidence of malformation of the skull, cleft lip, stenotic nares or cleft palate. The mucous membranes should be light pink and moist. The teeth, if present, should be examined for periodontal disease and occlusion problems. Periodontal disease generally begins in dogs when the first teeth appear in the mouth and continues in variable degrees throughout the animal's life. Frequent dental examinations as part of the preventive health program convey to the owner the need for regularly performed prophylactic dentistry, the importance of providing the right type of food for the control of periodontal disease and the importance of brushing even a young dog's teeth on a regular basis. Routine dental care and dental surgery are discussed in Chapter 15.

The skin and ears should be inspected for wounds, state of hydration, completeness of hair cover and condition of foot pads. When necessary, the dermatological examination may also require such diagnostic procedures as exfoliative cytology, bacterial culture and sensitivity testing, skin scrapings, and dermatophyte culture and identification of external parasites (such as ear mites, fleas, ticks and chiggers). When the observation and basic inspection phase has been completed, the animal is assessed according to specific body systems. Detailed information concerning the history and physical examination is found in Chapter 2.

Vaccinations

In the general outline of the preventive program, the statement "vaccinate with DA₂PL-PC vaccine" refers to the use of a vaccine to protect against the following: D—canine distemper; A₂ (canine adenovirus type 2)—infectious canine hepatitis; P—canine parainfluenza; L—leptospirosis; P—canine parvovirus type 2 disease; and C—canine coronavirus disease. A listing

of some vaccines currently available is presented in Table 31–2. In addition, a fourth office visit may be desired at 20 weeks of age for an additional canine parvovirus-2 vaccine booster in some puppies, especially Doberman Pinscher and Rottweiler breeds.

In addition to regularly scheduled DA₂PL-PC and rabies vaccinations, other immunizations can be incorporated into the preventive health program, as detailed below.

Infectious Tracheobronchitis Vaccine. Vaccination can be an effective means for preventing or, at least, reducing the incidence of infectious tracheobronchitis (kennel cough) in dogs of all ages (Wagnener et al., 1984). Intranasal vaccination, in particular, provides rapid, long-term protection against *Bordetella bronchiseptica* and parainfluenza virus infection and disease (Table 31–2). Puppies can be vaccinated intranasally (Intra-Trac-II, Schering-Plough Animal Health; Naramune-2, Bio-Ceutic Laboratories) as early as 2 to 4 weeks of age without interference from maternal antibody, or they can be revaccinated when they receive their first DA₂PL-PC vaccination. One dose is effective for a full year. Adult dogs can receive a one-dose intranasal vaccination at the same time as their puppies or at the time they receive their annual vaccinations. Puppies being prepared for shipment or entering a boarding kennel or veterinary hospital should be vaccinated at least 1 to 2 weeks before admission or shipping. Other infectious tracheobronchitis vaccines available include inactivated *Bordetella bronchiseptica* parenteral vaccine (CoughGuard B or CoughGuard BP, SmithKline Beecham Animal Health; Bronchicine, Fermenta Animal Health). Parenteral vaccines are administered as two doses 2 to 4 weeks apart. When dogs younger than 4 months of age are being vaccinated, they should be revaccinated after reaching the age of 4 months. Initial vaccination of puppies with parenteral vaccines is recommended at or about 6 to 8 weeks of age.

Canine Lyme Disease Vaccine. Canine *Borrelia burgdorferi* vaccine, available as killed bacteria product (LymeVax, Fort

Table 31–5
GENERAL OUTLINE OF A PREVENTIVE HEALTH PROGRAM FOR HORSES

First Quarter: January to March

All Horses

Deworm—minimum of every 8 weeks. Exercise care in choice of anthelmintics for mares in the third trimester. Begin deworming foals at 2 months of age.

Trim feet—every 6 weeks. More frequently in foals requiring limb correction.

Dentistry—check adults twice yearly and float as needed. Remove wolf teeth in 2-year-olds and retained caps in 2-, 3- and 4-year-olds. Immunize for respiratory disease: influenza, strangles and rhinopneumonitis.

Stallions

Perform complete breeding examination. Maintain stallions under lights if being used for early breeding.

Pregnant Mares

Immunize with tetanus toxoid, and open sutured mares 30 days prepartum. Develop a colostrum bank. Ninth-day breeding only for mares with normal foaling history and normal reproductive tract. Wash udders of foaling mares.

Open Mares

Maintain under lights if being used for early breeding. Perform daily teasing. Perform reproductive tract examination during estrus. Mares should not be too fat but in gaining condition during breeding season.

Newborn Foals

Dip navel in disinfectant. Carefully, give a cleansing enema at birth. Administer tetanus prophylaxis if indicated by history.

Second Quarter: April to June

All Horses

Deworm—minimum of every 8 weeks.

Trim feet—every 6 weeks. Don't forget the foals and yearlings.

Dentistry—check teeth and remove or float teeth as needed.

Immunize for equine encephalomyelitis. Administer appropriate vaccine boosters.

Stallions

Maintain an exercise program. Monitor the semen quality.

Brood Mares

Palpate at 21, 42 and 60 days after successful breeding.

Foals

Creep feed the foals and provide free-choice minerals. Immunize at 3 months of age. Group the foals by sex and size when weaned.

Third Quarter: July to September

All Horses

Deworm—minimum of every 8 weeks. Clip and sweep the pastures.

Trim feet—every 6 weeks. Continue corrective trimming on foals.

Dentistry—check teeth and remove or float teeth as needed.

Stallions

Maintain an exercise program.

Brood Mares

Administer rhinopneumonitis boosters to pregnant mares according to manufacturer's labeled directions. Administer appropriate vaccine boosters to foals and yearlings. Check condition of mare's udder at weaning and reduce the amount of feed given until milk flow is reduced.

Foals

Administer all appropriate immunizations. Provide free-choice minerals. Maintain a protein supplement in creep feeders.

Fourth Quarter: October to December

All Horses

Deworm—minimum every 8 weeks. Select anthelmintics appropriate for season.

Trim feet—every 6 weeks. Continuous corrective trimming on foals.

Dentistry—check teeth and remove or float teeth as needed.

Stallions

Continue the exercise program. Check immunizations. Perform breeding examination.

Brood Mares

Confirm pregnancy. Begin treating the open mares. Check immunizations.

Table 31–6
EQUINE VACCINES*

Vaccine	Manufacturer	Type‡	EE	WE	VEE	EVA	A1	A2	EHV	TT	TAT	RB	ST	ANX	PHF
Anthrax Vaccine	Colorado Serum													X	
Arvac	Fort Dodge Laboratories	MLV				X									
Cephalovac EWT	Coopers Animal Health	I	X	X						X					
Cephalovac VEW	Coopers Animal Health	I	X	X	X										
Cephalovac VEWT	Coopers Animal Health	I	X	X	X					X					
Encephaloid I.M.	Fort Dodge Laboratories	I	X	X											
Encephalomyelitis Vaccine	Colorado Serum	I	X	X											
Encevac with Havlogen	Haver	I	X	X											
Encevac-T with Havlogen	Haver	I	X	X						X					
Encevac TC-4 with Havlogen	Haver	I	X	X			X	X		X					
Equibac II	Fort Dodge Laboratories											X			
Equicine II with Havlogen	Haver	I					X	X							
Equi-flu	Coopers Animal Health	I					X	X							
Equiloid	Fort Dodge Laboratories	I	X	X						X					
Fluvac	Fort Dodge Laboratories	I					X	X							
Fluvac EWT	Fort Dodge Laboratories	I	X	X			X	X		X					
Fluvac EHV-1	Fort Dodge Laboratories	I					X	X	X						
Fluvac-T	Fort Dodge Laboratories	I					X	X		X					
Imrab	Pitman-Moore	I										X			
Inflogen	Solvay	I					X	X							
Inflogen-T	Solvay	I					X	X		X					
PHF-Vax	Schering Animal Health	I													X
Pneumabort-K	Fort Dodge Laboratories	I							X						
Rabguard-TC	SmithKline Beecham	I										X			
Rhinomune	SmithKline Beecham	MLV							X						
Strepguard with Havlogen	Haver	I											X		
Strepvax II	Coopers Animal Health	I											X		
Super-Tet Tetanus Toxoid with Havlogen	Haver	I								X					
Tetanus Toxoid	Fort Dodge Laboratories	I								X					
Tetnogen	Solvay	I								X					
Tetanus Antitoxin	Sanofi	Antitoxin									X				
Tetanus Antitoxin	Fort Dodge Laboratories	Antitoxin									X				
Tetanus Antitoxin	Haver	Antitoxin									X				

Table continued on following page

Table 31–7
GENERAL OUTLINE OF A PREVENTIVE HEALTH PROGRAM FOR BEEF CATTLE

Cow-Calf Herd Recommendation*

At Birth
Ingestion of colostrum within the first few hours after birth is an important factor in baby calf survival. Immunize with oral bovine rotavirus and coronavirus enteric disease vaccine if a calf diarrhea problem exists in the herd.

One- to Three-Month-Old Calves
Immunize for *Clostridium chauvoei* and *Clostridium septicum* or a seven-way clostridial diseases product. Deworm with commercial product that is safe for calves.

Preweaning Calves
Deworm with broad-spectrum commercial dewormer and immunize as follows:

IMMUNIZING VACCINE	AGE FOR VACCINE ADMINISTRATION
Brucella abortus, strain 19 (calfhood vaccination—replacement heifers only)	5–6 months of age (dependent upon federal and state regulations)
Clostridial diseases *Clostridium perfringens* types C & D, *chauvoei, novyi, septicum* and *sordelli*	5–6 months of age
Infectious bovine rhinotracheitis (IBR) and parainfluenza-3 (PI-3) respiratory diseases (inactivated vaccines only)	5–6 months of age, booster at 12–13 months of age
Bovine virus diarrhea (BVD) (inactivated vaccines only)	5–6 months of age, booster at 12–13 months of age

Weaning Calves
Deworm with broad-spectrum commercial dewormer and treat for lice and grubs. Castrate the bull calves. Immunize with *Pasteurella* (optional) and *Haemophilus* (optional) vaccines.

Prebreeding Replacement Heifers
Deworm with broad-spectrum commercial dewormer and treat for lice. Immunize as follows:

IMMUNIZING VACCINE	TIME OF VACCINE ADMINISTRATION
Infectious bovine rhinotracheitis (IBR) and parainfluenza-3 (PI-3) respiratory diseases	10–12 months of age
Clostridial diseases *Clostridium perfringens* types C & D, *chauvoei, novyi, septicum,* and *sordelli*	10–12 months of age
Bovine virus diarrhea (BVD)	10–12 months of age
Leptospirosis	10–12 months of age
Vibrosis	10–12 months of age

Prebreeding Cows
Deworm with broad-spectrum dewormer and treat for lice. Immunize for leptospirosis and vibrosis.

Precalving Cows
Immunize as follows:

IMMUNIZING VACCINE	TIME OF VACCINE ADMINISTRATION
Infectious bovine rhinotracheitis (IBR) and parainfluenza-3 (PI-3) respiratory diseases (inactivated vaccines only)	Prior to calving
Bovine virus diarrhea (BVD) (inactivated vaccines only)	Prior to calving
Bovine rotavirus and coronavirus enteric diseases	Prior to calving
Escherichia coli enteric disease	Prior to calving
Clostridial disease *Clostridium perfringens* types C & D	Prior to calving

Bulls
Deworm annually with broad-spectrum dewormer and treat for lice and grubs. Immunize as recommended for prebreeding replacement heifers annually (see the above section).

Feedlot Recommendations†

On Arrival into the Feedlot
Deworm with a broad-spectrum dewormer and immunize for infectious bovine rhinotracheitis (IBR), parainfluenza-3 (PI-3), bovine virus diarrhea (BVD) and clostridial diseases (use seven-way vaccine). Inactivated infectious bovine rhinotracheitis, parainfluenza-3, and bovine virus diarrhea vaccines are the safest.

Three to Four Weeks After Arrival into the Feedlot
Implant a commercial implant product. Treat for lice and grubs. Administer booster immunizations if necessary. Abort the heifers if necessary. Castrate and dehorn if necessary.

*Other optional vaccines that may be incorporated into the immunization program, depending on individual herd needs and/or diseases endemic to the area, include anthrax and anaplasmosis.
†Other optional vaccines that may be incorporated into the immunization program, depending on individual herd needs and/or diseases endemic to the area, include *Haemophilus somnus, Pasteurella* spp., respiratory syncytial virus, leptospirosis and anthrax.

Table 31–8

GENERAL OUTLINE OF A PREVENTIVE HEALTH PROGRAM FOR DAIRY CATTLE*

Calves

At Birth
Immunize with bovine rotavirus and coronavirus enteric disease vaccine† and administer orally *Escherichia coli* enteric disease vaccine.

Weaning Age (about 2 months of age) to Breeding Age (about 15 months of age)

IMMUNIZING VACCINE	AGE FOR VACCINE ADMINISTRATION
Brucella abortus, strain 19 (calfhood vaccination—replacement heifers only)	4–8 months of age optimal time (dependent upon federal and state regulations)
Clostridial diseases	2–4 months of age
Clostridium perfringens types C & D, *chauvoei, novyi, septicum* and *sordelli*	
Infectious bovine rhinotracheitis (IBR) and parainfluenza-3 (PI-3) respiratory diseases	4–6 months of age, booster at 12–13 months of age
Bovine virus diarrhea (BVD)	6–8 months of age, booster at 12–13 months of age
Leptospirosis	4–6 months of age, booster in 2 weeks
Vibriosis (if natural breeding)	4–6 months of age, booster at 12–13 months of age

Fresh Cows and Heifers

IMMUNIZING VACCINE	TIME OF VACCINE ADMINISTRATION
Infectious bovine rhinotracheitis (IBR) and parainfluenza-3 (PI-3) respiratory diseases (inactivated vaccines only)	30 days postpartum
Bovine virus diarrhea (BVD) (inactivated vaccines only)	30 days postpartum
Leptospirosis	30 days postpartum
Vibrosis	30 days postpartum

Dry Cows and Bred Heifers

The goal of dry cow immunization is to provide for optimal protection for the newborn calf.

IMMUNIZING VACCINE	TIME OF VACCINE ADMINISTRATION
Leptospirosis	At time of dry off
Bovine rotavirus and coronavirus enteric diseases†	At time of dry off, booster in 2–3 weeks
Escherichia coli enteric disease†	At time of dry off, booster in 2–3 weeks
Clostridial disease	At time of dry off, booster in 2–3 weeks
Clostridium perfringens types C & D	

*Other vaccines that may be incorporated into the vaccination program, depending on individual herd needs and/or diseases endemic to the area, include *Haemophilus somnus, Pasteurella* spp., *Salmonella* spp., *Clostridium haemolyticum*, anthrax and anaplasmosis.
†Use if problem of neonatal calf diarrhea exists on the farm.

Table 31–9
CATTLE VACCINES*

Vaccine Components†

Vaccines	Manufacturer	Type‡	IBR	PI3	BVD	BRVS	HAEMOPHILUS	PASTEURELLA	LEPTOSPIROSIS	CLOSTRIDIUM CHAUVOEI	CLOSTRIDIUM SEPTICUM	CLOSTRIDIUM NOVYI	CLOSTRIDIUM SORDELLII	CLOSTRIDIUM HEMOLYTICUM	CLOSTRIDIUM PERFRINGENS C & D	CAMPYLOBACTER	TRICHOMONAS	ESCHERICHIA COLI	CORONOVIRUS	ROTAVIRUS	MORAXELLA	TETANUS	ANAPLASMOSIS	ANTHRAX	BRUCELLA	RABIES
5-Way Leptospirosis Vaccine	Sanofi	I							X																	
7-Way Clostridium	B.V.I	I								X	X	X	X		X											
Anaplaz	Fort Dodge	L																					X			
Anthrax Spore Vaccine	Colorado Serum	L																						X		
Bar Somnus	Anchor	I					X																			
Bar Somnus-2P	Anchor	I					X	X																		
Bar-1 BVD	Anchor	I			X																					
Bar-1 BVD	Bio-Ceutic	I			X																					
Bar-3	Anchor	I	X	X	X																					
Bar-3/Somnus	Anchor	I	X	X	X		X																			
Bar-4	Anchor	I	X	X	X																					
Bar-4/Somnus	Anchor	I	X	X	X		X																			
Bar-Vac-7	Anchor	I								X	X	X	X		X											
Bar-Vac 7/Somnus	Anchor	I					X			X	X	X	X		X											
Bar-Vac-8	Anchor	I								X	X	X	X	X	X											
Bar-Vac-CD/T	Anchor	I													X							X				
Blacklegol 4 with Spur	Cutter	I								X	X	X	X													
Blacklegol 7 Somnus with Spur	Cutter	I					X			X	X	X	X		X											
Blacklegol 7 with Spur	Cutter	I								X	X	X	X		X											
Blacklegol 8 with Spur	Cutter	I								X	X	X	X	X	X											
Bovac 3	SmithKline Beecham	I	X	X	X																					
Boveye	SmithKline Beecham	I																			X					
Bovine Pili Shield	Grand	MLV																X								
Bovine Rhinotracheitis Vaccine with Leptospira Pomona Bacterin	Sanofi	MLV/1	X						X																	
Bovine Rhinotracheitis-Parainfluenza-3 Vaccine	Sanofi	MLV	X	X																						
Bovine Rhinotracheitis-Parainfluenza-3 Vaccine with Pasteurella Haemolytica-Multocida Bacterin	Sanofi	MLV/1	X	X				X																		
Bovine Rhinotracheitis-Virus Diarrhea Vaccine	Sanofi	MLV	X		X																					
Bovine Rhinotracheitis-Virus Diarrhea-Parainfluenza-3 Vaccine	Colorado Serum	MLV	X	X	X																					
Bovine Rhinotracheitis-Virus Diarrhea-Parainfluenza-3 Vaccine	Sanofi	MLV	X	X	X																					

Product	Manufacturer	Type
Bovine Rhinotracheitis-Virus Diarrhea Vaccine with Leptospira Pomona Bacterin	Sanofi	MLV/I
Bovine Rhinotracheitis-Virus Diarrhea-Parainfluenza-3 Vaccine with Pasteurella Haemolytica-Multocida Bacterin	Sanofi	MLV/I
Bovine Virus Diarrhea Vaccine	Sanofi	MLV
Bovira B	Coopers	MLV
Bovira I	Coopers	MLV
Bovira IB	Coopers	MLV
Bovira IBL5	Coopers	MLV
Bovira IBP	Coopers	MLV
Bovira IBPL5	Coopers	MLV/I
Bovira IL	Coopers	MLV/I
Bovishield 3	SmithKline Beecham	MLV
Bovishield 4	SmithKline Beecham	MLV
Bovishield 4 + L5	SmithKline Beecham	MLV/I
Bovishield 4 + L5 (BVD-K)	SmithKline Beecham	MLV/I
Bovishield 4 (BVD-K)	SmithKline Beecham	MLV/I
Bovishield IBR-BRSV-LP	SmithKline Beecham	MLV/I
Bovishield IBR-BVD-BRSV-LP	SmithKline Beecham	MLV/I
Bovishield IBR-BVD-LP	SmithKline Beecham	MLV/I
Bovishield IBR-P13-BRSV	SmithKline Beecham	MLV
BRD-1	Franklin	I
Breed-Back-7/Pinkeye	Anchor	I
Breed-Back-10	Anchor	MLV/I
Breed-Back-10	Bio-Ceutic	MLV/I
BRSV	SmithKline Beecham	MLV
BRSV Vac	Cutter	MLV
BRSV Vac	Haver/Diamond Scientific	MLV
BRSV Vac 3	Cutter	MLV
BRSV Vac 3	Haver/Diamond Scientific	MLV
BRSV Vac 4	Cutter	MLV
BRSV Vac 4	Haver/Diamond Scientific	MLV
BRSV Vac 9	Cutter	MLV/I
BRSV Vac 9	Haver/Diamond Scientific	MLV/I
BRSV-KV	Anchor	I
BRSV-KV	Bio-Ceutic	I
Brucella Abortus Vaccine	Colorado Serum	Strain 19 Live
Brucellosis Vaccine	Coopers	Strain 19 Live
Calf-Guard	SmithKline Beecham	MLV
CattleMaster 3	SmithKline Beecham	I
CattleMaster	SmithKline Beecham	MLV/I
CattleMaster 4 + L5	SmithKline Beecham	MLV/I
CattleMaster 4 + VL5	SmithKline Beecham	MLV/I
CattleMaster BVD-K	SmithKline Beecham	I
Clostri Shield 7	Grand	I
Clostri Shield 8	Grand	I
Clostri Shield C	Grand	I
Clostridial-4-Way	Lextron	I
Clostridial-7-Way	AgriLabs	I
Clostridial-7-Way	Lextron	I
Clostridial-7-Way plus Somnumune	AgriLabs	I
Clostridial-8-Way	AgriLabs	I
Clostridium Chauvoei-Septicum Bacterin	Colorado Serum	I
Clostridium Chauvoei-Septicum-Pasteurella Haemolytica-Multocida Bacterin	Colorado Serum	I

Table 31–9
CATTLE VACCINES* *Continued*

Vaccine Components†

Vaccines	Manufacturer	Type‡	IBR	PI3	BVD	BRVS	*HAEMOPHILUS*	*PASTEURELLA*	LEPTOSPIROSIS	*CLOSTRIDIUM CHAUVOEI*	*CLOSTRIDIUM SEPTICUM*	*CLOSTRIDIUM NOVYI*	*CLOSTRIDIUM SORDELLII*	*CLOSTRIDIUM HEMOLYTICUM*	*CLOSTRIDIUM PERFRINGENS C & D*	*CAMPYLOBACTER*	*TRICHOMONAS*	*ESCHERICHIA COLI*	*CORONOVIRUS*	*ROTAVIRUS*	*MORAXELLA*	*TETANUS*	*ANAPLASMOSIS*	*ANTHRAX*	*BRUCELLA*	*RABIES*
Clostridium Haemolyticum Bacterin	Colorado Serum	I												X												
Clostridium Perfringens Types C&D-Tetanus Toxoid	Colorado Serum	I													X							X				
Clostridium Perfringens Types C&D Toxoid	Colorado Serum	I													X											
Coli-Bovis/CD	SmithKline Beecham	I													X			X								
Combi-Lep 5	Franklin	I							X																	
Coopervax 3-Way	Coopers	I								X	X	X	X													
Coopervax 5-Way	Coopers	I								X	X	X	X	X												
Coopervax 5-Way Plus Lepto	Coopers	I							X	X	X	X	X	X												
Coopervax 8-Way	Coopers	I								X	X	X	X	X	X											
Coopervax C&D	Coopers	I													X											
Cow-Vac 9	AgriLabs	MLV/I	X	X	X				X							X										
Cow-Vac 9	Lextron	MLV/I	X	X	X				X							X										
Defender IBR-BVD-PI3	Lextron	I	X	X	X																					
Defender IBR-BVD-PI3-BRSV	Lextron	I	X	X	X	X																				
Defender IBR-BVD-PI3-L5	Lextron	I	X	X	X				X																	
Defender IBR-BVD-PI3-SomnuMune	Lextron	I	X	X	X		X																			
Defender (Killed BVD)	Lextron	I			X																					
Discovery-3	Franklin	I	X	X	X																					
Discovery-3L5	Franklin	I	X	X	X				X																	
Discovery-3 VL5	Franklin	I	X	X	X				X							X										
Discovery-4	Franklin	I	X	X	X	X																				
Discovery-4L5	Franklin	I	X	X	X	X			X																	
Discovery-4 + PH	Franklin	I	X	X	X	X		X																		
Discovery-4 + Somnus	Franklin	I	X	X	X	X	X																			
Discovery BRSV-Kv	Franklin	I				X																				
Ecoli Guard	Haver/Diamond Scientific	I																X								
Ecoli-Guard Cow-Sow	Cutter	I																X								
Electroid 7	Coopers	I								X	X	X	X		X											
Electroid 7 Plus H.S.	Coopers	I					X			X	X	X	X		X											
Electroid D	Coopers	I													X											
Elite 4	Anchor	I	X	X	X	X																				
Elite 4	Bio-Ceutic	I	X	X	X	X																				
Elite 4-HS	Anchor	I	X	X	X	X	X																			
Elite 4-HS	Bio-Ceutic	I	X	X	X	X	X																			
Fermicon CD/T	Bio-Ceutic	I													X							X				
Fermicon-7	Bio-Ceutic	I								X	X	X	X		X											

Product	Manufacturer	Type
Fermicon-7/MB	Bio-Ceutic	I
Fermicon-7/Somugen	Bio-Ceutic	I
Fringol C&D with Spur	Cutter	I
Haemophilus Somnus Bacterin	Cutter	
Herd-Vac 9	Fermenta	MLV/I
Horizon I	Cutter	I
Horizon I	Haver/Diamond Scientific	
Horizon I + Vac 3	Cutter	MLV/I
Horizon I + Vac 3	Haver/Diamond Scientific	MLV/I
Horizon IV	Cutter	MLV/I
Horizon IV	Haver/Diamond Scientific	MLV/I
Horizon IX	Cutter	MLV/I
Horizon IX	Haver/Diamond Scientific	MLV/I
IBR Vaccine	Lextron	MLV
IBR-BVD	Fermenta	MLV
IBR-BVD Vaccine	Lextron	MLV
IBR-BVD-L	Fermenta	MLV/I
IBR-BVD-Lepto P	AgriLabs	MLV/I
IBR-BVD-Lepto P	Lextron	MLV/I
IBR-BVD-PI3	AgriLabs	MLV
IBR-BVD-PI3	B.V.I.	MLV
IBR-BVD-PI3	Fermenta	MLV
IBR-BVD-PI3	Lextron	MLV
IBR-BVD-PI3/Bar Somnus-2P	Anchor	MLV/I
IBR-BVD-PI3-Lepto 5	Fermenta	MLV/I
IBR-BVD-PI3-Lepto 5 8 Way	AgriLabs	MLV/I
IBR-BVD-PI3-Lepto P	Lextron	MLV/I
IBR-BVD-PI3-Sommumune	AgriLabs	MLV/I
IBR-BVD-PI3-Sommumune	Lextron	MLV/I
IBR-BVD-PI3-Somnutech	Fermenta	MLV/I
IBR-PI3	B.V.I.	MLV
IBR-PI3	Fermenta	MLV
IBR-PI3	Lextron	MLV
IBR-PI3/Bar Somnus-2P	Anchor	MLV/I
IBR-PI3-L	Fermenta	MLV/I
IBR-PI3-Lepto P	Lextron	MLV/I
IBR-PI3/Somnugen-2P	Bio-Ceutic	MLV/I
Immu-Coli-B	Sanofi	I
Imrab	Rhone Merieux	I
Jencine B	Coopers	MLV
Jencine I	Coopers	MLV
Jencine IB	Coopers	MLV
Jencine IBL5	Coopers	MLV/I
Jencine IBP	Coopers	MLV
Jencine IBPL5	Coopers	MLV/I
Jencine IL	Coopers	MLV/I
Jencine K99	Coopers	I
K Brand BVD	Sanofi	I
K Brand IBR-BVD	Sanofi	I
K Brand IBR-BVD-PI3-Lepto 5	Sanofi	I
KL Brand IBR BVD PI3	Sanofi	MLV/I
Leptavoid 5	Coopers	I
Lepto 5	AgriLabs	I
Lepto-5	Colorado Serum	I
Lepto 5	Fermenta	I

Table 31-9
CATTLE VACCINES* *Continued*

Vaccine Components†

Vaccines	Manufacturer	Type‡	IBR	PI3	BVD	BRVS	HAEMOPHILUS	PASTEURELLA	LEPTOSPIROSIS	CLOSTRIDIUM CHAUVOEI	CLOSTRIDIUM SEPTICUM	CLOSTRIDIUM NOVYI	CLOSTRIDIUM SORDELLII	CLOSTRIDIUM HEMOLYTICUM	CLOSTRIDIUM PERFRINGENS C & D	CAMPYLOBACTER	TRICHOMONAS	ESCHERICHIA COLI	CORONOVIRUS	ROTAVIRUS	MORAXELLA	TETANUS	ANAPLASMOSIS	ANTHRAX	BRUCELLA	RABIES
Lepto 5	Lextron	I							X																	
Lepto P	Lextron	I							X																	
Lepto Shield 5	Grand	I							X																	
Leptoferm-5	SmithKline Beecham	I							X																	
Leptomune-5	SmithKline Beecham	I							X																	
Leptospira Pomona Bacterin	Sanofi	I							X																	
Nasalgen IP	Coopers	MLV	X	X																						
Nasal-Ject I.P.	AgriLabs	MLV	X	X																						
Nasavac IP	Coopers	MLV	X	X																						
Navalep 5	Coopers	I							X																	
Pasteurella Haemolytica Multocida Bacterin	Colorado Serum	I						X																		
Pasteurella Haemolytica Multocida Bacterin	Sanofi	I						X																		
Pasturpro	Coopers	MLV						X																		
Piliguard E. Coli-1	Schering-Plough	I																X								
Piliguard Pinkeye 1	Schering-Plough	I																			X					
Pilivib Shield	Grand	I														X		X								
Pneumosyn-H	Franklin	I						X																		
Preg-Guard 9	SmithKline Beecham	MLV/I	X	X	X				X							X										
Preg-Guard 9 + BRSV	SmithKline Beecham	MLV/I	X	X	X	X			X							X										
Pregsure 9	SmithKline Beecham	MLV/I	X	X	X				X							X										
Premier	Fermenta	I		X	X																					
Premier 3	Fermenta	I	X	X	X																					
Premier 3-Somutech	Fermenta	I	X	X	X		X																			
Premier 4	Fermenta	I	X	X	X	X																				
Premier 8	Fermeta	I			X																					
Presponse	Langford	I						X																		
Pre-Vent 6	AgriLabs	I			X																					
Pro-Vac 3	Bio-Ceutic	I	X	X				X	X							X										
Quadraplex/Somnugen	Bio-Ceutic	I	X	X			X		X																	
Rabguard-TC	SmithKline Beecham	I																								X
Redwol with Spur	Cutter	MLV												X												
Respirvac	SmithKline Beecham	I						X																		
ResProMune 3 I-B-P	AgriLabs	I	X	X	X																					
ResProMune 4 IBP-BRSV	AgriLabs	I	X	X	X	X																				
ResProMune 8 IBP-Lepto 5	AgriLabs	I	X	X	X				X																	
Resvac 2/Somnubac	SmithKline Beecham	MLV/I	X	X			X																			
Resvac 3/Somnubac	SmithKline Beecham	MLV/I	X	X	X		X																			

Product	Manufacturer	Type
Resvac 3/Somnubac-P	SmithKline Beecham	MLV/I
Resvac 4/Somnubac	SmithKline Beecham	MLV/I
Scourguard 3 (K)	SmithKline Beecham	I
Scourguard 3 (K)/C	SmithKline Beecham	I
Septimune PH-K	Fort Dodge	I
Shipguard	Coopers	MLV
Siteguard G	Coopers	I
Siteguard L	Coopers	I
Siteguard M	Coopers	I
Siteguard ML	Coopers	I
Siteguard ML Plus Novalep P	Coopers	I
Siteguard MLG	Coopers	I
Somnu Shield	Grand	I
Sommu Shield + 7 Way	Grand	I
Sommu Shield XT	Grand	I
SommuMune	AgriLabs	I
SommuMune	Lextron	I
Sommutech	Fermenta	I
Sommubac	SmithKline Beecham	I
Sommubac-P	SmithKline Beecham	I
Staybred VL5	SmithKline Beecham	I
Syn Shield	Grand	I
Tetanus Toxoid	Colorado Serum	I
Tetanus Toxoid-Concentrated	Colorado Serum	I
Tetnogen	Solvay	I
Thraxol-2	Cutter	L
Triangle 1	Fort Dodge	I
Triangle 2	Fort Dodge	I
Triangle 3	Fort Dodge	I
Triangle 4	Fort Dodge	I
Triangle 4 + PH-K	Fort Dodge	I
Triangle 8	Fort Dodge	I
Triangle 9	Fort Dodge	I
Triangle BRSV-K	Fort Dodge	I
Trichomonus Foetus Vaccine	Fort Dodge	I
Trichomonus Foetus Vaccine	Franklin	I
TriPreg 9	Fort Dodge	I
TriVib	Fort Dodge	I
TriVib 5L	Fort Dodge	I
TSV-2	SmithKline Beecham	MLV
Ultilep 5	Fort Dodge	I
Ultrabac 7	SmithKline Beecham	I
Ultrabac 7/Somnubac	SmithKline Beecham	I
Ultrabac 8	SmithKline Beecham	I
Ultrabac CD	SmithKline Beecham	I
Ultrabac CS	SmithKline Beecham	I
Ultrabac CSNS	SmithKline Beecham	I
Ultrabac CSNS/Somnubac	SmithKline Beecham	I
Ultrabac CSP	SmithKline Beecham	I
Unitox	Coopers	I
Vib Shield	Grand	I
Vib Shield L5	Grand	I
Vib Shield Plus	Grand	I
Vibo-5/Somnugen	Bio-Ceutic	I
Vibralone-H-L5	Cutter	I

Table 31–9
CATTLE VACCINES* *Continued*

Vaccine Components†

Vaccines	Manufacturer	Type‡	IBR	PI3	BVD	BRVS	HAEMOPHILUS	PASTEURELLA	LEPTOSPIROSIS	CLOSTRIDIUM CHAUVOEI	CLOSTRIDIUM SEPTICUM	CLOSTRIDIUM NOVYI	CLOSTRIDIUM SORDELLII	CLOSTRIDIUM HEMOLYTICUM	CLOSTRIDIUM PERFRINGENS C & D	CAMPYLOBACTER	TRICHOMONAS	ESCHERICHIA COLI	CORONOVIRUS	ROTAVIRUS	MORAXELLA	TETANUS	ANAPLASMOSIS	ANTHRAX	BRUCELLA	RABIES
Vibralone-L5	Cutter	I							X							X										
Vibri-Lep 5	Franklin	I							X							X										
Vibrin	SmithKline Beecham	I														X										
Vibrio-Lepto 5	AgriLabs	I							X							X										
Vibrio-Lepto-5	Anchor	I							X							X										
Vibrio-Lepto 5	Fermenta	I							X							X										
Vibrio-Lepto 5	Lextron	I							X							X										
Vibrio-Lepto-5/Somnus	Anchor	I					X		X							X										
Vibrio/Leptoferm-5	SmithKline Beecham	I							X							X										
Vibromune/5L	SmithKline Beecham	I							X							X										
Vira Shield 2	Grand	I	X		X																					
Vira Shield 3	Grand	I	X	X	X																					
Vira Shield 4	Grand	I	X	X	X																					
Vira Shield 4 + L5	Grand	I	X	X	X				X																	

*Compiled with the assistance of Compendium of Veterinary Products, 1st ed., Port Huron, MI, North American Compendiums Inc., 1991.

†IBR = infectious bovine rhinotracheitis; PI3 = parainfluenza-3 virus; BVD = bovine virus diarrhea; BRSV = bovine respiratory syncytial virus.

‡L = live; I = inactivated (killed); MLV = modified live virus (attenuated); MLV/I = combinations of modified live virus (attenuated) and inactivated.

genital tract often causes early embryonic death resulting in temporary infertility, repeat breeding, delayed conception and a prolonged calving interval. *Campylobacter fetus* may be transmitted during coitus or by artificial insemination with contaminated semen. Inactivated vaccines are available for its prevention. Vaccination of breeding stock is highly recommended.

Trichomoniasis Vaccine. Trichomoniasis, caused by *Trichomonas foetus,* is a venereal protozoal disease of cattle that manifests as infertility, relatively early abortions or pyometra. It causes virtually no systemic illness, so its presence within a herd may go undetected for long periods of time, resulting in substantial economic losses. The bull serves as an asymptomatic carrier, and the organism may be spread by natural breeding or artificial insemination with contaminated semen (Bon-Durant, 1985). Inactivated protozoal vaccines are now commercially available to aid in prevention of the disease.

Leptospirosis Vaccine. Leptospirosis is a common bacterial disease of cattle that may cause hemolytic anemia, nephritis, decreased milk production and late-term abortion. The abortions are probably the most economically significant effect of the disease. Regular vaccination of breeding animals for leptospirosis is strongly encouraged.

Brucellosis Vaccine. Brucellosis is caused by the organism *Brucella abortus.* Infection in the cow can result in late-term abortion, usually around 5 months or more into gestation, and shedding of the *Brucella* organisms in the milk. In bulls, infection results in orchitis, impaired fertility, and shedding of *Brucella* organisms in the semen. Brucellosis is a serious human health hazard, and known *Brucella*-positive reactors must be culled from the herd and vaccination of replacement heifers performed. Vaccination of females only is accomplished using a strain 19 live culture vaccine. Age of vaccination of heifers is critical and usually determined by federal and state regulations. Care must always be exercised when using *Brucella abortus* vaccine, since accidental injection, ingestion or exposure through broken skin or mucous membranes can result in human brucellosis.

Anthrax Vaccine. Anthrax is caused by the bacterium *Bacillus anthracis* and is characterized by septicemia and sudden death. Many times, affected animals are simply found dead without any prior signs of illness. Typically, the dead animal exhibits blood oozing from body orifices, failure of blood to clot and absence of rigor mortis. Differential diagnosis of sudden death in cattle may include anthrax, lightning strike, clostridial diseases and anaplasmosis. Vaccination for anthrax is recommended 4 weeks prior to anticipated exposure only in those areas where the disease has historically been a problem

Clostridial Vaccines. Clostridial infections are caused by bacteria that live as spores in the soil. These spores may be ingested by cattle as they graze or may enter the body via wound contamination. The more common clostridial infections encountered in cattle are briefly described in the following paragraphs.

Infections with *Clostridium chauvoei* (the causative agent of blackleg), *Clostridium septicum* (the causative agent of malignant edema) and *Clostridium sordellii* primarily affect striated muscles. The spores of these organisms are deposited in muscles by the circulation after ingestion or via wound contamination. When conditions of reduced oxygen tension within these muscles exist (such as trauma during handling, transporting, butting or riding), the spores vegetate and the resulting organisms multiply. Toxins released by the multiplying organisms rapidly destroy the muscles and cause death through destructive effects on vital organs. Death may occur suddenly, as early as 12 hours after onset of infection.

Infections with *Clostridum novyi* type B and *Clostridium haemolyticum* (also known as *Clostridium novyi* type D) primarily affect the liver. These spores are usually ingested and travel by the circulation to the liver, where they remain latent until some form of liver damage occurs that allows the spores to vegetate and the resulting organisms to multiply. Predisposing conditions that may activate the spores in the liver include liver flukes, migrating parasites, abscesses, bacterial hepatitis, fatty infiltration and various hepatotoxins. Potent toxins produced by the multiplying bacteria are absorbed systemically and cause death through destructive effects on vital organs and blood vessels. Death may occur suddenly, as early as 24 hours after onset of infection.

Infections with *Clostridium perfringens* types B, C and D affect primarily the gastrointestinal tract. These organisms are normal inhabitants of the gastrointestinal tract of cattle and tend to proliferate under conditions of reduced oxygen tension created by consumption of large quantities of concentrate feed or when sudden changes in feed occur. With favorable conditions, the organisms multiply rapidly and produce toxins that can cause several intestinal lesions leading to a hemorrhagic, necrotic enteritis and sudden death, particularly in young animals.

Clostridium tetani is the clostridial organism responsible for tetanus. *Clostridium tetani* is a soil inhabitant that commonly gains entry through contaminated wounds or through uterine infection after calving. Multiplying organisms produce a neurotoxin that affects the central nervous system. The neurotoxin causes tonoclonic spasms and muscle rigidity that, if untreated, can lead to prostration, convulsions and death.

Because these clostridial infections commonly occur in cattle, routine vaccination for clostridial infections is highly recommended.

Anaplasmosis Vaccine. Anaplasmosis in the United States is a common rickettsial disease of cattle and is caused by the intra-erythrocytic parasite *Anaplasma marginale.* Affected red blood cells are destroyed by the liver and spleen, resulting in a severe anemia. Clinical signs due to an acute anemia may include pale mucous membranes, weakness, depression or aggressive behavior and increased heart and respiratory rates. Anaplasmosis often causes sudden death and must be differentiated from anthrax and the clostridial diseases.

An anaplasmosis vaccine is currently available that helps to reduce severe clinical illness and death. One risk in using this vaccine in brood cows is neonatal isoerythrolysis (Luther et al., 1985). Neonatal isoerythrolysis is an anemic syndrome initiated by antibodies in the colostrum that, when absorbed, destroy the red blood cells of some newborn calves. When making a decision on whether to vaccinate brood cows for anaplasmosis, the protective benefits of the vaccination should be weighed against potential risks of neonatal isoerythrolysis.

Bovine Respiratory Disease Complex Vaccines. There are several viruses and bacteria that are widespread in the cattle population and are considered to be the major contributors to the bovine respiratory disease complex. Multiple infections may occur with these viruses, and secondary infections with these bacteria often exacerbate the primary diseases produced (Kiorpes et al., 1988).

Parainfluenza-3 (PI-3) virus causes a mild respiratory disease that is often associated with shipment of cattle to the feedlot (and, thus, commonly referred to as "shipping fever"). Clinical signs may include fever, serous to mucopurulent nasal discharge, coughing, increased respiratory rate, weakness, depression and weight loss.

Infectious bovine rhinotracheitis (IBR) virus causes high fever, nasal discharge, conjunctivitis, increased respiratory rate, coughing, dyspnea, and severe hyperemia of the muzzle (commonly referred to as "red nose").

Bovine virus diarrhea (BVD) virus can cause respiratory disease and is often confused with or obscured by the other viruses of this complex. In addition to the respiratory disease, the virus may also cause a mild transient diarrhea and may be associated with abortions and birth of malformed or weak calves if the primary infection occurs during pregnancy. The chronic form of bovine virus diarrhea, known as mucosal disease, often results in ulcerative lesions throughout the alimentary tract, causing persistent diarrhea and usually death. In general, attenuated (modified live virus) vaccines containing infectious bovine rhinotracheitis and/or bovine virus diarrhea should *not* be administered intramuscularly to pregnant cows or to calves being nursed by pregnant cows since abortion may result. Intranasal attenuated infectious bovine rhinotracheitis vaccines *are* safe, however, for pregnant cows or calves being nursed by pregnant cows.

Bovine respiratory syncytial virus (BRSV) has been recognized in recent years as a major viral component of the bovine respiratory disease complex (Baker and Velicer, 1991). Infection typically causes anorexia, coughing, increased respiratory rate, serous ocular and nasal discharge, fever, pulmonary edema and emphysema and subcutaneous edema of the neck and throat. Death may occur rapidly, as early as 48 hours after onset of infection (Baker, 1986).

The bacteria *Pasteurella multocida* and *Pasteurella haemolytica* are normal inhabitants of the bovine respiratory tract and therefore are common secondary bacterial invaders in cases of primary viral pneumonia in cattle. In addition, these bacteria contribute to a primary fibrinous pneumonia and pleuritis that are readily apparent at necropsy. Clinical signs associated with these *Pasteurella* organisms may include fever, coughing, dyspnea, mucopurulent nasal discharge, depression, anorexia and, in severe cases, death.

The bacterium *Haemophilus somnus* is another bacterial pathogen that can be a part of the bovine respiratory disease complex. It ranks second to *Pasteurella haemolytica* as the most frequent isolate from acute cases of fibrinopurulent pneumonia. *Haemophilus somnus* infection often develops as a septicemia, which can progress into fibrinous pleuritis, pericarditis, polyarthritis and/or thromboembolic meningoencephalitis (also known as TEME or Sleeper syndrome).

Many vaccines are currently available for these virus- and bacteria-induced bovine respiratory diseases. The vaccines contain these agents in various combinations and in the attenuated (modified live virus) or inactivated forms. Their routine use will depend on the needs of the herds and herdsman.

Enteric Disease Vaccine. Bovine rotavirus and coronavirus as well as enterotoxigenic bacterial strains of *Escherichia coli* are often isolated from calves with diarrhea. These organisms may occur in combination or with other bacterial, viral or protozoal pathogens. The combination of enterotoxins produced by *Escherichia coli* and the cytopathogenic effects of rotavirus and coronavirus induces secretion of large amounts of fluid and electrolytes into the lumen of the gut, resulting in diarrhea, dehydration and, in severe cases, death (Naylor, 1990). Vaccines are currently available for immunization of pregnant heifers or cows before calving. Some of these vaccines are also designed for oral administration to the newborn calf.

Moraxella Vaccine. *Moraxella bovis* is the principal cause of infectious bovine keratoconjunctivitis (IBK). Infection may result in characteristic clinical signs including epiphora, blepharospasm, photophobia, corneal ulcers, corneal edema and chemosis. Healing may occur at any stage, but occasionally, with or without appropriate treatment, an affected cornea may perforate, resulting in loss of vision (George, 1984). Several inactivated vaccines are now available for protection against infection by *Moraxella bovis*.

External and Internal Parasites

Control of external parasites, especially lice and grubs, may be done with repeated applications of approved insecticidal sprays or pour-on products or with the use of ivermectin. Many commercial products are currently available for effective treatment of lice and grubs. Always follow the manufacturer's labeled instructions completely and closely observe the slaughter and milk withdrawal times when using these products. Some products are not recommended for use in Brahmans, Brahman crosses or exotic cattle breeds.

The most common internal parasites of beef and dairy cattle are the barber's pole worm (*Haemonchus* spp.), the brown stomach worm (*Ostertagia* spp.), the bankrupt worm (*Trichostrongylus* spp.), the hookworm (*Bunostomum* spp.), Cooper's worm (*Cooperia* spp.), the intestinal worm (*Nematodirus* spp.), the nodular worm (*Oesophagostomum* spp.), the lungworm (*Dictyocaulus* spp.) and the liver fluke (*Fasciola* spp.). In general, it is a good idea to deworm calves at least once before weaning and again at weaning. Cows, heifers and bulls should be dewormed as needed. Many commercial dewormers are currently available. Product choice depends on the parasite(s) diagnosed by fecal examinations within a herd and resistance patterns of those parasites. Cattle raised in locales where liver flukes exist should be treated in the spring and fall with clorsulon (Curatrem, MSD AGVET; Ivomec-F, MSD AGVET) or albendazole (Valbazen, SmithKline Beecham). Chapter 5 contains additional information on parasitology and specific drug therapy.

Several commercial implants are currently available for beef cattle that are designed to improve feed efficiency and increase feed savings. Most implants contain anabolic agents, such as estradiol, progesterone, testosterone, zeranol or various combinations of these agents. The type of implant and its scheduled use depends on the sex and age of calves implanted as well as the needs of the herdsman. Ruminant nutrition is discussed in Chapter 21.

Management Recommendations for Dairy Calves

The ultimate goal in raising replacement heifers is to produce a healthy heifer that will calve and enter the milking herd by 24 months of age (see Table 31–8). Probably the single most important factor in successful rearing of baby calves is to see that the calves ingest colostrum soon after birth (Aldridge et al., 1992). If the calf does not nurse on its own shortly after birth, the herdsman should administer at least 2 liters of warm colostrum to the calf within the first hour. During the first 3 days of life, continue to feed colostrum at 10 percent of the calf's body weight daily, split into two feedings (as an example, a 40-kg calf should receive 2 liters of colostrum twice daily).

After this time, the calf can be switched to whole milk or a good-quality commercial milk replacer administered at 10 percent of its body weight daily divided into two feedings. For the neonatal calf, it is important to use a milk replacer that contains 20 to 22 percent crude protein, all of which is milk derived, and 18 to 20 percent crude fat. Fresh water should be provided at all times, and grain (18 to 20 percent protein) and hay should be offered free choice beginning at 7 to 14 days of age.

Calves should be housed in individual huts until weaned. Separating calves helps to control direct transmission of disease, prevents post-feeding sucking among calves, reduces stress of competition and allows for assessment of individual feed intake and fecal consistency. Most dairy calves should be weaned by 50 to 60 days of age.

PREVENTIVE HEALTH PROGRAM FOR SWINE

An effective and economical preventive health program is an essential part of successful swine production. Preventive health programs should be individually designed by the consulting veterinarian and based on the specific needs of the swine herd and the producer. The preventive health programs should include immunization programs for disease prevention, well-proven methods for external and internal parasite control, recommendations for appropriate nutrition and improvements in general management and sanitation procedures. A general approach to preventive health programs for swine herds and its implementation is presented in Table 31–10.

Vaccinations

Vaccines that may be incorporated in preventive health programs for swine herds can be obtained from manufacturers as individual components or in various combinations. A listing of some vaccines currently available is presented in Table 31–11. Diseases for which vaccines are commonly used in preventive health programs are described below.

Leptospirosis Vaccine. Leptospirosis is an important bacterial disease that affects domestic animals as well as humans and wildlife. Leptospirosis in swine is characterized by poor production, anemia, kidney disease and abortions. Abortions are especially common after infection during late pregnancy. Routine vaccination of the breeding swine (such as gilts, sows, and boars) 2 to 4 weeks before breeding has proved to be effective in its prevention. Since immunity is short lived, semiannual revaccination is generally recommended (Thacker and Gonzalez, 1988).

Porcine Parvovirus Vaccine. Porcine parvovirus (PPV) is believed to be the most common cause of infectious reproductive failure in swine (Thacker and Gonzalez, 1988). Infection of pregnant sows and gilts can result in stillbirths, mummified

Table 31–10
GENERAL OUTLINE OF A PREVENTIVE HEALTH PROGRAM FOR SWINE

Prebreeding Recommendations for Boars
Purchase boars 60 days before intended use. Quarantine the new boars for 30 days, then allow fence line contact with gilts and sows for 30 days before breeding. Immunize boars for leptospirosis and erysipelas. Treat for external and internal parasites before breeding.

Prebreeding Recommendations for Sows and Gilts
Immunize for leptospirosis, porcine parvovirus infection,* and pseudorabies* 2 to 4 weeks before breeding. Flush gilts by increasing feed (energy) intake before breeding to increase ovulations. Treat for external and internal parasites before breeding

Prefarrowing Recommendations for Sows and Gilts
Limit feed intake to about 4 pounds per head per day or feed according to condition to avoid overweight sows or gilts at farrowing. Immunize for colibacillosis,* atrophic rhinitis, erysipelas, transmissible gastroenteritis (TGE), porcine rotavirus infection* and *Clostridium perfringens* type C* according to the manufacturer's labeled instructions. Treat for external and internal parasites before farrowing with approved products.

Farrowing Recommendations
Gradually increase feed intake so lactating swine are receiving full feed at peak milk production. (Rule of thumb: Feed daily 1 pound of feed for every pig being nursed [e.g., a lactating sow with a litter of 12 pigs should receive at least 12 pounds of feed daily].)

General Recommendations for Pigs
At Birth
Perform newborn pig procedures (e.g., clip needle teeth, dock tails, castrate, ear notch and inject iron dextran).
One Week of Age
Immunize for transmissible gastroenteritis (TGE)* orally and for atrophic rhinitis.
Three Weeks of Age
Immunize for porcine rotavirus infection.*
Four to Five Weeks of Age
Weaning occurs at this time. Immunize for atrophic rhinitis, erysipelas, *Haemophilus* infection* and swine dysentery.*
Six to Eight Weeks of Age
Treat for external and internal parasites with approved products.
Older Than Eight Weeks of Age
Repeated treatments for external and internal parasites with approved products may need to be done during the growing-finishing period.

*Dependent on problems in the individual swine herd.

fetuses, embryonic death and infertility (formerly referred to as SMEDI). Prebreeding vaccination is recommended in swine herds experiencing porcine parvovirus infections.

Transmissible Gastroenteritis Vaccine. Transmissible gastroenteritis (TGE) is a common viral disease of swine. Transmissible gastroenteritis affects swine of all ages but is most devastating to pigs younger than 10 days of age. Clinical signs in very young pigs may include anorexia, vomiting, profuse watery diarrhea and dehydration, which often progresses to death (Biehl and Hoefling, 1986). Older swine can exhibit similar but milder symptoms, and death loss is rare.

Vaccination of prefarrowing sows and gilts may be necessary for herds in which transmissible gastroenteritis has been diagnosed as a cause of neonatal diarrhea. In addition, vaccination of pigs within the first week of life may assist in the prevention of post-weaning scours.

Text continued on page 628

Table 31-11
SWINE VACCINES*

Vaccines	Manufacturer	Type†	Bordetella	Pasteurella	Haemophilus	Mycoplasma	Erysipelas	Clostridium	Escherichia coli	Rotavirus	TGE†	Leptospirosis	Parvovirus	Pseudorabies	Salmonella	Treponema	Streptococcus	EMC†
AR-Pac-P	Schering-Plough	I	X	X														
AR-Pac-P + D	Schering-Plough	I	X	X														
AR-Pac-P + ER	Schering-Plough	I	X	X			X											
AR-Pac-PD + ER	Schering-Plough	I	X	X			X											
Atrobac 3	SmithKline Beecham	I	X	X														
Borde Shield 4	Grand	I	X															
Bordegen	Rhone Merieux	I	X															
Bordetella Bronchiseptica Vaccine	MVP	MLV	X															
BordeTech-P.E.	Fermenta	I	X	X														
BratiVac	SmithKline Beecham	I					X											
BratiVac-6	SmithKline Beecham	I					X					X						
Breed Sow 6	AgriLabs	I					X					X	X					
Breed Sow 7	AgriLabs	I					X					X	X					
Clostri Shield C	Grand	I						X										
Clostridium Bac with Imugen II	O.V.L.	I						X										
Clostridium Perfringens Types C&D Toxoid	Colorado Serum	I						X										
Colimix	Central Biologics	I							X									
Colipig	Sanofi	I							X									
Coli-Suis	SmithKline Beecham	I							X									
Combi-Lep 5	Franklin	I										X						
Concord V	Haver/Diamond Scientific	I		X	X													
E-Bac	O.V.L.	I							X									
Ecoli Guard	Haver/Diamond Scientific	I						X	X									
Ecoli-Guard Cow-Sow	Cutter	I						X	X									
EMC-Vac	O.V.L.	I																X
Emulsibac H.P.	MVP	I		X	X													
Er Bac	SmithKline Beecham	I					X											
Er Bac/Leptoferm-5	SmithKline Beecham	I					X					X						
Erocon	Fermenta	I					X											
Ery Shield	Grand	I					X											
Erycell	Grand	MLV					X											
Ery-Mune C	Anchor	I					X											
Erysipelas	Lextron	I					X											
Erysipelothrix Rhusiopathiae Bacterin	AgriLabs	I					X											
Erysipelothrix Rhusiopathiae Bacterin	Colorado Serum	I					X											
Erysipelothrix Rhusiopathiae Bacterin	Sanofi	I					X											
Eva	SmithKline Beecham	A					X											
Farrowsure	SmithKline Beecham	I					X					X	X					
Farrowsure B	SmithKline Beecham	MLV/I					X					X	X					
Farrowsure B-PRV	SmithKline Beecham	MLV/I					X					X	X	X				
Farrowsure PRV	SmithKline Beecham	I					X							X				
Genesis B-P + D	AgriLabs	I	X	X														

Product	Manufacturer	Type
Haemo Shield P	Grand	I
Hydrovac/AVE	Anchor	MLV
Hydrovac/AVE	Bio-Ceutic	MLV
Hy-Guard with Havlogen	Haver/Diamond Scientific	I
Leptavoid	Coopers	I
Lepto 5	AgriLabs	I
Lepto 5	Colorado Serum	I
Lepto 5	Fermenta	I
Lepto 5	Lextron	I
Lepto Shield 5	Grand	I
Leptoferm 5	SmithKline Beecham	I
Leptospira Pomona Bacterin	Sanofi	I
Neo-Vac 7	Cutter	I
Neo-Vac 7	Haver/Diamond Scientific	I
Novalep 5	Coopers	I
Omnimark PRV	Fermenta	MLV
Para Shield	Grand	I
Parapleuro Shield P	Grand	I
Parvo Shield L5	Grand	I
Parvo Shield L5E	Grand	I
Parvo-Lepto Vac	O.V.L.	I
Parvoplex-6 Way	Lextron	I
Parvotech-Lepto 5	Fermenta	I
Parvo-Vac	SmithKline Beecham	I
Parvo-Vac/Leptoferm 5	SmithKline Beecham	I
Pilimune	O.V.L.	I
Pleuro Ban	A.A.H.	I
Pleuro Ban E	A.A.H.	I
Pleuroguard 3	SmithKline Beecham	I
Pleuroguard 4	SmithKline Beecham	I
Pleuromune PRV with Imugen II	O.V.L.	I
Pleuromune with Imugen II	O.V.L.	I
Pleuromune-S with Imugen II	O.V.L.	I
Pneu Pac	Schering-Plough	I
Pneu Pac-ER	Schering-Plough	I
Pneumosuis III	SmithKline Beecham	I
Pneumotox	Sanofi	I
Porcimune	Rhone Merieux	I
Porcimune B	Rhone Merieux	I
Porcine Pili Shield	Grand	I
Porsibac 1	Fort Dodge	I
Porsibac 2	Fort Dodge	I
Porsibac 3	Fort Dodge	I
Porsibac H	Fort Dodge	I
Porsibac HHP	Fort Dodge	I
Porsivac Pv5L	Fort Dodge	MLV
Porsivac T.G.E.	Fort Dodge	MLV
ProSystem 1	Ambico	MLV
ProSystem 2	Ambico	MLV
ProSystem 2*1	Ambico	MLV/I
ProSystem 2*1*3	Ambico	MLV/I
ProSystem 2*1*4*3	Ambico	MLV/I
ProSystem 2*1*4*3/B*P*E	Ambico	MLV/I
ProSystem 2*3	Amico	MLV/I
ProSystem 2*4*3	Ambico	MLV/I

Table 31–11

SWINE VACCINES* Continued

Vaccines	Manufacturer	Type‡	Bordetella	Pasteurella	Haemophilus	Mycoplasma	Erysipelas	Clostridium	Escherichia coli	Rotavirus	TGE‡	Leptospirosis	Parvovirus	Pseudorabies	Salmonella	Treponema	Streptococcus	EMC‡
ProSystem 3	Ambico	I						X	X									
ProSystem 4*3	Ambico	I							X									
ProSystem B*P	Ambico	I	X	X														
ProSystem B*P*E	Ambico	I	X	X			X											
Pr-Vac	SmithKline Beecham	MLV												X				
Pr-Vac-Killed	SmithKline Beecham	–												X				
PRV/Marker	Syntrovet	MLV												X				
PRV/Marker-KV	Syntrovet	–												X				
PRV/Marker L5	Syntrovet	MLV/I										X		X				
PRV/Marker Parvo Lepto 5	Syntrovet	MLV/I										X	X	X				
Prv-Mune with Imugen II	O.V.L.	–												X				
Pseudo Cell IN IM	Grand	MLV												X				
Pseudorabies Vaccine	Bio-Ceutic	MLV												X				
Respogen	O.V.L.	–							X									
Rhi-Co-Pig D	Sanofi	–	X	X														
Rhinicell	Grand	MLV	X															
Rhinicell + E	Grand	MLV	X				X											
Rhinipig D	Sanofi	–	X	X														
Rhini Tech—P.E.	AgriLabs	–	X	X			X											
Rhini Tech—P.E.	Lextron	–	X	X			X											
Rhinobac 3	SmithKline Beecham	–	X	X														
Rhinogen CT 5000	O.V.L.	–	X	X														
Rhinogen CTE 5000	O.V.L.	–	X	X			X											
Rhinogen P	O.V.L.	–	X	X														
Rhinogen PE	O.V.L.	–	X	X			X											
Rhusigen	Rhone Merieux	–					X											
Rotamune with Imugen II	O.V.L.	MLV								X								
Rota-Vac TGE	SmithKline Beecham	MLV								X	X							
RT-Mune	Schering-Plough	MLV/I								X	X							
Salmo Shield 2	Grand	–													X			
Salmo Shield C	Grand	–													X			
Salmonella Bacterin	SmithKline Beecham	–													X			
Scourmune	Schering-Plough	–							X									
Scourmune/AR-Pac-P	Schering-Plough	–	X	X					X									
Scourmune—C	Schering-Plough	–						X	X									
Scourmune—CR	Schering-Plough	–						X	X	X								
Scourmune—CRT	Schering-Plough	MLV/I						X	X	X	X							
ScourShield	SmithKline Beecham	MLV/I						X	X	X	X							
Sow Bac-E	O.V.L.	–					X											
Strep Bac with Imugen II	O.V.L.	–															X	
Strep Shield	Grand	–															X	
Suvaxyn GestaFend 6	Solvay	–										X	X					

Product	Manufacturer	Type	1	2	3	4	5	6	7	8	9
Suvaxyn HerdFend PrV	Solvay	I	X								
Suvaxyn MaternaFend 4	Solvay	I				X	X		X		
Suvaxyn MaternaFend 7	Solvay	I				X	X		X		
Suvaxyn RespiFend 2D	Solvay	I							X		
Suvaxyn RespiFend 3D	Solvay	I							X	X	
Suvaxyn RespiFend HP	Solvay	I									X
Suvaxyn RespiFend MH	Solvay	I						X			
Swine Master 8	AgriLabs	MLV/I			X	X	X	X	X	X	
Swine Master B-P + D/M	AgriLabs	I				X	X	X	X		
Swine Master B-P-E + D	AgriLabs	I				X	X	X	X		
Swine Master B-P-E + D/C-E	AgriLabs	I					X	X	X		
Swine Master H/P	Rhone Merieux	I						X			
Swine Master—R	AgriLabs	MLV				X	X	X	X		
Swine Master—R.T.	AgriLabs	MLV				X	X	X	X		
Swine Master—R.T.C.E.	AgriLabs	MLV/I				X	X	X	X		
Swine Master—T	AgriLabs	MLV					X	X			
Swine Vac 3 Way	Franklin	I						X	X		
Swine Vac E. Coli	Franklin	I							X		
Swine Vac HPP	Franklin	I				X					
Swine Vac Par-5	Franklin	I						X			
Swine Vac Triple P	Franklin	I					X	X	X		
Swine-Plex 2	Bio-Ceutic	I			X		X	X	X		
Swivax 8	Rhone Merieux	I			X	X	X	X	X	X	
TG-Emune Rota with Imugen II	O.V.L.	MLV						X	X		
TG-Emune with Imugen II	O.V.L.	I						X	X		
TGE Vaccine	SmithKline Beecham	MLV						X			
TGE/Ecoli Vac 4-C	Cutter	MLV/I				X	X	X	X		
TGE/Ecoli Vac 4-C	Haver/Diamond Scientific	MLV/I				X	X	X	X		
TGE/Neo-Vac 7	Cutter	MLV/I				X	X	X	X		
TGE/Neo-Vac 7	Haver/Diamond Scientific	MLV/I				X	X	X	X		
TGE Vac	Haver/Diamond Scientific	MLV						X	X		
TGE Vac C	Haver/Diamond Scientific	MLV/I					X	X	X		
Titan 3	Rhone Merieux	I				X	X	X	X		
Tolvid	UpJohn	MLV						X			
Toxivac AD	NOBL	I				X	X				
Toxivac AD + E	NOBL	I				X	X	X			
Triplogen H/P	Rhone Merieux	I						X	X		
True-Vac-2	Anchor	I									X
Ultilep 5	Fort Dodge	I									
WeanGuard	SmithKline Beecham	MLV						X	X		X
Weanvac 3	SmithKline Beecham	I			X		X	X	X		

*Compiled with the assistance of Compendium of Veterinary Products, 1st ed., Port Huron, MI, North American Compendiums Inc., 1991.

†TGE = transmissible gastroenteritis; EMC = encephalomyocarditis virus.

‡I = inactivated (killed); A = avirulent, live; MLV = modified live virus (attenuated); MLV/I = combination of modified live virus (attenuated) and inactivated.

Porcine Rotavirus Vaccine. Porcine rotavirus infection causes a gastroenteritis that may be characterized by vomiting, watery diarrhea, dehydration and death in young pigs. It is generally difficult to differentiate porcine rotavirus infection from transmissible gastroenteritis (TGE) (Biehl and Hoefling, 1986). Porcine rotavirus infection commonly occurs in both nursing and weaned pigs, and many swine herds have serological evidence of its presence. Vaccination of prefarrowing sows and gilts, nursing pigs and pigs 7 to 10 days before weaning is recommended for the prevention of post-weaning scours in herds where porcine rotavirus infection has been diagnosed as a cause of enteric disease in young pigs.

Clostridium perfringens Type C Vaccine. The bacterium *Clostridium perfringens* type C can cause enteric disease in young pigs. In peracute infection, there is a rapid onset of bloody diarrhea and death within the first 2 days of life. Acutely infected young pigs usually develop a red-brown liquid feces and die within 2 days after onset of enteric disease. The subacute infection may result in persistent diarrhea, emaciation and death after 5 to 7 days of age. In chronic infections, a gray mucoid diarrhea occurs that lasts for about 7 days. Some of these patients will die, while others survive and typically become chronic poor doers (Bergeland, 1986).

Vaccination of prefarrowing sows and gilts effectively assists in the control of *Clostridium perfringens* type C infections in nursing pigs.

Neonatal Porcine Colibacillosis Vaccine. Neonatal porcine colibacillosis is caused by bacterial enterotoxigenic strains of *Escherichia coli*. The results are diarrhea, dehydration and, in severe cases, death (Biehl and Hoefling, 1986). Vaccination of healthy, pregnant sows and gilts provides good protection against neonatal colibacillosis in their nursing pigs.

Swine Dysentery Vaccine. Swine dysentery is caused by the enteric bacterium *Treponema hyodysenteriae*. Swine dysentery affects pigs of all ages and occurs more commonly in pigs during the post-weaning and early fattening periods. Clinical signs begin as a mucoid diarrhea that often progresses to dysentery with blood, mucus and fibrin. The major economic loss associated with swine dysentery is due to death, reduced performance and continuous medication cost (Larsen, 1987). A formaldehyde-inactivated vaccine is currently available that may be utilized in herds where exposure is imminent.

Bordetella, Pasteurella and Haemophilus Vaccines. *Bordetella bronchiseptica* is considered to be the major cause of atrophic rhinitis in swine. In young pigs, atrophic rhinitis is characterized by acute rhinitis that results in destruction of the nasal turbinates. Destruction of the turbinates leads to impaired filtering of air in the nasal passages, decreased rate of weight gain and increased incidence of respiratory infections, including pneumonia. Vaccination of pregnant swine and nursing pigs can often reduce the incidence of clinical atrophic rhinitis. *Pasteurella multocida* is a common bacterial pathogen of the respiratory tract of swine. In combined infections, *Pasteurella multocida* and *Bordetella bronchiseptica* can cause a more severe form of atrophic rhinitis than in cases where either agent occurs alone (Barfod and Pedersen, 1982). Several inactivated vaccines containing *Pasteurella multocida* are currently available.

Haemophilus pleuropneumoniae is also a bacterial pathogen of the respiratory tract of swine that causes fibrinopurulent bronchopneumonia and fibrinous pleuritis. Acute *Haemophilus* infections can cause death within 24 hours after the onset of clinical signs (such as coughing, cyanosis and blood-tinged nasal discharge). However, some individuals may die suddenly without development of clinical signs. Chronic infections are usually subclinical and are characterized by decreased performance and an extended finishing period (Lewis and Schwartz, 1987).

Erysipelas Vaccine. Erysipelas is caused by the bacterium *Erysipelothrix rhusiopathiae*, which can occur as acute septicemia, skin discoloration (commonly known as "diamond skin disease"), chronic arthritis and vegetative endocarditis. Erysipelas is extremely common among swine herds, and therefore routine vaccination of gilts and sows prefarrowing and of pigs at weaning is highly recommended.

Pseudorabies Vaccine. Pseudorabies is a viral disease of swine that is characterized by fever, vomiting, encephalitis and sudden death in nursing pigs, and abortion, stillbirths or mummies in pregnant swine. Vaccines are currently available, but their use is limited by federal or state regulations.

Streptococcus Vaccine. *Streptococcus suis* is a primary cause of meningitis and septicemia in post-weaning pigs. It has also been associated with pneumonia and arthritis in pigs and abortion and infertility in sows and gilts. Peracute cases may die suddenly, while less severe cases exhibit CNS signs often followed by death. *Streptococcus suis* can pose a significant human health hazard. Available vaccines may help to reduce the losses caused by *Streptococcus suis*.

External and Internal Parasites

Control of external parasites, especially lice (*Haemophilus suis*) and mange mites (*Sarcoptes scabiei* var. *suis*), may be done with repeated applications of approved insecticidal sprays or pour-on products or with the use of ivermectin. Treatment of external parasites should be done at the same time as treatment for internal parasites; however, always read the manufacturer's labeled instructions, since some types of sprays and pour-on products cannot be used simultaneously with dewormers or may not be used safely in pregnant or young nursing swine.

The most common internal parasites of swine are the roundworm (*Ascaris suum*), the whipworm (*Trichuris suis*), the threadworm (*Strongyloides* spp.), the nodular worm (*Oesophagostomum* spp.), the lungworm (*Metastrongylus* spp.), the red stomach worm (*Hyostrongylus rubidus*), and the kidney worm (*Stephanurus dentatus*). Many commercial dewormers are currently available (Primm et al., 1990). Product choice should depend on the parasites diagnosed by fecal examinations within a herd, convenience of administration and cost-effectiveness. In general, it is a good idea to deworm adults before breeding, sows and gilts before farrowing and pigs once or twice after weaning and once during the growing-finishing period. Chapter 5 contains additional information on parasitology and specific drug therapy.

PREVENTIVE HEALTH PROGRAM FOR SMALL RUMINANTS

In North America, sheep and goats are managed under a wide variety of conditions including extensive range operations, semi-confinement, total confinement and hobby farm systems, and as backyard pets. One primary task of the small ruminant veterinarian and veterinary technician is to educate the producer about the value of careful observation, animal identification and record-keeping for improvement of herd/flock health and productivity (Sherman and Robinson, 1983). With adequate information, the veterinarian and veterinary technician can then make sound recommendations concerning nutrition, vaccination, parasite control and management geared to the needs of a particular herd or flock.

Vaccinations

Many commercial vaccines are labeled for use in sheep only; however, small ruminant veterinarians have used several of these vaccines safely and effectively in goats (Robinson and Wolf, 1991). Use of vaccines depends upon the disease incidence within a given herd or flock, but vaccination for enterotoxemia and tetanus should be included in every herd/flock health program (Table 31–12).

Enterotoxemia Vaccine. Toxins produced by *Clostridium perfringens*, types C and D, may cause enterotoxemia in young sheep and goats. The organism is present in the gastrointestinal tract of healthy animals but may overgrow and produce potent toxins in the presence of rich ingesta and bowel stasis. Enterotoxemia is most likely to occur in young animals nursing from dams that are heavy milk producers or in animals receiving heavy grain rations as in feedlot situations. It is for this reason that the disease is called "overeating" disease. Enterotoxemia is easily prevented by vaccination of the dams before lambing/kidding and vaccination of lambs/kids several times at 2- to 4-week intervals beginning at 6 to 8 weeks of age. Vaccination for enterotoxemia is effective and should be a part of all herd health programs.

Tetanus Vaccine. Tetanus is caused by a toxin produced by the anaerobic organism *Clostridium tetani*, a bacteria that may be carried into wounds or surgery sites. Clinical signs may include muscular stiffness ("sawhorse" stance), difficulty in swallowing ("lockjaw"), prolapse of the third eyelids, labored breathing and exaggerated response to external stimuli. Since small ruminants are particularly susceptible to infection, vaccination for tetanus at the time of vaccination for enterotoxemia is vital (combination products are available). In addition, booster vaccination is recommended any time an animal is wounded or has undergone any surgical procedure (such as dehorning, castration or tail docking).

Contagious Ecthyma Vaccine. Contagious ecthyma (soremouth, orf) is a viral infection of goats. Kids are primarily affected but may spread the disease to the udder of the doe. Clinical signs include papules, vesicles, pustules and scabs on the lips, muzzle, eyelids, oral cavity, udder, teats and feet. Affected kids usually exhibit a decrease in feed consumption, and some kids become depressed, anorectic and febrile (Scott and Smith, 1984). Contagious ecthyma is transmissible to humans, and so it is advisable to wear gloves when handling infected animals. Effective live-virus vaccines are available but are not recommended for closed herds that are not experiencing contagious ecthyma.

Foot Rot Vaccine. *Bacteroides nodosus* is the primary causative agent of foot rot in sheep. It is a highly contagious disease and is probably the most common disease of sheep in the United States, causing more economic loss than any other disease.

Lameness in one or more feet is the most obvious clinical sign. The development of foot rot is facilitated by wet environmental conditions. A vaccine is available that, when combined with regular foot trimming and foot baths, significantly reduces the incidence of disease within a flock (Bulgin et al., 1986).

Bluetongue Vaccine. Bluetongue is a viral disease of ruminants; however, clinical disease is largely restricted to sheep. Clinical signs may include oral ulcers; edema of the face, lips, muzzle and ears; excessive salivation; cyanosis of the tongue (thus the name, bluetongue); and lameness caused by coronitis. Teratogenic effects include abortions, stillbirths, and weak, live "dummy lambs" (Bulgin, 1986). An attenuated live virus vaccine is available for prebreeding vaccination of healthy sheep and goats; vaccination of pregnant females may produce teratogenic effects.

Vibriosis Vaccine. Vibriosis is caused by *Campylobacter fetus* subsp. *fetus* and *Campylobacter jejuni*. The principal clinical sign with this disease is abortion, which usually occurs in the last 6 weeks of pregnancy. Losses from abortion may be substantial in individual flocks. Vaccines for *Campylobacter* alone, or in combination with *Chlamydia*, are now available for prevention of abortion in sheep.

Chlamydia Vaccine. *Chlamydia psittaci*, the cause of enzootic abortion of ewes (EAE), is a major cause of abortion in sheep and goats. Abortions or stillbirths with placentitis usually occur in the fourth or fifth month of gestation; other animals in the flock or herd may concurrently show signs of arthritis or pneumonia. Vaccines for *Chlamydia* alone, or in combination with *Campylobacter*, are now available for prevention of abortion in sheep.

Foot Care

Foot rot is one of the most common diseases of sheep and goats. It is highly contagious, and infection can result in lameness in a significant number of animals within a herd or flock. Frequent foot trimming combined with foot baths, foot soaks and/or vaccination is important in the control of the disease. Repeated foot soaking alone is an economical, practical and effective treatment for foot rot in large commercial operations where hoof trimming is impractical. Products typically used for foot baths or foot soaks include zinc sulfate, copper sulfate and formalin (Bulgin et al., 1986). There is some evidence of genetic susceptibility to development of foot rot in sheep; therefore, culling of animals with recurring infections may be helpful (Bulgin, 1986).

Nutrition

Sheep and goats should be fed a good-quality commercial feed labeled for that particular species. Feeding horse or cattle feeds to small ruminants may result in copper toxicity since the copper levels in those feeds are much higher than normally tolerated by sheep and goats. Feed commercial feeds according to the manufacturer's recommendations and based on the needs and use of the animal. Good-quality roughage may be fed free choice. Since castrated lambs and kids (wethers) are predisposed to the development of urinary calculi, it may be advisable to supplement their feed with salt and a urinary acidifier such as ammonium chloride (see Chapter 17).

Table 31-12
OVINE VACCINES

Vaccines	Manufacturer	Type	C. Chauvoei	C. Septicum	C. Novyi	C. Sordellii	C. Haemolyticum	C. Perfringens C & D	Escherichia Coli	Leptospira	Pasteurella	Tetanus	Bacteroides Nodosus	Bluetongue	Campylobacter	Chlamydia	Ecthyma	Epididymitis	Rabies
Bar-Vac-7	Anchor	I	X	X	X	X		X											
Bar-Vac-8	Anchor	I	X	X	X	X	X	X											
Bar-Vac-CD/T	Anchor	I						X				X							
Blacklegol 4 with Spur	Cutter	I	X	X	X	X													
Blacklegol 7 with Spur	Cutter	I	X	X	X	X		X											
Blacklegol 8 with Spur	Cutter	I	X	X	X	X	X	X											
Bluetongue Vaccine	Colorado Serum	MLV												X					
Campylobacter Fetus Bacterin	Colorado Serum	I													X				
Campylobacter Fetus-Chlamydia Psittaci-	Grand	I													X	X			
Escherichia Coli Bacterin	Colorado Serum	I							X										
Chlamydia Psittaci Bacterin	Grand	I														X			
Clostri Shield 7	Grand	I	X	X	X	X		X											
Clostri Shield 8	Grand	I	X	X	X	X	X	X											
Clostri Shield C	Lextron	I						X											
Clostridial-4-Way	AgriLabs	I	X	X	X	X													
Clostridial 7-Way	Lextron	I	X	X	X	X		X											
Clostridial-7-Way	AgriLabs	I	X	X	X	X		X											
Clostridial 8-Way	AgriLabs	I	X	X	X	X	X	X											
Clostridium Chauvoei-Septicum Bacterin	Colorado Serum	I	X	X															
Clostridium Chauvoei-Septicum-Pasteurella Haemolyticum-Multocida Bacterin	Colorado Serum	I	X	X							X								
Clostridium Perfringens Types C&D	Colorado Serum	I						X											
Tetanus Toxoid	Colorado Serum	I										X							
Clostridium Perfringens Types C&D Toxoid	Colorado Serum	I						X											
Coopervax 3-Way	Coopers	I	X	X		X		X											
Coopervax 5-Way	Coopers	I	X	X	X	X	X	X											
Coopervax 5-Way Plus Lepto	Coopers	I	X	X	X	X	X	X		X									
Coopervax 8-Way	Coopers	I	X	X	X	X	X	X											
Coopervax C&D	Coopers	I						X											
Covexin 8	Coopers	I	X	X	X	X	X	X				X							
Electroid 7	Coopers	I	X	X	X	X		X											
Electroid D	Coopers	I						X											
Enzabort Eae-Vibrio	Colorado Serum	I													X	X			
Fermicon CD/T	Bio-Ceutic	I		X	X	X		X				X							
Fermicon-7	Bio-Ceutic	I	X																
Footvax	Coopers	I											X						
Fringol C&D with Spur	Cutter	I						X											

Product	Manufacturer	Type	1	2	3	4	5	6	7	8	9	10	11	12	13
Fringol CDT with Spur	Cutter	I	X			X									
Imrab	Rhone Merieux	I			X										
Ovine Ecthyma Vaccine	Colorado Serum	L			X										
Ovine Ecthyma Vaccine	Cutter	L		X											
Ovine Pili Shield	Grand	I	X				X		X						
Pasteurella Haemolytica-Multocida Bacterin		I													
Rabguard-TC	SmithKline Beecham	I				X		X							
Ram Epididymitis Bacterin	Colorado Serum	I		X											
Redwol with Spur	Cutter	I				X			X						
Siteguard G	Coopers	I								X					
Siteguard L	Coopers	I						X	X	X	X	X			
Siteguard M	Coopers	I							X	X	X	X	X	X	X
Siteguard ML	Coopers	I				X		X	X	X	X	X	X	X	X
Siteguard ML Plus Novalep P	Coopers	I				X		X	X	X	X	X	X	X	X
Siteguard MLG	Coopers	I						X	X	X	X	X	X	X	
Super-Tet with Havlogen	Haver/Diamond Scientific	I				X									
Tetanus Toxoid	Colorado Serum	I				X									
Tetanus Toxoid	Fort Dodge	I				X									
Tetanus Toxoid-Concentrated	Colorado Serum	I				X									
Tetnogen	Solvay	I				X									
T-Toxol with Spur	Cutter	I				X									
Ultrabac 7	SmithKline Beecham	I						X	X	X	X	X	X	X	
Ultrabac 8	SmithKline Beecham	I						X	X	X	X	X	X	X	X
Ultrabac CD	SmithKline Beecham	I									X	X	X	X	X
Ultrabac CS	SmithKline Beecham	I									X	X	X		
Ultranbac CSNS	SmithKline Beecham	I									X	X	X		
Ultranbac CSP	SmithKline Beecham	I					X				X	X	X		
Unitox	Coopers	I				X									

External and Internal Parasites

There are few effective anthelmintics labeled for use in small ruminants. Most small ruminant veterinarians utilize cattle dewormers for the treatment of external and internal parasites in sheep and goats. Products commonly used include ivermectin, fenbendazole and albendazole. Caution should be exercised when using these products in lactating does and animals intended for slaughter. Recommendations for extra label use of these products and suggested milk and slaughter withdrawal times may be obtained from the Food Animal Residue Avoidance Data Bank.

Frequency of deworming varies according to several factors including concentration of animals in a given area and environmental conditions. Severe gastrointestinal parasitism can be life-threatening, especially in subtropical climates, where it may be necessary to deworm small ruminants as often as every 4 weeks during the hot, humid summer months. Routine fecal examinations, either individual or composite samples, may be useful to determine the frequency of deworming and the effectiveness of various anthelmintics. See Chapter 5 for more information.

Recommended Reading

Dogs and Cats

Hoskins JD: Preventive health program for cats. Vet Technician 9(5):273–278, 1988.

Hoskins JD: Feline infectious peritonitis: A current update. Vet Technician 12:193–201, 1991a.

Hoskins JD: Tick-borne zoonoses: Lyme disease, ehrlichiosis, and Rocky Mountain spotted fever. Sem Vet Med Surg (Small Animal) 6(3):236–243, 1991b.

Hoskins JD: The puppy's first veterinary examination: Physical examination and preventive health program. Vet Technician 12:521–528, 1991c.

Scott FW: Feline immunization. *In* Kirk RW (editor): Current Veterinary Therapy VIII. Philadelphia, WB Saunders Co., 1983, p 1127.

Wagnener JS, Sobonya R, Minnich L et al.: Role of canine parainfluenza virus and *Bordetella bronchiseptica* in kennel cough. Am J Vet Res 45:1862, 1984.

Horses

Beeman GM: Care of the teeth. *In* Robinson NE (editor): Current Therapy in Equine Medicine. 2nd ed. Philadelphia, WB Saunders Co., 1987, p 6.

Beeman GM: Medical examination of horses for purchase. Proceedings of the 33rd Annual Convention Am Assoc Equine Pract, 1988, p 217.

George LW: Diseases of the nervous system. *In* Smith BP (editor): Large Animal Internal Medicine. St. Louis, Mosby–Year Book, 1990, pp 917, 1023.

Herd RP: A new look at equine worm control. Proceedings of the 33rd Annual Convention Am Assoc Equine Pract, 1988, p 55.

Hintz HF: Feeding programs. *In* Robinson NE (editor): Current Therapy in Equine Medicine. 2nd ed. Philadelphia, WB Saunders Co., 1987, p 412.

Martens JG and Martens RJ: Equine herpesvirus type 1: Its classifications, pathogenesis, and prevention. Vet Med 86:936, 1991.

Messer NT, IV: The use of biologics in the prevention of infectious diseases. *In* Smith BP (editor): Large Animal Internal Medicine. St. Louis, Mosby–Year Book, 1990, p 1478.

Steckel RR: Puncture wounds, abscesses, thrush, and canker. *In* Robinson NE (editor): Current Therapy in Equine Medicine. 2nd ed. Philadelphia, WB Saunders Co., 1987, p 266.

Timoney JF, Gillespie JH, Scott FW and Balough JE: Hagan and Bruner's Microbiology and Infectious Diseases of Domestic Animals. 8th ed. Ithaca, NY, Comstock Publishing Associates, 1988.

Wilson JH and Erickson DM: Neurological syndrome of rhinopneumonitis. Proceedings of the Am Coll Vet Int Med Forum, 1991, p 419.

Cattle

Aldridge B, Garry F and Adams R: Role of colostral transfer in neonatal calf management: Failure of acquisition of passive immunity. Comp Cont Educ Pract Vet 14:265–270, 1992.

BonDurant RH: Diagnosis, treatment, and control of bovine trichomoniasis. Comp Cont Educ Pract Vet 7:S179–S188, 1985.

Baker JC and Velicer LF: Bovine respiratory syncytial virus vaccination: current status and future vaccine development. Comp Cont Educ Pract Vet 13:1323–1335, 1991.

Baker JC: Bovine respiratory syncytial virus: Pathogenesis, clinical signs, diagnosis, treatment, and prevention. Comp Cont Educ Pract Vet 8:F31-F40, 1986.

George LW: Clinical infectious bovine keratoconjunctivitis. Comp Cont Educ Pract Vet 6:S712–S724, 1984.

Kiorpes AL, Dubielzig RR and Beck KA: Enzootic pneumonia in calves: clinical and morphologic features. Comp Cont Educ Pract Vet 10:248—261, 1988.

Luther DG, Cox HU and Nelson WO: Screening for neonatal isohemolitic anemia in calves. Am J Vet Res 46:1078, 1985.

Naylor JM: Diarrhea in neonatal ruminants. *In* Smith BP (editor): Large Animal Internal Medicine. St. Louis, Mosby–Year Book, 1990, p 348.

Spire MF: Bovine immunizations. The Bovine Practitioner 16:101, 1981.

Swine

Barfod K and Pedersen KB: Synergism between *Bordetella bronchiseptica* and a toxin-producing strain of *Pasteurella multocida* in the causation of atrophic rhinitis in SPF pigs. International Pig Vet Congress, 1982, p 112.

Bergeland ME: Clostridial infections. *In* Leman AD, Straw B, Glock RD, et al. (editors): Diseases of Swine. 6th ed. Ames, IA, Iowa State University Press, 1986, p 557.

Biehl LG and Hoefling DC: Diagnosis, treatment, and prevention of diarrhea in 7- to 14-day-old pigs. J Am Vet Assoc 188:1144, 1986.

Larsen LP: Eradication of swine dysentery. Proceedings of the Am Assoc Swine Practitioners, 1987, p 563.

Lewis DH and Schwartz WL: *Haemophilus pleuropneumoniae* in swine. Comp Cont Educ Pract Vet 9:F7–F13, 1987.

Primm ND, Friendship RM and Hall WF: Deworming strategies for swine. Part II. Anthelmintics and their use in the control of endoparasites. Comp Cont Educ Pract Vet 12:889–896, 1990.

Thacker BJ and Gonzalez PL: Infectious reproductive disease in swine. Comp Cont Educ Pract Vet 10:669–680, 1988.

Small Ruminants

Bulgin MS: Diagnosis of lameness in sheep. Comp Cont Educ Pract Vet 8(12):F122–F128, 1986.

Bulgin MS, Lincoln SD, Lane VM et al: Comparison of treatment methods for the control of contagious ovine foot rot. J Am Vet Med Assoc 184:194–196, 1986.

Robinson A and Wolf C: American Association of Small Ruminant Practitioners survey of biologic usage. Symposium on Health and Disease of Small Ruminants, 1991, pp 197–214.

Scott DW and Smith MC: Caprine dermatology. Part II. Viral, nutritional, environmental, and congenitohereditary disorders. Comp Cont Educ Pract Vet 6(8):S473–S484, 1984.

Sherman DM and Robinson RA: Sheep and goat medicine. Clinical examination of sheep and goats. Vet Clin North Am (Large Animal Pract) 5(3):409–426, 1983.

Appendix

Common Abbreviations Used in Veterinary Medicine

AAHA	American Animal Hospital Association	BRSV	Bovine respiratory syncytial virus
AC	Before meals	BSP	Bromsulphalein
ACD	Acid-citrate-dextrose	BT	Blue tongue
ACTH	Adrenocorticotropic hormone	BUN	Blood urea nitrogen
AD	Right ear	BUTE	Phenylbutazone
AD LIB	Freely, as wanted	BV	Bronchovesicular
ADR	Active defense reflex	BVD	Bovine virus diarrhea
AF	Atrial fibrillation	c̄	With
A-G	Albumin-globulin ratio	C & S	Culture and sensitivity
AGID	Agar gel immunodiffusion	C-S	Coughing/sneezing
AL	Left ear	C-SPINE	Cervical spine
ALB	Albumin	Ca	Calcium
ALK PHOS	Alkaline phosphatase	CA	Carcinoma
ALP	Alkaline phosphatase	CAE	Caprine arthritis-encephalitis
ALT	Alanine transaminase	CAV-1	Canine adenovirus type 1
AM	Antemortem	CBC	Complete blood count
AMA	Against medical advice	CC	Chief complaint
AMP	Ampule	CCM	Congestive cardiomyopathy
ANA	Antinuclear antibody	CD	Canine distemper
ANS	Autonomic nervous system	CEA	Canine erythrocyte antigen
AP	Anterior posterior	CEM	Contagious equine metritis
APC	Atrial premature contraction	CFJ	Coxofemoral joint
APTT	Activated partial thromboplastin time	CGP	Circulating granulocyte pool
ARF	Acute renal failure	CHD	Canine hip dysplasia
ARR	Arrhythmia	CHF	Congestive heart failure
AS	Aortic stenosis	CHOL	Cholesterol
ASAP	As soon as possible	CHV	Canine hepatitis virus
ASD	Atrial septal defect	CI	Cardiac insufficiency
ASIF	Association for the Study of Internal Fixation	CID	Combined immunodeficiency
AST	Aspartate aminotransferase	CIN	Chronic interstitial nephritis
AU	Each ear	CITE	Concentration immunoassay technology
AV	Atrioventricular	Cl	Chloride
AV BLOCK	Atrioventricular as in first-, second-, third- degree AV block	CM	Cardiomyopathy
		CMT	California Mastitis Test
B & A	Bright and alert	CNE	Canine distemper encephalitis
BAER	Brain stem auditory-evoked response	CNS	Central nervous system
BE	Barium enema colon only	COB	Care of body
BID	Twice daily	CODE E	Used in emergency for cardiac arrest
BLD	Blood	CPA	Cardiopulmonary arrest
BLV	Bovine leukosis virus	CPD	Citrate-phosphate-dextrose
BM	Bowel movement	CPK	Serum creatine phosphokinase
BMR	Basal metabolic rate	CPR	Cardiopulmonary resuscitation
BOL	Large pill (hora)	CPU	Central processing unit
BP	Blood pressure	CREAT	Creatinine
BRD	Bovine respiratory disease	CRF	Chronic renal failure

CRT	Capillary refill time; cathode-ray tube
CSF	Cerebrospinal fluid
CSM	Cervical stenotic myelopathy
CTZ	Chemoreceptor trigger zone
CVP	Central venous pressure
CVS	Cardiovascular system
CWT	Hundred weight
CXR	Chest x-ray
D BILI	Direct bilirubin
D/S	Dextrose in saline
D_5W	5 percent dextrose in water
DDX	Differential diagnosis
DEC	Decrease; diethylcarbamazine
DES	Diethylstilbestrol
DHL	Canine distemper-hepatitis-leptospirosis vaccine
DIC	Disseminated intravascular coagulation
DJD	Degenerative joint disease
DLH	Domestic longhair
DMSO	Dimethyl sulfoxide
DOA	Dead on arrival
DOS	Disc operating system
DS	Dose or days not acceptable
DSH	Domestic shorthair
DTM	Dermatophyte test medium
DV	Dorsal ventral
DX	Diagnosis
EAE	Enzootic abortion of ewes
ECG OR EKG	Electrocardiogram
ECHO	Echocardiogram
EDTA	Ethylenediaminetetraacetic acid
EEE	Eastern equine encephalomyelitis
EEG	Electroencephalogram
EENT	Eyes, ears, nose, throat
EHV	Equine herpesvirus
EIA	Equine infectious anemia
EM	Electron microscopy
EMD	Electromechanical dissociation
EMG	Electromyogram
ER	Emergency room
ERG	Electroretinogram
F-A	Fecal analysis
FA	Fluorescent antibody
FB	Foreign body
FD	Feline distemper
FeLV	Feline leukemia virus
FIP	Feline infectious peritonitis
FIV	Feline immunodeficiency virus
FPV	Feline panleukopenia virus
FUO	Fever of unknown origin
FUS	Feline urological syndrome
FVR	Feline viral rhinotracheitis
Fx	Fracture
g	Gram
gal	Gallon
GAS	General adaptation syndrome
GDV	Gastric dilatation volvulus
GGT	Gamma glutamyl transferase
GI	Gastrointestinal
gtt	Drops (guttae)
GU	Genitourinary
GUI	Graphical-user interface
H	Hour
HB	Hemoglobin
HBC	Hit by car
HBS	Harsh bronchial sounds
HC	Health certificate
HIS	Hospital information systems
HS	At bedtime (hora somni)
HSA	Hemangiosarcoma
HX	History
I BILI	Indirect bilirubin
IBK	Infectious bovine keratoconjunctivitis
IBR	Infectious bovine rhinotracheitis
IC	Intracardiac
ICH	Infectious canine hepatitis
ICU	Intensive care unit
IM	Intramuscular
IP	Intraperitoneal
ISE	Ion-selective electrodes
IT	Intratracheal
IV	Intravenous
IVD	Intervertebral disk disease
IVP	Intravenous pyelogram
K	Potassium
K-9	Canine
Kcal	Kilocalorie
KCS	Keratoconjunctivitis sicca
Kg	Kilogram
L or LT	Left
LBBB	Left bundle branch block
LDA	Left displaced abomasum
LDH	Lactate dehydrogenase
LN	Lymph node
LR	Left ear
LRS	Lactated Ringer's solution
LSA	Lymphosarcoma
m^2	Meter squared
MAC	Minimum alveolar concentration
MAP	Mean arterial pressure
mcg or μg	Microgram
μl	Microliter
MCH	Mean corpuscular hemoglobin
MCHC	Mean corpuscular hemoglobin concentration
MCT	Mast cell tumor
MCV	Mean corpuscular volume
MEA	Mean electrical axis
Mg	Magnesium
MGP	Marginated granulocyte pool
MI	Mitral insufficiency or myocardial insufficiency
MIC	Minimal inhibitory concentration
MIP	Mare's immunological pregnancy test
MLV	Modified live virus
MM	Mucous membrane
Na	Sodium
NC	No change
NCC	Nucleated cell count
NON REP	Do not repeat
NPL	No palpable lesions
NPO	Nothing per os (nothing by mouth)
NR	Not remarkable
NRBC	Nucleated red blood cell
NRC	National Research Council

NSF	No significant findings
NSR	Normal sinus rhythm
NVL	No visible lesions
OB	Obstetrics
OCD	Osteochondritis dissecans
OD	Right eye (oculus dexter)
OD or SID	Once daily
OFA	Orthopedic Foundation for Animals
OHE	Ovariohysterectomy (spay)
OPP	Ovine progressive pneumonia
OS	Left eye (oculus sinister)
OSA	Osteosarcoma
OU	Both eyes
P3	Third phalanx or coffin bone
PAC	Premature atrial contraction
PAT	Paroxysmal atrial tachycardia
PC	After meals
PCV	Packed cell volume
PDA	Patent ductus arteriosus
PDQ	Pretty darned quick
PDR	Passive defense reflex
PEA	Phenylethyl alcohol
PER OS	Orally, by mouth
PER R	Per rectum, rectally
PGA	Polyglycolic acid
Phos	Phosphorus
PI3	Parainfluenza-3
PK	Pigmentary keratitis
PM	Postmortem
PO	Postoperative
POVMR	Problem-oriented veterinary medicine record
PPH	Pertinent past history
PPM	Persistent pupillary membrane
PPV	Porcine parvovirus
PRA	Progressive retinal atrophy
PRAA	Persistent right aortic arch
PRN	As necessary
PRV	Pseudorabies virus
PS	Pulmonic stenosis
PTA	Prior to admission
PTH	Parathyroid hormone
PTS	Put to sleep
PU	Penile urethrostomy
PVC	Premature ventricular contraction
PWD	Powder
Q 2 H	Every 2 hours
Q 6 H	Every 6 hours
QBC	Quantitative buffy coat
QD	Every day
QH, OH	Every hour
QID	Four times a day
QNS	Quantity not sufficient
QOD	Every other day
QS	Quantity sufficient
R or RT	Right
RACL	Ruptured anterior cruciate ligament
RADS	Radiographs
RAM	Random access memory
RAS	Reticular activating system
RBBB	Right bundle branch block
RBC	Red blood cell

RDA	Right displaced abomasum
RER	Resting energy requirement
RETIC	Reticulocyte
RHF	Right heart failure
RID	Radial immunodiffusion
R/O	Rule out
RTG	Ready to go
RV	Rabies vaccination
RX	Take thou of (prescription)
s̄	Without (sine)
SC OR SQ	Subcutaneous
SCC	Squamous cell carcinoma
SDH	Sorbitol dehydrogenase
SG	Specific gravity
SGOT	Serum glutamic-oxaloacetic transaminase
SGPT	Serum glutamic-pyruvic transaminase
SIG	Directions, instructions
SIM	Sulfide-indole-motility (medium)
SMEDI	Stillbirths, mummified fetuses, embryonic death and infertility
SOAP	Subjective, objective, assessment, plan
SOB	Shortness of breath
S/P	Status post
SP	Species
SR	Suture removal
STAT	Statum (immediately)
Sx	Signs, symptoms
T BILI	Total bilirubin
TAT	Tetanus antitoxin
TDN	Total digestible nutrients
TEME	Thromboembolic meningoencephalitis
TGC	Time gain compensation
TGE	Transmissible gastroenteritis
TGEV	Transmissible gastroenteritis virus
TI	Tricuspid insufficiency
TID	Thrice daily
T-L	Thoracolumbar vertebra
TLC	Tender loving care
TP	Total protein
TPR	Temperature, pulse, respiration
TR	Trace
TRIG	Triglycerides
TS-FIPV	Temperature-sensitive feline infectious peritonitis virus
TSH	Thyroid-stimulating hormone
TSI	Triple sugar iron
TT	Tetanus toxoid
TX	Treatment
U	Unit
UA	Urinalysis
UG	Urogenital
UGI	Upper gastrointestinal (includes stomach and intestine)
UNG	Ointment
UO	Urinary obstruction
URI	Upper respiratory infection
US	Ultrasound
USG	Urine specific gravity
UT DICT	As directed (ut dictum)
UTI	Urinary tract infection
V TACH	Ventricular tachycardia
VD	Ventral dorsal

V-D	Vomiting and diarrhea	VS	Vital signs
VECCS	Veterinary Emergency and Critical Care Society	VSD	Ventricular septal defect
		VSV	Vesicular stomatitis virus
VER	Visual evoked response	WBC	White blood cell
VES	Ventricular extrasystole	WEE	Western equine encephalomyelitis
VMDB	Veterinary medical data base	WNL	Within normal limits
VPC	Ventricular premature contraction	XRT	Radiation therapy

INDEX

Note: Page numbers in *italics* refer to illustrations; page numbers followed by t refer to tables.